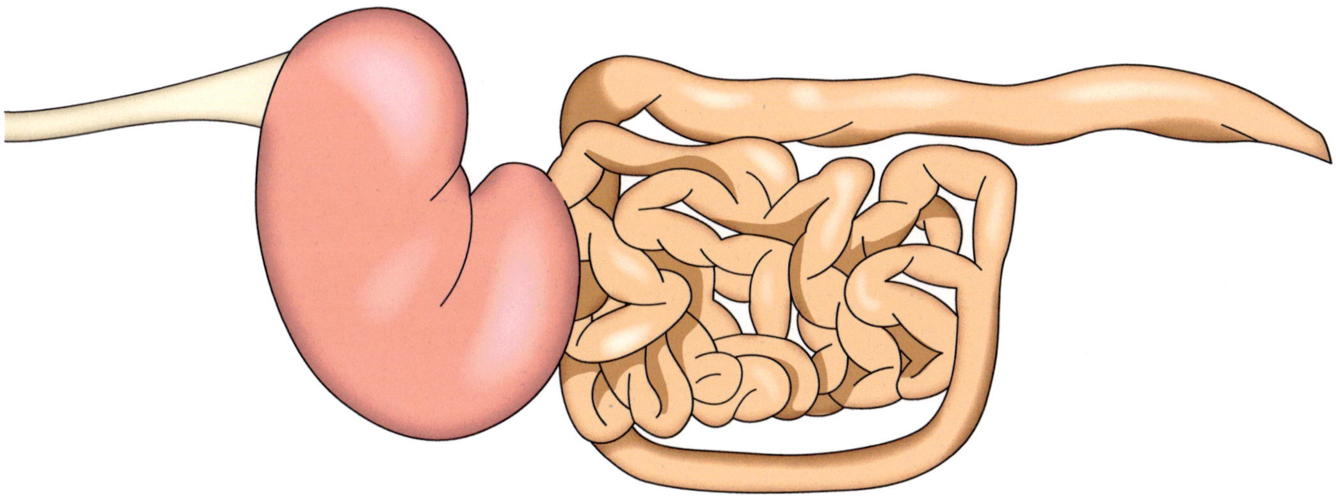

VETERINARY INTERNAL MEDICINE SERIES - Edward Feldman, Federico Fracassi. Editors-in-chief.
Edward Hall - Canine gastroenterology

ISBN: 978-1-962679-43-5
eISBN: 978-1-962679-79-4

Book Publishing Manager: Costanza Smeraldi

Cover: Laura Barzacca

Layout: T&T studio s.a.s, Milano

Copyediting: Melissa Testa and Jorge Viejo, Grupo Asìs; TDI Digital Solutions Inc., New York

edra
PUBLISHING

Edra Publishing US LLC
3309 Northlake Boulevard
Suite 203, Palm Beach Gardens
FL, 33403
EIN: 844113980
info@edrapublishing.com
www.edrapublishing.com

Printed in Italy by "Kosmoprint" S.r.l. Rimini (RN)

Series editors

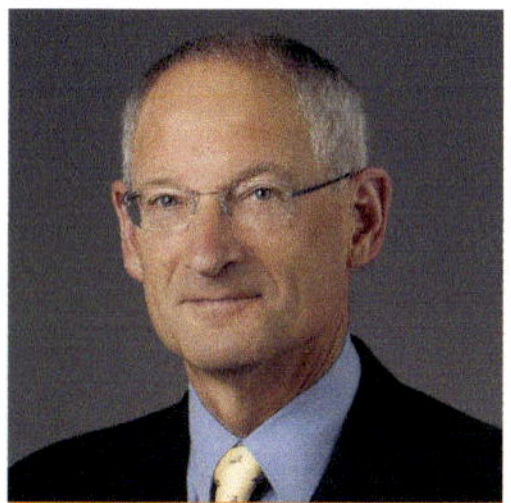

Edward C. Feldman
DVM, ACVIM Diplomate (SAIM), Emeritus Professor of Small Animal Internal Medicine,
University of California, Davis, USA

Dr. Feldman earned his DVM from the University of California in 1973. He joined the Davis faculty in 1979 after an internship at the Animal Medical Center in New York City, a Residency with Dr. Stephen Ettinger in the world's first referral only private veterinary practice in Berkeley California, a year in general practice and another on faculty at the University of Saskatchewan, in Canada. He has authored more than 160 peer-reviewed scientific publications, 110 scientific abstracts, and 75 book chapters.
Dr. Feldman has coedited the last six editions of The Textbook of Veterinary Internal Medicine with Dr. Stephen Ettinger and the last two also with Dr. Etienne Côté. He coauthored the four editions of Canine and Feline Endocrinology with Dr. Richard Nelson and the 4th edition also with Drs. Claudia Reusch, Catharine Scott-Moncrieff, and Ellen Behrend. He coedited Feline Endocrinology with Dr. Fracassi and Dr. Peterson.
Dr. Feldman has lectured in more than 45 of the 50 United States and 43 countries.

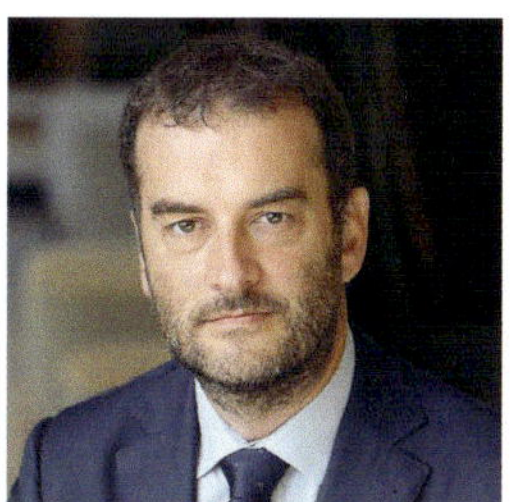

Federico Fracassi
DVM, ECVIM Diplomate (SAIM)
Professor of Small Animal Internal Medicine
University of Bologna, Italy

Dr. Fracassi graduated in Veterinary Medicine (DVM) at the University of Bologna, Italy. In 2005 he defended his PhD thesis and then completed a Residency in Internal Medicine at the University of Zurich, Switzerland.
He is now an Associate Professor of Veterinary Internal Medicine at the University of Bologna. His publication list consists of more than 100 journal articles.
He is the editor of "Veterinaria", a peer-reviewed journal and associate editor of JSAP. He coedited Feline Endocrinology with Dr. Feldman and Dr. Peterson. He has edited the book "Diagnostic and therapeutic algorithms in internal medicine for dogs and cats".
Dr. Fracassi has lectured in 22 countries.

Book editor

Edward Hall

MA, Vet MB, PhD, DECVIM-CA, FRCVS

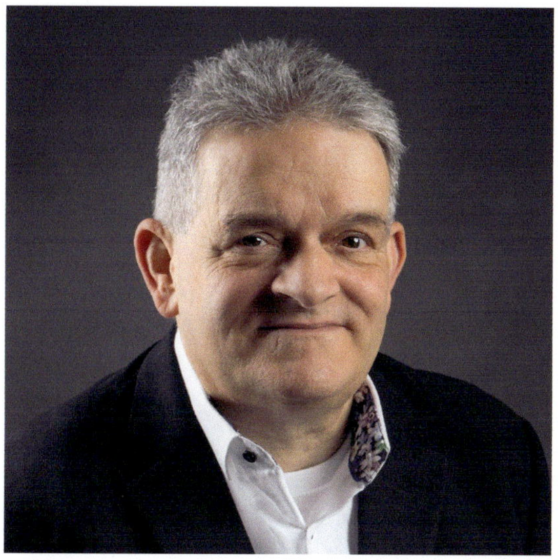

After graduating from Cambridge in 1979, Ed undertook a Rotating Internship at the University of Pennsylvania in Philadelphia. After two years in private practice in the UK, he returned to Penn to complete a Medicine Residency. Then, back in the UK, he studied for a Wellcome-funded PhD in Liverpool defining gluten-sensitive enteropathy in Irish setters, followed by a post-doctoral Fellowship investigating intestinal permeability in canine enteropathies. His subsequent research career has focussed on the interaction of the intestinal mucosa and its immune system with luminal bacteria and food, publishing widely as well as writing book chapters and editing textbooks. He was a member of the WSAVA GI Standardization Group that produced the ACVIM Consensus statement on the "Histopathological standards for the diagnosis of gastrointestinal inflammation in endoscopic biopsy samples".

Ed moved to Bristol Veterinary School in 1995, being promoted to Senior Lecturer then Professor of Small Animal Internal Medicine. He became Head of the Division of Companion Animal Studies, and then Deputy Head of School. Ed is a Diplomate of the European College of Veterinary Internal Medicine, a RCVS Recognised Specialist in Small Animal Medicine (Gastroenterology), a Fellow of the RCVS, and a Past President of the British Small Animal Veterinary Association. He retired from the University of Bristol in 2021, becoming Emeritus Professor of Small Animal Internal Medicine and was awarded a PhD *honoris causa* by the University of Helsinki in 2023.

He continues to teach gastroenterology and flexible endoscopy to veterinary practitioners.

Contributors

Sophie Adamantos, BVSc, CertVA, DACVECC, DECVECC, FHEA, MRCVS
Paragon Referrals
Wakefield, UK

Fergus Allerton, BSc, BVSc, CertSAM, DECVIM-CA, FRCVS
Willows Veterinary Centre
Shirley, UK

Sarah Caddy, MA, VetMB, PhD, DACVM, FRCVS
Baker Institute for Animal Health, College of Veterinary Medicine
Cornell University
Ithaca, NY, USA

Tawny Chandler, MS, PhD
Baker Institute for Animal Health, College of Veterinary Medicine
Cornell University
Ithaca, NY, USA

Andrea Corsini, DVM, PhD, DECVIM-CA
Department of Veterinary Science
University of Parma
Parma, Italy

Marta Costa, DVM, MSc, FRCPath, DECVCP, MRCVS
IDEXX Laboratories
Wetherby, UK

Francesca Del Baldo, DVM, MRCVS, PhD, DECVIM-CA
Department of Veterinary Medical Sciences
Alma Mater Studiorum - University of Bologna
Ozzano Emilia (BO), Italy

Florent Duplan, DVM, MSc, AFHEA, DECVIM-CA, MRCVS
Internal Medicine Department
Bristol Vet Specialists
Vet Oracle Telemedicine
Bristol, UK

Hany M. Elsheikha, BVSc, MSc, PhD, PGCHE, DEVPC, FHEA
School of Veterinary Medicine and Science
Faculty of Medicine and Health Sciences
University of Nottingham
Loughborough, UK

Samuel Fowlie, BSc(Hons), BVSc(Hons), MVM, DECVIM-CA, MRCVS
Southfields Veterinary Specialists
Basildon
Essex, UK

Marie-Aude Genain, MA, DMV, MSc, FHEA, PGCTLHE, DECVDI, MRCVS
The Queen's Veterinary School Hospital
University of Cambridge
Cambridge, UK

Stefania Golinelli, DVM, PhD
Department of Veterinary Medical Sciences
Alma Mater Studiorum - University of Bologna
Ozzano Emilia (BO), Italy

Sara M. Gould, BVetMed, DSAM, FRCVS
Langford Vets
University of Bristol
Langford, UK

Megan Grobman, DVM, MS, PhD, DACVIM (SAIM)
Department of Clinical Sciences, College of Veterinary Medicine
Auburn University
Auburn, AL, USA

Mara Holz, Dr. med. vet.
Clinic for Small Animal Internal Medicine, Vetsuisse Faculty
University of Zurich
Zürich, Switzerland

Sara Jablonski, DVM, PhD, DACVIM (SAIM)
Department of Small Animal Clinical Sciences,
College of Veterinary Medicine
Michigan State University
East Lansing, MI, USA

Aarti Kathrani, BVetMed(Hons), PhD, DACVIM (SAIM & Nutrition), FHEA, MRCVS
Department of Clinical Science and Services
The Royal Veterinary College
University of London
Hertfordshire, UK

John McGarry, MSc, PhD, SFHEA
Institute of Infection, Veterinary & Ecological Sciences,
Faculty of Health and Life Sciences
University of Liverpool
Liverpool, UK

Jo Murrell, BVSc(Hons), PhD, DECVAA, MRCVS
Anaesthesia & Analgesia Department
Bristol Vet Specialists
Bristol, UK

Sarah O'Shaughnessy, BVetMed(Hons), PGCert (HPE), PGDip (clinical practice), FHEA, MRCVS
School of Veterinary Science
University of Bristol
Langford, UK

Kostas Papasouliotis, DVM, PhD, DECVCP, MRCVS
Vet In Progress Plus Veterinary Laboratories
Agia Paraskevi
Athens, Greece

Mark G. Papich, DVM, MS, DACVCP
College of Veterinary Medicine
North Carolina State University
Raleigh, NC, USA

Andrea Petrelli, DVM, AFHEA, DECVIM-CA, MRCVS
Internal Medicine Department
ChesterGates Veterinary Specialists
Chester, UK

Marco Pietra, DVM
Department of Veterinary Medical Sciences
Alma Mater Studiorum - University of Bologna
Ozzano Emilia (BO), Italy

Simon L. Priestnall, BSc(Hons), BVSc,PhD, PGC(VetEd), FHEA, FRSB, DACVP, FRCPath, FRCVS
Department of Pathobiology & Population Sciences,
The Royal Veterinary College
University of London
Hertfordshire, UK

Cameron Prior, BVSc, MSc, PgCert CertAVP, DECVIM-CA, MRCVS
Willows Veterinary Centre & Referral Service
Solihull
West Midlands, UK

Fabio Procoli, DMV, MVetMed, DACVIM (SAIM), DECVIM-CA, MRCVS
AniCura Veterinary Hospital I Portoni Rossi
Bologna, Italy

Jenny Reeve, BVSc, DECVIM-CA, FHEA, MRCVS
Langford Vets, Small Animal Referral Hospital
University of Bristol
North Somerset, UK

Craig Ruaux, BVSc (Hons I), PhD, DACVIM (SAIM)
University Veterinary Teaching Hospital, Sydney
Sydney School of Veterinary Science
The University of Sydney
Sydney, Australia

Beatrice Ruggerone, DVM, PhD, DECVIM-CA
AniCura Veterinary Hospital I Portoni Rossi
Bologna, Italy

Guillaume C. Ruiz, DVM, CEAV-MI, DECVIM-CA, MRCVS
Internal Medicine Department
Bristol Vet Specialists
Bristol, UK

Silke Salavati Schmitz, Dr.med.vet., PhD, DECVIM-CA, FHEA, FRCVS
Hospital for Small Animals, Royal (Dick) School of Veterinary Studies and The Roslin Institute, University of Edinburgh
Midlothian, UK

Sonia Sanchez-Redondo, LdaVet, MSc, CSAVP (Internal Medicine), DACVP (Clinical Pathology), MRCVS
Diagnostic Laboratories, Langford Vets
University of Bristol
Langford, UK

Alejandro Suarez-Bonnet, DVM, MVetMed (Distinction), PhD(Hons), DipRCPath, DACVP, MRCVS
Department of Pathobiology & Population Sciences
The Royal Veterinary College
University of London
Hertfordshire, UK

Alyssa M. Sullivant, DVM, MS, DACVIM (SAIM)
College of Veterinary Medicine
Mississippi State University
Mississippi State, MS, USA

Katie Tolbert, DVM, PhD, DACVIM (SAIM & Nutrition)
Department of Small Animal Clinical Sciences (VSCS)
Texas A&M College of Veterinary Medicine & Biomedical Sciences
College Station, TX, USA

Linda Toresson, DVM, Swedish Spec. Small Anim. Intern Med, PhD
Evidensia Specialist Animal Hospital
Helsingborg, Sweden

Stefan Unterer, DVM, Dr Med Vet, Dr Habil, DECVIM-CA
Clinic for Small Animal Internal Medicine, Vetsuisse Faculty
University of Zurich
Zürich, Switzerland

Ferran Valls Sanchez, DVM, DECVIM-CA, MRCVS
WeYouVets
Ingrave, UK

Nathaniel Whitley, BVMS, PhD, CertVC, DACVIM (SAIM), DECVIM-CA, FRCVS
Davies Veterinary Specialists
Hertfordshire, UK

Ian Wright, BVMS, BSc, MSc, MRCVS
Mount Veterinary Practice
Fleetwood, Lancashire, UK

Series preface

"Oh! You are a veterinarian? I (or my brother, my sister, my son, my daughter...) always wanted to be a veterinarian." All of us, as veterinary students and later as veterinarians, have often heard comments like this. Becoming a veterinarian seems to be such a wonderful career to non-veterinarians: helping helpless dogs and cats. Veterinarians should be happy and satisfied in their *chosen* profession because they are able to earn a living by caring for loved pets. The journey to satisfaction and happiness for veterinarians, however, never seems to follow an obvious, straight, or level path.

The 1950s witnessed a dramatic growth in the popularity of pet dogs and in the number of veterinarians who cared exclusively for pets. The popularity of cats soon followed. Today, more dogs and cats are considered "members of the family" than ever before in human history, and their owners want to protect their family members from illness or to resolve any illness. There are more veterinarians who care for dogs and cats currently than ever before in human history. Veterinary medicine has evolved remarkably to meet the ever-growing medical care expectations and demands of dog and cat owners.

When learning of a diagnosis, prognosis, treatment, and/or the cost of care for their ill pet, some owners become distressed. These emotions are often directed at the "messenger" of the bad news: the veterinarian. The veterinarian, in turn, may not respect their own knowledge and feel inadequate. One reason that a veterinarian may feel inadequate is the realization that it is impossible for anyone in general practice to be expert and current on all the canine and feline conditions encountered in a day, week, or month: everything from orthopedics to oncology, from vaccinology to dermatology, from ophthalmology to cardiology. Nor is it possible for an internal medicine specialist to be expert and current in each condition they encounter, from endocrinology to gastroenterology or from respiratory conditions to chronic kidney disease. Further, it is clear that cats are not small dogs. Perceived "knowledge deficiencies" can cause veterinarians to feel they are failing to meet their clients' expectations.

The internal medicine textbooks in this new series offer one approach for enjoying veterinary practice. We encourage colleagues to embrace developing expertise in one area. By focusing on and studying one organ system in either the dog or cat, one can achieve greater knowledge and skills and, in turn, greater confidence. Each book in this series offers a clear path to learning current opinions on pathophysiology, diagnosis, treatment, prognosis, and costs associated with illnesses involving one system in one species. Confidence gained in a focused area can be sensed by devoted owners. Further, confidence in one area of internal medicine also creates confidence in sharing limitations: "I am extremely confident in diagnosing and managing some conditions but I lack that level of expertise in all other conditions".

The books in this series have been constructed to help build expertise in one organ system in either the dog or the cat. Each book is edited by one or two specialists with outstanding international credentials. Each editor was tasked with building a text that contains all the information found in general internal medicine textbooks, but with much more in-depth discussions on each condition. Each book has early chapters focusing on differential diagnoses of owner concerns, physical examination findings, and laboratory and/or imaging results. These are excellent for students as they begin to apply their basic knowledge to clinical cases. These chapters also provide a quick review for experienced general practitioners and specialists. Each chapter provides at least one algorithm designed to take the reader from a vague owner concern, physical examination finding, or laboratory abnormality to a specific diagnosis with step-by-step instructions. The "techniques section" in each text teaches currently employed procedures, most with videos. In-depth chapters on known illnesses comprise 70 to 80% of each book's content. The editors have provided a larger number of chapters, a larger number of expert contributors, and greater depth on each organ system than any general textbook can supply. The material has a level of credibility that no internet site can claim. Each book can guide the reader through a more complete journey of understanding than is available in any other veterinary resource.

Edward Feldman
Federico Fracassi

Preface

So why do we need a new textbook about veterinary gastroenterology?

It has been forty years since I began my clinical and research career in canine gastroenterology: veterinary endoscopy was in its infancy; folate and cobalamin were still being measured by bioassay; and the canine TLI test had only just been developed. A lot has changed since then and this book aims to bring together the latest information. Also, there has never been a textbook dedicated solely to *Canine Gastroenterology*. There is an excellent book on *Feline Gastroenterology* published by Edra, but dogs are not large cats!

When I started my PhD, documenting gluten-sensitive enteropathy in Irish setters, the focus of gastrointestinal (GI) research was on biochemical changes in the digestive process. Since then, there has been an exponential increase in relevant research and publications, but with the focus changing over time. First, the role of altered intestinal permeability in intestinal diseases was investigated. Subsequent elucidation of the innate and adaptive immune pathways in the gut helped our understanding of intestinal inflammation, complementing the WSAVA Guidelines on the interpretation of inflammation in endoscopic biopsies. Most recently, molecular techniques have led to our understanding of the importance of host genetics and the intestinal microbiome in health and disease.

Originally called *chronic enteritis*, then *inflammatory bowel disease*, and now renamed *chronic inflammatory enteropathy*, we still don't know the whole story, However, the summation of the research so far strengthens the hypothesis that intestinal inflammation (and possibly alimentary lymphoma) is a consequence of alterations in the interactions between the mucosal barrier, the mucosal immune system and the microbiome, with both genetic and environmental factors influencing its expression. Clinically, we now know the importance of cobalamin supplementation and the role of diet in managing chronic enteropathies. Furthermore, new methods of modulating the microbiome, such as prebiotics, probiotics, postbiotics, and fecal microbiota transplantation, offer new treatment options.

So when I was asked to edit this book by Professors Feldman and Fracassi, I saw the opportunity to invite the best clinician researchers to write something that would not only be helpful to practitioners but also stimulate further research. The target audience ranges from the undergraduate veterinary students, through primary care clinicians, Residents, and Specialists to academic researchers.

This book is divided into six sections, starting with the diagnostic approach to specific clinical presentations that may or may not be due to GI disease, with each chapter including an algorithmic pathway. A section on diagnostic methods is followed by sections about the management of GI diseases and non-specific and specific drug treatments. The fifth section covers diffuse inflammatory, infectious and neoplastic diseases of the GI tract. Specific diseases of each area of the tract from oesophagus to large intestine are found in the final section. Although diseases of the liver and pancreas are critical to normal GI function, they are discussed in detail in "*Canine Hepatobiliary and Exocrine Pancreatic Diseases*", also published by Edra.

Finally, great thanks are due to the many authors who have been so kind in contributing to this book for all their efforts and for educating me. Thanks are also due to Ed Feldman for his constant support and periodic weather reports from sunny California. Finally, I must thank Costanza Smeraldi of Edra Publishing for her guidance and encouragement throughout the publication process and for the production of such a high-quality book of which I am rightly proud.

Edward Hall

Abbreviations

AChR acetylcholine receptor
ACTH adrenocorticotropic hormone
ACTHst adrenocorticotropic hormone stimulation test
Ag antigen
AHDS acute hemorrhagic diarrhea syndrome
AL alimentary lymphoma
ALARA as low as reasonably achievable
ALP alkaline phosphatase
ALT alanine aminotransferase
AP aspiration pneumonia
aPTT activated partial thromboplastin time
ARE antimicrobial-responsive enteropathy
AST aspartate aminotransferase
BA bile acids
BAst bile acid stimulation test
BCS body condition score
BIPS barium-impregnated polyethylene spheres
BMBT buccal mucosal bleeding time
BOAS brachycephalic obstructive airway syndrome
BW body weight
CaAstV canine astrovirus
CBC complete blood count
CCD charge-coupled device
CCECAI canine chronic enteropathy clinical activity index
CDV canine distemper virus
CE chronic enteropathy
CECoV canine enteric coronavirus
CFU colony-forming units
CHPG chronic hypertrophic pylorogastropathy
CIE chronic inflammatory enteropathy
CILBD chronic idiopathic large bowel diarrhea
CIPO chronic intestinal pseudoobstruction
CK creatine kinase
CKD chronic kidney disease
CM congenital megaesophagus
CMO craniomandibular osteopathy
CMOS complementary metal-oxide-semiconductor
CNS central nervous system
CNV canine norovirus
COX cyclo-oxygenase
CPMA canine parvovirus monoclonal antibody
CPV canine parvovirus
CRI continuous rate infusion
CRP C-reactive protein
CRTZ chemoreceptor trigger zone
CSF cerebrospinal fluid
CT computed tomography
cTSH canine thyroid-stimulating hormone
DFs dietary fibers
DI dysbiosis index
DSF de Simone formulation
EATL-2 Enteropathy-associated T-cell lymphoma
EDTA ethylenediaminetetraacetic acid
EERD extraesophageal reflux disease
EF Enterococcus faecium
EGJ esophageal gastric junction
ELISA enzyme-linked immunosorbent assay
EMG electromyography
EndoFLIP endoluminal functional lumen imaging probe
EPI exocrine pancreatic insufficiency
FBs foreign bodies
FCoV feline coronavirus
FISH fluorescence *in situ* hybridization
FLOTAC flotation technique for accurate cyst analysis
FMT fecal microbiota transplantation
FNA fine-needle aspiration
FRE food-responsive enteropathy
FUO fever of unknown origin
GABA γ-amino butyric acid
GDV gastric dilatation-volvulus
GEI gastroesophageal intussusception
GERD gastroesophageal reflux disease
GGT γ-glutamyl transferase
GH growth hormone
GHG giant hypertrophic gastritis
GHLO gastric Helicobacter-like organisms
GI gastrointestinal
GIST gastrointestinal stromal tumor
GLDH glutamate dehydrogenase
GOLPP geriatric onset laryngeal paralysis polyneuropathy
GRVs gastric residual volumes
HCT hematocrit
HCY homocysteine
Hgb hemoglobin
HGE hemorrhagic gastroenteritis
IBD inflammatory bowel disease
IBS irritable bowel syndrome
ICC idiopathic chronic colitis
ICC/FC immunocytochemistry/flow cytometry
IF intrinsic factor
IgA immunoglobulin A
IgE immunoglobulin E
IGF insulin-like growth factor
IgG immunoglobulin G
IHC immunohistochemistry
IL intestinal lymphangiectasia
IM intramuscular
IRE immunosuppressant-responsive enteropathy

IV intravenously
IVFT intravenous fluid therapy
LAB lactic acid bacteria
LES lower esophageal sphincter
LI large intestine
LMND lower motor neuron disease
LN lymph node
LPE lymphoplasmacytic enteritis
LP-PNC laryngeal paralysis–polyneuropathy complex
MAC minimum alveolar concentration
MCHC mean corpuscular hemoglobin concentration
MCS muscle condition scoring
MCT mast cell tumor
MCV mean corpuscular volume
MDR1 multidrug resistance mutation
ME megaesophagus
MG myasthenia gravis
MIFC merthiolate–iodine–formalin-concentration
MLV modified live virus
MMA methylmalonic acid
MPV mean platelet volume
MRI magnetic resonance imaging
MrMRE microbiota-related modulation-responsive enteropathy
NCV nerve conduction velocity
NFE nitrogen-free extract
NLR neutrophil-to-lymphocyte ratio
NMDA N-methyl-D-aspartate
NRE nonresponsive enteropathy
NSAIDS nonsteroidal anti-inflammatory drugs
PARR polymerase chain reaction for antigen receptor rearrangements
PCR polymerase chain reaction
PCV packed cell volume
PD polydipsia
PEG percutaneous endoscopic gastrostomy
PEG polyethylene glycol
PGE_1 prostaglandin E_1
PGs inflammatory prostaglandins
PLE protein-losing enteropathy
PLI pancreatic lipase immunoreactivity
PLR platelet-to-lymphocyte ratio
PN parenteral nutrition
PO per os
POCUS point-of-care ultrasound scan
POMC pro-opiomelanocortin
PPE personal protective equipment
PPI proton pump inhibitor
PT prothrombin time
PTH parathyroid hormone
PTHrp parathyroid hormone–related protein
PU polyuria
RBC red blood cell count
rCDI recurrent Clostridioides difficile
RCTs randomized controlled trials
RER resting energy requirement
RI reference interval
SAFC sodium acetate–acetic acid–formalin-concentration
SARDS sudden acquired retinal degeneration syndrome
SBA serum bile acids
SBS short bowel syndrome
SC subcutaneous
SCFAs short-chain fatty acids
SDMA symmetric dimethylarginine
SHH sliding hiatal hernia
SI small intestine
SLAM signaling lymphocyte activation molecule
SOP standard operating procedure
Spec cPL specifically measure lipases of pancreatic origin
SRE steroid-responsive enteropathy
T_4 serum total thyroxine
TC transcobalamin
TE thromboembolic
TEG thromboelastogram
TGEV transmissible gastroenteritis virus of swine
TGFβ transforming growth factor beta
THF tetrahydrofolate
TKIs tyrosine kinase inhibitors
TLI trypsin-like immunoreactivity
TP total protein
TSH thyroid-stimulating hormone
UES upper esophageal sphincter
UPC urine protein-to-creatinine ratio
USG urine specific gravity
VCM viscoelastic coagulation monitoring
VFSSs videofluoroscopic swallow studies

Table of contents

SECTION I Diagnostic approach to presenting complaints

SECTION IV Nonspecific drug therapy

SECTION V Diffuse gastrointestinal diseases

SECTION VI Specific organ systems

Diagnostic approach to gastrointestinal disease

Edward J. Hall
MA, VetMB, PhD, DECVIM-CA, FRCVS

The gastrointestinal (GI) tract is a complex organ that has paradoxical roles of digesting and absorbing food whilst acting as a barrier to pathogens. It is the largest immune organ in the body and surveys ingested food antigens, reacts to potential pathogens, and interacts with a population of commensal microbes (the microbiome) that appears critical to the overall health of the animal. Complex connections between the central, autonomic, and enteric nervous systems and many hormones coordinate motility, secretion, and absorption along the GI tract and the activity of adjunctive organs such as the pancreas and gallbladder. Other hormones, some of which (e.g., cholecystokinin, ghrelin) are derived from the GI tract, mediate the sensations of hunger and satiety. Considering the complexity of the GI tract, it is not surprising that minor variations in stool quality are seen and are of no clinical significance.

The cardinal signs of GI dysfunction, namely vomiting and diarrhea, have been shown to be one of the most common reasons for the presentation of dogs to UK primary care veterinary practices, a situation which is likely to be the same worldwide, with infectious causes more likely in countries with a low uptake of vaccination and deworming. In a survey of 148,741 dogs attending 93 clinics in the UK, a total of 10.5% of cases were presented because of vomiting (4.1%) or diarrhea (6.4%), similar to the number of presentations for otitis externa (10.2%) or periodontal disease (9.3%), with a further 2.6% classified as having gastroenteritis.[1] However, most cases are mild and self-limiting, and many never seek veterinary attention.[2] Thus, whilst GI dysfunction is a common presenting complaint, it is only severe acute cases and chronic cases that require in-depth investigations to either reach a definitive diagnosis or choose appropriate empirical treatment. Most acute cases presented to veterinary practices never receive a definitive diagnosis and only require supportive care, of which fluid therapy to prevent dehydration is most important.

It is also crucial to understand that signs of GI dysfunction may not be the result of a primary GI problem. Diseases in other organ systems may secondarily cause GI signs, so the GI tract could be considered to be suffering collateral damage. For example, hypoadrenocorticism can manifest as diarrhea and weight loss, while coagulopathies may cause GI bleeding. Systemic diseases may also involve the GI tract, although other signs are likely to be present (e.g., respiratory and neurological signs in patients with distemper infection; see Chapter 36). The clinician must rule out conditions secondarily affecting the GI tract before investing time and money looking for a primary GI disease. The diagnostic approach to dogs presenting with signs potentially related to GI disease is detailed in Chapters 2–16, each with a problem-solving algorithm. Throughout, attention to the hydration status of the patient is obligatory, as any loss from the enormous flux of fluid passing through the GI tract can cause rapid and severe dehydration (see Chapter 24).

As with the investigation of all medical conditions, the diagnostic pathway starts with the history and physical examination, which may be sufficient to rule in/out primary GI disease. Key information about vaccination and deworming status, appetite (see Chapters 2 and 3), and travel and dietary history (see Chapter 25) are as important as the actual signs and any disease progression. The physical examination (see Chapter 17) may identify weight loss (see Chapter 4) and abdominal enlargement or pain (see Chapters 5 and 6), and a digital rectal examination may confirm the presence of diarrhea and/or bleeding (see Chapters 11, 12, and 14).

If there are concerns about the patient's condition, and the owner agrees, a minimum database of hematology and serum biochemistry will help quantify the degree of dehydration or any anemia (see Chapter 18) and identify a protein-losing enteropathy (see Chapter 13). Importantly, it will also identify potential non-GI causes. A fecal examination for parasites is recommended in all patients with diarrhea (see Chapters 19, 39, and 40). Stool culture is often more confusing than helpful but is recommended in dogs fed a raw meat diet (see Chapter 37). Determination of the *dysbiosis index* (i.e., quantification of key bacteria in the feces as a proxy for identifying dysbiosis) may be helpful in assessing disease severity and directing and monitoring treatment.[3] Further laboratory testing for a range of biomarkers may be indicated in chronic disease to provide indirect assessment of disease severity, whilst measurement of serum folate and cobalamin concentrations may also identify a need for supplementation (see Chapter 20).

TABLE 1.1 Criteria of concern in chronic enteropathies.

- Abnormal palpation and/or imaging findings
- Anorexia
- Hypoalbuminemia (protein-losing enteropathy)
- Persistent vomiting
- Profuse gastrointestinal bleeding
- Severe weight loss

Indications for further investigations (potentially including biopsy) rather than empirical treatment trials with parasiticides and diet.

Imaging in GI disease is most useful for identifying surgical conditions of the GI tract (e.g., foreign bodies, intussusceptions, solid neoplasms) and extra-GI diseases such as pancreatitis (see Chapter 21). Whilst plain radiography and abdominal ultrasound are complementary, the latter is most useful in imaging the structure of the GI wall and is now often complemented by computed tomography.

There is rarely any indication for intestinal biopsy in dogs with acute GI disease, especially as the majority have self-limiting disease, but may be indicated in chronic disease. However, most chronic enteropathies are inflammatory in nature.[4] Therefore, if there are no criteria of concern (Table 1.1), the current diagnostic approach is to perform a series of empirical treatment trials—i.e., parasiticides (see Chapter 30), exclusion diet (see Chapter 25), and even immunosuppressants (see Chapter 34)—before biopsy.[4,5] Empirical trials with antibacterials are not recommended (see Chapter 29).[6] Endoscopic biopsy is the preferred method because it is minimally invasive (see Chapter 22), but it has diagnostic limitations as described in Chapter 23.

Presentations other than vomiting and/or diarrhea may require specific investigations, such as a barium swallow in dogs with drooling, dysphagia, or regurgitation (see Chapters 7–9). However, all investigations should start with a history and physical examination, and dehydration should be addressed. Once a diagnosis is suspected or confirmed, either empirical or definitive treatment, respectively, can commence.

References

1. O Neill DG, Church DB, McGreevy PD, et al. Prevalence of disorders recorded in dogs attending primary-care veterinary practices in England. *PLoS One* 9(3):e90501, 2014.
2. Hubbard K, Skelly BJ, McKelvie J, Wood JL. Risk of vomiting and diarrhoea in dogs. *Vet Rec* 161(22):755–757, 2007.
3. AlShawaqfeh MK, Wajid B, Minamoto Y, et al. A dysbiosis index to assess microbial changes in fecal samples of dogs with chronic inflammatory enteropathy. *FEMS Microbiol Ecol* 93(11), 2017.
4. Volkmann M, Steiner JM, Fosgate GT, et al. Chronic diarrhea in dogs— retrospective study in 136 cases. *J Vet Intern Med* 31(4):1043–1055, 2017.
5. Dandrieux JR. Inflammatory bowel disease versus chronic enteropathy in dogs: are they one and the same? *J Small Anim Pract* 57(11):589–599, 2016.
6. Cerquetella M, Rossi G, Suchodolski JS, Schmitz SS, Allenspach K, Rodriguez-Franco F, et al. Proposal for rational antibacterial use in the diagnosis and treatment of dogs with chronic diarrhoea. Journal of Small Animal Practice. 2020;61(4):211-5.

CHAPTER 2

Anorexia/decreased appetite

Andrea Corsini
DVM, PhD, DECVIM-CA

Pathophysiology

Decreased appetite is a nonspecific finding and a common reason for an owner to seek medical care for their pet. A complete lack of appetite is referred to as anorexia, while the term hyporexia better signifies a partial decrease in appetite. Dysorexia defines altered eating patterns, including eating only palatable food and refusing prescribed diets. Decreased appetite must be distinguished from an inability to eat, as seen in diseases causing pain in opening the mouth, dental diseases, or oral dysphagia. This distinction is crucial but is not always straightforward for the owner to distinguish.

The regulation of food intake involves many internal and external stimuli, including sensory signals (e.g., olfaction, physical attributes of food, flavor), metabolic signals (e.g., orexigenic and anorexigenic factors), environmental signals (e.g., timing and location of meals, ambient noise level, the person offering the food, previous negative or positive associations), and previously learned behavior. Consequently, many diseases or conditions can negatively impact appetite. Patients with organ failure, neoplasia, inflammatory disease, and fever usually have increased circulation of anorexigenic factors (e.g., inflammatory cytokines, uremic toxins, or other substances that are generally metabolized by affected organs). Both pain and nausea, which are common in abdominal and GI diseases, result in anorexia/hyporexia.

The resolution of anorexia/hyporexia depends on the effective treatment of its etiology, which can sometimes be easily achieved. Anorexia/hyporexia due to chronic conditions or untreatable diseases is more challenging and critical because of the negative consequences of prolonged decreased food intake.[1] Indeed, even a few days of anorexia can significantly impact a patient's condition. For example, protein and fat catabolism markedly increase because both are used to perform gluconeogenesis in place of carbohydrates, which are depleted. This leads to immune system suppression, muscle and weight loss, and secondary organ dysfunction, which in turn worsens anorexia/hyporexia. Whenever anorexia/hyporexia is not resolved promptly, appetite stimulants or assisted feeding are warranted to counteract the negative impact of prolonged decreased food intake.

Diagnostic approach

A nondefinitive list of causes of decreased appetite is reported in Table 2.1. The approach to the diagnosis and treatment of patients with decreased appetite is depicted in Algorithm 2.1.

Algorithm 2.1 Note 1 Nonsteroidal anti-inflammatory drugs, opioid analgesics, proton pump inhibitors, antibiotics (beta-lactams, erythromycin, metronidazole, sulphonamides), chemotherapeutic agents, cardiac glycosides, penicillamine, and ferrous sulfate are some of the medications that can reduce appetite.

Algorithm 2.1 Note 2 A wide spectrum of diseases involving the oral cavity, skull, or nose can lead to anorexia. Common diseases to rule out are stomatitis, dental/periodontal disease, foreign body, neoplasia, fracture, osteomyelitis, temporomandibular joint problem, retrobulbar abscess, sinonasal aspergillosis.

Algorithm 2.1 Note 3 Masticatory myositis, trigeminal neuritis, and cranial nerve neoplasia affect mouth opening and swallowing, resulting in reduced food intake due to the inability to eat. Intention to eat, i.e., appetite, is often preserved in these cases.

Algorithm 2.1 Note 4 Orthopedic or neurologic diseases can lead to decreased appetite for a variety of reasons, including pain and/or discomfort. Common orthopedic diseases include osteoarthritis, panosteitis, septic arthritis, or immune-mediated polyarthritis. Common neurological diseases include intervertebral disc disease, steroid-responsive meningoarteritis, meningoencephalitis of unknown etiology, discospondylitis, vestibular diseases, and brain neoplasia.

Algorithm 2.1 Note 5 Renal diseases tend to cause anorexia when uremia or complications (e.g., nephrotic syndrome, metabolic acidosis) develop. Acute kidney injury, advanced (i.e., IRIS stage 3 or 4) chronic kidney disease (CKD), acute pyelonephritis, and severe glomerulopathies commonly cause decreased appetite, while appetite is usually unaffected in early CKD or chronic pyelonephritis.

TABLE 2.1 List of common causes for decreased appetite in dogs.

Gastrointestinal diseases	■ Acute gastroenteritis ■ Chronic inflammatory enteropathy ■ Esophageal diseases ■ Gastrointestinal neoplasia
Behavioral factors	■ Food aversion
Dietary or environmental factors	
Oropharyngeal/cranial disorders	■ Oral and periodontal diseases ■ Nasal diseases ■ Ocular disease ■ Skull and mandibular lesions

Extragastrointestinal abdominal diseases	■ Hepatobiliary diseases
	  ■ Congenital liver disease
	  ■ Acute hepatobiliary diseases
	  ■ Advanced chronic hepatitis
	  ■ Biliary tract diseases (e.g., gallbladder mucocele, cholecystitis)
	  ■ Hepatobiliary neoplasia
	■ Pancreatic diseases
	  ■ Acute or chronic pancreatitis
	  ■ Pancreatic neoplasia
	■ Peritoneal diseases
	■ Renal and urinary tract diseases
	  ■ Acute kidney injury
	  ■ Severe chronic kidney disease (IRIS stage 3 or 4)
	  ■ Nephrotic syndrome
	  ■ Urinary obstruction/rupture
	■ Reproductive diseases
	  ■ Acute prostatitis
	  ■ Pyometra

Endocrine diseases	■ Diabetic ketoacidosis ■ Hypoadrenocorticism
Orthopedic or neurological diseases	■ Brain neoplasia ■ Inflammatory diseases of the central nervous system ■ Intervertebral disk disease ■ Osteoarthritis ■ Septic arthritis or immune-mediated polyarthritis
Respiratory distress	■ Airway or lung diseases ■ Congestive heart failure ■ Mediastinal diseases ■ Pleural effusion
Chronic infectious/inflammatory diseases	
Fever of unknown origin (FUO)	
Lymphoproliferative neoplasia	
Medications	
Moderate to severe anemia	
Pain	

Algorithm 2.1 Note 6 Acute pancreatitis is a common cause of decreased appetite/anorexia in both dogs and cats, usually associated with vomiting and, especially in dogs, abdominal pain. Simultaneous evaluation of serum lipase concentration (i.e., canine pancreatic lipase immunoreactivity (PLI) and DGGR lipase) and abdominal ultrasound is the best available diagnostic approach.[2,3] Chronic pancreatitis may also cause decreased appetite or dysorexia but is more difficult to diagnose and requires histologic evaluation; therefore, the diagnosis is usually presumptive.

Algorithm 2.1 Note 7 Liver function is evaluated by measuring serum bile acids (SBA) and ammonia. Computed tomography angiography is helpful to identify macroscopic vascular anomalies. Liver cytology is an easy and inexpensive method to evaluate some neoplasms (e.g., round cell neoplasia). Percutaneous ultrasound-guided cholecystocentesis with bile culture and cytology is warranted whenever a bacterial infection is suspected.[4] A liver biopsy must be performed to confirm chronic hepatitis and gain information about etiology.

Algorithm 2.1 Note 8 Chronic enteropathies (CE) are common in dogs. Fecal examination and measurement of serum folate and cobalamin concentrations should always be performed. Serum basal cortisol, urinary cortisol to creatinine ratio, or an adrenocorticotropic hormone (ACTH) stimulation test can be considered to rule out hypoadrenocorticism.[5] Upper and lower GI endoscopy with biopsies is indicated for patients who fail to respond to diet trials and treatments aimed at modulating the microbiota, or when diffuse gastrointestinal neoplasia (e.g., intestinal lymphoma) is strongly suspected. Focal intestinal lesions are usually approached by performing full-thickness biopsies at laparotomy.

Algorithm 2.1 Note 9 Hypoadrenocorticism can present with normal serum concentrations of potassium and sodium (eunatremic, eukalemic hypoadrenocorticism) and an ACTH stimulation test should be considered in patients with suggestive clinical signs, even in absence of hyperkalemia and hyponatremia. To avoid false positive results, the history must be carefully assessed for exogenous glucocorticoid administration, and concurrent endogenous ACTH measurement should be considered.[6]

Algorithm 2.1 Note 10 Further testing should be considered based on the history and physical exam findings if a cause of anorexia is not apparent at this point. Lymph node cytology must be performed if lymphadenomegaly is present to assess for neoplasia (e.g., lymphoma) or infectious diseases (e.g., leishmaniosis). Infectious diseases should be tested based on clinical suspicion and epidemiological exposure. Total and ionized calcium concentrations must be measured because both hypocalcemia and hypercalcemia can decrease appetite. Advanced diagnostic imaging can help to identify neoplasia that is not apparent (e.g., intracranial neoplasia). Bone marrow aspirate is indicated if peripheral cytopenias are present or hemopoietic neoplasia (e.g., multiple myeloma) is suspected. Prostatic diseases (e.g., prostatitis) in male dogs and uterine disease in females must be ruled out.

ALGORITHM 2.1

Diagnostic approach to decreased appetite.

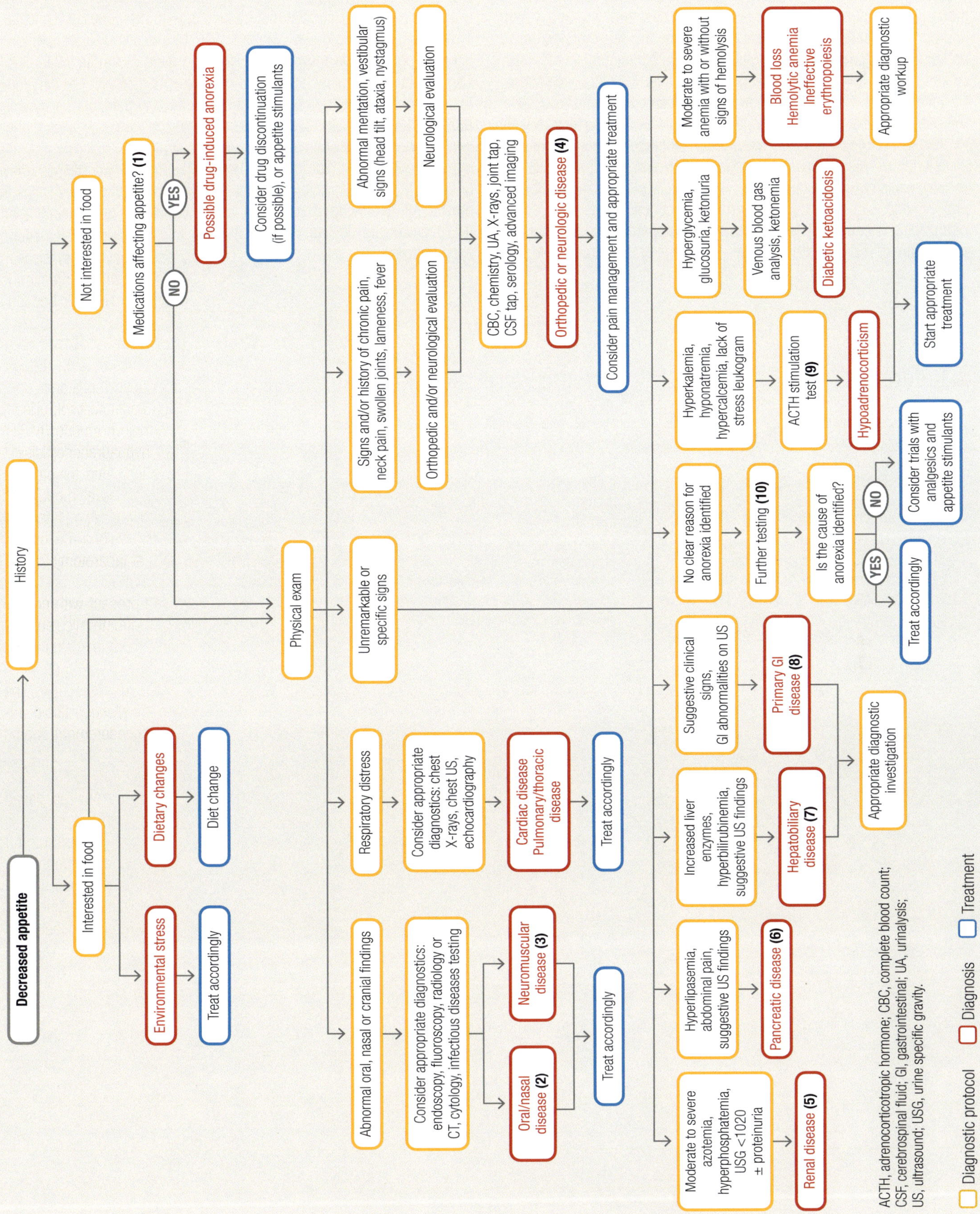

ACTH, adrenocorticotropic hormone; CBC, complete blood count; CSF, cerebrospinal fluid; GI, gastrointestinal; UA, urinalysis; US, ultrasound; USG, urine specific gravity.

Managing decreased appetite

A reason for decreased appetite is almost always identifiable after a thorough assessment. An analgesic trial may be warranted, and it is an appropriate treatment if pain is suspected to be the cause of decreased appetite. Symptomatic treatment with appetite stimulants should never substitute the effort to make a diagnosis and treat the underlying cause. However, a trial with appetite stimulants can be considered to support the patient during the diagnostic investigations or once extensive testing has failed to define a clear reason for decreased appetite. Appetite stimulants are also indicated in patients with decreased appetite due to irreversible chronic disease (e.g., neoplasia, chronic inflammation) to promote adequate caloric intake and counteract cachexia.[1]

Mirtazapine is commonly used in cats as an appetite stimulant but can also be used in dogs, although the effect is less predictable and less reliable. A 1.0 to 1.5 mg/kg q12–24h dosage has been suggested, but the ideal dose and frequency require further studies.[7] Alternatively, cyproheptadine (0.2 mg/kg PO q12h) can be used in dogs. Capromorelin is a ghrelin receptor agonist that causes growth hormone (GH) release, increases insulin-like growth factor 1 (IGF-1), and stimulates appetite. It is FDA-approved for appetite stimulation in dogs (3 mg/kg q24h PO).[8] Capromorelin oral solution proved effective and has demonstrated a wide margin of safety, but it is currently only licensed in the USA.

Assisted feeding by the placement of feeding tubes (i.e., nasoesophageal, esophagostomy tubes) should be considered if anorexia persists for more than 2–3 days if prompt intervention is required (e.g., parvovirosis) or when the condition causing decreased caloric intake is expected to persist for a prolonged period of time.[9] Resting energy requirement (RER) calculation is useful to assess the adequate caloric intake for each patient.

References

1. Johannes CM, Musser ML. Anorexia and the cancer patient. *Vet Clin North Am Small Anim Pract* 49:837–854, 2019.
2. Cridge H, Twedt DC, Marolf AJ, et al. Advances in the diagnosis of acute pancreatitis in dogs. *J Vet Intern Med* 35:2572–2587, 2021.
3. Forman MA, Steiner JM, Armstrong PJ, et al. ACVIM consensus statement on pancreatitis in cats. *J Vet Intern Med* 35:703–723, 2021.
4. Schiborra F, McConnell JF, Maddox TW. Percutaneous ultrasound-guided cholecystocentesis: complications and association of ultrasonographic findings with bile culture results. *J Small Anim Pract* 58:389–394, 2017.
5. Del Baldo F, Gerou Ferriani M, Bertazzolo W, et al. Urinary cortisol-creatinine ratio in dogs with hypoadrenocorticism. *J Vet Intern Med* 36:482–487, 2022.
6. Tardo AM, Del Baldo F, Leal RO, et al. Prevalence of eunatremic, eukalemic hypoadrenocorticism in dogs with signs of chronic gastrointestinal disease and risk of misdiagnosis after previous glucocorticoid administration. *J Vet Intern Med* 2023; 1–9.
7. Giorgi M, Yun H. Pharmacokinetics of mirtazapine and its main metabolites in Beagle dogs: A pilot study. *Vet J* 2012; 192:239–241.
8. Zollers B, Wofford JA, Heinen E, et al. A prospective, randomized, masked, placebo-controlled clinical study of capromorelin in dogs with reduced appetite. *J Vet Intern Med* 2016; 30:1851–1857.
9. Dumont R, Lemetayer J, Desquilbet L, et al. Tolerability of naso-esophageal feeding tubes in dogs and cats at home: Retrospective review of 119 cases. *J Vet Intern Med* 2023; 37:2315–2321.

CHAPTER 3

Polyphagia

Andrea Corsini
DVM, PhD, DECVIM-CA

Pathophysiology

Polyphagia is the excessive consumption of food, which can be physiological, pathological, or drug-induced. Food intake is regulated by several factors, including the central nervous system (CNS), the gastrointestinal (GI) tract, peripheral factors, and the environment. Gastrointestinal regulation is due to gastric distension, gastric emptying rate, various GI hormones (e.g., ghrelin, cholecystokinin), and nutrient absorption. Adipose tissue releases important hormones involved in appetite regulation, such as leptin and adiponectin. Peripheral factors such as insulin or the endocannabinoid system also play a role in appetite regulation. All these stimuli, together with environmental inputs processed by the cerebral cortex (e.g., smell, sight), are integrated within the CNS; this complex interplay takes place mainly in the hypothalamic nuclei, which define the feeding center and the satiety center.[1]

Insulin and leptin are potent stimulants of the satiety center, while ghrelin stimulates the feeding center. Serum concentrations of amino acids, glucose, and lipids affect hypothalamic regulation, stimulating the feeding center when they decrease.

Consequently, any condition affecting these mechanisms, both physiologic and pathologic, can induce increased food consumption. Primary polyphagia is due to conditions that affect CNS regulatory centers, such as increasing appetite despite normal energy stores. Secondary polyphagia derives from any conditions causing increased metabolic rate, decreased energy supply, or both, thus leading to a negative energy balance. The metabolic rate may increase both in physiologic (e.g., pregnancy, increased exercise) and pathologic conditions (e.g., hyperthyroidism). A decreased energy supply is likely the most common reason behind polyphagia in dogs and can be due to inadequate nutrient intake (e.g., low-calorie diet, megaesophagus), malabsorption/maldigestion (e.g., GI diseases or exocrine pancreatic insufficiency [EPI]), or inability to uptake nutrients within the cells (e.g., diabetes mellitus). Also, treatment with certain drugs (e.g., glucocorticoids) can cause polyphagia. Finally, the exact mechanisms responsible for polyphagia in certain diseases (e.g., Cushing's syndrome, liver diseases, suddenly acquired retinal degeneration syndrome) are multifactorial or not completely understood.

A list of the causes of polyphagia is reported in Table 3.1.

TABLE 3.1 Differential diagnoses for polyphagia.

Usually associated with weight gain	Usually associated with weight loss
■ Primary polyphagia	■ Small intestinal malabsorption
▪ Psychogenic (stress, gluttonous behavior)	▪ Chronic inflammatory enteropathy
▪ Hypothalamic diseases*	▪ Lymphangiectasia
■ Drug-induced polyphagia	▪ Intestinal parasitism
▪ Glucocorticoids	■ Exocrine pancreatic insufficiency
▪ Progestins	■ Portosystemic shunts/hepatic encephalopathy
▪ Phenobarbital	■ Congenital megaesophagus
▪ Capromorelin	■ Diabetes mellitus
▪ Benzodiazepines	■ Hyperthyroidism*
▪ Propofol	■ Inadequate feeding
▪ Cyproheptadine	■ Increased exercise
▪ Mirtazapine	
■ Cushing's syndrome	
■ Sudden acquired retinal degeneration syndrome	
■ Hypersomatotropism	
■ Insulinoma*	

*Uncommon cause of polyphagia in dogs.

Diagnostic approach

As described in Algorithm 3.1, the first step in assessing a polyphagic patient is establishing whether weight gain or loss has occurred or if body weight is unchanged. This assessment is extremely helpful in prioritizing steps in the diagnostic process. A careful evaluation of concurrent clinical signs is also very useful. Indeed, when polyphagia is the consequence of a disease, it is rarely the only clinical sign present.

Algorithm 3.1 Note 1 Once physiologic conditions (growth or pregnancy) have been excluded, weight gain points to primary polyphagia or specific endocrine diseases. Primary polyphagia is usually psychogenic due to gluttonous behavior, stress, or introduction of a new highly palatable food, but it can have an underlying

ALGORITHM 3.1

Diagnostic approach to polyphagia.

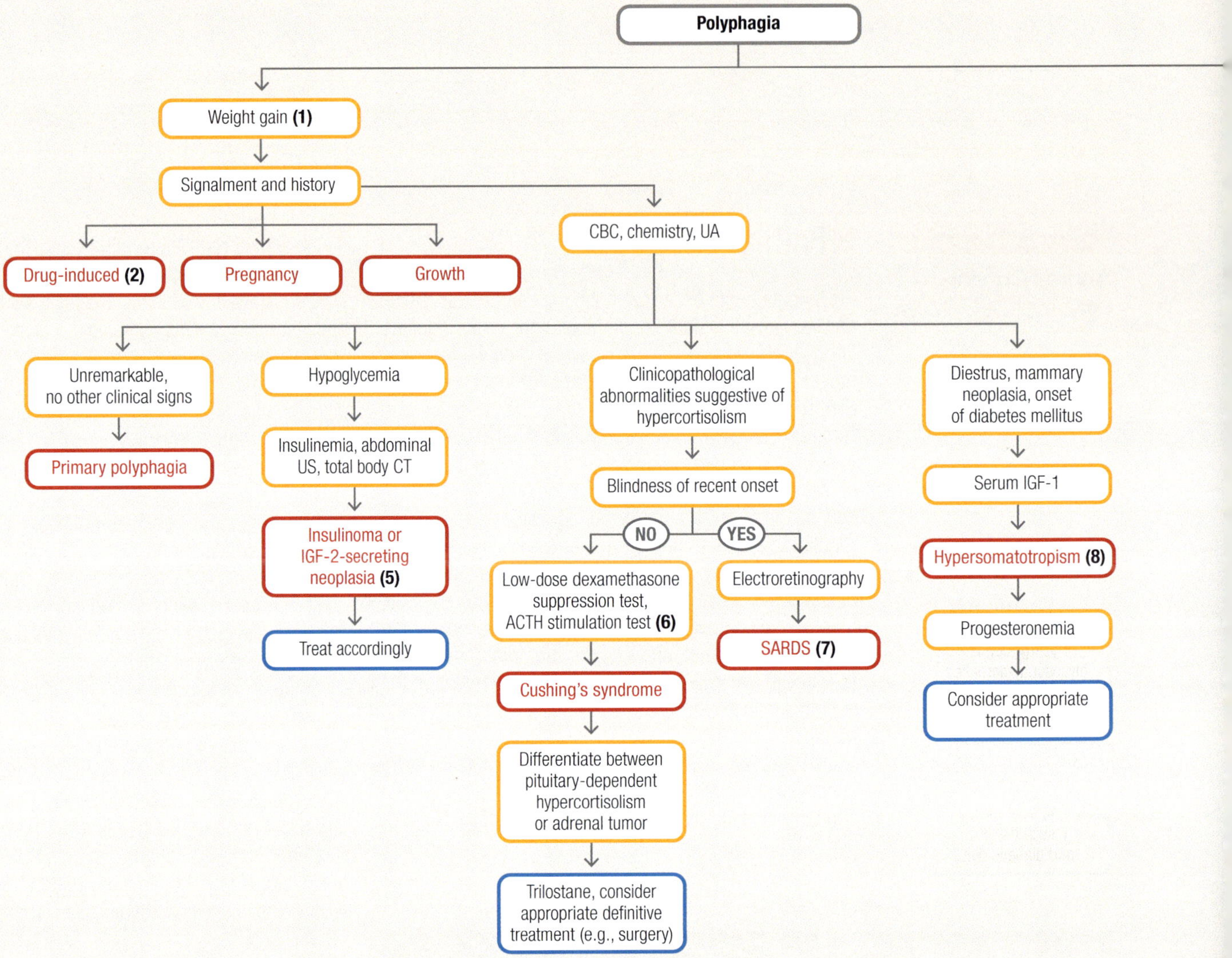

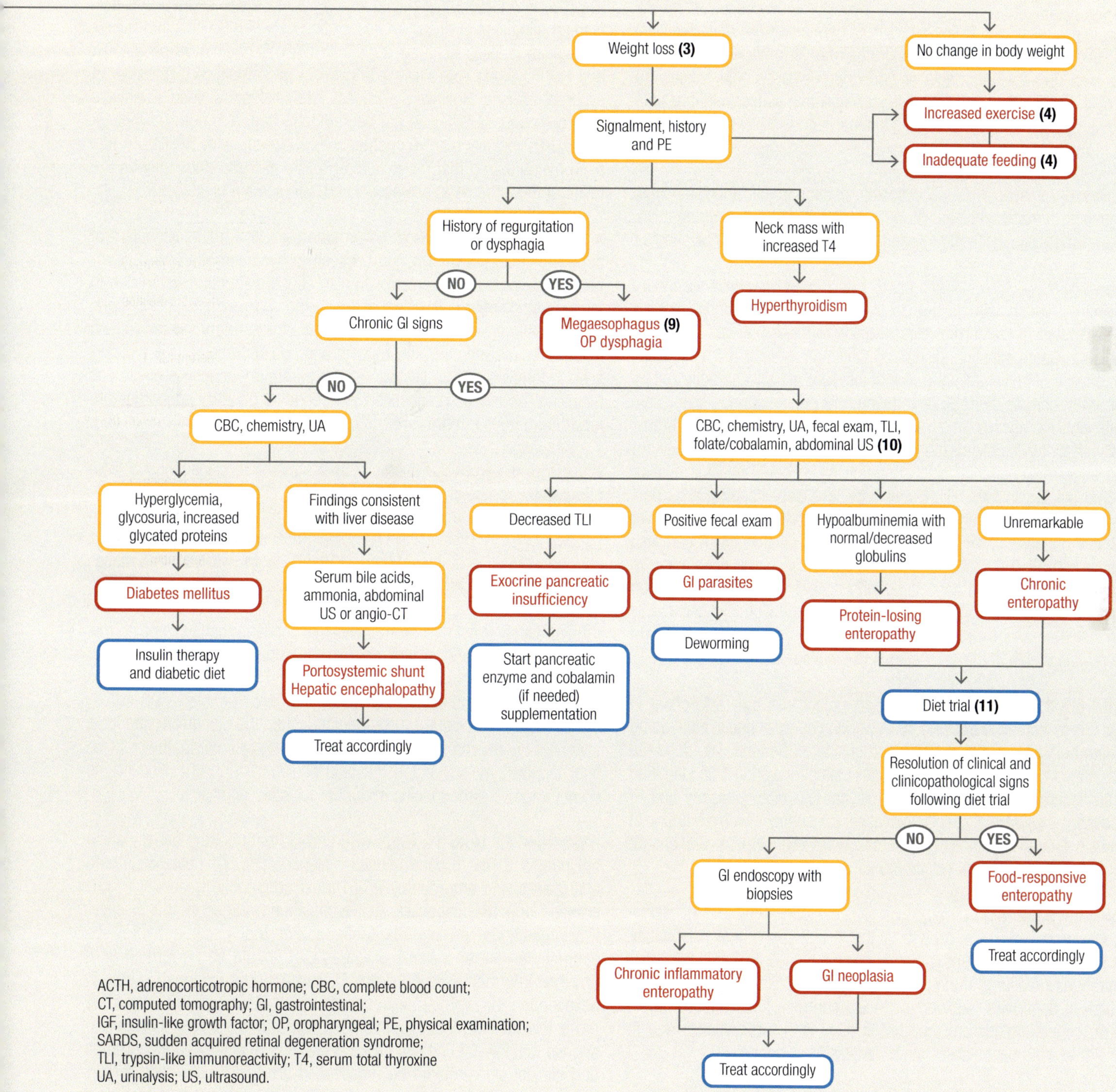

ACTH, adrenocorticotropic hormone; CBC, complete blood count; CT, computed tomography; GI, gastrointestinal; IGF, insulin-like growth factor; OP, oropharyngeal; PE, physical examination; SARDS, sudden acquired retinal degeneration syndrome; TLI, trypsin-like immunoreactivity; T4, serum total thyroxine UA, urinalysis; US, ultrasound.

Diagnostic protocol | Diagnosis | Treatment

genetic predisposition, e.g., a deletion in the pro-opiomelanocortin (POMC) gene in some Labrador Retrievers predisposes them to gluttony and obesity.[2] Thus, dogs with primary polyphagia can usually be easily identified through careful history, including lack of other clinical signs and unremarkable bloodwork. Rarely, primary polyphagia can be caused by diseases affecting the hypothalamic satiety center, but in this case, neurological signs are usually evident. Dogs with polyphagia and weight gain due to endocrine diseases almost invariably show concurrent clinical signs (e.g., polyuria/polydipsia [PU/PD], dermatological abnormalities) and abnormalities in bloodwork and urinalysis, or both. Of note, not all dogs with primary polyphagia or endocrine diseases gain weight; for example, dogs with hypercortisolism can maintain stable weight despite polyphagia and showing marked abdominal distension due to concurrent loss of muscle mass.

Algorithm 3.1 Note 2 Glucocorticoids, phenobarbital, antihistamines, progestins, benzodiazepines, propofol,[3] cyproheptadine, capromorelin, and mirtazapine are commonly used drugs that can induce polyphagia.[4]

Algorithm 3.1 Note 3 Weight loss is often associated with secondary polyphagia, which can be due to many different conditions, making the evaluation of concurrent clinical signs in these patients extremely important. Gastrointestinal disorders, which are among the most common causes of polyphagia and weight loss, are usually characterized by concurrent chronic diarrhea or vomiting: this presentation is suggestive of intestinal malabsorption or maldigestion as commonly seen in chronic GI diseases or EPI. Polyuria/polydipsia, along with polyphagia and weight loss, suggests endocrine diseases such as diabetes mellitus or liver disease leading to liver failure and hepatic encephalopathy (e.g., portosystemic shunt). Rarely, dogs with malabsorption can be polydipsic, probably because of an unsatisfied hunger. Hyperthyroidism can also present with PU/PD, polyphagia, and weight loss but is uncommon in dogs and is most often associated with thyroid neoplasia or raw food diets contaminated with the thyroid gland. Regurgitation is suggestive of megaesophagus or esophageal motility disorders, although body weight can remain stable in the early stages of the disease.

Algorithm 3.1 Note 4 Polyphagia and weight loss may also occur in dogs due to increased exercise, as in working dogs, or due to inadequate feeding both in terms of quantity and quality of the food, i.e., dogs fed unbalanced home-prepared diets. These situations should be identified by an accurate assessment of the clinical and dietary history and, if necessary, exclusion of specific diseases. Consultation with a nutritionist can help accurately define the patient's energy requirements and ensure that the diet meets these requirements.

Algorithm 3.1 Note 5 Chronic hypoglycemia caused by tumors secreting insulin or insulin-like growth factors (IGFs) can trigger polyphagia, but this is not a consistent finding in these patients. Serum insulin concentrations measured during hypoglycemia are inappropriately normal or high in dogs with insulinoma. On the contrary, low to undetectable insulin concentrations are reported in dogs with hypoglycemia due to IGF-2-secreting neoplasia or other neoplasia.[5]

Algorithm 3.1 Note 6 Polyphagia is only one of the many signs of hypercortisolism, albeit very common. In order to decrease the risk of false-positive results and misdiagnosis, dogs with polyphagia should be tested for Cushing's syndrome using dynamic hormonal tests only when other suggestive clinical (e.g., PU/PD, abdominal distension, dermatological abnormalities) and clinicopathological signs (e.g., thrombocytosis, mature neutrophilia, lymphopenia, increased alkaline phosphatase, alanine transaminase, and γ-glutamyltransferase activity, hyperlipasemia, hyperlipidemia, diluted urine, proteinuria) are present.[6]

Algorithm 3.1 Note 7 Sudden acquired retinal degeneration syndrome (SARDS) is an idiopathic retinal disease that causes sudden and permanent blindness in dogs. An association between SARDS and hypercortisolism is likely because dogs with SARDS often have polyphagia and PU/PD along with clinicopathological abnormalities suggestive of hypercortisolism. However, a causal relationship between Cushing's syndrome and SARDS has not been established, and both polyphagia and PU/PD usually resolve spontaneously in dogs with SARDS. It has been hypothesized that the hypercortisolism in these dogs may be the result of the extreme stress associated with sudden blindness.[7]

Algorithm 3.1 Note 8 Growth hormone (GH) is a potent stimulant of appetite. Thus, polyphagia can be seen in hypersomatotropism (acromegaly). Hypersomatotropism can also cause diabetes mellitus due to the marked diabetogenic effect of GH, further worsening the polyphagia. In dogs, this is usually due to an excess of mammary GH production induced by elevated serum progesterone concentrations. It is typically seen in females during diestrus or with mammary neoplasia or in dogs receiving exogenous progestins.[8] GH-secreting pituitary adenomas are reported in dogs but are rare.[9]

Algorithm 3.1 Note 9 Patients with congenital megaesophagus (CM) often show apparent polyphagia but with re-eating of food after regurgitation. Failure to thrive and poor general conditions are common in puppies with CM. Dyspnea is a common presenting sign in these patients as a consequence of aspiration pneumonia. Dogs with acquired megaesophagus usually have a normal or decreased appetite.

Algorithm 3.1 Note 10 Serum cobalamin concentrations can be normal or decreased in patients with chronic enteropathy or EPI (see Chapter 20). Parenteral or oral supplementation should be started whenever the serum cobalamin concentration is less than approximately 400 ng/L.[10] Abdominal ultrasonography is suggested when the bloodwork and fecal exam are unremarkable, and chronic inflammatory enteropathy or intestinal neoplasia are suspected. It should also be performed if clinical signs do not improve after specific treatment for other diseases.

Algorithm 3.1 Note 11 Dogs with chronic enteropathy usually show polyphagia if the disease causes malabsorption. Of note, dogs with a protein-losing enteropathy (PLE) most commonly present with decreased appetite, especially in the advanced stages of the disease. If examinations are unremarkable, a diet trial using a hydrolyzed commercial diet or a home-prepared diet should be performed as a first-line treatment (see Chapters 25 and 41). The response is usually assessed in the first 2–4 weeks of the trial. Dogs with PLE should be fed a low-fat diet, ideally containing less than 10% fats. Clinical response to a low-fat diet can be excellent; serum albumin concentration and clinical signs should be reassessed after 5–7 days, and further diagnostic evaluations are warranted if no improvement is detected. In dogs with PLE, endoscopy with biopsies is usually required to diagnose the disease causing the PLE (e.g., lymphoplasmacytic enteritis, primary lymphangiectasia, neoplasia).[11]

References

1. Ahima RS, Antwi DA. Brain regulation of appetite and satiety. *Endocrinol Metab Clin North Am* 37:811–823, 2008.
2. Raffan E, Dennis RJ, O'Donovan CJ, et al. A deletion in the canine POMC gene is associated with weight and appetite in obesity-prone Labrador Retriever dogs. *Cell Metab* 23:893–900, 2016.
3. Papageorgiou V, Ververidis C, Anagnostou T, et al. Use of propofol to induce food consumption by anorectic dogs following ovariohysterectomy. *J Am Vet Med Assoc* 259:56–61, 2021.
4. Johannes CM, Musser ML. Anorexia and the cancer patient. *Vet Clin North Am Small Anim Pract* 49:837–854, 2019.
5. Goutal CM, Brugmann BL, Ryan KA. Insulinoma in dogs: A review. *J Am Anim Hosp Assoc* 48:151–163, 2012.
6. Bennaim M, Shiel RE, Mooney CT. Diagnosis of spontaneous hyperadrenocorticism in dogs. Part 1: Pathophysiology, aetiology, clinical and clinicopathological features. *Vet J* 252:105342, 2019.
7. Komáromy AM, Abrams KL, Heckenlively JR, et al. Sudden acquired retinal degeneration syndrome (SARDS) –A review and proposed strategies toward a better understanding of pathogenesis, early diagnosis, and therapy. *Vet Ophthalmol* 19:319–331, 2016.
8. Fracassi F, Zagnoli L, Rosenberg D, et al. Spontaneous acromegaly: A retrospective case-control study in German Shepherd dogs. *Vet J* 202:69-75, 2014.
9. Steele MME, Lawson JS, Scudder C, et al. Trans-sphenoidal hypophysectomy for the treatment of hypersomatotropism secondary to a pituitary somatotroph adenoma in a dog. *J Vet Intern Med* 38:351–357, 2024.
10. Kather S, Grützner N, Kook PH, et al. Review of cobalamin status and disorders of cobalamin metabolism in dogs. *J Vet Intern Med* 34:13–28, 2020.
11. Craven MD, Washabau RJ. Comparative pathophysiology and management of protein-losing enteropathy. *J Vet Intern Med* 33:383–402, 2019.

CHAPTER 4

Weight loss

Francesca Del Baldo
DVM, MRCVS, PhD, DECVIM-CA

Pathophysiology

The maintenance of body weight reflects the balance between nutrient intake, absorption, and utilization (Table 4.1). Weight loss occurs when energy expenditure exceeds dietary energy intake. The predominant loss is adipose tissue; lean tissue loss is initially limited. However, lean tissue loss becomes inevitable if the energy deficit is severe (Fig. 4.1). The terms weight loss and cachexia are often used interchangeably, with cachexia usually referring to more severe weight loss that is associated with disease. However, cachexia is different from weight loss, being a metabolic disorder of increased energy expenditure that cannot be reversed by solely providing extra calories.[1] It differs from simple weight loss in that the normal physiological mechanisms supporting muscle preservation are lost despite increased energy demands.[2] Thus, in the cachexic animal, protein, as well as adipose tissue, provide energy, resulting in disproportionate muscle wasting. Cachexia occurs with severe debilitating disease, including renal failure, heart failure, malignancy, and chronic inflammatory diseases.[3] Although the pathogenesis of cachexia is not fully understood, proinflammatory cytokines and hormones such as cortisol, catecholamines, insulin, and glucagon have been implicated as mediators.[4] Systemic inflammation from cell injury or activation of the immune system can trigger the release of cytokines (e.g., interleukin-1 and -2, interferon-γ, tumor necrosis factor-α) into the circulation. These cytokines can activate proteolytic systems that cause hypercatabolism as well as activate tissue factors responsible for decreased protein synthesis and enhanced lipolysis.[5,6] The result of these processes is a negative energy balance, muscle wasting, and weight loss. A diagnosis of cachexia should be considered for any dog with marked weight loss, severe muscle loss (sarcopenia), and decreased appetite in the setting of a chronic inflammatory response or cancer.

Clinically relevant weight loss has not been defined for dogs; however, unintentional weight loss >5% is a reasonable benchmark. Common mechanisms leading to weight loss include decreased caloric intake, inability to absorb or utilize ingested calories, accelerated energy loss, or increased metabolic demand (Table 4.1). Etiologies determining weight loss typically act through several mechanisms, each of which should be evaluated if weight

TABLE 4.1 Differential diagnosis for weight loss.

Decreased caloric intake	Malabsorption/maldigestion	Increased metabolic demand

■ Inadequate intake of a nutritionally complete diet
■ Nutritionally incomplete or unbalanced diet
■ Decreased voluntary food intake
  ▪ Pain (e.g., oral or periodontal disease)
  ▪ Reduced appetite (e.g., nausea)
  ▪ Altered sense of smell (e.g., nasal cavity disease)
■ Problems with prehension, chewing, and swallowing of food
  ▪ Head trauma
  ▪ Oral disease (e.g., neoplasia, ulcers)
  ▪ Periodontal disease
  ▪ Cranial nerve lesions affecting swallowing function
  ▪ Cricopharyngeal achalasia
  ▪ Masticatory muscle myositis
■ Regurgitation
■ Repeated vomiting
	■ Small intestinal malabsorption
	  ▪ Chronic inflammatory enteropathy
	  ▪ Alimentary lymphoma
	  ▪ Lymphangiectasia
	  ▪ Intestinal parasitism
	■ Exocrine pancreatic insufficiency
	■ Liver disease
	■ Short bowel syndrome
		■ Excessive protein or calorie loss
		  ▪ Diabetes mellitus
		  ▪ Protein-losing enteropathy
		  ▪ Protein-losing nephropathy
		  ▪ Exudative skin disease
		■ Increased metabolic rate
		  ▪ Extreme exercise
		  ▪ Decreased ambient temperature
		  ▪ Pregnancy and lactation
		  ▪ Growth
		  ▪ Hyperthyroidism
		■ Metabolic derangement leading to cachexia
		  ▪ Neoplasia
		  ▪ Cardiac diseases
		  ▪ Chronic kidney disease
		  ▪ Chronic inflammatory disease
		  ▪ Hypoadrenocorticism
		  ▪ Prolonged glucocorticoid treatment

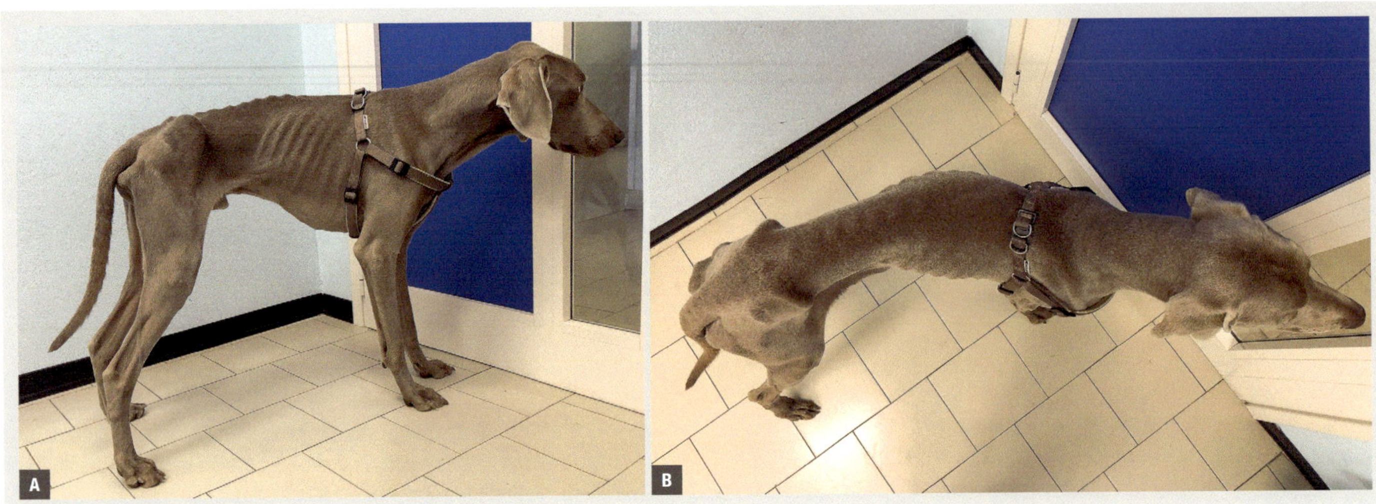

FIG. 4.1 (A) Lateral and (B) dorsal views of a 2-year-old male Weimaraner dog in extremely poor body condition (body condition score 2/9) and evidence of muscle wasting.

loss is to be understood and treated. Malabsorption/maldigestion and enteric protein loss are most relevant in gastrointestinal (GI) diseases.

Clinical signs

Weight loss is a well-recognized clinical sign in numerous disorders. It can be the primary or sole complaint or, more commonly, it accompanies other signs associated with an underlying condition. One of the most important clinical signs to evaluate in a dog presenting for weight loss is its appetite. Appetite may be reduced, normal, or increased in a dog showing weight loss. In cases of systemic illnesses, renal disease, cardiac diseases, or hypoadrenocorticism, the appetite can be reduced or suppressed completely (anorexia), leading to unintentional weight loss. In contrast, diseases that cause a loss of nutrients (e.g., diabetes mellitus), intestinal malabsorption (e.g., chronic enteropathy), or maldigestion (e.g., pancreatic exocrine insufficiency) are usually associated with an increased food intake in order to compensate for the energy loss.

Other signs identified in the history can help to direct the diagnostic approach; for example, GI signs (vomiting, diarrhea, nausea, and loss of appetite) are often present in primary GI disorders, hepatic disease, or endocrine diseases such as hypoadrenocorticism. Abnormalities in prehension and swallowing of food should raise the suspicion of oral diseases or dysphagia, while regurgitation is indicative of an esophageal disease. Polyuria and polydipsia are key signs in conditions such as renal diseases, diabetes mellitus, or hypercalcemia. Polydipsia may be seen in dehydrated GI patients and in cases of malabsorption, but polyuria is not typical in GI disease. Other clinical signs associated with weight loss can include coughing, dyspnea, and exercise intolerance, which may denote cardiac or respiratory diseases.

Diagnostic approach

The diagnostic algorithm provides additional details on weight loss and associated clinical signs based on the underlying disease. The approach to the diagnosis and treatment of patients with weight loss is depicted in Algorithm 4.1.

Algorithm 4.1 Note 1 Confirm true weight loss: the dog must be weighed on an accurate and appropriate scale (e.g., pediatric scales for small dogs) and, if possible, the same scale should be used at each visit. Weight loss can also result from dehydration, so before considering the weight loss to be relevant, the hydration status of the patient should be evaluated. If the dog is dehydrated, investigate possible causes and correct the hydration state by administering fluid therapy or augmenting water consumption.

Algorithm 4.1 Note 2 Take a history and perform a physical examination: determining whether appetite is increased, decreased, or unchanged can help refine the list of differential diagnoses. Other clinical signs important to explore during the anamnesis are the presence of GI signs, including swallowing difficulties and polyuria/polydipsia.

The body condition should be assessed using the nine-point body condition score (BCS) system.[7] These assessments mainly detect changes in peripheral body fat mass rather than lean tissue and also lack sensitivity because it typically takes an approximate 10% change in body weight before a change in BCS is noted. To identify more subtle changes and/or muscle mass loss in otherwise overweight dogs, muscle condition scoring (MCS) is recommended. A four-category MCS has been validated, and it is assessed by visualization and palpation of the spine, scapulae, skull, and wings of the ilia.[7]

Algorithm 4.1 Note 3 Take a dietary history: this should include all food currently fed and consumed, how the proportions are measured out, how the food is fed, and any recent dietary changes. If necessary, the owners should be asked to provide label information. For home-prepared food, it might be necessary to consult a veterinary nutritionist. It is also important to consider if the animal's energy demand is increased (e.g., due to extreme exercise or lactation). In this case, a specific diet should be administered, or alternatively, the dose of food should be increased to satisfy the increased energy demand.

Algorithm 4.1 Note 4 Assess potential cardiorespiratory disease: cardiac auscultation coupled with assessment of pulse quality and rate is important to determine whether the cardiac disease is present, as well as inspecting the rest of the body for other signs of cardiovascular

ALGORITHM 4.1

Diagnostic approach to weight loss.

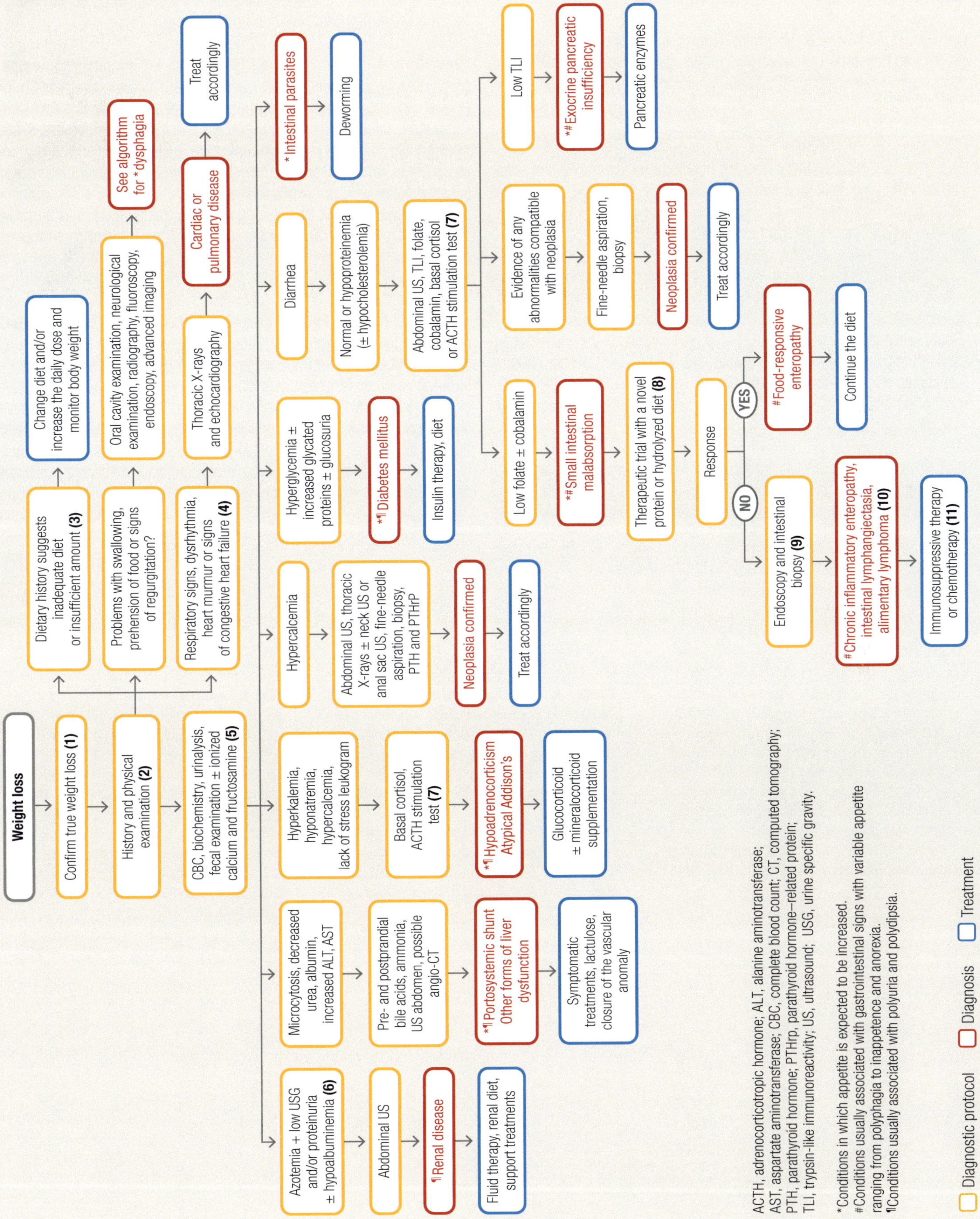

ACTH, adrenocorticotropic hormone; ALT, alanine aminotransferase; AST, aspartate aminotransferase; CBC, complete blood count; CT, computed tomography; PTH, parathyroid hormone; PTHrp, parathyroid hormone–related protein; TLI, trypsin-like immunoreactivity; US, ultrasound; USG, urine specific gravity.

*Conditions in which appetite is expected to be increased.
#Conditions usually associated with gastrointestinal signs with variable appetite ranging from polyphagia to inappetence and anorexia.
¶Conditions usually associated with polyuria and polydipsia.

Diagnostic protocol | Diagnosis | Treatment

diseases, such as ascites, subcutaneous edema, jugular distension, and temperature of the extremities. Thoracic auscultation is indicated to detect evidence of pulmonary or pleural disease.

Algorithm 4.1 Note 5 Minimum laboratory database: in endemic areas, and based on the presence of other clinical signs, screening for vector-borne diseases might be appropriate. In the presence of polyuria and polydipsia, evaluation of serum fructosamine and ionized calcium should be included in the initial blood tests.

Algorithm 4.1 Note 6 Protein-losing nephropathy: creatinine and urea can be within the reference range, and biochemistry usually shows low albumin and high cholesterol due to excessive albumin loss through the glomerulus and increased synthesis of lipoproteins.

Algorithm 4.1 Note 7 Rule in/out hypoadrenocorticism: if no causes of weight loss are found, it may be useful to carry out an adrenocorticotropic hormone (ACTH) stimulation test even in eunatremic and eukalemic dogs. Serum basal cortisol >55 nmol/L (>2 µg/dL) excludes hypoadrenocorticism. If the basal cortisol is <55 nmol/L (<2 µg/dL), an ACTH stimulation test should be performed to confirm or exclude the disease.[8] In the treatment of eunatremic, eukalemic hypoadrenocorticism, it is only necessary to administer glucocorticoids.

Algorithm 4.1 Note 8 Rule in/out a food-responsive enteropathy; by definition, idiopathic chronic inflammatory enteropathy is an exclusion diagnosis. A therapeutic diet trial is indicated, assuming the dog is not anorexic.

Algorithm 4.1 Note 9 Identify the cause of chronic enteropathy; if no causes of weight loss are found, it may be recommended to perform an endoscopy even if folate and cobalamin are normal, in particular in dogs that are presented with diarrhea and vomiting.

Algorithm 4.1 Note 10 Classify chronic inflammatory enteropathies; this is according to the predominant inflammatory cell type and anatomical location. Lymphoplasmacytic enteritis is seen most frequently, followed by eosinophilic enteritis; the granulomatous and neutrophilic forms occur less commonly.[9] Chronic inflammatory enteropathies, intestinal lymphangiectasia, and intestinal lymphoma can be associated with panhypoproteinemia (protein-losing enteropathies) due to excessive loss of proteins through the GI tract. In this case, biochemistry usually also shows low cholesterol and the hemogram shows lymphopenia.

Algorithm 4.1 Note 11 Glucocorticoids, typically prednisolone, are generally used as the first-line treatment in dogs with inflammatory bowel disease if the diet trial fails.[9] The recommended dose is 1–2 mg/kg q24h PO. In cases that appear refractory to glucocorticoids, adjunctive immunosuppressive therapy should be considered. Options include ciclosporin, azathioprine, and chlorambucil.[9]
In the case of small-cell intestinal lymphoma, a combination of steroids and alkylating agents (chlorambucil) is the first-line treatment. In the case of high-grade intestinal lymphoma, treatment with multiagent injectable chemotherapy protocol is recommended.[10]

References

1. Morley JE, Thomas DR, Wilson MM. Cachexia: pathophysiology and clinical relevance. *Am J Clin Nutr* 83(4):735–743, 2006.
2. Thomas DR. Distinguishing starvation from cachexia. *Clin Geriatric Med* 18(4):883-891, 2002.
3. Freeman LM. Cachexia and sarcopenia: emerging syndromes of importance in dogs and cats. *J Vet Intern Med* 26(1):3–17, 2012.
4. Tisdale MJ. Molecular pathways leading to cancer cachexia. *Physiology (Bethesda)* 20:340–348, 2005.
5. Shintani F, Nakaki T, Kanba S, et al. Role of interleukin-1 in stress responses. A putative neurotransmitter. *Mol Neurobiol* 10(1):47–71, 1995.
6. Ryden M, Arvidsson E, Blomqvist L, et al. Targets for TNF-alpha-induced lipolysis in human adipocytes. *Biochem Biophys Res Comm* 318(1):168–175, 2004.
7. Freeman L, Becvarova I, Cave N, et al. WSAVA Nutritional Assessment Guidelines Task Force Members. WSAVA Nutritional Assessment Guidelines. *J Small Anim Pract* 52(7):385–396, 2011.
8. Gold AJ, Langlois DK, Refsal KL. Evaluation of basal serum or plasma cortisol concentrations for the diagnosis of hypoadrenocorticism in dogs. *J Vet Intern Med* 30:1798–1805, 2016.
9. Dandrieux JR. Inflammatory bowel disease versus chronic enteropathy in dogs: are they one and the same? *J Small Anim Pract* 57(11):589–599, 2016.
10. Couto KM, Moore PF, Zwingenberger AL, et al. Clinical characteristics and outcome in dogs with small cell T-cell intestinal lymphoma. *Vet Comp Oncol* 16(3):337–343, 2018.

CHAPTER 5

Abdominal enlargement

Stefania Golinelli
DVM, PhD

Pathophysiology

Abdominal enlargement in dogs can arise from a variety of physiological and pathological processes (Table 5.1). Understanding the diverse pathophysiologic mechanisms underlying this problem is crucial for accurately diagnosing and effectively managing affected dogs.

The causes of abdominal enlargement can be categorized into organomegaly or abdominal mass, abdominal effusion (ascites), gas-related issues (bloat), and other conditions such as hypercortisolism (resulting in hepatomegaly and weak abdominal musculature), fat accumulation (obesity), pregnancy, and constipation. Physiologically, postprandial distension of the abdomen occurs due to the ingestion of food, leading to temporary enlargement that resolves after digestion. Bloating of the gastrointestinal (GI) tract can be secondary to aerophagia but may indicate obstruction, abnormal motility, or perforation with consequent pneumoperitoneum.

Organomegaly can be characterized as benign or neoplastic enlargement of abdominal organs such as the liver, spleen, or kidneys. Neoplasms originating from the GI or reproductive organs may also lead to abdominal enlargement. Additionally, fluid accumulation within the abdominal cavity, such as ascites resulting from conditions like heart failure or liver disease, or within the uterus (pyometra) are other causes of abdominal distension.

Abdominal fluid categories are determined by their underlying mechanisms, aiding in the refinement of the differential diagnosis list. Transudates may arise from alterations in plasma hydrostatic pressure or oncotic pressure. While previously classified as "pure" or "modified", a classification distinguishing between low- and high-protein transudates proves more beneficial in determining causative factors. Low-protein transudates typically result from severe hypoalbuminemia or presinusoidal portal hypertension, stemming from conditions such as protein-losing enteropathies, protein-losing nephropathies, liver vascular anomalies, hepatic cirrhosis, or burn injuries. Conversely, high-protein transudates often indicate sinusoidal or postsinusoidal portal hypertension, attributed to causes including congestive heart failure, pericardial tamponade, liver disease, caudal vena cava thrombosis, Budd–Chiari syndrome, or neoplasia.[1]

Exudates arise from increased vascular permeability due to inflammatory mediators or vessel or viscus injury/leakage, typically containing increased protein and cell counts. Infectious (bacterial, viral, fungal, protozoal) or noninfectious (pancreatitis, neoplasia, bile, urine, foreign body) disorders can lead to exudative fluid accumulation.[1]

The primary reported cause of chylous effusions in dogs is intra-abdominal neoplasia, notably carcinoma. Additional causes noted in dogs include right-sided heart failure and lymphatic obstruction, rupture, or leakage.

Hemorrhagic effusion, termed hemoperitoneum or hemoabdomen, may arise spontaneously or from trauma or rodenticide toxicosis. In dogs, spontaneous cases are predominantly linked to neoplasia. Notably, the etiology and source of hemorrhage vary between small and large dogs, with differences in the prevalence of splenic hemorrhage and hemorrhage from other sites. Anaphylaxis-induced hemoperitoneum has also been documented in dogs.[1]

Uroabdomen results from urinary tract rupture, most commonly occurring at the bladder, followed by the

TABLE 5.1 Main causes of abdominal enlargement.

Bloat	Ileus (functional or mechanical) Gastric dilatation/volvulus Gastrointestinal tract rupture Intestinal or mesenteric torsion Iatrogenic (postsurgical) Trauma Emphysematous bacterial infection
Liquids	Effusion Cyst Abscess Pyometra
Masses	Organomegaly not due to neoplasia Neoplasia Granuloma Intra-abdominal lymphadenomegaly
Others	Pregnancy Constipation Obesity Hypercortisolism

urethra, with renal or ureteral rupture being rare. Trauma, such as a vehicular accident, is the most common cause, alongside urinary tract obstruction, traumatic bladder expression or catheterization, bladder neoplasia, urethral catheterization, and postoperative leakage.[1]
Biliary effusion stems from biliary tract disruption, attributed to trauma or obstructive lesions, inflammation, mucocele rupture, or neoplasia.[1]

Clinical signs

Abdominal enlargement is a frequently observed clinical indicator of various diseases in dogs, necessitating a meticulous and methodical diagnostic approach. Pet owners may report abdominal distension or note other associated clinical signs such as exercise intolerance, weight gain, increased respiratory rate and effort, lethargy, weakness, decreased appetite, or signs specific to the underlying disease, such as collapse with cardiac tamponade or unproductive retching with gastric dilatation/volvulus. Prompt intervention may be necessary for certain patients with abdominal enlargement, underscoring the importance of a comprehensive medical history to evaluate the urgency of such actions and to establish a comprehensive list of potential diagnoses. Physical examination findings will vary depending on the cause and may encompass indications such as a fluid wave upon palpating the abdomen, abdominal or GI tract gas distension, abdominal pain, organomegaly, or detection of a soft tissue mass.[2]

Diagnostic approach

Algorithm 5.1 shows the diagnostic approach to abdominal enlargement in dogs.

Algorithm 5.1 Note 1 Abdominal enlargement often develops insidiously, and obesity, pregnancy, or constipation are often identified by the history and physical examination. However, abdominal enlargement may also be acute in onset, as with gas accumulation in the stomach in gastric dilatation/volvulus or bleeding from a ruptured splenic neoplasm. A thorough history is vital for assessing the need for emergency intervention and for developing a complete differential diagnosis list. The history should include a description of clinical signs and their duration, the pet's environment and its travel history, drug administration, and previous medical history. If the patient is relaxed and not obese, abdominal palpation may directly detect intra-abdominal masses, organomegaly, gas, or fluid accumulation.

Algorithm 5.1 Note 2 The abdomen can be imaged by a variety of methods (plain and contrast radiographs, ultrasound, computed tomography or magnetic resonance imaging scans). Abdominal ultrasound is probably the highest-yielding test if fluid or organomegaly is present, if hypercortisolism is suspected (e.g., enlarged adrenals), or if no abnormalities are detected on physical examination. An abdominal radiograph can identify the presence of free or intraluminal gas and gastric volvulus and confirm obesity, pregnancy, or constipation.

Algorithm 5.1 Note 3 Dogs and cats with abdominal masses or diffuse organomegaly should undergo a fine-needle aspiration or biopsy of the tissue(s) involved to identify the underlying abnormality (e.g., neoplasia, inflammation). Cytology is less invasive than a biopsy, does not require general anesthesia, and usually does not require a clotting study. However, although it may allow assessment of the cell types present, it will not identify structural changes in organs such as fibrosis, cirrhosis, dysplasia and hyperplasia, and it does not permit diagnosis of neoplasia if the cells involved do not exfoliate.

Algorithm 5.1 Note 4 Fluid analysis begins with assessing fluid color and ease of collection. Changes from clear to bloody or vice versa suggest blood contamination, while a continuous bloody appearance indicates hemorrhage. Similarity to blood may signal severe hemorrhage or organ aspiration. Differentiation involves transferring fluid to a nonanticoagulant tube. Clot presence supports in vivo hemorrhage; absence suggests contamination. Postcollection visual inspection aids further diagnostic steps such as fluid cytologic analysis, cell counts, and measurement of bilirubin, creatinine, and other variables.[3]

Algorithm 5.1 Note 5 In the case of a transudate, a serum total protein concentration equal to or greater than 25 g/dL serves as a distinguishing factor between low-protein (protein-poor or pure) and high-protein (protein-rich or modified) transudates. Low-protein transudate typically arises from prehepatic or hepatic pre- and early sinusoidal hypertension, leading to the leakage of low-protein intestinal lymph. Some liver diseases or protein-losing conditions commonly underlie this type. Conversely, high-protein transudate usually stems from late sinusoidal or postsinusoidal hypertension, resulting in the leakage of high-protein hepatic lymph. Liver disease, cancer, pericardial tamponade, and congestive heart failure are frequent causes of this variant.[3]

Algorithm 5.1 Note 6 Gas accumulation can cause abdominal distension and may occur within the abdominal organs or freely in the peritoneal or retroperitoneal spaces. Distension of the GI tract with gas can be seen with gastric dilatation/volvulus or mesenteric torsion. Gas accumulation in the GI tract can also be secondary to mechanical and/or functional ileus. Emphysematous bacterial infections can result in gas production within the liver, gallbladder, or urinary bladder. Lastly, free gas in the peritoneal and retroperitoneal spaces may result from GI perforation or perforating trauma, secondary to gas-producing bacteria in bacterial peritonitis, or can be iatrogenic in origin after surgical interventions.

Algorithm 5.1 Note 7 Progressive wasting and weakening of the abdominal musculature commonly occurs due to high concentrations of glucocorticoids (hypercortisolism). This can also cause hepatic enlargement as a result of glycogen accumulation in the liver. Muscle wasting and hepatic enlargement combine to produce the classical potbellied appearance in the patient. This is a major complaint with hypercortisolism but is typically associated with other signs such as polyuria/polydipsia, polyphagia, bilaterally symmetrical hair loss, thin skin, comedones, and excessive panting. Abdominal wall vessels often appear prominent.

Algorithm 5.1 Note 8 Antibiotics should only be used if an infection is present and the fluid or tissue culture test positive. The choice of antibiotics should be based on susceptibility tests.[1]

ALGORITHM 5.1

Diagnostic approach to abdominal enlargement in dogs.

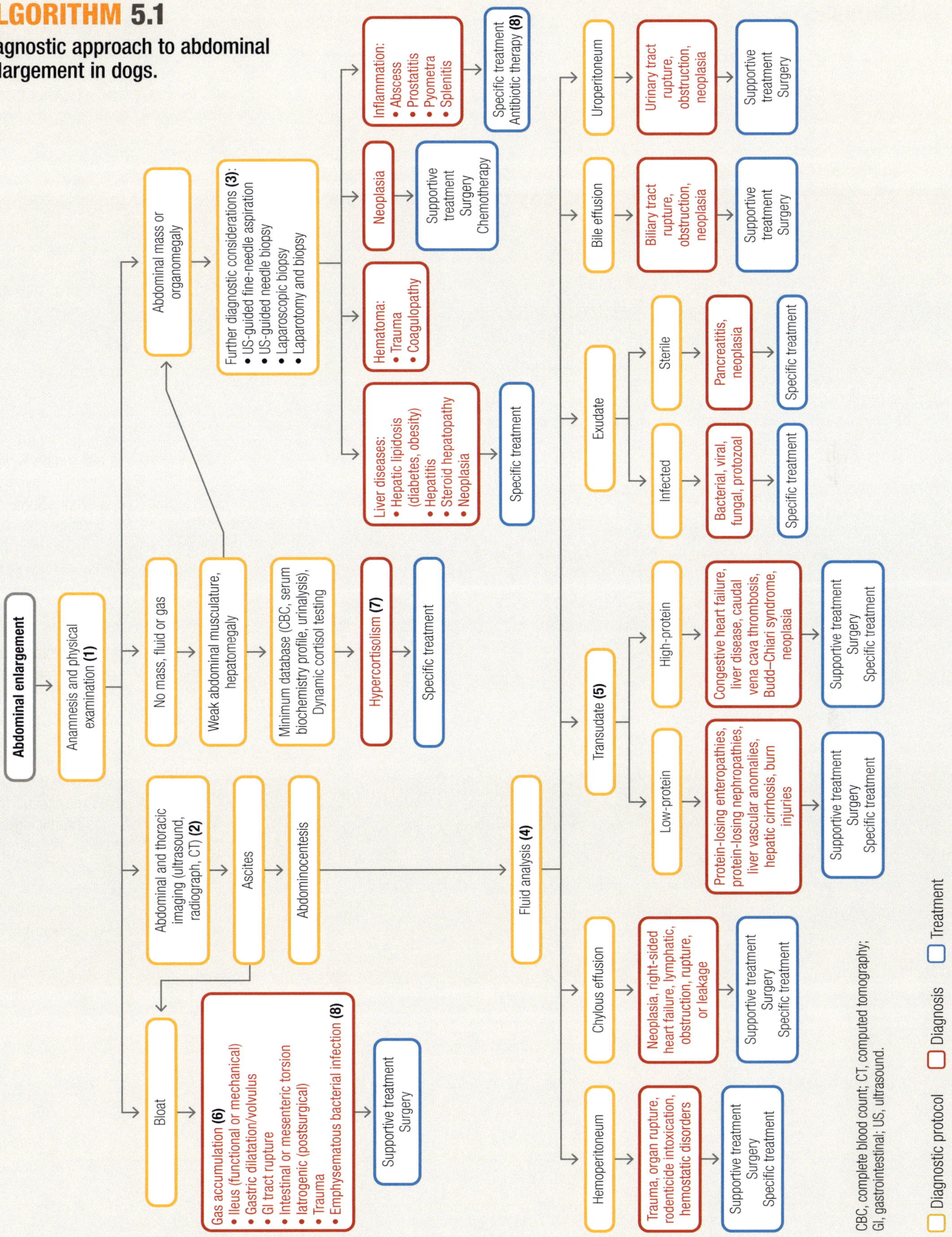

CBC, complete blood count; CT, computed tomography; GI, gastrointestinal; US, ultrasound.

References

1. Walter J. Abdominal enlargement. In: Ettinger SJ, Feldman EC, Côté E (editors). *Textbook of Veterinary Internal Medicine*, 8th edition. St. Louis, Elsevier, 2017, pp. 450–455.
2. Nelson RW, Couto CG. Clinical manifestations of gastrointestinal disorders. In: Nelson RW, Couto CG (editors). *Small Animal Internal Medicine*. St. Louis, Elsevier, 2013, pp. 388–389.
3. Stokol T. Fluid analysis: thoracic, abdominal, joint. In: Côté E, Ettinger SJ, Feldman EC (editors). *Ettinger's Textbook of Veterinary Internal Medicine*, 9th edition. St. Louis, Elsevier, 2024, pp. 340–352.

CHAPTER 6

Abdominal pain

Jo Murrell
BVSc(Hons), PhD,
DECVAA, MRCVS

When presented with a dog with abdominal pain, signs may reflect either somatic (body wall) pain or visceral pain, which is often associated with gastrointestinal (GI) diseases. In contrast to somatic pain, visceral pain has a poorly understood pathophysiology, reflecting the relative ease of studying cutaneous pain directly by applying noxious stimuli to the skin.

Pathophysiology of visceral pain

The GI tract has dual extrinsic innervation through the parasympathetic and sympathetic nervous systems, which transmit information from the brain to the gut (efferent system) and from the gut to the central nervous system (sensory afferents—vagal nerve and spinal afferent fibers). There are differences in the physiology of vagal and spinal afferents reflecting differences in receptive fields, projections, and receptor subtypes; however, they are predominantly A delta and C fibers that relay information in both vagal and spinal nerves.[1] Both vagal and spinal afferents carry information relating to visceral sensation and participate in reflexes controlling GI function, whereas only spinal afferents carry information relating to visceral pain.

Visceral sensations can be divided into two classes: vague sensations (e.g., hunger, fullness, nausea) that inform about the functional state of the GI tract and are not associated with pain and visceral pain sensations which inform about potentially tissue damaging events. Abdominal viscera are generally insensitive to stimuli that normally provoke profound pain when applied to the skin. Instead, stimuli to visceral organs that induce pain include distention, irritation of the serosa, torsion of the mesentery, inflammation, and hypoxemia of the tissues. One phenomenon that is frequently described for visceral pain sensations is referred pain, whereby pain arising from the viscera is referred to the skin of a different body part. This is explained by the convergence of visceral and cutaneous afferents onto the same viscerosomatic spinal neuron. Some spinal afferents also have free nerve endings with receptive fields that receive sensory information from more than one visceral structure, which may also explain the diffuse and poorly defined nature of visceral pain. The spinal afferents from different abdominal viscera enter the spinal cord in a rostrocaudal organization, with visceral afferents terminating predominantly in laminae I, V–VII, and X. This distribution in the laminae is very different from that of cutaneous afferents. Evidence suggests that there are two types of sensory neurons in the spinal cord, those that receive cutaneous input only and those that respond to both cutaneous and visceral stimulation. Therefore, visceral sensation can only be mediated by somatosensory pathways; there is no pathway specific for visceral nociception.

The visceral nociceptive pathway does not comprise one-way traffic to the central nervous system and higher brain centers; indeed, there are a number of mechanisms by which the pathway can be modulated to either increase or decrease the sensation of pain. In the central nervous system, these comprise emotional and cognitive factors, whereas the predominant mechanism in the spinal cord is the descending inhibitory system, which can become facilitatory under certain circumstances. In terms of descending modulation of visceral pain, similar structures that are important in the descending modulation of cutaneous pain have been identified.

Similar to somatic pain, central and peripheral sensitization occur in visceral pain disorders and are thought to underpin many functional GI disorders, such as irritable bowel syndrome, and interstitial cystitis. The hallmarks of sensitization are allodynia, where stimuli that are not normally painful (e.g., touch, stroking) start to elicit pain, and hyperalgesia, where stimuli that are normally painful elicit a greater level of pain than normal. Mechanisms of peripheral sensitization include awakening of silent visceral afferent nociceptors, which are mechanically insensitive afferent fibers that acquire mechanosensitivity after inflammation, lowering the threshold at which distention of a hollow viscera causes pain.[1] Central sensitization occurs primarily in the spinal cord and higher brain centers, with nociceptive discharges in visceral afferents provoking profound central changes resulting in increased excitability of viscerosomatic afferent fibers.[2] Descending inhibitory pathways can also become facilitatory, contributing to the maintenance of chronic pain states and stress and anxiety.

The interaction of the gut microbiome and the enteric nervous system in chronic visceral pain conditions is being increasingly recognized.[3] The enteric nervous system, supported by enteric glial cells that help to maintain the integrity of the intestinal barrier, plays a role in intestinal inflammation and interaction with the microbiome. Enteric sensory neurons also receive information via enteroendocrine and enterochromaffin cells and can generate enteric reflexes such as secretion, peristalsis, and perception of pain and inflammation.

The gut microbiome is also reported to play a role in neuroinflammatory responses in the gut driving chronic pain and central sensitization.[3] The microbes in the gut can also synthesize neurotransmitters and hormones that are involved in gut–brain communication. For example, glutamate, a major neurotransmitter involved in the pain pathway and synthesized by some bacteria, may regulate gut sensory and motor functions via receptors in the enteric nervous system.

In conclusion, visceral pain pathways are complex and relatively poorly understood compared with the cutaneous pain pathway. This may be a factor hindering the development of new therapeutics for the management of visceral pain.

Conditions causing visceral pain in dogs

Visceral pain is generally described as pain arising from any abdominal or thoracic viscera. The causes are numerous. Table 6.1 shows some examples of different conditions causing visceral pain in dogs.

Diagnostic approach to visceral pain

Diagnosis of any pain condition can be challenging, but this is particularly so for visceral pain, which is reported by humans to be diffuse and often nonspecific in nature and may be referred to different cutaneous regions on the body. It is currently recognized that changes in behavior are the most reliable way to assess pain, whereas changes in physiology (e.g., heart rate, respiratory rate, blood pressure) are generally considered to be unreliable. It is worth noting that conditions causing GI distention and pain are often associated with a relative bradycardia rather than with an increased heart rate, which might be assumed to be a more likely response.

TABLE 6.1 Examples of conditions causing visceral pain in dogs.

Underlying pathophysiology	Conditions
Inflammation	■ Esophagitis, gastritis, enteritis, colitis, peritonitis ■ Pancreatitis ■ Urinary tract infections: bacterial pyelonephritis, cystitis, prostatitis
Distention	■ Gastric dilation and volvulus ■ Tumors and foreign bodies causing obstruction of the gastrointestinal tract
Stretching of solid organs	■ Liver and kidney tumors
Ischemia	■ Mesenteric torsion or infarction ■ Ischemic pain related to hypotension in hypoadrenocorticism

The approach to the diagnosis and treatment of dogs with visceral pain is depicted in Algorithm 6.1.

Algorithm 6.1 Note 1 Knowledge of the animal's behavior before the onset of pain is useful because it is then easier to recognize any changes, but this is rarely possible unless the animal is hospitalized beforehand. However, this information may be obtained by questioning the owner about their pet's normal behavior.

Algorithm 6.1 Note 2 Observe the dog's behavior from a distance (e.g., from outside of the kennel) and look at their posture and facial expression. Animals with abdominal pain are often hunched or tucked up in their abdomen and rarely show normal sleeping behavior. Cranial abdominal pain (e.g., caused by severe pancreatitis) is classically associated with the patient adopting a praying position, characterized by the dog standing upright on the hind limbs while kneeling down or "praying" on the forelimbs. Animals may also turn to look at their flank more frequently when they present with abdominal pain. Facial expressions associated with pain have been well defined in cats but not in dogs. It is also important to assess the animal's demeanor; that is, if the animal is interested in and interactive with the environment. Changes in demeanor, such as depression and anxiety, are common signs of pain.

Algorithm 6.1 Note 3 If there is evidence of pain unrelated to the abdominal viscera on physical examination, investigate and treat appropriately. Beware of falsely interpreting pain due to lesions of the abdominal skin or subcutis (e.g., panniculitis) or musculature or spinal pain as visceral pain.

Algorithm 6.1 Note 4 Gently palpate the abdomen to detect signs of guarding (extreme muscle tension in the abdominal wall), turning to look at the flank during palpation, or, occasionally, vocalizing if the dog is experiencing severe pain.

Algorithm 6.1 Note 5 If the animal shows no sign of abdominal pain on physical examination, then continue to observe the dog for signs of abnormal behavior and repeat the physical examination if indicated.

Algorithm 6.1 Note 6 Use of pain scoring tools to quantify visceral pain can be really helpful to ensure that analgesic treatment is adequate to manage pain. It also aids in ensuring standardization in pain assessment between assessors and, therefore, better continuity of analgesic care. Finally, it can help guide decision-making about analgesic treatment, with analgesic drugs of greater efficacy being given to animals rated as having more severe pain.

There are no scoring tools that have been specifically developed to quantify visceral or abdominal pain. Most of the studies carried out to validate currently available pain scoring tools assessed dogs following surgery, which may result in them being relatively insensitive for the detection of visceral pain, particularly if the pain is diffuse in nature. These tools were also designed to measure acute rather than chronic pain. However, the author still recommends use of pain scoring tools to try and help quantify the severity of visceral pain in clinical patients.

The best validated and widely used pain scoring tool for acute pain in dogs is the short form of the Glasgow composite pain scale.[4] It comprises six questions that relate to the dog's demeanor and attitude, ability or willingness to walk, and response to palpation around a painful area or

ALGORITHM 6.1

Diagnostic approach to visceral pain in dogs.

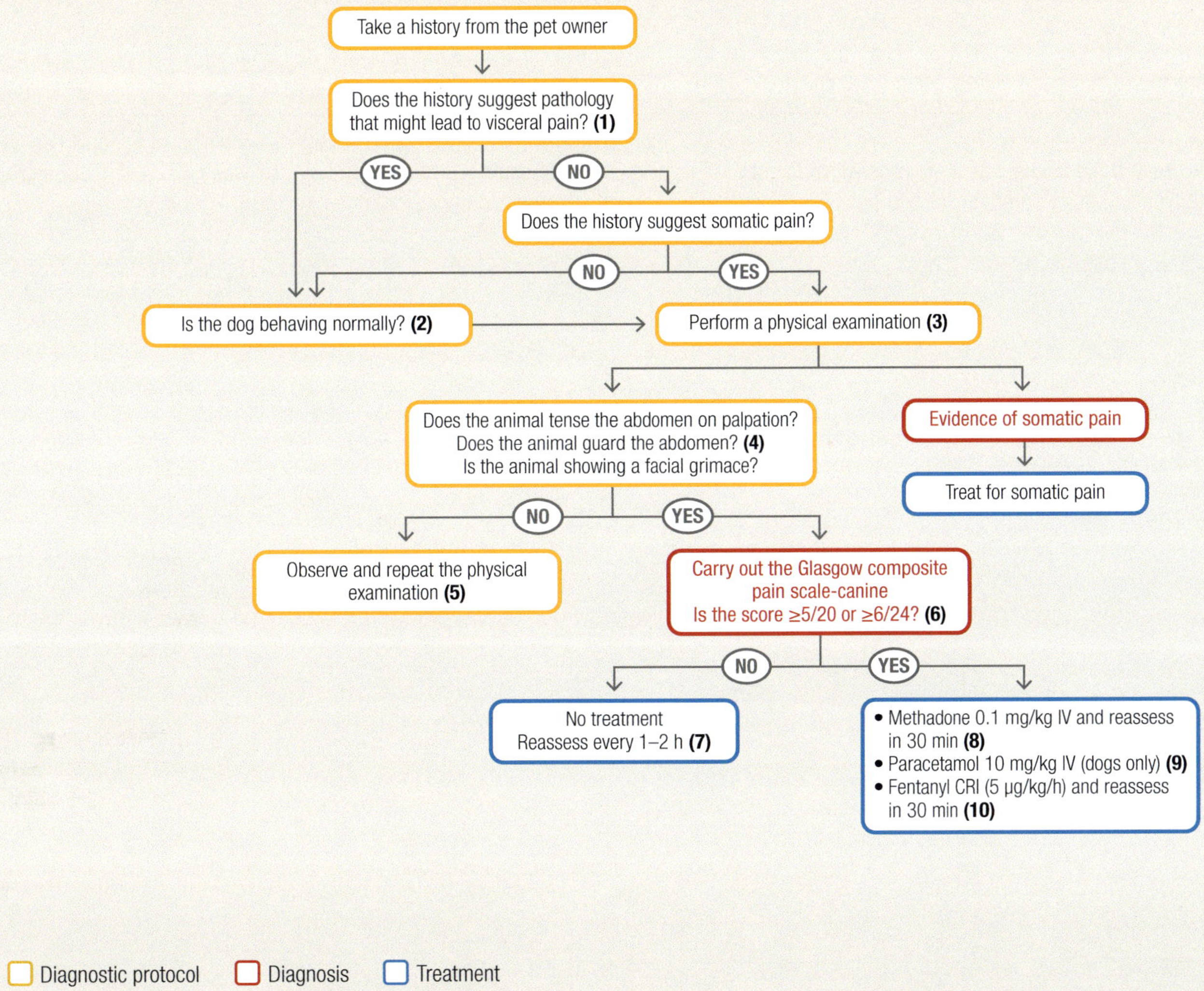

surgical wound. To detect abdominal visceral pain, abdominal palpation is a key and important feature of pain assessment. Importantly, this pain scoring tool provides validated cutoff points for the administration of rescue analgesia, with a score of ≥5 out of 20 or ≥6 out of 24 (the maximum score depends on whether the dog is ambulatory or not) indicating that further analgesia is needed.

Algorithm 6.1 Note 7 If the pain score is below the threshold for intervention, continue to score the animal using the same scale every 1–2 hours.

Algorithm 6.1 Note 8 If the animal has a pain score that is above the threshold for intervention, an appropriate starting point for analgesia is methadone 0.1 mg/kg IV. Reassess the animal 30 minutes later using the same scale to confirm that this dose is sufficient. Methadone can be topped up if the pain level remains above the threshold for intervention 30 minutes later. If a total dose of methadone of 0.3 mg/kg IV is needed for analgesia and the dog remains above the threshold for intervention, switch to a constant rate infusion of fentanyl.

Algorithm 6.1 Note 9 Paracetamol at 10 mg/kg IV can be given at the same time as methadone.

Algorithm 6.1 Note 10 The constant rate infusion of fentanyl can be adjusted, depending on the pain score, between 2.5 and 10 µg/kg/h, making changes to the infusion rate in 2.5 µg/kg/h intervals.

References

1. Gebhart GF. Visceral pain—peripheral sensitisation. *Gut* 47 Suppl 4(Ch 4):iv54–iv55, 2000.
2. Cervero F. Visceral pain—central sensitisation. *Gut* 47 Suppl 4(Ch 4):iv56–iv57, 2000.
3. Ustianowska K, Ustianowski Ł, Machaj F, et al. The role of the human microbiome in the pathogenesis of pain. *Int J Mol Sci* 23(21):13267, 2022.
4. Testa B, Reid J, Scott ME, et al. The short form of the Glasgow composite measure pain scale in post-operative analgesia studies in dogs: a scoping review. *Front Vet Sci* 8:751949, 2021.

CHAPTER 7

Drooling/ptyalism

Andrea Petrelli
DVM, DECVIM-CA, MRCVS

Pathophysiology

True ptyalism is medically defined as an increase in saliva production, which manifests as drooling. However, drooling can also be caused by the inability to swallow saliva, a condition referred to as pseudoptyalism. In certain large breeds of dogs, such as the Saint Bernard, Dogue de Bordeaux, and Mastiff, and also in other brachycephalic dogs and Cocker Spaniels, drooling can be considered an expected trait as a consequence of their lip or jaw conformation.

Saliva is a viscous protein-based, bicarbonate-rich fluid produced and secreted by the salivary tissues, predominantly composed of discrete glands but also diffusely throughout the buccal cavity. Dogs have four major pairs of salivary glands: parotid, zygomatic, mandibular, and sublingual.[1]

Saliva serves multiple functions: it works as a lubricant, initiating the breakdown of ingesta, and plays a protective role for the oral soft tissues. The secretion of saliva from the salivary glands is increased by both parasympathetic and sympathetic stimuli. The rate of salivary secretion is controlled by parasympathetic postganglionic cholinergic nerve fibers. Sympathetic stimulation promotes saliva flow through masticatory muscle contractions around the salivary ducts.

Ptyalism is normal in dogs anticipating feeding but can be caused by a variety of conditions originating from different etiologies (Table 7.1). These include diseases of the oral cavity, esophagus, and other parts of the alimentary tract, as well as within the salivary glands themselves. Hypersalivation can also occur due to extragastrointestinal causes, which include systemic or neurological conditions such as seizures (Video 7.1), and exposure to toxins.[2]

Clinical signs

Ptyalism can vary in intensity, ranging from a mild to a severe condition, and its occurrence can be intermittent or continuous. The clinical sign of ptyalism can appear suddenly or may be observed as a gradual or chronic condition. Macroscopically, the saliva may have a clear appearance, or it could be mixed with blood or purulent exudate, depending on the etiology. Other potential clinical signs such as vomiting, regurgitation, anorexia, pain, and oral inflammatory lesions can be related to the primary cause of drooling.[3] The treatment should aim to resolve the primary cause that has elicited hypersalivation. However, symptomatic treatment with antinausea medication can be started before proceeding with diagnostic investigations in order to relieve the patient from this sign. A particular mention should be reserved for rabies infection: this is an important zoonosis and dogs suspected to have this condition should be isolated immediately.

TABLE 7.1 Causes of hypersalivation in dogs, according to anatomical location or etiology.

Oral diseases	Esophageal diseases	Gastric diseases	Metabolic diseases	Neurological diseases	Intoxication	Iatrogenic
■ Stomatitis/dental disease ■ Oral foreign body ■ Oral neoplasia	■ Megaesophagus ■ Mass/foreign body ■ Esophagitis ■ Stricture ■ Vascular ring anomaly	■ Nausea ■ Gastric carcinoma	■ Uremia	■ Phenobarbital-responsive sialadenosis ■ Brainstem/forebrain/vestibular lesion ■ Facial/trigeminal nerve paralysis ■ Pseudorabies (Aujeszky's disease) ■ Rabies	■ Toxic substances, e.g., organophosphate ■ Caustic substance ■ Irritants, e.g., processionary moth caterpillars	■ Bitter medications ■ Chemotherapy

Video 7.1

Dog during a seizure with autonomic activity. A 7-year-old female neutered English Bulldog diagnosed with structural epilepsy (glioma) during a focal epileptic seizure with motor activity (twitching of facial musculature) and autonomic activity (hypersalivation) with unimpaired consciousness.

Diagnostic approach

Algorithm 7.1 shows the approach to drooling/ptyalism. Dogs of any age, sex, or breed can develop drooling, which may be either true ptyalism or pseudoptyalism.

Algorithm 7.1 Note 1 Due to the numerous causes for drooling, a comprehensive history, signalment, and physical examination can facilitate the distinction between true and pseudoptyalism and aid localization of the underlying reason. Recent administration of medications, the possibility of toxin exposure, or the presence of other signs, for example, loss of consciousness and tonic-clonic movements in the case of seizures, help to direct the next investigations. Age and breed are also key factors to take into account: a young patient might be more likely to be in contact with toxins or have an underlying congenital condition compared to an adult dog with acute signs and a history of foreign body ingestions.

Algorithm 7.1 Note 2 In the case of organophosphate intoxication, treatment should aim to prevent further absorption (activated charcoal, bathing) and control muscarinic and nicotinic clinical signs.

Algorithm 7.1 Note 3 Nausea can be caused by several conditions. Treatment should aim to resolve the primary cause. However, this sign can cause hyporexia/anorexia and vomiting. While investigating the primary cause, starting with symptomatic treatment (e.g., maropitant 1 mg/kg IV q24h) is recommended.

Algorithm 7.1 Note 4 Rabies should always be suspected in dogs that suddenly develop profound behavior changes or features of lower motor neuron paralysis if they live in an area endemic for rabies. Unvaccinated animals should be euthanized or put in quarantine in a secure enclosure for a period specified by relevant national guidelines, avoiding contact with other animals or humans. Clinical signs usually progress rapidly over 4–7 days.[4]

Algorithm 7.1 Note 5 This is a rare idiopathic disease described in dogs. Animals can be presented for retching and gulping with bilateral enlargement of the mandibular salivary glands, causing swallowing difficulties. Diagnostic examinations are required to rule out the most important systemic etiologies, as there is no specific test to diagnose this condition. Diagnosis is confirmed clinically by a rapid and dramatic improvement of clinical signs after the institution of phenobarbital treatment (initial dose, 2.5 mg/kg PO q12h).[5]

Algorithm 7.1 Note 6 As it is a dynamic problem, radiography (even with contrast) has a poor sensitivity for esophageal dysmotility. It should be evaluated using contrast media mixed with food of different consistencies (dry, wet-soft, and liquid) during a fluoroscopic swallow study.[7] In fact, dysmotility can be more evident only with certain consistencies. The history might provide some clues regarding the consistency that is not tolerated (e.g., regurgitation after drinking water or regurgitation after eating dry food).

Algorithm 7.1 Note 7 Balloon dilatation can be performed by progressively increasing the diameter of balloons. An alternative approach is the placement of an indwelling esophageal balloon dilatation feeding tube.[8] Following the dilatation, mild to moderate mucosal hemorrhage may be present.

Algorithm 7.1 Note 8 The therapy should support animals' alimentation, reducing as much as possible any clinical signs and resolving, if possible, any primary cause present. Affected animals should be fed a high-calorie diet, in small frequent feedings, from an elevated or upright position. Dietary consistency should be formulated based on the single individual. A response to sildenafil citrate, which can reduce the lower esophageal sphincter tone, improving the clinical signs when used at 1 mg/kg PO bid, supports a diagnosis of achalasia causing congenital idiopathic megaesophagus.[9]

Algorithm 7.1 Note 9 Vascular ring anomalies are malformations that entrap the esophagus, causing regurgitation following weaning. Persistence of the right aortic arch is the most reported clinical case. Other total or partial ring anomalies can be present, such as double aortic arch, right-sided ligamentum arteriosum with normal left aortic arch (described in German Shepherd dogs, Irish Setters, Great Danes, and German Pinschers,[10] persistent right ductus arteriosus, aberrant left subclavian artery, aberrant left subclavian artery with persistence of the right aortic arch, and aberrant right subclavian artery. Their anatomy is best clarified with CT angiography.

ALGORITHM 7.1

Diagnostic approach to drooling and ptyalism.

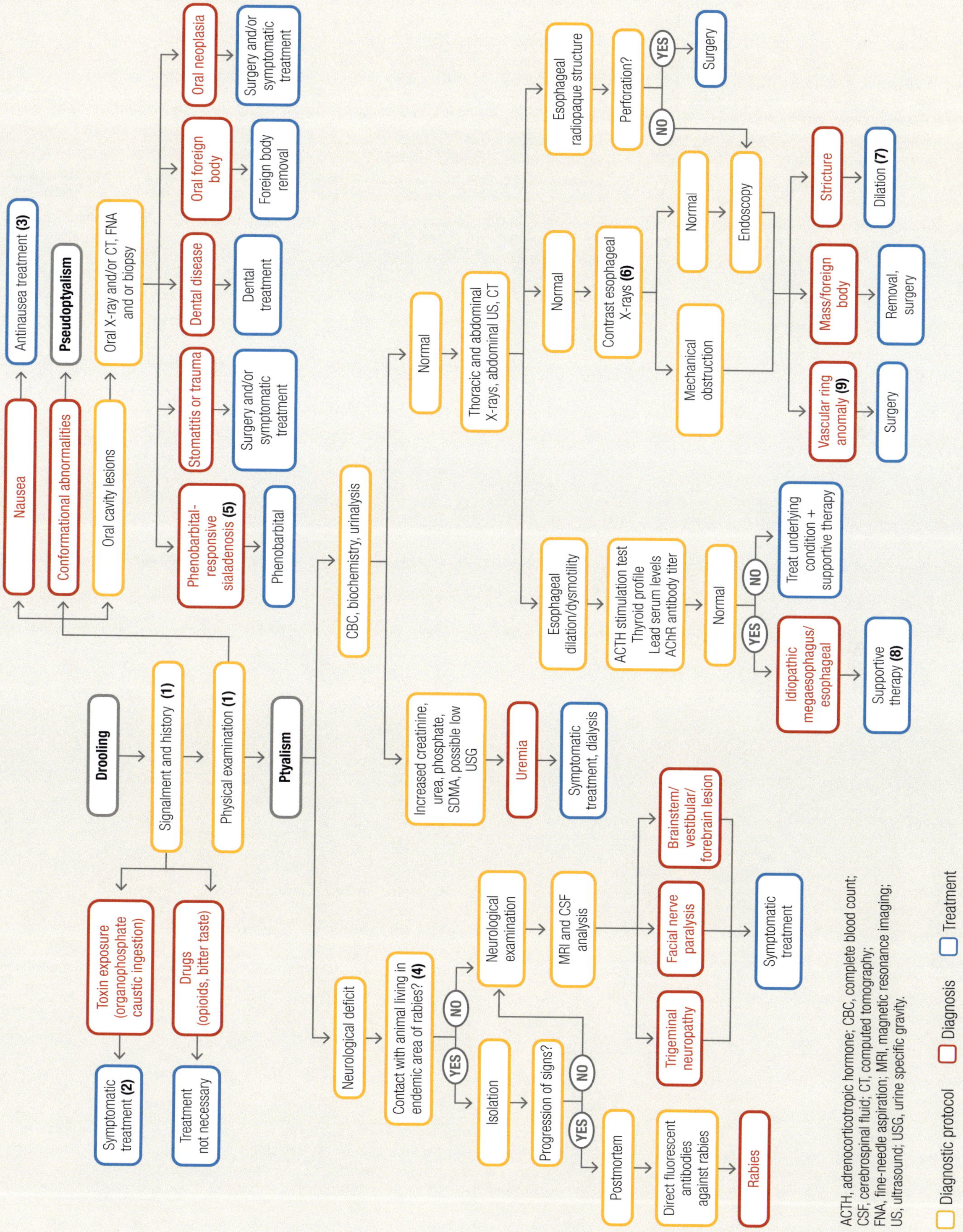

ACTH, adrenocorticotropic hormone; CBC, complete blood count; CSF, cerebrospinal fluid; CT, computed tomography; FNA, fine-needle aspiration; MRI, magnetic resonance imaging; US, ultrasound; USG, urine specific gravity.

References

1. Taney K. Oropharynx. In: Washabau RJ, Day MJ (editors). *Canine and Feline Gastroenterology*. St Louis, Elsevier, 2013, pp. 540–569.
2. Heinze C, Niemiec BA. Ptyalism and halitosis. In: Ettinger SJ, Feldman EC, Côté E (editors). *Textbook of Veterinary Internal Medicine*, 8th edition. St Louis, Elsevier, 2017, pp. 146–151.
3. Furman R, Niemiec BA. Salivation. In: Washabau RJ, Day MJ (editors). *Canine and Feline Gastroenterology*. St Louis, Elsevier, 2013, pp. 162–166.
4. Chomel BB, Sykes JE. Rabies. In: Sykes JE (editor). *Greene's Infectious Diseases of the Dog and Cat*, 5th edition. St Louis, Elsevier, 2023, pp. 260–270.
5. Alcoverro E, Tabar MD, Lloret A, et al. Phenobarbital-responsive sialadenosis in dogs: case series. *Top Companion Anim Med* 29(4):109–112, 2014.
6. Harris RA, Grobman ME, et al. Standardization of a videofluoroscopic swallow study protocol to investigate dysphagia in dogs. *J Vet Intern Med* 31(2):383-393, 2017.
7. Tan DK, Weisse C, Berent A, et al. Prospective evaluation of an indwelling esophageal balloon dilatation feeding tube for treatment of benign esophageal strictures in dogs and cats. *J Vet Intern Med* 32(2):693–700, 2018.
8. Quintavalla F, Menozzi A, Pozzoli C, et al. Sildenafil improves clinical signs and radiographic features in dogs with congenital idiopathic megaoesophagus: a randomised controlled trial. *Vet Rec* 180(16):404, 2017.
9. Kyles AE, Huck JL. Esophagus. In: Johnston SA, Tobias KM (editors). *Veterinary Surgery of Small Animals*, 2nd edition. St Louis, Elsevier, 2018, pp. 1684–1687.
10. Niek J. Beijerink, Mark A. Oyama, John D. Bonagura. Congenital Heart Disease. In: Ettinger SJ, Feldman EC, Côté E (editors). Textbook of Veterinary Internal Medicine, 8th edition. St Louis, Elsevier, 2017, pp. 1207–1248.

CHAPTER 8

Swallowing abnormalities

Samuel Fowlie
BSc(Hons), BVSc(Hons), MVM, DECVIM-CA, MRCVS

Pathophysiology

The medical term for an abnormality or difficulty in swallowing is *dysphagia*, and it can be a diagnostic challenge. The causes of dysphagia can be broadly divided into functional (i.e., secondary to neurological or muscular disease) or structural (i.e., secondary to an injury, stricture, foreign body, or neoplasia). Dysphagia may also be associated with pain when swallowing, termed *odynophagia*.

Observing an animal's ability to drink water and eat foods of different consistencies can help narrow down the differential diagnoses. Structural dysphagia typically occurs with more solid foods, whereas functional dysphagia usually occurs with both solids and liquids.

Dysphagia can be further characterized by the phase of swallowing affected as follows:[1]

- Oral preparatory dysphagia involves difficulty with the prehension, mastication, lubrication, and transportation of food from the tongue to the pharynx.
- Pharyngeal dysphagia occurs when there is a problem with movement of the bolus from the oropharynx into the proximal esophagus. This includes cricopharyngeal dysphagia when passage of the bolus through the upper esophageal sphincter is affected: cricopharyngeal achalasia (structural) and cricopharyngeal asynchrony (functional).
- Esophageal dysphagia happens when there are abnormalities in the movement of the bolus down the esophagus, through the lower esophageal sphincter, and into the stomach. This includes gastroesophageal dysphagia, such as with hiatal hernia and gastroesophageal reflux disease (see Chapter 9).

TABLE 8.1 Causes of dysphagia and associated clinical signs in dogs.

	Phase of swallowing		
	Oral preparatory	**Pharyngeal**	**Esophageal**
Functional dysphagia	■ Masticatory myositis ■ Peripheral neuropathy ■ CNS disease ■ Cranial nerve V, VII, and XIII dysfunction	■ Cricopharyngeal achalasia (increased sphincter tone) ■ Cricopharyngeal asynchrony ■ Botulism ■ Tetanus ■ Polyradiculoneuritis ■ Peripheral neuropathy ■ Polymyositis ■ Myasthenia gravis ■ CNS disease ■ Cranial nerve V, VII, X, and IX dysfunction	■ Megaesophagus ■ Botulism ■ Tetanus ■ Distemper ■ Polyradiculoneuritis ■ Peripheral neuropathy ■ CNS disease ■ Polymyositis ■ Myasthenia gravis
Structural dysphagia	■ Dental disease ■ Stomatitis ■ Oronasal fistula ■ Cleft palate ■ Foreign body ■ Mass/neoplasia ■ Fractures	■ Cricopharyngeal achalasia (stricture) ■ Foreign body ■ Mass/granuloma ■ Neoplasia ■ Pharyngitis	■ Foreign body ■ Hiatal hernia ■ Mass/granuloma ■ Neoplasia ■ Esophagitis ■ Stricture ■ Vascular ring anomaly
Clinical signs	■ Abnormal prehension* ■ Dropping food* ■ Halitosis ■ Ptyalism ■ Cough	■ Repeated attempts to swallow* ■ Odynophagia ■ Gagging/retching ■ Halitosis ■ Ptyalism ■ Cough	■ Regurgitation* ■ Lip-licking ■ Halitosis ■ Ptyalism ■ Cough

CNS, central nervous system. * Common clinical signs.

The various causes of dysphagia and associated clinical signs are illustrated in Table 8.1. The prognosis depends on the severity of the clinical signs and the extent to which the underlying cause can be managed. Secondary aspiration pneumonia is a common complication and often the reason for euthanasia.

History and clinical signs

The patient's signalment and clinical signs may help narrow down the differential diagnoses, so taking a detailed history is important. Young dogs are much more likely to have congenital abnormalities, such as cricopharyngeal achalasia or vascular ring anomalies, which may become apparent at weaning. Those with acquired disease tend to be middle-aged or older, whilst geriatric dogs may exhibit progressive neuropathies with pharyngeal weakness and associated dysphagia. Other aspects of the clinical history such as known ingestion of foreign bodies or caustic agents, administration of certain oral medications (e.g., doxycycline), recent general anesthesia, vomiting, previous esophageal trauma, or radiotherapy can give clues to suggest the possibility of obstruction, esophagitis, or stricture. Geographic location in, or travel history to, a country with *Spirocera lupi* parasitism or endemic rabies should also be excluded.

Certain breeds have a predisposition for dysphagia, including the Cocker and Springer Spaniel and Miniature Wire-haired Dachshund (cricopharyngeal achalasia), Golden Retriever (pharyngeal weakness), Cavalier King Charles Spaniel and Bouvier des Flandres (muscular dystrophy), German Shepherd and Irish Setter (vascular ring anomalies), English Bulldog (esophageal dysmotility), Boston Terrier, French Bulldog, and Pug (hiatal hernia), and Boxer (inflammatory myopathy).[2]

Diagnostic approach

Algorithm 8.1 shows the diagnostic approach to dogs with swallowing abnormalities. Investigations should follow a logical approach, starting from the least invasive and progressing towards more invasive testing as diseases are excluded. Investigations may progress down different pathways sequentially or simultaneously. Some tests that are used in humans, such as esophageal manometry (to evaluate esophageal pressure and motor function) and nuclear scintigraphy (to assess mucociliary clearance and detect reflux and aspiration events), are largely research tools in dogs and are not commonly used clinically.[3,4]

Treatment is focused on the underlying cause if possible, but frequently there is no specific treatment available and management relies on symptomatic medications and changes to diet consistency (e.g., slurry vs. meat balls), meal frequency, and position of feeding (i.e., postural feeding—"feeding from a height", so that the mouth is higher than the stomach and then holding up the dog more vertically after a meal). Enteral feeding tubes may be necessary in animals that cannot meet their daily calorie or water requirements, but the ethics and feasibility of this need to be judged on an individual patient and owner basis.

Algorithm 8.1 Note 1 It is essential to watch dysphagic animals eating and drinking. Owner-acquired videos may be helpful in patients that will not do this in the clinic. Oral dysphagia, with food either not prehended or dropping from the mouth after chewing, can often be diagnosed by doing so in conjunction with a thorough oral and neurological examination. Pharyngeal dysphagia is more challenging to diagnose, but cases often present with gagging, retching, and repeated gulping attempts at swallowing. Esophageal dysphagia typically involves regurgitation (see also Chapter 9).

Algorithm 8.1 Note 2 Physical examination should include an assessment of the patient's respiratory rate and effort and any coughing noted, as concurrent aspiration pneumonia is common. Weight loss and/or dehydration should also be noted. Careful examination of the mouth, tongue, and throat should be performed to look for any trauma, anatomical abnormalities (e.g., cleft palate), obstructions (e.g., foreign body, mass), or inflammation (e.g., stomatitis, dental disease) but may need to be performed under sedation or general anesthesia, in which case laryngeal function can also be assessed (e.g., polyneuropathy). Palpation of the neck is important to assess for any masses, asymmetry, or pain.

Algorithm 8.1 Note 3 Cranial nerve assessment should be performed to assess the gag reflex, jaw tone, and tongue sensation. The lack of a gag reflex can be normal and should not be overinterpreted as evidence of cranial nerve dysfunction.

Algorithm 8.1 Note 4 A minimum database (hematology, biochemistry including electrolytes, and urinalysis) should be performed to rule out systemic disease and to assess the dog's general health prior to further investigations, but it is often unremarkable. Blood lead concentrations can be measured if there is a history of exposure or suspicion on blood smear review (nucleated red blood cells despite normal packed cell volume, basophilic stippling).

Algorithm 8.1 Note 5 Measurement of creatine kinase (CK) and aspartate aminotransferase (AST) may help assess for neuromuscular disease, although normal values do not exclude it. Further testing should be based on the patient's signalment, history, and anatomical localization of dysphagia.

Algorithm 8.1 Note 6 Patients with neuromuscular weakness, including laryngeal paralysis (and/or megaesophagus), should have thyroid function testing (total thyroxine, TT_4; canine thyroid-stimulating hormone, cTSH) performed to rule out hypothyroidism, although the link between hypothyroidism and functional dysphagia is tenuous.

Algorithm 8.1 Note 7 Patients with acquired megaesophagus should have a basal cortisol or adrenocorticotropic hormone (ACTH) stimulation test performed to exclude hypoadrenocorticism, even if electrolytes are within reference ranges.

Algorithm 8.1 Note 8 In patients with pharyngeal dysphagia and/or megaesophagus for which no other cause has been identified, measurement of acetylcholine receptor (AChR) autoantibodies should be performed to identify myasthenia gravis.

Algorithm 8.1 Note 9 Megaesophagus is present in around 84% of dogs with generalized myasthenia gravis, and positive titers are found in ~98% of cases, with a smaller percentage of positives in dogs with focal myasthenia gravis. Antibody titers may be falsely negative early in disease or if corticosteroids were administered prior to testing. Therefore, retesting after 1–2 months is recommended when myasthenia gravis is still suspected.

Algorithm 8.1 Note 10 Diagnostic imaging should include a minimum of cervical and three-view thoracic radiographs to assess for signs of structural dysphagia (e.g., masses, foreign bodies, vascular ring anomalies, megaesophagus) and aspiration pneumonia. Assessment for megaesophagus should be performed on radiographs taken in conscious patients. In dogs with myasthenia gravis, cranial mediastinal masses, usually thymomas, may be seen in a small proportion (3.4%) of cases. In some instances, it may be more appropriate to perform computed tomography angiography if available (see Chapter 21).

Algorithm 8.1 Note 11 A magnetic resonance imaging scan with or without cerebrospinal fluid analysis may take priority over other tests if cranial nerve or brain stem lesions are suspected, so they could be performed earlier in the diagnostic pathway. Thoracic imaging is still worthwhile if there is a concern of aspiration pneumonia or primary or metastatic neoplastic disease.

Algorithm 8.1 Note 12 Electrodiagnostics and muscle and nerve biopsies may be considered in a referral setting to further investigate and characterize myopathies and neuromuscular disease. Since electromyography and biopsies require general anesthesia and take some time to complete, the patient's general health should be considered prior to biopsy collection. These investigations can potentially be combined with other tests (e.g., endoscopy) and management (e.g., feeding tube placement). Muscle and nerve biopsies should be sent to a laboratory with expertise in processing and interpreting them.

Algorithm 8.1 Note 13 Videofluoroscopic swallowing studies are vital for assessing the swallowing reflex, particularly the pharyngeal and esophageal phases of swallowing, and may detect hiatal hernias and gastroesophageal reflux disease.[5,6] These conditions are commonly associated with brachycephalic obstructive airway syndrome.[7] Videofluoroscopic swallowing studies involve feeding a barium suspension and barium-laced foods (ideally wet and dry) to animals, with real-time capture of X-ray images for analysis, but they are generally only available in referral centers. Care should be taken in dogs that are likely to aspirate barium, and any benefits should be weighed against the risk of performing the study. It is worth noting that esophageal motility in young animals may continue to develop up until 1 year of age, so this fact should be considered if mild abnormalities are found in this population.[8]

Algorithm 8.1 Note 14 Endoscopy under general anesthesia allows for the removal of foreign bodies and assessment of the esophagus for signs of esophagitis, strictures, masses, and hiatal hernias. It may also be necessary to take biopsies or perform balloon dilatation of strictures and allows for the placement of esophagostomy or gastrotomy tubes.

Algorithm 8.1 Note 15 Esophageal neoplasia is rare in dogs, although leiomyomas, carcinomas, and sarcomas are reported. For patients in certain geographic areas or with a relevant travel history, *Spirocerca lupi* granulomas and associated neoplasia should be considered.

Algorithm 8.1 Note 16 The most common vascular ring anomaly is a persistent right aortic arch, which develops from the right rather than the left fourth aortic arch, trapping the esophagus between the aorta, pulmonary artery, ligamentum arteriosum, and trachea. Treatment involves surgical transection of the ligamentum arteriosum. However, irreversible esophageal damage may have already occurred, leading to some clinical signs persisting in up to 70% of patients, with no improvement in 13% of cases.[9]

ALGORITHM 8.1

Diagnostic approach to swallowing abnormalities in dogs.

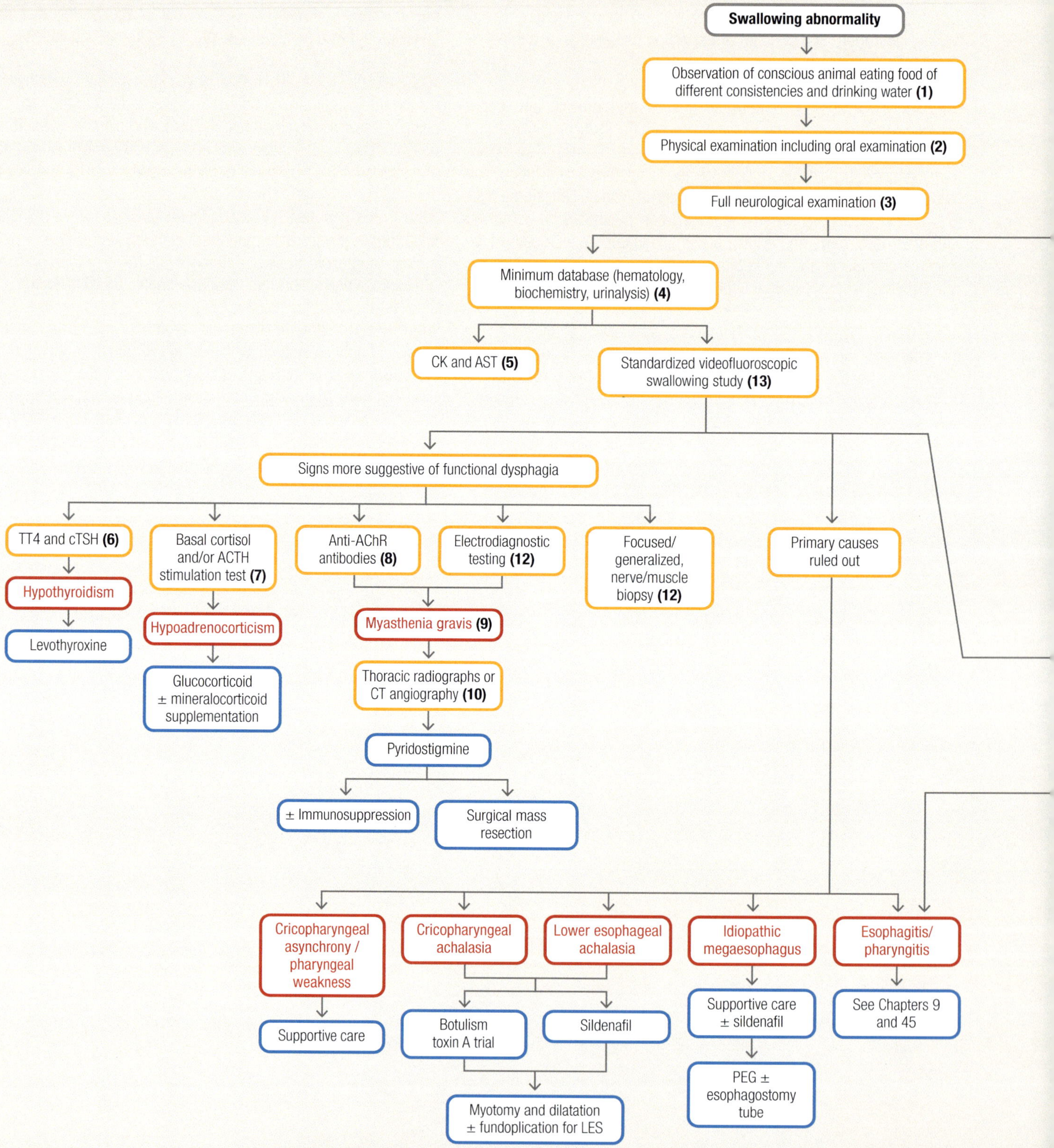

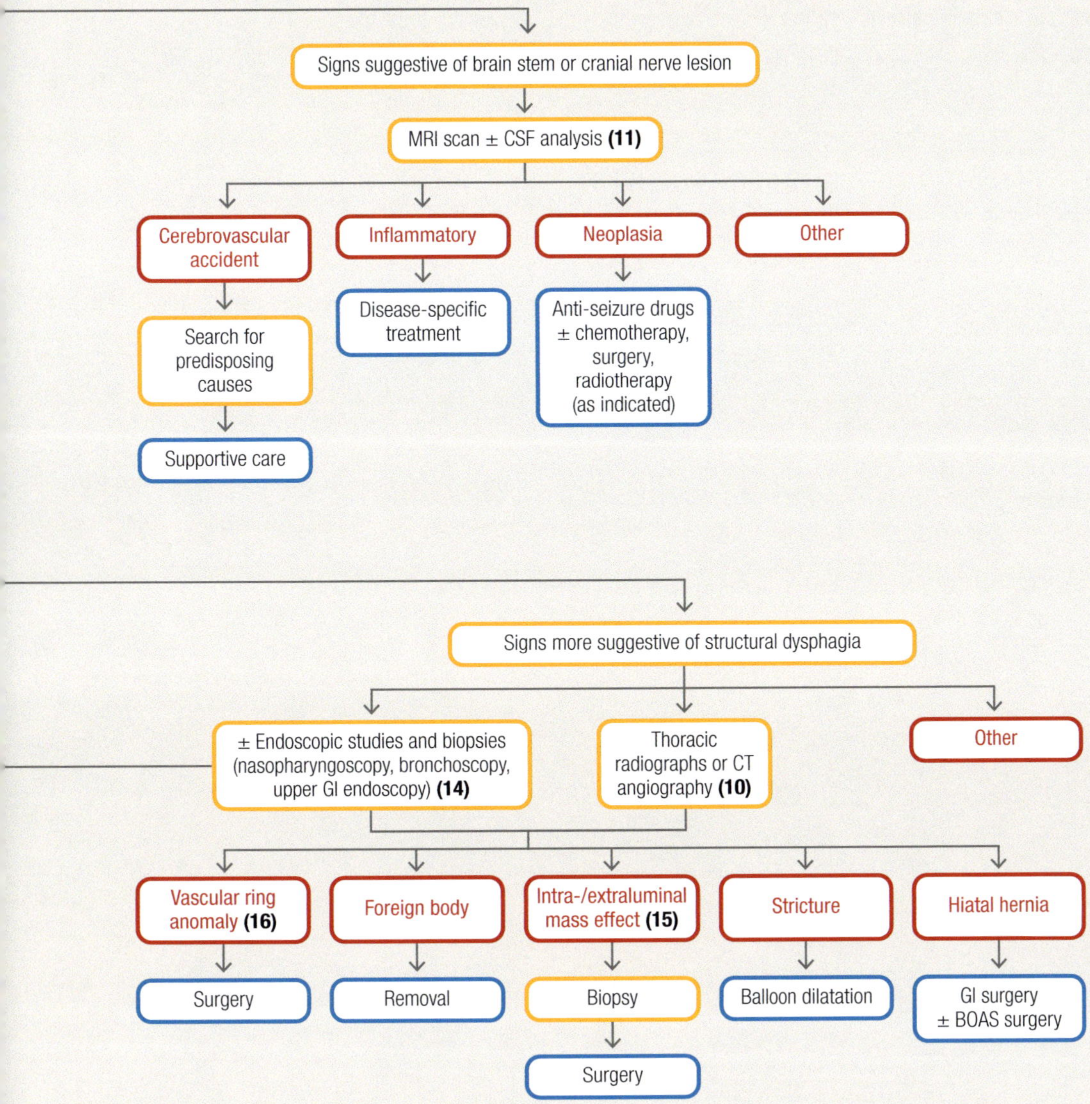

AChR, acetylcholine receptor; ACTH, adrenocorticotropic hormone; AST, aspartate aminotransferase; BOAS, brachycephalic obstructive airway syndrome; CK, creatine kinase; CSF, cerebrospinal fluid; CT, computed tomography; cTSH, canine thyroid-stimulating hormone; GI, gastrointestinal; LES, lower esophageal sphincter; MRI, magnetic resonance imaging; PEG, percutaneous endoscopic gastrostomy TT_4, total thyroxine.

Source: Adapted from Swales.[10]

Diagnostic protocol | Diagnosis | Treatment

References

1. Grobman M, Reinero C. A One Health review of aerodigestive disease in dogs. *J Vet Intern Med* 37(3):817–834, 2023.
2. Ullal TV, Marks SL, Belafsky PC, et al. A comparative assessment of the diagnosis of swallowing impairment and gastroesophageal reflux in canines and humans. *Front Vet Sci* 9:889331, 2022.
3. Kempf J, Heinrich H, Reusch CE, Kook PH. Evaluation of esophageal high-resolution manometry in awake and sedated dogs. *Am J Vet Res* 74(6):895–900, 2013.
4. Grobman ME, Maitz CA, Reinero CR. Detection of silent reflux events by nuclear scintigraphy in healthy dogs. *J Vet Intern Med* 34(4):1432-1439, 2020.
5. Harris RA, Grobman ME, Allen MJ, et al. Standardization of a videofluoroscopic swallow study protocol to investigate dysphagia in dogs. *J Vet Intern Med* 31(2):383–393, 2017.
6. Pollard RE, Marks SL, Cheney DM, Bonadio CM. Diagnostic outcome of contrast videofluoroscopic swallowing studies in 216 dysphagic dogs. *Vet Radiol Ultrasound* 58(4):373–380, 2017.
7. Eivers C, Chicon Rueda R, Liuti T, Salavati Schmitz S. Retrospective analysis of esophageal imaging features in brachycephalic versus non-brachycephalic dogs based on videofluoroscopic swallowing studies. *J Vet Intern Med* 33(4):1740–1746, 2019.
8. Bexfield NH, Watson PJ, Herrtage ME. Esophageal dysmotility in young dogs. *J Vet Intern Med* 20(6):1314–1318, 2006.
9. Krebs IA, Lindsley S, Shaver S, MacPhail C. Short- and long-term outcome of dogs following surgical correction of a persistent right aortic arch. *J Am Anim Hosp Assoc* 50(3):181–186, 2014.
10. Swales H. Dysphagia. In: Fracassi F (ed.). *Diagnostic and Therapeutic Algorithms in Internal Medicine for Dogs and Cats*. Palm Beach Gardens: Edra Publishing; 2022. pp. 89–92.

CHAPTER 9

Regurgitation

Megan Grobman
DVM, MS, PhD,
DACVIM (SAIM)

Pathophysiology

Regurgitation, the passive retrograde expulsion of food and/or liquids from the esophagus because of dysmotility or mechanical obstruction, is the most commonly recognized clinical manifestation of esophageal dysphagia. Grossly, the esophagus is a muscular tube comprised of various proportions of smooth and striated muscle depending on the species; in dogs, it is composed entirely of striated muscle. The esophagus is bracketed by the high-pressure zones of the upper esophageal sphincter (UES) and the lower esophageal sphincter (LES). In a healthy dog, the esophageal phase of swallowing is involuntary and irreversible once triggered. Pharyngeal swallowing stimulates primary esophageal peristalsis and conduction of the bolus through the LES and into the stomach. Residual material within the esophagus, not cleared by a primary peristaltic wave, is cleared by secondary peristalsis, which is triggered by esophageal distension and augmented by chemosensory stimulation. Any disruption of bolus flow may result in regurgitation.[1]

It should be noted that diseases of the esophageal–gastric junction (EGJ), such as sliding hiatal hernia, gastroesophageal reflux disease, and extraesophageal reflux disease (i.e., extension of refluxed material from the stomach to beyond the UES with accompanying clinical signs), may also result in regurgitation.[1,2] Decreases in LES tone (e.g., sliding hiatal hernia, sedation, anesthesia) or impaired gastrointestinal motility (e.g., gastroparesis) may predispose dogs to reflux, esophagitis, and subsequent regurgitation. In some cases of extraesophageal reflux disease, the refluxate may extend so far as to leave the oral cavity and be clinically indistinguishable from esophageal regurgitation.[1]

Regurgitation carries a high risk of aspiration.[3] Airway protective mechanisms present during retching or vomiting, including apnea, glottal closure, UES closure, nasopharyngeal closure, and laryngeal elevation, are diminished or absent during regurgitation.[1] Critically, aspiration events may not be witnessed, and respiratory diseases may go unrecognized as consequences of esophageal dysphagia, particularly in dogs with more subtle esophageal dysfunction.[1]

TABLE 9.1 Clinical or historical features used to differentiate regurgitation and vomiting.

Clinical Signs	Regurgitation	Vomiting
Prodromal Signs (e.g., Food Aversion, Lip Smacking, Ptyalism)	Rare	Common
Abdominal Effort/Retching	No	Yes
Presence of Bile	Rare	±
Esophageal Bulge	±	No
Time after Eating	Variable	Variable
Shape	Variable	Variable
Volume	Variable	Variable
pH	Variable	Variable

Clinical signs

Dogs with regurgitation have evidence of passive expulsion of food, water, or saliva from the esophagus. This may be accompanied by weight loss, weakness, polyphagia, halitosis, nasal discharge, painful swallowing, and signs consistent with aspiration (e.g., cough, respiratory distress). Nervous system abnormalities may be present for some causes of esophageal dysphagia and regurgitation (e.g., myasthenia gravis). Dogs should be carefully evaluated for cranial nerve deficits and generalized neuromuscular dysfunction. In some dogs with megaesophagus (ME), a fluid-filled esophagus "bulging" at the neck may be observed.

Diagnostic approach

Algorithm 9.1 shows the diagnostic approach to patients with regurgitation. It is critical to first distinguish regurgitation from vomiting, the active retrograde expulsion of gastric and occasionally proximal small intestinal contents (Table 9.1). Vomiting is a commonly encountered clinical complaint and is often indistinguishable from regurgitation to pet owners. However, differential diagnoses, diagnostic approaches, and clinical interventions are often markedly different between these two clinical complaints. It should be noted that both conditions can occur in the same dog. Careful questioning of the owner and observation/filming of feeding behaviors or episodes may provide important clarifying information. A thorough history and physical examination are critical and may identify concurrent illnesses and potential exposures underlying or accompanying esophageal dysfunction and regurgitation (see Chapter 42).[1]

Thoracic (three views) and lateral cervical radiographs are important first-line diagnostic tests to assess for ME (focal or generalized), evidence of aspiration, or signs consistent with obstruction (e.g., by a vascular ring anomaly or esophageal foreign material). However, it is important to recognize that esophageal dysfunction, regurgitation, and even aspiration can occur in the absence of overt radiographic abnormalities.[1,4] Transient esophageal dilation secondary to aerophagia may be observed in some dogs. This must be distinguished from ME, which is characterized by esophageal dilation with concurrent esophageal dysmotility. Contrast radiography may be beneficial when standard radiographs are nondiagnostic, or to assess for esophageal perforation. Despite the utility of radiographs, they are often insufficient to identify functional dysmotility and frequently underestimate the extent and severity of respiratory pathology. Videofluoroscopic swallow studies (VFSSs) are often needed to characterize the extent and type of esophageal dysphagia (e.g., LES achalasia-like syndrome[5]) and diseases of the EGJ (e.g., reflux, sliding hiatal hernia). A thorough diagnostic evaluation of dogs with esophageal dysfunction is important, as some causes may respond to interventions for disease and/or specific targets (e.g., LES achalasia-like syndrome). Endoscopy may be diagnostic and therapeutic in cases of suspected esophageal strictures or foreign bodies, and it also allows for sample collection if esophageal masses or other gross lesions are identified.

Thoracic computed tomography may be beneficial to classify the extent and type of aspiration-associated respiratory disease.[6] Functional upper airway examinations may also be recommended in some dogs to assess for respiratory conditions (e.g., brachycephalic obstructive airway syndrome, laryngeal paralysis) which are associated with concurrent esophageal dysfunction and/or disorders of the EGJ.[1]

The minimum database, including complete blood count, serum biochemical profile, and urinalysis, may be unremarkable, or it may be suggestive of systemic causes of esophageal dysfunction (e.g., basophilic stippling in lead toxicity). Disease-specific tests, such as serum lead concentration, thyroid testing, adrenocorticotropic hormone stimulation testing, and acetylcholine receptor antibody testing, should be considered in dogs with esophageal dysfunction if appropriate (see Chapter 42). The association between ME and hypothyroidism is unclear, although frequently referenced. Care should be taken when interpreting total thyroxine concentrations in dogs out of concern for euthyroid sick syndrome.[7]

Algorithm 9.1 Note 1 The absence of esophageal dilation on radiographs does not rule out esophageal dysfunction. In a dog with regurgitation and normal thoracic and cervical radiographs, assessment for a functional motility disorder, EGJ abnormality, or mechanical obstruction not readily identified by radiographs (e.g., stricture, radiolucent material) is recommended.

Algorithm 9.1 Note 2 A VFSS is distinct from contrast radiography. In some countries, VFSSs have traditionally been performed in lateral recumbency with force feeding. However, upright and free-fed protocols are now advocated, as they allow for physiologically relevant bolus sizes and consistencies (e.g., liquid, canned, kibble), feeding position, and minimized risk of aspiration.

Algorithm 9.1 Note 3 VFSSs or contrast radiography may be helpful to rule in or out perforation if conventional radiography is inconclusive.

Algorithm 9.1 Note 4 LES achalasia-like syndrome is a recently identified cause of regurgitation in which the LES fails to relax in response to pharyngeal swallow (see Chapter 42). Diagnosis in dogs is typically made by VFSSs.

Algorithm 9.1 Note 5 Delayed esophageal maturation, manifesting as esophageal dysmotility without ME, may be seen in some puppies. Esophageal motility may continue to improve up to approximately 1 year of age.

Algorithm 9.1 Note 6 Physiological reflux is observed in approximately 40% of normal dogs. Pathological reflux (reflux marginating beyond the distal third of the esophagus) may be clinically significant.[1,8]

Algorithm 9.1 Note 7 Dogs with regurgitation and a normal VFSS should be evaluated for intermittent conditions often localized to the EGJ (e.g., sliding hiatal hernia, reflux).

Algorithm 9.1 Note 8 The absence of obvious esophageal lesions on endoscopy does not rule out reflux/esophagitis as a potential cause of regurgitation (e.g., nonerosive esophagitis).

Algorithm 9.1 Note 9 Dogs with LES achalasia-like syndrome have been demonstrated to respond to interventions targeting the LES, including botulinum toxin A injections with mechanical dilation, and/or Heller myotomy with Dor fundoplication. Whether sildenafil has any efficacy in LES achalasia-like syndrome is yet to be clarified.[9]

Algorithm 9.1 Note 10 Dogs with esophageal dysfunction may benefit from upright feeding, small frequent meals, and feeding trials with various feed consistencies. The response to treatment for esophagitis may be variable depending on the underlying cause of regurgitation. In some dogs, percutaneous endoscopic gastrostomy tubes or surgically placed gastrostomy tubes may be needed to maintain body condition and reduce the risk of aspiration.

Algorithm 9.1 Note 11 Several conditions (e.g., myasthenia gravis, Addison's disease, lead toxicity) have been implicated in esophageal dysfunction and regurgitation (see Chapter 42).

Algorithm 9.1 Note 12 Balloon esophagostomy tubes may be considered for some dogs.

Algorithm 9.1 Note 13 A multimodal approach is recommended to treat dogs with reflux and esophagitis.[10] A combination of antacids, prokinetics, and dietary changes (e.g., low-fat diet) can be used to address the content of the refluxate and the frequency of reflux events. Sucralfate is recommended for dogs with confirmed or strongly suspected esophageal erosions, but it is not considered preventative against esophageal erosions/ulcers. Treatment trials for reflux may take up to 6–8 weeks to show effect (see Chapter 42).

ALGORITHM 9.1

Diagnostic approach to regurgitation in dogs.

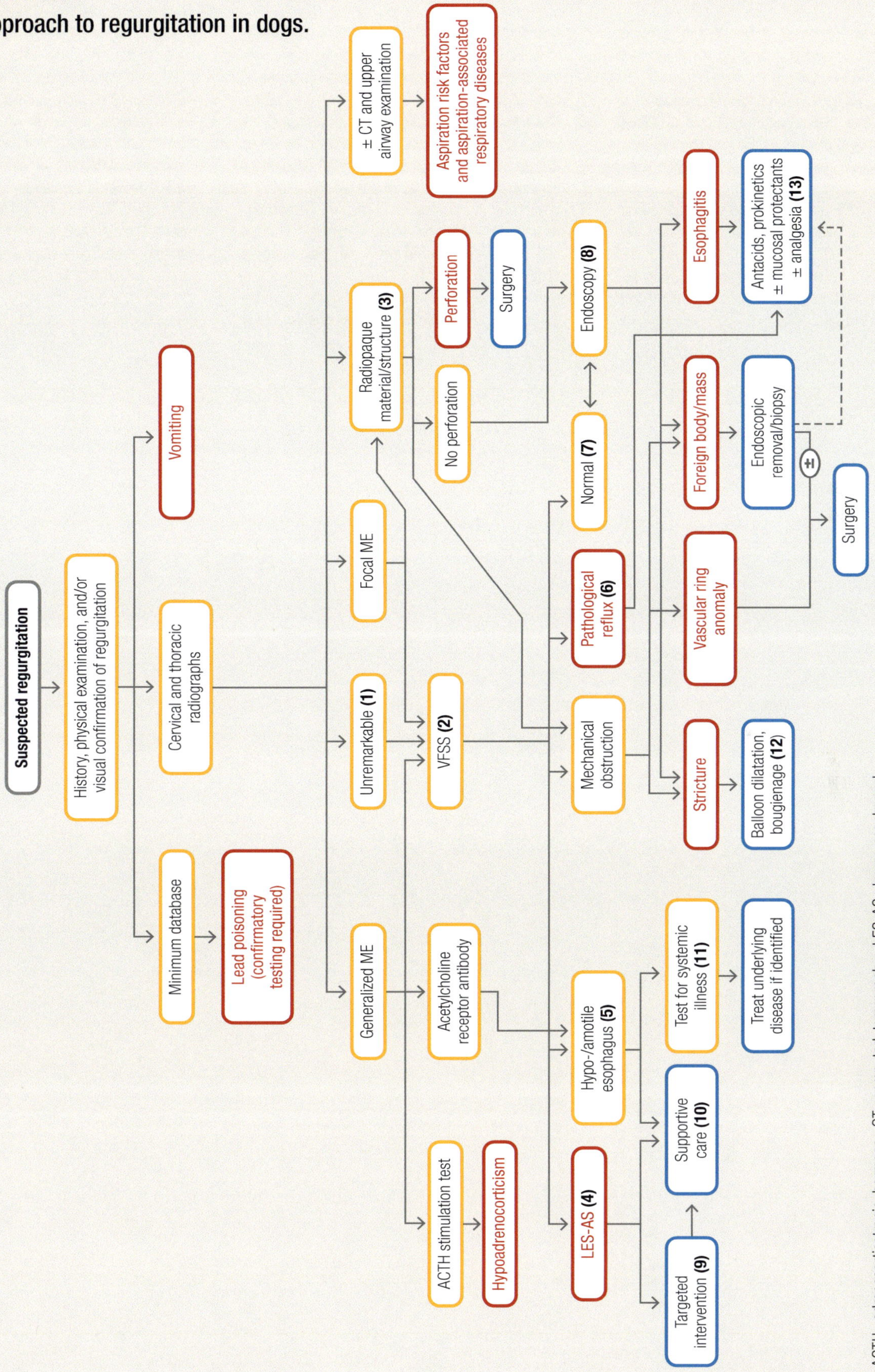

ACTH, adrenocorticotropic hormone; CT, computed tomography; LES-AS, lower esophageal sphincter achalasia-like syndrome; ME, megaesophagus; VFSS, videofluoroscopic swallow study.

Diagnostic protocol | Diagnosis | Treatment

References

1. Grobman M, Reinero C. A One Health review of aerodigestive disease in dogs. *J Vet Intern Med* 37(3):817–834, 2023.
2. Luciani E, Reinero C, Grobman M. Evaluation of aerodigestive disease and diagnosis of sliding hiatal hernia in brachycephalic and nonbrachycephalic dogs. *J Vet Intern Med* 36(4):1229–1236, 2022.
3. Sherman R, Karagiannis M. Aspiration pneumonia in the dog: a review. *Top Companion Anim Med* 32(1):1–7, 2017.
4. Bexfield NH, Watson PJ, Herrtage ME. Esophageal dysmotility in young dogs. *J Vet Intern Med* 20(6):1314–1318, 2006.
5. Grobman ME, Schachtel J, Gyawali CP, et al. Videofluoroscopic swallow study features of lower esophageal sphincter achalasia-like syndrome in dogs. *J Vet Intern Med* 33(5):1954–1963, 2019.
6. Masseau I, Reinero CR. Thoracic computed tomographic interpretation for clinicians to aid in the diagnosis of dogs and cats with respiratory disease. *Vet J* 253:105388, 2019.
7. Whitehead K, Cortes Y, Eirmann L. Gastrointestinal dysmotility disorders in critically ill dogs and cats. *J Vet Emerg Crit Care (San Antonio)* 26(2):234–253, 2016.
8. Harris RA, Grobman ME, Allen MJ, et al. Standardization of a videofluoroscopic swallow study protocol to investigate dysphagia in dogs. *J Vet Intern Med* 31(2):383–393, 2017.
9. Grobman ME, Hutcheson KD, Lever TE, et al. Mechanical dilation, botulinum toxin A injection, and surgical myotomy with fundoplication for treatment of lower esophageal sphincter achalasia-like syndrome in dogs. *J Vet Intern Med* 33(3):1423–1433, 2019.
10. Marks SL, Kook PH, Papich MG, et al. ACVIM consensus statement: Support for rational administration of gastrointestinal protectants to dogs and cats. *J Vet Intern Med* 32(6):1823–1840, 2018.

CHAPTER 10

Vomiting

M. Katherine Tolbert
DVM, PhD, DACVIM
(SAIM & Nutrition)

Pathophysiology

Vomiting, the expulsion of ingesta and digestive secretions from the small intestine and/or stomach through the mouth, is a common chief complaint reported by owners of dogs presented to the veterinarian for evaluation. Vomiting is not specific for gastrointestinal (GI) disease and involves a complex pathway with stimuli originating from at least four major areas, including the abdominal viscera (e.g., pancreas, liver, GI tract), chemoreceptor trigger zone, vestibular apparatus, and central nervous system. Stimuli from these areas terminate in the vomiting center of the medulla oblongata, where they summate to trigger the vomiting reflex. The type and number of receptors that lead to a proemetic or antiemetic stimulus varies by anatomical location and by species. Causes of vomiting range from toxin ingestion or dietary indiscretion to metabolic disturbances or neoplasia. Acute vomiting is characterized by clinical signs less than 2 weeks in duration. Chronic vomiting is characterized by persistent or intermittent vomiting of variable frequency and character greater than 2 weeks in duration.

Clinical signs

Vomiting is a common clinical sign but can be easily misinterpreted by pet owners as regurgitation or even coughing and retching. Prior to embarking on a diagnostic approach for vomiting, the owner should be asked to describe the process to ensure that the problem is truly vomiting (Table 10.1). Vomiting can be the only clinical sign reported or can be accompanied by additional GI signs (e.g., diarrhea, dysorexia, nausea, regurgitation) or systemic signs (e.g., polyuria, seizures).

Physical examination findings in vomiting dogs can vary. Dogs can have a history of mild signs and no abnormalities on examination or have severe signs with multiple physical examination abnormalities such as hunched posture, poor body condition or hair coat, abdominal pain, dehydration, ptyalism, thickened bowel, or palpable masses or foreign objects. Cranial abdominal pain may be appreciated on physical examination in cases of foreign body ingestion, gastric dilatation–volvulus, pancreatitis, or GI ulceration. Rectal and fecal examination should be performed to evaluate for the presence of frank blood, tarry stools, and parasites. Examination of the vomitus for the presence of blood or parasites is also recommended. Body and muscle condition scores are expected to be normal in cases of acute vomiting and are often normal in animals with chronic vomiting in the absence of comorbidities or additional GI signs such as dysorexia or diarrhea.

TABLE 10.1 General guideline to help differentiate regurgitation from vomiting.

Clinical sign	Nausea	Marked abdominal effort	Bile-stained	pH of fluid
Regurgitation	±	–	–	>4
Vomiting	+	+	±	Variable, but <4 suggests gastric contribution

Diagnostic approach

Algorithms 10.1 and 10.2 show the approach to the dog with acute and chronic vomiting, respectively.

Algorithm 10.1 Note 1 Pet owners should be questioned to confirm that the presenting complaint is truly vomiting. Asking owners to bring videos of the problem, if possible, can be helpful, especially in dogs where the diagnostic results (e.g., megaesophagus visualized on radiographs) are not well explained by the presenting problem.

Algorithm 10.1 Note 2 Once the act of vomiting is confirmed, the signalment and history of the dog are considered. Owners should be questioned regarding the possibility of exposure of their dog to foreign objects (e.g., toys, clothing, kitchen items), trash, household chemicals, new foods or treats, or drugs (including medications for pets or their owners, such as nonsteroidal anti-inflammatory drugs). Owners should be asked if any objects have gone missing from the household. Intoxications secondary to chocolate (theobromine), macadamia nuts, mycotoxins (e.g., mushrooms, molds), sago palms, blue-green algae, and marijuana should be considered in dogs exhibiting vomiting in association with an acute onset of neurological abnormalities. Viral etiologies are rarely causes of vomiting alone but should be suspected when there is an outbreak of GI signs in multiple dogs from the same shelter or household or when signs are severe, particularly in young animals. Owners should also be questioned about the presence of additional clinical signs such as those that point to either diffuse GI or systemic disease.

Algorithm 10.1 Note 3 Particular attention should be paid to the dog's body and muscle condition. Unless comorbidities are present, animals with acute vomiting should be in good body condition with adequate muscle mass and a good hair coat. Particular attention should be paid to the animal's mentation, vital parameters, hydration status, and presence of abdominal pain, masses, foreign objects, distension, and lymphadenopathy. Dogs with gastric dilatation–volvulus will often display unproductive retching, which the owners might call "vomiting", and a tympanitic, distended abdomen.

Algorithm 10.1 Note 4 Vomiting dogs with a good appetite, normal hydration status, normal vital parameters, and normal energy levels, and if gastric dilatation–volvulus, foreign object, toxin, or drug exposure is not suspected, can be treated supportively with an 8–12-hour restriction of food followed by introduction of a highly digestible diet with reduced fat content. When possible, small, frequent meals consisting of high-moisture content (i.e., canned food or moistened dry food) are recommended to enhance gastric emptying. Antiemetics should be withheld if foreign material or toxin ingestion cannot be ruled out.

Algorithm 10.1 Note 5 Dogs that improve following introduction of a highly digestible, reduced-fat diet should continue to eat the diet for a minimum of 3–5 days followed by slow transition to the dog's maintenance diet. If a more chronic history is suspected or the dog has other risk factors for GI disease, it might be prudent to continue the diet for a longer period.

Algorithm 10.1 Note 6 Dogs with mild signs that do not improve with supportive care or dogs presenting with more severe signs or abnormalities detected on physical examination should undergo further diagnostic evaluation. The diagnostic tests should be selected based on review of the dog's signalment, history, and physical examination findings and might include fecal testing, complete blood count, serum biochemistry panel, urinalysis, abdominal radiography, abdominal ultrasound, evaluation of serum canine pancreatic lipase immunoreactivity, and/or hypoadrenocorticism testing (i.e., baseline cortisol, urine cortisol:creatinine, adrenocorticotropic hormone—ACTH—stimulation test).

Algorithm 10.1 Note 7 If a small gastric or proximal duodenal foreign body is confirmed or suspected and vomiting will not cause harm, emesis can be attempted. If emesis is not successful and there is concern for obstruction with natural passage, the foreign body should be removed by endoscopy or surgery. If no foreign bodies are identified at the time of endoscopy or surgical exploration, GI biopsies should be performed to further evaluate the cause of vomiting.

Algorithm 10.1 Note 8 Dogs presenting with history, physical examination, or blood work findings including but not limited to prolonged hyporexia (≥72 hours), intractable vomiting or retching, distended abdomen, persistent hematemesis, hypotension and/or pulse deficits, pale mucous membranes, abdominal pain, altered mentation, severe anemia, severe electrolyte or acid-base derangements, severe neutropenia, azotemia, and/or moderate to severe hepatopathy benefit from hospitalization and targeted intervention to identify and correct the sequelae of vomiting.

Algorithm 10.1 Note 9 For dogs presenting with clinical or biochemical signs of GI bleeding (e.g., hematemesis, melena, anemia, hypoproteinemia, thrombocytosis, thrombocytopenia, increased blood urea nitrogen), additional diagnostic testing, such as coagulation evaluation and parasitic and region-specific infectious disease testing should be considered (see Chapter 14). If upper GI bleeding is suspected, treatment with proton pump inhibitors and cytoprotectants should be initiated.[1,2]

Algorithm 10.1 Note 10 If vomiting and/or GI bleeding cannot be resolved with supportive care, additional therapeutics (e.g., antiemetics, promotility drugs – see Chapters 31 and 32) and diagnostics (e.g., endoscopy, abdominal computed tomography) should be considered. Assisted feeding (e.g., small bolus or constant rate infusion diet via nasoenteric, esophageal or gastric tube, postpyloric feeding, parenteral nutrition) should be considered for dogs consuming <50% of their resting energy requirement for ≥3 days (see Chapter 25).

ALGORITHM 10.1

Diagnostic approach to acute vomiting in dogs.

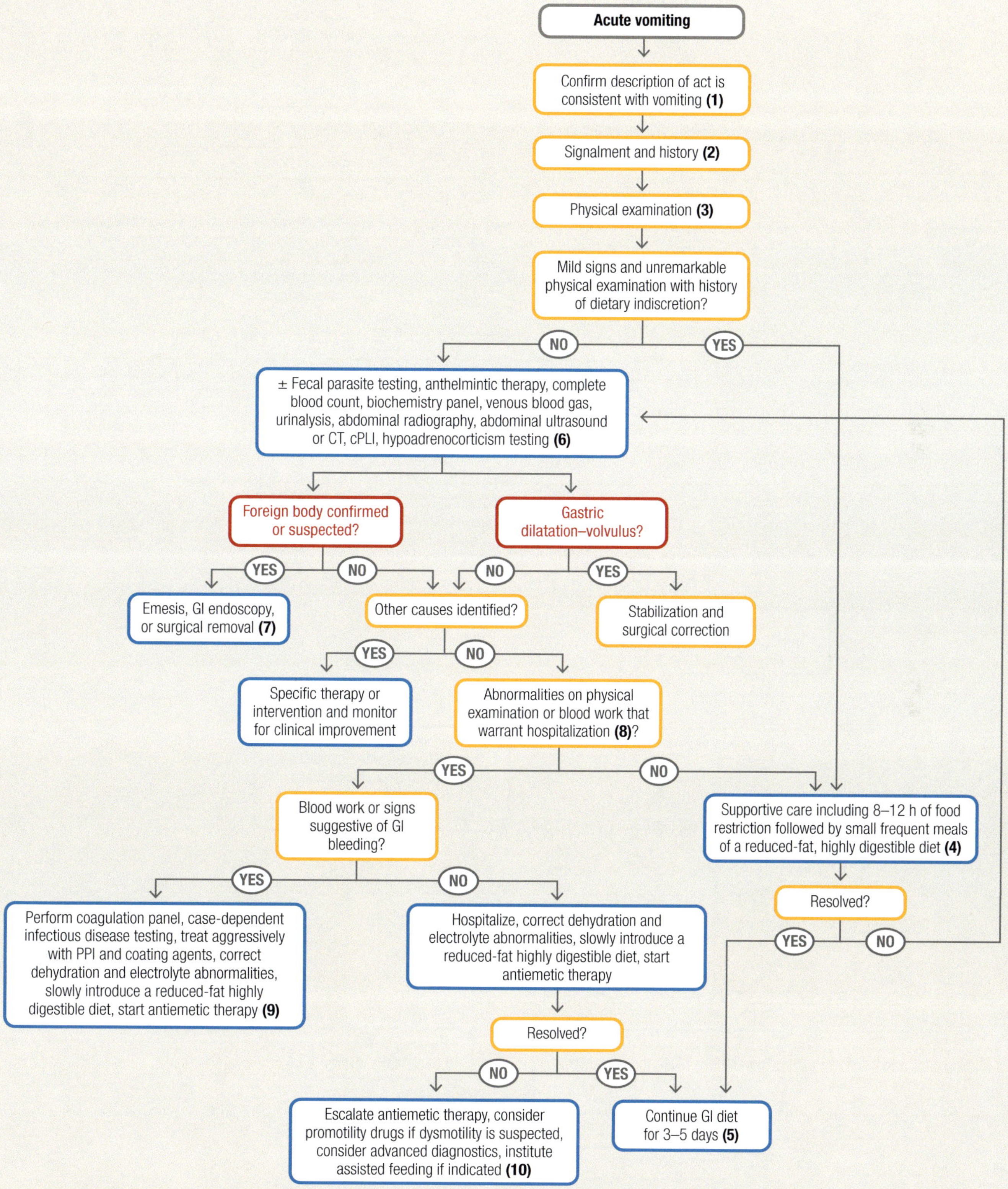

PPI, proton pump inhibitor

Diagnostic protocol | Diagnosis | Treatment

ALGORITHM 10.2

Diagnostic approach to chronic vomiting in dogs.

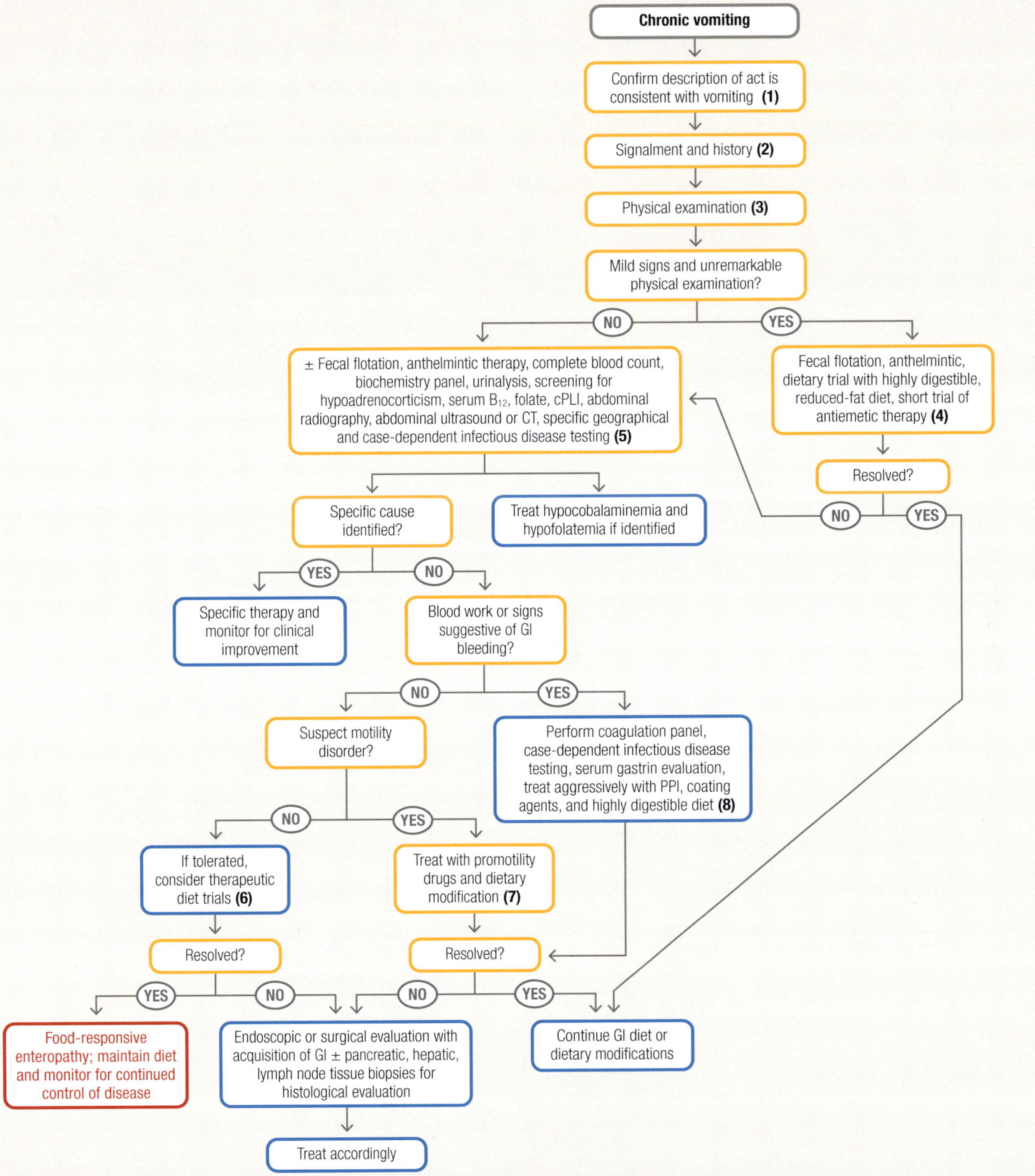

cPLI, canine pancreatic lipase immunoreactivity

Algorithm 10.2 Note 1 Pet owners should be questioned to confirm that the presenting complaint is truly vomiting. Asking owners to bring videos of the problem, if possible, can be helpful, especially in dogs where the diagnostic results (e.g., megaesophagus visualized on radiographs) are not well explained by the presenting problem.

Algorithm 10.2 Note 2 Once the act of vomiting is confirmed, the signalment and history of the dog, including dietary history, are considered. Although foreign bodies and drug/toxin exposure are uncommon causes of chronic vomiting, a complete history including information about the possibility of exposure of the patient to foreign objects, household chemicals, new foods or treats, or drugs (including medications for pets or their owners) should be obtained. Owners should also be questioned about the presence of additional clinical signs, such as those that suggest either diffuse GI or systemic disease.

Algorithm 10.2 Note 3 A thorough physical examination should be performed, including assessment of the dog's body condition, muscle mass index, and hair and skin condition. The presence, severity, and location of pain and/or discomfort on abdominal palpation should be noted rather than just describing the abdomen as "tense" (see Chapter 17). Vomiting dogs with a normal appetite and activity level as well as an ideal body and muscle condition may undergo a simplified diagnostic approach. Dogs presenting for evaluation of chronic GI signs that are experiencing lethargy, weight or muscle loss, hematemesis, changes in appetite (decreases, increases, or absence of appetite), and/or presence of abdominal pain or a palpable abdominal mass require more extensive diagnostic investigations.

Algorithm 10.2 Note 4 Fecal flotation and/or anthelmintic therapy, and a dietary trial with a highly digestible, reduced-fat diet, can be pursued in dogs with mild signs. In patients in which foreign material is not suspected, a short course of antiemetic therapy can also be provided to help with the transition to the new diet.

Algorithm 10.2 Note 5 Dogs with mild signs that do not improve with supportive care or dogs presenting with more severe signs or abnormalities detected on physical examination should undergo further diagnostic evaluation. The diagnostic tests should be selected based on review of the dog's signalment, history, and physical examination findings and might include fecal testing, complete blood count, serum biochemistry panel, urinalysis, abdominal radiography, abdominal ultrasound, evaluation of serum folate, cobalamin, and canine pancreatic lipase immunoreactivity, hypoadrenocorticism testing (i.e., baseline cortisol, urine cortisol:creatinine, adrenocorticotropic hormone (ACTH) stimulation test), and/or geographic-specific infectious disease testing.

Algorithm 10.2 Note 6 If no underlying cause is identified, a motility disorder is not suspected, and the severity of the signs do not necessitate endoscopy or exploratory surgery, multiple dietary trials based on review of the patient's clinical signs and dietary history are recommended for treatment of possible food-responsive enteropathy.

Algorithm 10.2 Note 7 If a dysmotility is suspected,[3] treatment with promotility drugs (see Chapter 31) and targeted dietary modification (e.g., increased feeding frequency, reduced volume of feeding, alteration of dietary fiber content) should be pursued. Dogs with vomiting following a prolonged fast might have bilious vomiting syndrome and benefit from a treat or small meal between larger meals to prevent vomiting secondary to an empty stomach.[4] If there is no resolution with that course of therapy or the signs are severe and warrant further exploration, endoscopic or surgical evaluation with acquisition and examination of tissue biopsies should be performed. Full-thickness biopsies are recommended if a motility disorder or a nonepithelial neoplasm is suspected.[5]

Algorithm 10.2 Note 8 For dogs presenting with clinical or biochemical signs of GI bleeding (e.g., hematemesis, melena, anemia, hypoproteinemia, thrombocytosis, thrombocytopenia, increased blood urea nitrogen), additional diagnostic testing, such as coagulation evaluation, serum gastrin evaluation, and parasitic and region-specific infectious disease testing should be considered. If upper GI bleeding is suspected, treatment with proton pump inhibitors and cytoprotectants should be initiated after the sample for serum gastrin is collected. A highly digestible, high-moisture gastroenteric diet might be beneficial.

References

1. Marks SL, Kook PH, Papich MG, et al. ACVIM consensus statement: Support for rational administration of gastrointestinal protectants to dogs and cats. *J Vet Intern Med* 32(6):1823–1840, 2018.
2. Kuhl A, Odunayo A, Price J, et al. Comparative analysis of the effect of IV administered acid suppressants on gastric pH in dogs. *J Vet Intern Med* 34(2):678–683, 2020.
3. Husnik R, Gaschen F. Gastric motility disorders in dogs and cats. *Vet Clin North Am Small Anim Pract* 51(1):43–59, 2021.
4. Ferguson L, Wennogle SA, Webb CB. Bilious vomiting syndrome in dogs: retrospective study of 20 cases (2002–2012). *J Am Anim Hosp Assoc* 52(3):157–161, 2016.
5. Zacuto AC, Pesavento PA, Hill S, et al. Intestinal leiomyositis: a cause of chronic intestinal pseudo-obstruction in 6 dogs. *J Vet Intern Med* 30(1):132–140, 2016.

CHAPTER 11

Acute and hemorrhagic diarrhea

Jenny Reeve
BVSc, DECVIM-CA, MRCVS, FHEA

Pathophysiology

Acute diarrhea, characterized by increased fecal fluidity, is a common presenting sign in dogs. The term "acute diarrhea" refers to sudden onset diarrhea of less than one week duration, and certainly less than 3 weeks' duration, beyond which the diarrhea is considered chronic and necessitates consideration of a completely different set of prioritized differentials and clinical and diagnostic approach. Regardless of the underlying etiology, there are typically multiple ensuing pathophysiological mechanisms (osmotic, secretory, motility-related), contributing to the development of the diarrhea. The resultant fluid losses can vary from mild and fully clinically compensated, through to marked losses with associated hypovolemia and/or dehydration. Related electrolyte derangements can be variable and may reflect excess water loss, with associated hypernatremia, hyperchloremia, and (mild) hypercalcemia. Alternatively, considerable electrolyte deficits may be apparent, with many patients presenting with hypokalemia due to a combination of reduced intake and gastrointestinal (GI) losses. Some patients will present with the collective triad of hypokalemia, hyponatremia, and hypochloremia, and while this pattern of electrolyte deficits is more classically associated with upper GI obstruction, the marked functional small intestinal ileus that can accompany acute insults can result in the same electrolyte derangements. Metabolic acidosis is a common accompanying feature and may be multifactorial—due to bicarbonate losses in diarrhea or hypoperfusion and associated hyperlactatemia, among other causes.

Acute hemorrhagic diarrhea reflects a marked GI insult that has resulted in either superficial erosions (partial epithelial loss with a retained, intact, muscularis mucosa) or ulceration (more extensive epithelial denudation with lesions extending deep to the muscularis mucosa), which may sometimes be accompanied by mucosal sloughing. While acute hemorrhagic diarrhea reflects the severity of the insult rather than a particular etiology, the pathophysiological mechanisms associated with certain disease processes or insults (e.g., the predilection of parvovirus for the germinal epithelial cells in intestinal crypts; the inhibition of the homeostatic and GI protective mechanisms of prostaglandins by nonsteroidal anti-inflammatory drugs) increase the incidence of a hemorrhagic component of the diarrhea with certain etiologies. The syndrome previously referred to as hemorrhagic gastroenteritis (HGE) has recently been renamed *acute hemorrhagic diarrhea syndrome* (AHDS) due to histopathological demonstration of necrotic enterocolitis without gastritis. It warrants a particular mention as although the underlying pathophysiological process is not definitively characterized, current evidence supports a role of the pore-forming *Clostridium perfringens* type A netF toxin, with resultant marked GI fluid losses, hemorrhagic diarrhea, hemoconcentration, and hypovolemia.[1] See also Chapter 35.

Diseases causing acute and hemorrhagic diarrhea may have extra-GI and wider systemic clinical presentations, either due to a truly multisystemic nature of the underlying etiology (e.g., hypoadrenocorticism, distemper), or consequences of the primary disease process (e.g., systemic inflammatory response secondary to acute pancreatitis, neutropenia and sepsis accompanying parvovirosis, bacterial translocation or gut-derived sepsis arising from marked GI insults).

Differential diagnoses for acute and hemorrhagic diarrhea include primary GI and extra-GI disease; dietary indiscretion, intoxication (including anticipated or idiosyncratic adverse therapeutic drug reaction), and infectious disease are among the most common (Table 11.1).

Clinical signs

Diarrhea may display features of small intestinal (increased fecal volume, borborygmi, flatus) or large intestinal (increased defecation frequency, urgency, tenesmus, mucus, hematochezia) origin. Mixed pattern diarrhea is common and will display features of both.

Accompanying GI signs may include inappetence and vomiting; in toxic or infectious ingested insults, the clinical signs may appear to affect the GI tract sequentially, progressing from vomiting, through small intestinal, to large intestinal diarrhea. Clinical consequences of diarrhea are commonly directly related to the ensuing fluid deficit and associated clinical signs, which may range from mild lethargy, through weakness, to overt collapse, depending on the magnitude of dehydration, hypovolemia, or overt shock (hypovolemic, less commonly distributive or septic) present.

TABLE 11.1 Causes of acute diarrhea in dogs according to their pathophysiological classification.

Nutritional	Toxic	Infectious/inflammatory	Metabolic	Vascular
■ Abrupt dietary change ■ Dietary indiscretion (gluttony) ■ Dietary intolerance ■ Dietary hypersensitivity	■ Dietary indiscretion: scavenging spoiled food *vs.* contaminated food items (e.g., aflatoxins, mycotoxins) *vs.* non-food items (e.g., plants: *Cyclamen* spp., *Gladiola* spp., *Iris* spp.), foreign items, intoxication (e.g., methylxanthines, xylitol) ■ Therapeutics: **nonsteroidal anti-inflammatory drugs, steroids**, immunosuppressives (e.g., mycophenolate, ciclosporin), chemotherapeutics, tyrosine kinase inhibitors, antimicrobials, antithyroidal drugs, trilostane; many other therapeutic compounds ■ Type 1 hypersensitivity reactions	■ Gastrointestinal infections ▪ Viral: **canine parvovirus (CPV)**, canine distemper virus, enteric coronavirus, other viral (rarely of primary clinical significance) ▪ **Bacterial: *Salmonella* spp., *Campylobacter* spp., *Escherichia coli*, *Clostridium* spp.**, *Providencia alcalifaciens*,[2] *Yersinia* spp. ▪ **Acute hemorrhagic diarrhea syndrome** ▪ Parasitic*: hookworms (*Anyclostoma* spp., *Uncinaria stenocephala*), whipworms (*Trichuris vulpis*), threadworms (*Strongyloides stercoralis*) ▪ Protozoal: giardiasis, *Cystisospora* spp., *Cryptosporidium*, *Ameba* spp. ■ Extra-gastrointestinal infections ▪ Abdominal sepsis ▪ Intra-abdominal infections (e.g., pyometra, pyelonephritis, prostatitis, cholangiohepatitis) ▪ Systemic infections (sepsis) ■ Sterile inflammatory ▪ **Acute pancreatitis**	■ **Hypoadrenocorticism** ■ Acute kidney injury ■ Acute hepatic injury ■ **High catecholamine states** (e.g., extreme exercise)	■ Intussusception ■ **Acute hypoperfusion or ischemic event** ■ **Mesenteric thrombus, torsion, strangulation**

* More often cause chronic disease.
Conditions likely to cause hemorrhagic diarrhea are shown in bold.

Diagnostic approach

Frequently, canine acute diarrhea is self-limiting; many patients do not require diagnostic or therapeutic interventions. For clinically bright, appetent, euhydrated, euvolemic patients without a hemorrhagic component to their diarrhea and no abnormal findings on examination, the passage of time (3–5 days) may be all that is required for spontaneous resolution. Ongoing enteral nutrition with a highly digestible diet, with or without the addition of fiber or nutraceuticals (pre-/pro-/synbiotics) is recommended.[3,4]

Algorithm 11.1 shows the diagnostic approach to acute diarrhea.

Algorithm 11.1 Note 1 Both wholly unvaccinated dogs and those less than 1 year of age, whose most recent vaccination was before 16 weeks of age (considered at risk of incomplete vaccination due to persistence of maternally derived antibodies at the time of vaccination), should be evaluated for parvovirus.[5]

Algorithm 11.1 Note 2 Point-of-care enzyme-linked immunosorbent assays (ELISAs) for fecal canine parvovirus (CPV) antigen are readily available. Sensitivity varies between assays but is generally relatively low, and serial daily testing is therefore warranted when there is an initial negative result in the presence of high clinical suspicion; specificity is generally high, although false positives may occur after modified live virus (MLV) vaccination. Quantitative PCR (qPCR) assays are available, with comparable performance across pharyngeal or rectal swabs and blood samples. Sensitivity and specificity vary between assays but are generally higher with PCR than with antigen ELISAs; false positives may persist for days to weeks beyond MLV vaccination.[6] While it is important to be mindful of false-positive results, pragmatically, a recently vaccinated patient presenting with acute, especially hemorrhagic diarrhea, with a positive parvovirus antigen ELISA or PCR is more likely to have clinical parvovirus than a false-positive diagnostic assay, unless another cause for their presenting signs is readily apparent.

Algorithm 11.1 Note 3 Despite the viral etiology, parvovirus reflects one of the few instances of acute diarrhea in dogs in which broad-spectrum antimicrobials are often indicated as part of management. Concurrent mucosal denudation (as evidenced by hemorrhagic diarrhea) and neutropenia increase the risk for bacterial translocation and gut-derived sepsis.

Algorithm 11.1 Note 4 When coccidian parasites (*Cystoisospora*, *Cryptosporidium*) are identified, these are most commonly carried asymptomatically. Other organisms, when present, are likely of greater pathogenic significance and warrant treating first. Coccidian parasites can cause clinically significant disease, especially in puppies from unsanitary environments, and warrant treatment when the diarrhea is not self-limiting and other causes are not readily apparent. See also Chapter 39.

Algorithm 11.1 Note 5 When multiple dogs in the same household, social, or daycare group are affected, an environmental cause is overwhelmingly most likely—this may be a common source dietary indiscretion or infectious agent.

Algorithm 11.1 Note 6 Due to the high incidence of subclinical carriage of potentially pathogenic bacteria by clinically healthy dogs and the consequent challenges in the interpretation of positive fecal cultures, only when bacteremia/sepsis is a considerable concern (e.g., hemorrhagic diarrhea, pyrexia, neutropenia) is fecal culture warranted, or when other causes of the acute diarrhea have been excluded and/or epidemiological factors suggest an infectious agent.

Algorithm 11.1 Note 7 If the patient is presenting with hemorrhagic diarrhea and other bleeding diatheses are either reported by the owner or apparent on examination, then the primary problem is most likely an underlying coagulopathy. Primary coagulopathies (thrombocytopenia, thrombocytopathia, von Willebrand disease, vasculopathies) are much more likely to cause mucosal surface bleeding than secondary coagulopathies. Uncommonly, markedly inflammatory causes of acute diarrhea (e.g., acute pancreatitis) may secondarily result in disseminated intravascular coagulation and subsequent clinical presentation of a consumptive coagulopathy; these patients will often be severely systemically compromised.

Algorithm 11.1 Note 8 Prior to clinical examination or admission to the clinic, consider the risk for an infectious etiology and barrier nurse as appropriate until a diagnosis is confirmed to better guide ongoing care needs. Pending a diagnosis, clear owner communication, in particular regarding the potential zoonotic nature of bacterial differentials, is important. Rectal examination should be included as part of a full physical examination.

Algorithm 11.1 Note 9 Bradycardia in dogs with significant GI disease is often benign sinus bradycardia as a result of increased vagal tone, although awareness of pathological causes (e.g., hyperkalemia in hypoadrenocorticism) is important.

Algorithm 11.1 Note 10 Basal cortisol >55 nmol/L (>2 µg/dL) likely excludes hypoadrenocorticism, although when there is high clinical suspicion, this should not be used as an absolute cutoff. Evaluating delta cortisol with adrenocorticotropic hormone (ACTH) stimulation testing is required for definitive diagnosis. In the presence of post-ACTH cortisol <55 nmol/L (<2 µg/dL), rule out a recent history of exogenous glucocorticoid administration (systemic, topical), trilostane, mitotane, or ketoconazole; all of which may cause iatrogenic adrenal suppression.

Algorithm 11.1 Note 11 Pyrexia most likely alludes to an inflammatory (sterile, e.g., acute pancreatitis, or infectious) or neoplastic (less likely) underlying etiology. Pyrexia may sometimes be due to a complication of an underlying non-inflammatory disease (e.g., perforation of a GI ulcer resulting in abdominal sepsis). Rarely, non-inflammatory or non-neoplastic diseases or interventions can result in pyrexia (e.g., hepatic encephalopathy, opioid use).

Algorithm 11.1 Note 12 Considering the self-limiting nature of many causes of acute diarrhea in dogs, particular attention should be paid in the initial assessment to any finding which indicates that either achieving a definitive diagnosis or further therapeutic support is required. For clinically well patients without concerning examination findings, providing a fecal sample pot for the owners to start collecting a pooled fecal sample, in case the diarrhea does not show signs of improvement over the next 3–5 days, may save time further down the line.

Algorithm 11.1 Note 13 AHDS typically, but not exclusively, affects small breed dogs. Vomiting may precede the diarrhea, and hemoconcentration is considered a hallmark feature of this disease, although recent evidence suggests this is not as prevalent as once thought. In the absence of neutropenia or signs of sepsis, antimicrobials are not indicated, and therapy is supportive, primarily with fluids, although probiotics may also be beneficial. Individuals may suffer repeat events, and an AHDS episode may be a harbinger for more chronic GI disease.

Algorithm 11.1 Note 14 Neutropenia has diagnostic and therapeutic relevance. Neutropenia may reflect lack of production (e.g., in hypoadrenocorticism or parvovirosis), sequestration, or consumption (e.g., sepsis associated with parvovirus or acute bacterial enteritis). Broad-spectrum antimicrobial cover (e.g., clavulanate-potentiated amoxicillin) is considered appropriate in the presence of either signs of sepsis (classically pyrexia, hypothermia, or fluid refractory hypotension—although examination findings with sepsis may be highly variable) or an absolute neutrophil count $<0.5\text{–}1\times10^9$/L.[7]

Algorithm 11.1 Note 15 Abdominal point-of-care ultrasound scan (POCUS) should form part of the initial triage of both unstable patients and those with palpable abdominal abnormalities, to facilitate timely identification of abdominal emergencies, particularly sepsis. Complete abdominal imaging (abdominal computed tomography and/or ultrasound) may be required to achieve a definitive diagnosis after stabilization.

ALGORITHM 11.1

Diagnostic approach to patients with acute diarrhea.

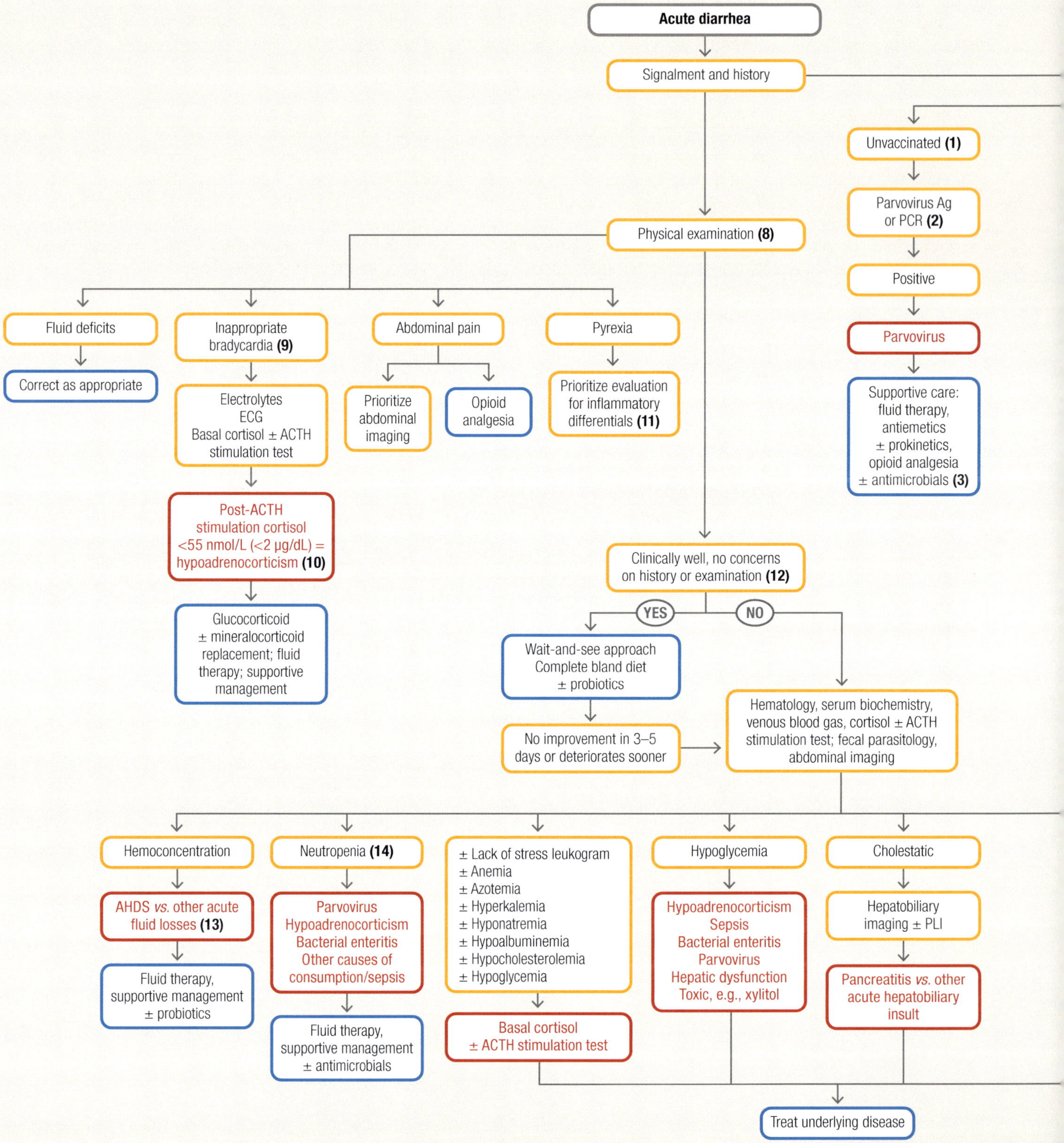

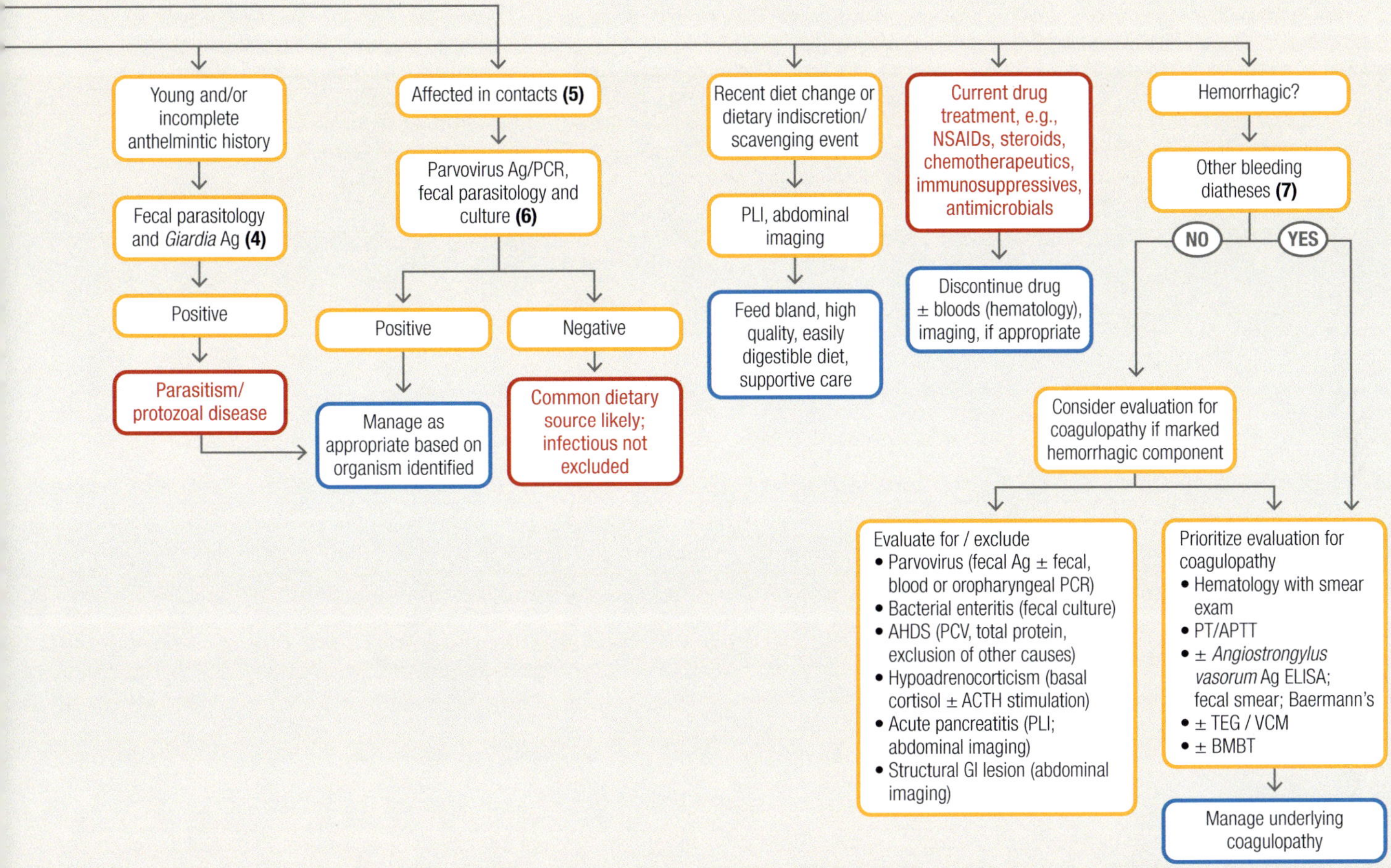

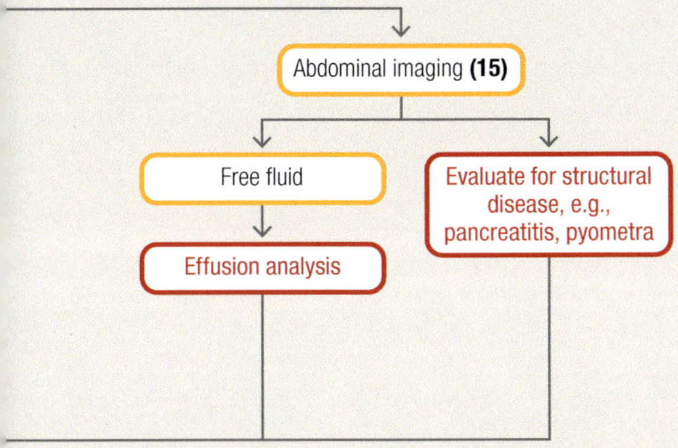

ACTH, adrenocorticotrophic hormone; AHDS, acute hemorrhagic diarrhea syndrome; Ag, antigen; aPTT, activated partial thromboplastin time; BMBT, buccal mucosal bleeding time; CT, computed tomography; ECG, electrocardiogram; ELISA, enzyme-linked immunosorbent assay; GI, gastrointestinal; MCT, mast cell tumor; NSAIDS, nonsteroidal anti-inflammatory drugs; PLI, pancreatic lipase immunoreactivity; PCR, polymerase chain reaction; PCV, packed cell volume; PT, prothrombin time; TEG, thromboelastogram; TKIs, tyrosine kinase inhibitors; VCM, viscoelastic coagulation monitoring.

Diagnostic protocol Diagnosis Treatment

References

1. Gohari IM, Unterer S, Whitehead AE, et al. NetF-producing *Clostridium perfringens* and its associated diseases in dogs and foals. *J Vet Diagn Investig* 32:230–238, 2020.
2. Jørgensen HJ, Valheim M, Sekse C, et al. An Official Outbreak investigation of acute haemorrhagic diarrhoea in dogs in Norway points to *Providencia alcalifaciens* as a likely cause. *Animals* 11:3201, 2021.
3. Scahill K, Jessen LR, Prior C, et al. Efficacy of antimicrobial and nutraceutical treatment for canine acute diarrhoea: A systematic review and meta-analysis for European Network for Optimization of Antimicrobial Therapy (ENOVAT) guidelines. *Vet J* 303, 106054, 2024.
4. Ziese AL, Suchodolski J, Hartmann K, et al. Effect of probiotic treatment on the clinical course, intestinal microbiome, and toxigenic Clostridium perfringens in dogs with acute hemorrhagic diarrhea. *PLoS ONE* 13:e0204691, 2018.
5. Squires RA, Crawford C, Marcondes M, et al. 2024 guidelines for the vaccination of dogs and cats – compiled by the Vaccination Guidelines Group (VGG) of the World Small Animal Veterinary Association (WSAVA). *J Small Anim Pr* 65:277–316, 2024.
6. Segev G, Yaaran T, Maurice S, et al. Effect of sampling site on the diagnosis of canine parvovirus infection in dogs using polymerase chain reaction. *J Vet Intern Med* 36:591–598, 2022.
7. National Institute for Health and Care Excellence. *Nice Guideline. Suspected sepsis: recognition, diagnosis and early management.* [Internet] July 2016, updated March 2024. Cited 21st April 2024. https://www.nice.org.uk/guidance/ng51/resources/suspected-sepsis-recognition-diagnosis-and-early-management-pdf-1837508256709

CHAPTER 12

Chronic diarrhea

Sara Jablonski
DVM, PhD, DACVIM (SAIM)

Pathophysiology

Diarrhea is characterized by increased frequency, volume, and fluid content of bowel movements and may or may not occur with other alterations of the character of the stool (color changes, presence of mucus or blood). It occurs as a consequence of processes that alter intestinal absorption, permeability, secretion, or motility. While diarrhea is the most common clinical sign associated with small and large intestinal disease, it also occurs secondary to disease outside the gastrointestinal (GI) tract.[1,2] Thus, a systematic approach to determining the cause of diarrhea is necessary. However, the diagnostic approach should take into consideration the overall health of the dog, as well as the duration of clinical signs. If diarrhea has been persistently present or episodically occurring for ≥3 weeks, it is classified as chronic. Causes of chronic diarrhea include infectious (parasitic, protozoal, fungal, algal, and bacterial), neoplastic, endocrine, structural, and noninfectious inflammatory disorders (GI and extragastrointestinal). Dogs with chronic diarrhea should undergo a systematic diagnostic evaluation according to the characteristics of their diarrhea and their other clinical findings.

Clinical findings

The presence of diarrhea should be confirmed with an available fecal scoring chart.[3] Establishing a baseline will also be useful when evaluating response to therapy. In many cases, chronic diarrhea is the only clinical sign reported, and the dog is noted to be otherwise well. In cases where there are other clinical signs, weight loss, changes in appetite (increased, decreased, or absent), and vomiting are most frequently reported. Importantly, if extragastrointestinal signs are reported (e.g., cough, respiratory difficulty, blindness, "redness" of eyes, neurologic signs) strong consideration should be given to systemic disorders that may be affecting the GI system. A thorough physical exam should be performed to include careful assessment of hydration status, body, and muscle condition, and evaluation for detection of abdominal pain, a fluid wave indicating ascites, abdominal masses, and/or abdominal or multicentric lymphadenopathy. A thorough evaluation for evidence of dermatologic disease should be performed as the presence of cutaneous signs may support an underlying GI food sensitivity. Digital rectal examination should be performed in all cases for assessment of intra- or extraluminal lesions, anal sac abnormalities, or prostatic disease and assessment of fecal consistency and color. It is important to note that the physical examination may be unremarkable, even in dogs with profuse diarrhea.

Diagnostic approach

The initial diagnostic approach includes careful consideration of the patient's signalment, complete clinical history, and degree of illness. First, consideration should be given to breed-related disorders that may influence the diagnostic approach (e.g., exocrine pancreatic insufficiency [EPI] in the German Shepherd dog, Rough Coated Collie, Cavalier King Charles Spaniel, and other breeds;[4] *E. coli*-associated granulomatous colitis in Boxers[5] and French Bulldogs[6]). Chronic enteropathies often present in early adulthood to middle age, while neoplasia is most likely to present in older dogs. It is important to identify if other clinical signs are present (e.g., regurgitation, polyuria/polydipsia, cough) and consider how they may change the diagnostic approach. Clinical history-taking should also include a detailed account of current and previous diets fed and the response to those diets, questions aimed at determining whether the problem appears to be small, large, or mixed bowel in origin (Table 12.1), travel history, exposure to other animals in and outside of the household, and the use of parasite preventatives. Finally, the degree of illness will influence the diagnostic approach as unstable dogs will require that the cause of their clinical signs is rapidly identified to be appropriately treated quickly, and anorexic dogs may not be accepting of initial treatment plans suitable for more stable dogs with chronic diarrhea.

TABLE 12.1 Differentiation between small vs. large bowel diarrhea*.

	Small bowel	Large bowel
Frequency of stool	≤3 times daily	>3 times daily
Volume of stool	Normal to increased	Decreased
Urgency to defecate	Rare	Common
Tenesmus during defecation	Rare	Common
Fecal blood	Rare; if present, melena	Common; usually hematochezia
Fecal mucus	Rare	Common
Weight loss	Common	Rare
Vomiting	Common	Rare

* Mixed pattern diarrhea is common.

Diagnosis

Algorithm 12.1 shows the approach to the dog with chronic diarrhea.

Algorithm 12.1 Note 1 If the diarrhea localizes to the large bowel (Table 12.1), repeat the rectal exam and ensure local disease is not detected. Diagnostic investigations and treatment trials may differ depending on the localization of diarrhea to the small vs. large bowel. However, the majority of dogs with chronic enteropathies have a mix of small and large bowel diarrhea.

Algorithm 12.1 Note 2 Dogs with diarrhea who maintain a normal appetite, body weight, and energy level would be considered clinically stable. A more measured diagnostic approach can be initially pursued. Dogs presenting for evaluation of chronic GI signs experiencing lethargy, weight loss, and changes in appetite (decreases, increases, or absence of appetite) require more extensive diagnostic investigation.

Algorithm 12.1 Note 3 Routine fecal testing is recommended in stable patients to exclude intestinal parasitism as the cause of their signs. Consideration can then be given to the exclusion of secondary causes of GI signs via a complete blood count, chemistry profile, urinalysis, and screening for hypoadrenocorticism. However, this may not be necessary in all cases of stable dogs and cats presenting for evaluation of chronic GI signs.

Algorithm 12.1 Note 4 Dogs with serum albumin <25 g/L (<2.5 g/dL) should receive more extensive diagnostic investigations. The diagnostic approach may also differ in a dog with chronic diarrhea and hypoalbuminemia, and the reader is referred to Chapter 13.

Algorithm 12.1 Note 5 The diagnostic investigations selected will depend on complete case information. Some diagnostics may be prioritized based on the localization of diarrhea. For example, serum trypsin-like immunoreactivity, B_{12}, and folate evaluation should be prioritized in dogs with small or mixed bowel chronic diarrhea vs. dogs with large bowel diarrhea. Fecal-based polymerase chain reaction (PCR) testing or culture is often unrewarding in cases of chronic diarrhea. Identifying an organism in the feces of a dog with diarrhea does not imply causation, and there is considerable overlap in positive findings in healthy dogs and dogs with diarrhea.[7,8] Thus, fecal enteropathogen detection is typically reserved for unique circumstances or outbreak situations.

Algorithm 12.1 Note 6 The majority of dogs with chronic diarrhea not caused by extragastrointestinal or infectious, neoplastic, or structural GI disorders will have improvement in response to a specific diet change.[9,10] A variety of dietary strategies are available for patients with chronic diarrhea, and there is no robust evidence to suggest that one dietary approach is better than the other. In addition, with the exception of a few discrete circumstances, we do not have good predictors of which specific diet or dietary approach may be best in an individual patient. Dietary considerations include type of diet (hydrolysate vs. limited ingredient vs. novel protein vs. elemental vs. home-cooked), fiber content, fat content, and digestibility.[11] Previous studies have demonstrated clinical improvement in dogs with chronic diarrhea in response to hydrolysate, highly digestible, and single-source protein diets. Home-cooked diets formulated by a board-certified veterinary nutritionist have also been used successfully in cases of chronic diarrhea. A fiber-enriched diet or supplemental fiber (e.g., psyllium husk powder) would be preferred for dogs with large bowel localizing signs. In order to measure success, the diet should be fed exclusively for the trial period. Improvement in clinical signs is typically seen within 7–14 days when a food trial is going to be successful.[11] See Chapters 25 and 41.

Algorithm 12.1 Note 7 Failure to respond to a single therapeutic diet trial does not indicate that the dogs' chronic diarrhea will not be food-responsive. If the dog was not responsive to the first dietary trial but remains clinically stable, implementing a new dedicated food trial with a differing approach (e.g., if a hydrolyzed diet trial is not successful, a fiber-enriched, highly digestible, home-cooked, novel protein or combination hydrolyzed/low-fat diet should be tried) is recommended.[12]

Algorithm 12.1 Note 8 Dogs with food-responsive enteropathy may remain clinically stable long-term or may experience relapse of clinical signs despite continued administration of the initially successful diet. If relapse occurs and the dog is otherwise clinically stable, attempting an alternative therapeutic diet trial should be considered. If relapse occurs and the dog is clinically unwell, full diagnostic investigations are indicated.

Algorithm 12.1 Note 9 If the result of diagnostic testing fails to determine a specific cause and, if appropriate, multiple appropriately conducted therapeutic diet trials fail to result in improvement in diarrhea, intestinal biopsy with histopathologic evaluation can be considered as the next diagnostic step. Intestinal biopsy can exclude infectious or neoplastic causes of chronic diarrhea and confirm inflammatory infiltrates, resulting in a diagnosis of chronic inflammatory enteropathy. Notably, inflammatory intestinal infiltrates are common and nonspecific, so it is important that other causes of chronic diarrhea (e.g., intestinal parasitism, hypoadrenocorticism, EPI, etc.) are definitively excluded prior to intestinal biopsy.[2] In some cases, additional testing of tissue may be necessary including tissue culture and fluorescence *in situ* hybridization (FISH) for detection of adherent or invasive bacteria in cases of suspected *E. coli*-associated granulomatous colitis. Occasionally, further characterization of intestinal tissue with immunophenotyping and/or PCR for antigen receptor rearrangement (PARR) may be necessary if

ALGORITHM 12.1

Diagnostic approach to chronic diarrhea.

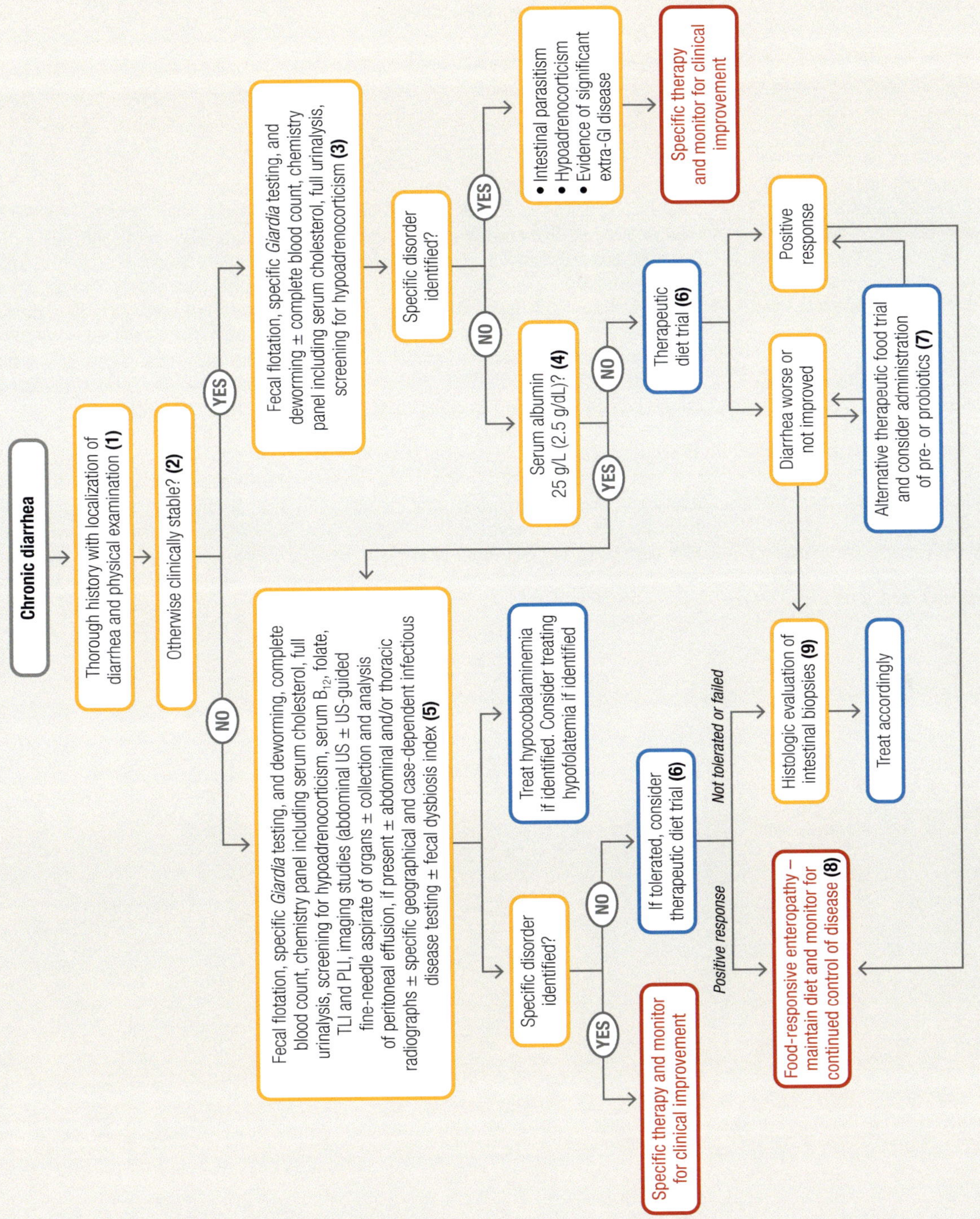

GI, gastrointestinal; PLI, pancreatic lipase immunoreactivity; TLI, trypsin-like immunoreactivity; US, ultrasound.

Diagnostic protocol | Diagnosis | Treatment

inflammation cannot be conclusively distinguished from a neoplastic population of cells. Flexible endoscopy for the collection of biopsies offers many advantages and is generally the preferred biopsy method for the collection of GI tissue in dogs with chronic diarrhea. Both esophago-gastro-duodenoscopy and recto-colono-ileoscopy are recommended for collection of both duodenal and ileal tissue since the pathologic process can differ by location.[13] See Chapter 22.

Laparotomy is preferred only if focal lesions are identified on prebiopsy imaging or if there is a desire to collect additional tissue, such as the liver or lymph node. If laparotomy is performed, representative sections of the duodenum, jejunum, and ileum should be collected. Surgical biopsy of the colon is not recommended. The placement of an esophageal feeding tube should be considered under the same anesthetic procedure for anorexic patients.

References

1. Tams T. Gastrointestinal symptoms. In: Tams TR (editor). *Handbook of Veterinary Gastroenterology*, 2nd edition. St. Louis, Elsevier Saunders, pp. 1–50, 2003.
2. Manchester A. Diarrhea. In: Côté E, Ettinger SJ, Feldman EC (editors). *Ettinger's Textbook of Veterinary Internal Medicine*, 9th edition. St. Louis, Elsevier, 2024, pp. 233–237.
3. Purina Fecal Score Chart [Internet]. Available from: https://www.proplanveterinarydiets.ca/wp-content/uploads/2016/04/PPPVD-Fecal-Scoring-Chart-EN-FINAL.pdf. [cited 2024 Apr 16].
4. Cridge H, Williams DA, Barko PC. Exocrine pancreatic insufficiency in dogs and cats. *J Am Vet Med Assoc* 262(2):246–255, 2024.
5. Craven M, Mansfield CS, Simpson KW. Granulomatous colitis of boxer dogs. *Vet Clin North Am Small Anim Pract* 41(2):433–445, 2011.
6. Manchester AC, Hill S, Sabatino B, et al. Association between granulomatous colitis in French Bulldogs and invasive *Escherichia coli* and response to fluoroquinolone antimicrobials. *J Vet Intern Med* 27(1):56–61, 2013.
7. Marks SL, Rankin SC, Byrne BA, Weese JS. Enteropathogenic bacteria in dogs and cats: diagnosis, epidemiology, treatment, and control. *J Vet Intern Med* 25(6):1195–208, 2011.
8. Sabshin SJ, Levy JK, Tupler T, et al. Enteropathogens identified in cats entering a Florida animal shelter with normal feces or diarrhea. *J Am Vet Med Assoc* 241(3):331–337, 2012.
9. Volkmann M, Steiner JM, Fosgate GT, et al. Chronic diarrhea in dogs –retrospective study in 136 cases. *J Vet Intern Med* 31(4):1043–1055, 2017.
10. Allenspach K, Culverwell C, Chan D. Long-term outcome in dogs with chronic enteropathies: 203 cases. *Vet Rec* 178(15):368, 2016.
11. Tolbert MK, Murphy M, Gaylord L, Witzel-Rollins A. Dietary management of chronic enteropathy in dogs. *J Small Anim Pract* 63(6):425–434, 2022.
12. Kathrani A. Dietary and nutritional approaches to the management of chronic enteropathy in dogs and cats. *Vet Clin North Am Small Anim Pract* 51(1):123–136, 2021.
13. Procoli F, Mõtsküla PF, Keyte SV, et al. Comparison of histopathologic findings in duodenal and ileal endoscopic biopsies in dogs with chronic small intestinal enteropathies. *J Vet Intern Med* 27(2):268–274, 2013.

CHAPTER 13

Protein-losing enteropathies

Sara Jablonski
DVM, PhD, DACVIM (SAIM)

Pathophysiology

Canine protein-losing enteropathy (PLE) is a syndrome characterized by excessive and uncompensated protein loss across the enteric mucosa. Protein-losing enteropathy purportedly occurs as a result of direct mucosal erosion or ulceration and secondary loss of protein, increased intestinal permeability and decreased protein uptake, and/or in association with altered lymphatic function and leakage or rupture of lymphatics leading to direct loss of protein-rich lymph. Given the varied pathophysiologic mechanisms that may result in this syndrome, PLE can occur as a consequence of a wide variety of disorders, including inflammatory, infectious, neoplastic, mechanical, and miscellaneous processes (Table 13.1). The most common disorders identified to cause canine PLE include chronic inflammatory enteropathies (CIE) and intestinal lymphangiectasia (IL).[1] Alimentary lymphoma would be the next most likely diagnosis in those geographic regions without intestinal fungal or hookworm infections.

TABLE 13.1 Causes of protein-losing enteropathy in the dog.

Diseases that alter intestinal permeability and/or cause mucosal injury	Lymphatic disease

■ Chronic enteropathies
■ Intestinal ulceration
■ Infectious enteropathies
  ■ Fungal (histoplasmosis, pythiosis)
  ■ Parasitic (hookworm, schistosomiasis)
  ■ Viral (parvovirus)
  ■ Bacterial—rare (*Campylobacter*, Salmonellosis)
■ Chronic obstruction of the intestine
  ■ Foreign body
  ■ Intussusception
■ Neoplasia
  ■ Intestinal lymphoma (solitary or diffuse)
  ■ Intestinal adenocarcinoma
■ Intestinal crypt disease (unknown if primary disorder or secondary change)
■ Hypoadrenocorticism (Addison's disease)
	■ "Primary" lymphangiectasia (suspected genetic predisposition)
	■ "Secondary" lymphangiectasia:
	  ■ Common
	    – Chronic enteropathies
	    – Intestinal neoplasia
	  ■ Suspected (unconfirmed in veterinary medicine)
	    – Right heart failure
	    – Constrictive pericarditis
	    – Portal hypertension
	■ Focal lipogranulomatous lymphangitis

Clinical findings

Signalment

Dogs with PLE may present at any age, and there is no known sex predilection. Any breed of dog can develop PLE. However, breeds with the highest frequency of PLE reported in the scientific literature include the Border Collie, German Shepherd dog, mixed breeds, Rottweiler, and Yorkshire Terrier. Additionally, the Chinese Shar-Pei, Maltese, Norwegian Lundehund, Rottweiler, Soft Coated Wheaten Terrier, and Yorkshire Terrier are considered specifically predisposed to IL.[1,2]

History and physical exam

Dogs with PLE are most commonly presented to veterinarians for progressive or chronic relapsing gastrointestinal (GI) signs, including diarrhea, vomiting, weight loss, changes in appetite, and/or signs associated with hypoalbuminemia (e.g., abdominal and/or pleural effusion, subcutaneous edema). Rarely, dogs may present with signs associated with a thromboembolic (TE) event; signs are variable but can include difficulty breathing, neurologic signs, and hind end weakness). Physical exam findings are variable but may include decreases in body and muscle conditioning, abdominal distension, abnormal rectal mucosa, and diarrheic feces on rectal examination.

Initial laboratory abnormalities

Hypoalbuminemia with serum albumin concentration <25 g/L (<2.5 g/dL) is the hallmark biochemical finding in dogs with PLE. Concurrent hypoglobulinemia is common and is an important differentiator for other causes of hypoalbuminemia in dogs. However, some dogs with PLE have normal or even increased serum globulin concentrations. Additional common findings on a serum biochemistry test include hypocholesterolemia, decreased serum creatinine, increased liver enzyme activities (usually mild), and decreased total serum calcium and magnesium. Frequent abnormalities in complete blood count in dogs with PLE include lymphopenia, thrombocytosis, and various types and degrees of leukocytosis. Ionized hypocalcemia may also occur secondary to decreases in vitamin D metabolites, and secondary hyperparathyroidism may be present in these cases. Hypocobalaminemia, hypofolatemia, and mild increases in canine pancreatic lipase immunoreactivity are also frequently observed.

Diagnostic approach

The first step in the diagnostic investigation of dogs with suspected PLE involves careful consideration and exclusion of non-GI causes of hypoalbuminemia (Table 13.2). At a minimum, this part of the investigation should include collection of urine for urinalysis and, if necessary, urine protein-to-creatinine ratio, and consideration of liver insufficiency as the cause of hypoalbuminemia, particularly in dogs with normal serum concentrations of globulin.

When necessary, measuring fecal alpha 1-proteinase inhibitor can confirm that protein loss through the GI tract is occurring, although false positives and negatives can occur. This assay is currently only available in North America.

Diagnosis

Once other causes of hypoalbuminemia are excluded, Algorithm 13.1 shows the approach to the dog with a PLE.

Algorithm 13.1 Note 1 Following the exclusion of other causes of hypoalbuminemia and prior to the recommendation of an intestinal biopsy, a thorough diagnostic evaluation is recommended to assess for non-GI causes of signs and comorbidities and to exclude: intestinal parasitism; eukalemic/eunatremic hypoadrenocorticism (serum basal cortisol >55 nmol/L [>2 μg/dL] excludes hypoadrenocorticism; if serum basal cortisol is <55 nmol/L [<2 μg/dL], an adrenocorticotropic hormone [ACTH] stimulation test should be performed to exclude hypoadrenocorticism); exocrine pancreatic insufficiency (canine trypsin-like immunoreactivity); focal or extraluminal lesions of the GI tract that may change the recommended diagnostic approach; and, depending on the specific case details and geographic location, specific screening for *Histoplasma capsulatum* and *Pythium insidiosum*. Diagnostic investigations should also include screening for consequences of the underlying disease, including peritoneal or pleural effusion, hypocobalaminemia, decreased serum vitamin D concentrations, ionized hypocalcemia, and, in some cases, TE. Sampling effusions may not be worthwhile if there is severe hypoalbuminemia (<15 g/L) that explains the effusion; if sampled, fluid analysis and cytologic examination should be performed.

TABLE 13.2 Nongastrointestinal causes of hypoalbuminemia and exclusionary tests.

Disorder	Test(s) for exclusion
Liver insufficiency/dysfunction	■ Dynamic bile acid testing
Protein-losing nephropathy	■ Urinalysis ± urine protein-to-creatinine ratio
Pancreatic insufficiency	■ Fasting serum trypsin-like immunoreactivity
Hemorrhage evaluation	■ Physical exam with rectal exam, for cavity effusions
Dilution or redistribution of albumin	■ Evaluation for renal and cardiac disease ■ Evaluation for evidence of vasculitis or effusions

Algorithm 13.1 Note 2 As cobalamin is important for GI health and function, a deficiency in this vitamin should be treated. Treatment is recommended for dogs with significant ionized hypocalcemia. It is unknown at this time whether dogs with PLE and hypofolatemia or hypovitaminosis D and normocalcemia would benefit from administration of folic acid or vitamin D products, respectively.

Algorithm 13.1 Note 3 Diet as the sole therapy in dogs with PLE has been shown to be successful in Yorkshire Terriers[3] and dogs of various breeds.[4] One study suggests that dogs with PLE are more likely to respond to dietary therapy without the need for glucocorticoids if their canine chronic enteropathy clinical activity index (CCECAI)[5] score is <8.6.[6]

Algorithm 13.1 Note 4 Diet choice will somewhat depend on availability and patient acceptance. However, the best diet for a dog with PLE is based on the complete integration of historical information (including previous diets fed and responses), signalment (including age and breed), and complete diagnostic testing, including intestinal histopathology. In the absence of complete information, considering that many dogs with PLE have some components of both CIE and IL,[7] a low-fat, hydrolyzed diet would be the best initial choice if available.

Algorithm 13.1 Note 5 According to the Rational Use of Antithrombotics in Veterinary Critical Care (CURATIVE) guidelines, dogs with PLE are considered at risk for thrombosis. The mechanism for developing thrombosis is not completely understood but is likely related to the loss of anticoagulant proteins and systemic inflammation. The CURATIVE guidelines recommend antithrombotic therapy for all dogs with PLE unless the risks are deemed to outweigh the potential benefit.[8]

A complete response would include improvement in CCECAI score to <3 and serum albumin to >25 g/L (2.5 g/dL). However, an improvement in the CCECAI score to <3 and stable serum albumin between 20–25 g/L (2–2.5 g/dL) could be considered an acceptable response.

Algorithm 13.1 Note 6 Intestinal biopsy can exclude infectious or neoplastic causes of PLE. Biopsy will also help to determine whether the dog is affected by CIE, IL or both, and if both, which process appears to predominate. Surgical exploration for biopsies provides the advantages of identifying focal areas of disease to biopsy and the ability to biopsy all segments of the small intestine, as well as other tissues, as indicated. However, flexible endoscopy is generally the preferred biopsy method

ALGORITHM 13.1

Diagnostic approach to protein-losing enteropathies.

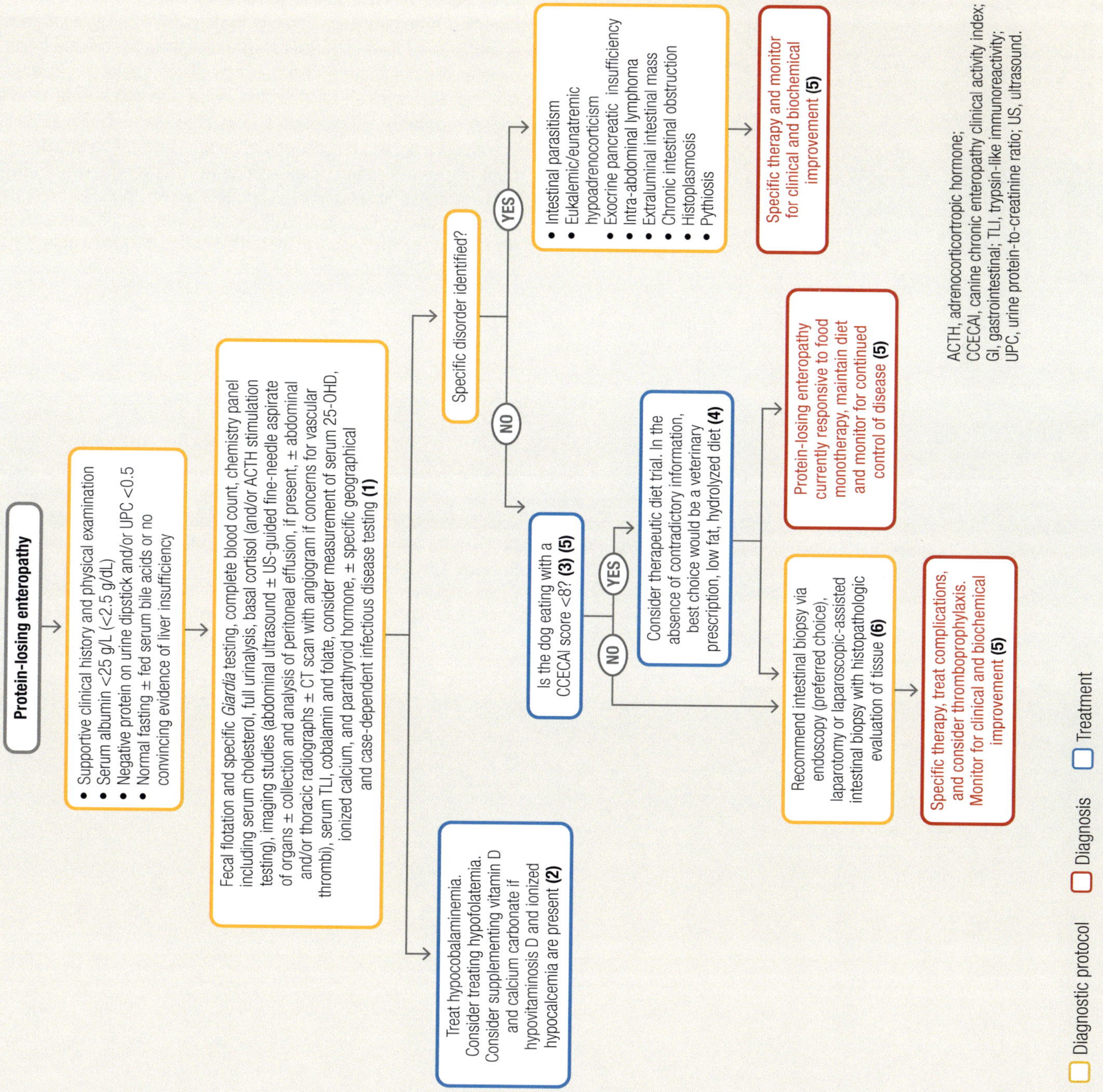

ACTH, adrenocorticotropic hormone; CCECAI, canine chronic enteropathy clinical activity index; GI, gastrointestinal; TLI, trypsin-like immunoreactivity; UPC, urine protein-to-creatinine ratio; US, ultrasound.

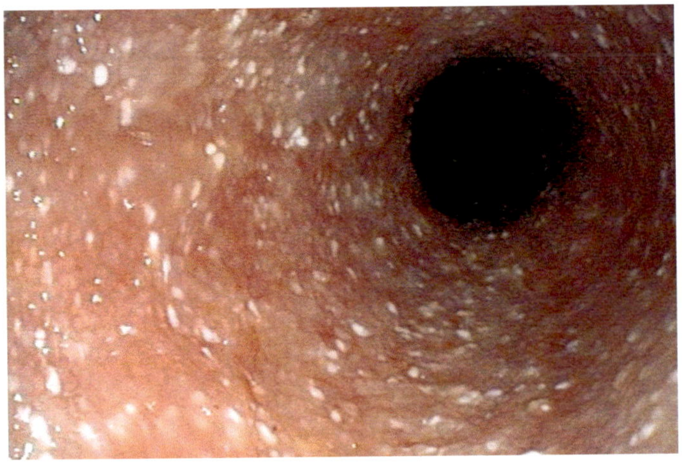

FIG. 13.1 Presence of small intestinal pinpoint to coalescing "white spots" consistent with dilated lacteals in a 5-year-old male castrated English Bulldog with histologically diagnosed moderate intestinal lymphangiectasia and the clinical syndrome of protein-losing enteropathy.

as it is considered equivalent diagnostically and safer and less invasive compared to laparotomy. The endoscopist should look for "white spots" on the mucosa (Fig. 13.1), which have been associated with intestinal lymphangiectasia. Pathology can differ between sections of the intestine; therefore, it is recommended that both esophago-gastro-duodenoscopy ("upper") and recto-colono-ileoscopy ("lower") endoscopy be performed. Importantly, endoscopy has limitations including the potential to miss lesions in regions that cannot be sampled.

Common histopathologic findings in dogs with PLE include mucosal edema, villus blunting, intestinal lymphangiectasia, diverse types and degrees of inflammatory infiltrates, and dilated, cystic crypts. Intestinal lymphangiectasia can be detected in the villi and lamina propria in endoscopic intestinal biopsies and in all layers of the small intestine in surgical biopsies. If concern for bacterial adherence/invasion arises from biopsy evaluation, fluorescence *in situ* hybridization (FISH) can be considered to evaluate for bacteria within formalin-fixed tissue. Immunohistochemistry and PCR for antigen receptor rearrangements (PARR) may be necessary to help distinguish intestinal lymphoma from inflammatory infiltrates.

References

1. Craven MD, Washabau RJ. Comparative pathophysiology and management of protein-losing enteropathy. *J Vet Intern Med* 33(2):383-402, 2019.
2. Jablonski SA. Pathophysiology, diagnosis, and management of canine intestinal lymphangiectasia: A comparative review. *Animals (Basel)* 12(20):2791, 2022.
3. Rudinsky AJ, Howard JP, Bishop MA, et al. Dietary management of presumptive protein-losing enteropathy in Yorkshire terriers. *J Small Anim Pract* 58(2):103–108, 2017.
4. Myers M, Martinez SA, Shiroma JT, et al. Prospective evaluation of low-fat diet monotherapy in dogs with presumptive protein-losing enteropathy. *J Am Anim Hosp Assoc* 59(2):74–84, 2023.
5. Allenspach K, Wieland B, Gröne A, Gaschen F. Chronic enteropathies in dogs: evaluation of risk factors for negative outcome. *J Vet Intern Med* 21(4):700–708, 2007.
6. Nagata N, Ohta H, Yokoyama N, et al. Clinical characteristics of dogs with food-responsive protein-losing enteropathy. *J Vet Intern Med* 34(2):659–668, 2020.
7. Jablonski Wennogle SA, Priestnall SL, Suárez-Bonnet A, et al. Lymphatic endothelial cell immunohistochemical markers for evaluation of the intestinal lymphatic vasculature in dogs with chronic inflammatory enteropathy. *J Vet Intern Med* 33(4):1669–1676, 2019.
8. Sharp CR, Blais MC, Boyd CJ, et al. 2022 Update of the Consensus on the Rational Use of Antithrombotics and Thrombolytics in Veterinary Critical Care (CURATIVE) Domain 6: Defining rational use of thrombolytics. *J Vet Emerg Crit Care (San Antonio)* 32(4):446–470, 2022.

CHAPTER 14

Gastrointestinal bleeding

Jenny Reeve
BVSc, DECVIM-CA,
FHEA, MRCVS

Pathophysiology

Gastrointestinal (GI) bleeding arises either due to structural pathology of the GI tract or as a result of an underlying coagulopathy. Coagulopathies that result in mucosal bleeds are typically disorders of primary hemostasis (thrombocytopenia, thrombocytopathies, von Willebrand disease, vasculopathies), and due to the inherent multisystemic nature of a coagulopathy, they will typically result in multifocal sites of hemorrhage, rather than being isolated to the GI tract alone.

Structural GI pathology resulting in bleeding may be macroscopic or microscopic and occurs due to loss of normal mucosal integrity.[1,2] Mucosal lesions are characterized as superficial erosions (partial epithelial loss with a retained, intact, muscularis mucosa) or ulceration (more extensive epithelial denudation with lesions extending deep to the muscularis mucosa). Gastrointestinal pathology resulting in bleeding may either arise due to primary disease of the GI tract itself (e.g., gastric adenocarcinoma with associated ulceration) or as a consequence of extra-GI disease (e.g., GI erosions or ulceration in hypoadrenocorticism, due to the absence of the multifaceted physiological glucocorticoid protective effect on the mucosal barrier).

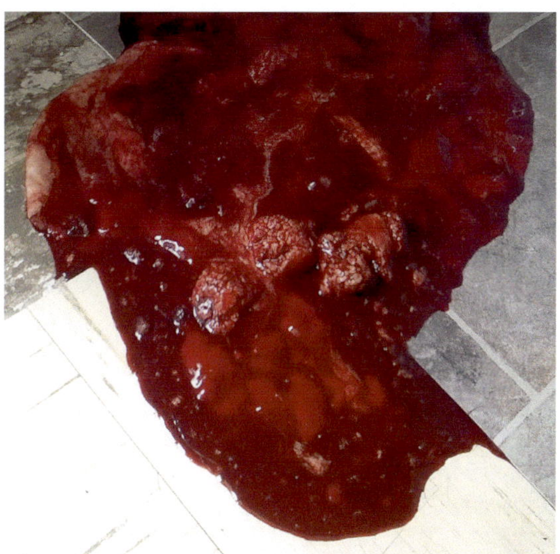

FIG. 14.1 Hematemesis can vary from minimal to profound. This is from a 7-year-old male Labrador with a 9-month history of intermittent marked hematemesis. Having excluded extragastrointestinal causes, endoscopy identified multifocal gastric erosions and underlying marked lymphoplasmacytic and mild eosinophilic gastroduodenitis. Sustained (>5 years) complete remission was achieved following institution of an exclusion diet (and an initial course of omeprazole and sucralfate). Image courtesy of Sally Shovelton.

Upper GI tract bleeding will typically manifest as hematemesis (fresh [Fig. 14.1] or digested coffee ground appearance) or melena (dark tarry stool, due to the digested blood component). Lower intestinal bleeding (aboral to the ileocecocolic valve) typically manifests as hematochezia (the rectal passage of fresh blood); this can be with or without concurrent diarrhea, depending on whether there is diffuse lower intestinal disease or a focal bleeding lesion leaving streaked blood on feces, respectively. The distinction between upper and lower GI bleeding causing melena and hematochezia is not absolute, as transit time through the GI tract will influence the extent of change of the blood. An acute, large-volume, upper GI bleed may be cathartic with a resultant rapid intestinal transit time, thus leading to hematochezia rather than melena, whereas colonic bleeding occurring in the presence of delayed intestinal transit time may appear as melena. Most cases of hematochezia will be due to bleeding of the cecum, colon, or rectum. Anal or perianal bleeding may be mistaken as hematochezia.

Due to many shared pathophysiological processes, there is considerable overlap in the differential diagnoses for hematemesis, melena, and hematochezia, although due to variances in applied physiology (including GI secretions, vascular supply and drainage) and predilection sites for infectious and neoplastic disease, important distinctions remain.

For causes of acute hemorrhagic diarrhea, the reader is referred to Chapter 11.

Clinical signs

Gastrointestinal bleeding may be readily apparent or occult. Many patients with GI bleeding due to structural GI disease will present with other signs referrable to the

TABLE 14.1 Causes of upper gastrointestinal bleeding in dogs according to their pathophysiological classification.

Drugs/toxins	Inflammatory/ infectious	Neoplastic	Metabolic	Vascular	Anomalous
■ Nonsteroidal anti-inflammatory drugs (NSAIDs) ■ Corticosteroids ■ Chemotherapeutic cytotoxics ■ Tyrosine kinase inhibitors (TKIs) ■ Immunosuppressants	Sterile inflammatory ■ Acute pancreatitis ■ Diffuse inflammatory enteropathies (typically eosinophilic) Gastrointestinal infections ■ Parasitic (*Ancylostoma* spp., *Uncinaria stenocephala*, *Spirocerca lupi*, *Physaloptera* spp.) ■ Fungal (e.g., *Pythium insidiosum*, *Histoplasma capsulatum*)	■ Adenocarcinoma ■ Lymphoma ■ Leiomyo(sarco)ma ■ Gastrointestinal stromal tumor (GIST) ■ Mast cell tumor/ mastocytosis ■ Extramedullary plasmacytoma ■ Hemangiosarcoma	■ Hypoadrenocorticism ■ Portal hypertension ■ Uremic gastritis ■ Hyperacidity syndromes (mast cell tumor, gastrinoma)	■ Vascular ectasia/ angiodysplasia ■ Arteriovenous fistula ■ Postmesenteric hypoperfusion/ ischemic event/torsion ■ Intrahepatic portosystemic shunt ■ Vascular aberrancy (e.g., Dieulafoy's lesion)	■ Foreign body ■ Intussusception ■ Stress (e.g., racing sled dogs) ■ Post-GI surgery

TABLE 14.2 Causes of lower gastrointestinal bleeding in dogs according to their pathophysiological classification.

Drugs/toxins	Inflammatory/ infectious	Neoplastic	Metabolic	Vascular	Anomalous
■ Chemotherapeutic cytotoxics ■ Tyrosine kinase inhibitors (TKIs) ■ Immunosuppressants ■ Nonsteroidal anti-inflammatory drugs (NSAIDs) ■ Corticosteroids	Sterile inflammatory ■ Diffuse inflammatory enteropathies – typically eosinophilic ■ Idiopathic colitis ■ Acute pancreatitis Gastrointestinal infections ■ Granulomatous colitis ■ Parasitic (*Trichuris vulpis*) ■ Fungal (e.g., *Pythium insidiosum*, *Histoplasma capsulatum*) ■ Algal (*Prototheca* spp.)	■ Adenocarcinoma ■ Lymphoma ■ Leiomyo(sarco)ma ■ Gastrointestinal stromal tumor (GIST) ■ Mast cell tumor / mastocytosis ■ Extramedullary plasmacytoma ■ Hemangiosarcoma	■ Hypoadrenocorticism	■ Vascular ectasia / angiodysplasia ■ Arteriovenous fistula	■ Colorectal adenomatous polyps ■ Foreign body ■ Penetrating pelvic fracture ■ Rectoanal strictures ■ Stress (e.g., racing sled dogs) ■ Ileocolic intussusception ■ Cecal inversion (cecocolic intussusception) ■ Post-GI surgery ■ Anal furunculosis

GI tract, which may include vomiting or diarrhea and often broader, nonspecific signs (e.g., inappetence, weight loss, or poor coat condition), associated with underlying GI malabsorptive disease.

Depending on the clinical course of the blood loss, patients may present with or without anemia, and they may either be clinically compensated or display a spectrum of clinical signs attributable to anemia and hypovolemic shock due to blood loss. These signs can range from mild lethargy through compensated shock (mild tachycardia, with hyperdynamic pulses) to overt collapse due to decompensated hypovolemic shock. Rarely, intermittent acute bleeds may result in a more chronic history of partial collapse or syncopal events.

Clinical signs outside the GI tract may include pedal pruritus (e.g., *Uncinaria* infection or concurrent food-responsive dermatopathy/enteropathy), cutaneous signs or lesions (due to systemic mycoses or paraneoplastic syndromes), and polyuria/polydipsia (e.g., hypoadrenocorticism, liver disease, kidney disease). When present, such signs can considerably facilitate prioritization of the differential diagnoses list.

Diagnostic approach

Prior to proceeding with a diagnostic pathway for GI bleeding, care should be taken to evaluate for and exclude the possibility of a systemic coagulopathy, swallowed blood of non-GI sources, or ingested pigmented or blood-containing products, any of which may masquerade as primary GI hemorrhage.

Occult GI blood loss can present a diagnostic challenge; a considerable volume of blood may be lost before hematemesis, melena, or hematochezia may be overtly apparent. Estimates in people indicate that an upper GI bleed of up to 1.5–2 mL/kg can occur without a change to fecal appearance. Occult GI hemorrhage should always be a differential diagnosis for anemia (regenerative or nonregenerative) or a regenerative erythrogram (regardless of hematocrit), as a regenerative response may avert the development of anemia until either iron deficiency develops or an acute large volume hemorrhage cannot be compensated for.

Fecal occult blood testing is rarely a valuable diagnostic test; false positives occur in the presence of red meat diets or peroxidases from other dietary items (including some plant-based items) or bacteria, while false negatives occur alongside intermittent blood loss. When performed, a meat-free diet (e.g., soy-based commercial diet) should be fed, and rectal interventions (thermometer, digital examination) should be avoided for at least 3 days prior to collection of a pooled fecal sample.

If a gastric ulcer is clinically suspected, it is reasonable to administer GI protectants including acid blockers (proton pump inhibitors) and coating agents (sucralfate) during investigation.[3] However, the latter should be delayed until after imaging and/or endoscopy so as not to obscure mucosal lesions.

The recommended diagnostic approach to hematemesis/melena is described in Algorithm 14.1.

Algorithm 14.1 Note 1 A comprehensive anamnesis should evaluate for the ingestion of activated charcoal, iron supplements, bismuth-containing medications or ingestion of significant quantities of liver, red meats, or blueberries, which may be a cause of apparent melena or darkly pigmented stool.

Algorithm 14.1 Note 2 True hematemesis or melena may arise from swallowed blood, which can be of oral, nasal, pharyngeal, esophageal, or respiratory origin. Comprehensive interrogation for the presence of extra-GI signs, alongside a thorough physical examination, should facilitate exclusion of these mimics of primary GI bleeding.

Algorithm 14.1 Note 3 Coagulopathic processes resulting in GI hemorrhage will typically be a primary bleeding disorder and exhibit multifocal sites of hemorrhage. Key sites of consideration during history taking include the urinary tract and respiratory tract, including epistaxis, which may be retrograde, swallowed, and not outwardly apparent. Care should be taken during examination to search for other evidence of mucosal bleeding—especially the gingival margin, internal pinnae, inguinal region, and other accessible mucosal surfaces (penis, prepuce, vulva). Overwhelmingly, the most common cause of primary coagulopathies in dogs is thrombocytopenia. Von Willebrand disease and vasculopathies are rarely reported as causes of GI hemorrhage in dogs, although they are important recognized causes in people. Where there is any question over the possibility of a coagulopathy, diagnostics should be performed to interrogate for this, ahead of invasive diagnostics.

Algorithm 14.1 Note 4 This may include exposure to an appropriate dose or overdose of therapeutic agents (e.g., aspirin, clopidogrel, rivaroxaban, low molecular weight heparin, unfractionated heparin) as well as toxin exposure (e.g., anticoagulant rodenticides).

Algorithm 14.1 Note 5 Further diagnostics may include, for example, PT and aPTT and/or a toxin screen to support a diagnosis of possible rodenticide exposure and guide specific therapy.

Algorithm 14.1 Note 6 Both orally administered and topical NSAIDs are reported to result in a comparable incidence of GI hemorrhage.[4]

Algorithm 14.1 Note 7 Geographic location, travel history, and lifestyle will guide targeted diagnostic testing for infectious disease. Hookworms (*Anyclostoma* spp., *Uncinaria stenocephala*) have a worldwide distribution (which varies between subspecies for *Ancylostoma* spp.); *A. caninum* causes markedly greater blood loss per worm compared to other species. *Spirocerca lupi* (esophageal worm) has a primarily tropical and subtropical distribution across Africa, the Middle East, the Caribbean, Brazil, and the southern United States. *Physaloptera* spp. (stomach worms) of canine importance are distributed primarily across North America, although feline subspecies, which have the potential to cause disease in dogs, have a worldwide distribution. *Pythium insidiosum*, a pathogenic dimorphic oomycete, is primarily of tropical and subtropical distribution, extending from the Gulf Coast of the United States to Brazil, southern Asia, and Eastern Australasia. *Histoplasma capsulatum* has a global distribution and is particularly reported from central and eastern United States, around the Ohio and Mississippi River Valleys, but it has a patchy distribution across all other continents (except Antarctica).

Algorithm 14.1 Note 8 Gastrointestinal parasitism is a relatively uncommon but simple and readily treatable cause of GI hemorrhage and should be considered and evaluated for, ahead of other more extensive investigation.

Algorithm 14.1 Note 9 If cutaneous mast cell disease is identified, this should be treated to evaluate for resolution of GI clinical signs before more extensive investigation.

Algorithm 14.1 Note 10 Hematological changes may include a regenerative erythrogram, with or without anemia, in the presence of acute or hematologically compensated GI hemorrhage. With chronic GI hemorrhage, an evolution from normocytic, normochromic anemia to microcytic, hypochromic, and ultimately nonregenerative iron-deficient anemia $\pm$ thrombocytosis will occur over time. Concurrent increased serum urea on a fasted sample, in the absence of a suspicion of renal disease, may further support a diagnosis of GI blood loss.

Algorithm 14.1 Note 11 Multiple pathophysiological mechanisms can result in GI hemorrhage in patients with liver disease.[5] Marked acute or chronic liver disease can be associated with significant hepatic dysfunction and concurrent reduced production of clotting factors. Some primary hepatobiliary diseases (e.g., infectious canine hepatitis, leptospirosis) may be associated with thrombocytopenia (either consumptive or immune-mediated). Otherwise, portal hypertension, either chronic and irreversible as a consequence of hepatic fibrosis and reduced hepatic compliance, or potentially reversible due to portal obstructive diseases (e.g., portal thrombi) may result in downstream mesenteric venous congestion, GI edema, reduced perfusion, and erosions/ulceration. Gastric and esophageal varices, although common sequelae of chronic liver disease in people, are not yet clearly recognized entities in dogs. Computed tomography (CT) angiography is an invaluable noninvasive diagnostic tool for evaluating hepatic perfusion, portal vasculature, and acquired shunting associated with portal hypertension.

Algorithm 14.1 Note 12 The diagnostic utility of cobalamin and folate in the setting of GI disease is primarily in looking for supporting evidence of malabsorptive disease and requirement to supplement as part of a wider therapeutic strategy (see Chapter 20).

Algorithm 14.1 Note 13 Basal cortisol >55 nmol/L (>2 µg/dL) likely excludes hypoadrenocorticism, although it should not be used as an absolute cutoff if the clinical suspicion is high. Evaluating delta cortisol with adrenocorticotropic hormone (ACTH) stimulation testing is required for

ALGORITHM 14.1

Diagnostic approach to hematemesis/melena.

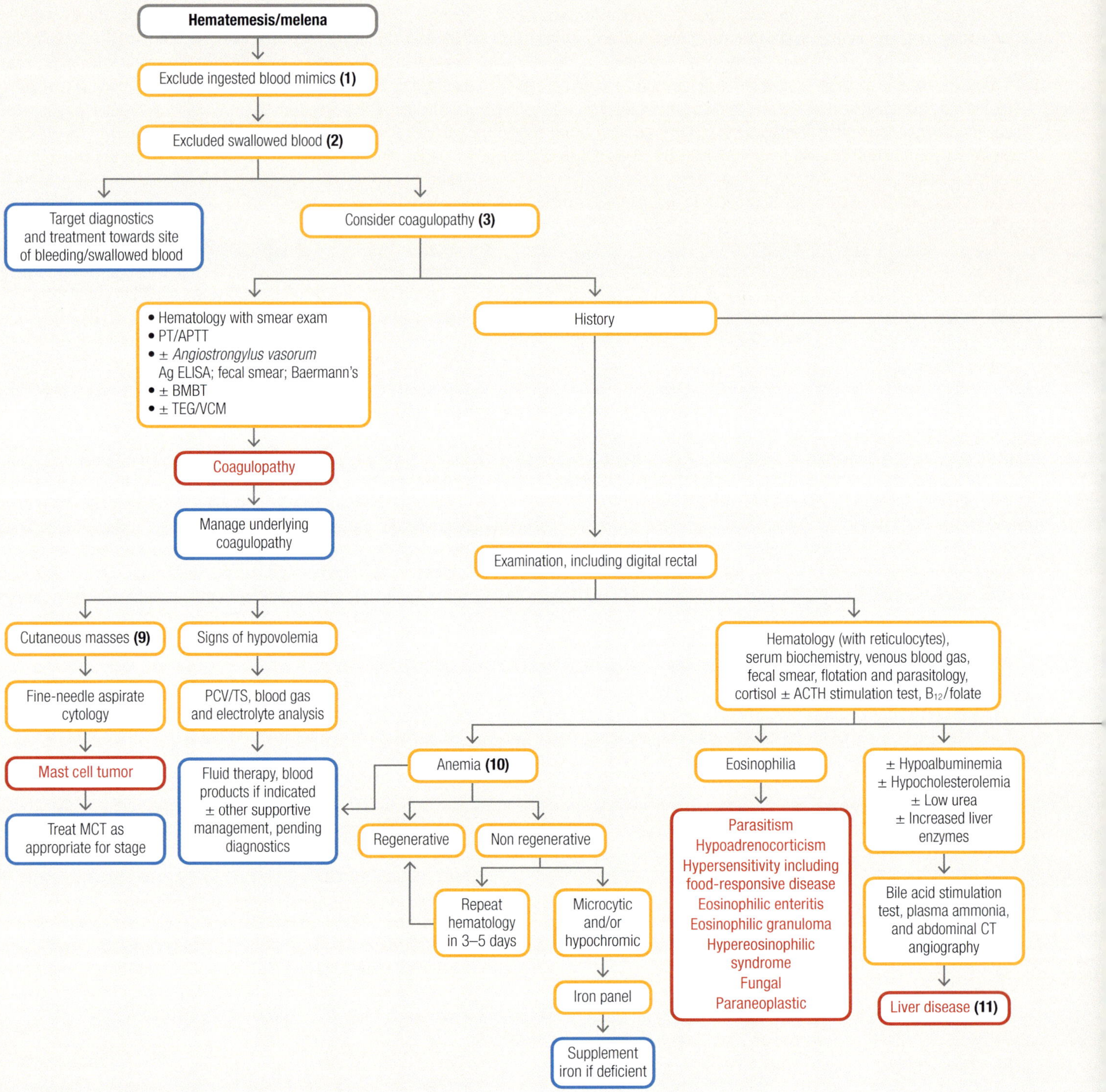

ACTH, adrenocorticotrophic hormone; Ag, antigen; aPTT, activated partial thromboplastin time; BMBT, buccal mucosal bleeding time; CT, computed tomography; ELISA, enzyme-linked immunosorbent assay; GI, gastrointestinal; MCT, mast cell tumor; NSAIDs, nonsteroidal anti-inflammatory drugs; PT, prothrombin time; TEG, thromboelastogram; TKIs, tyrosine kinase inhibitors; VCM, viscoelastic coagulation monitoring.

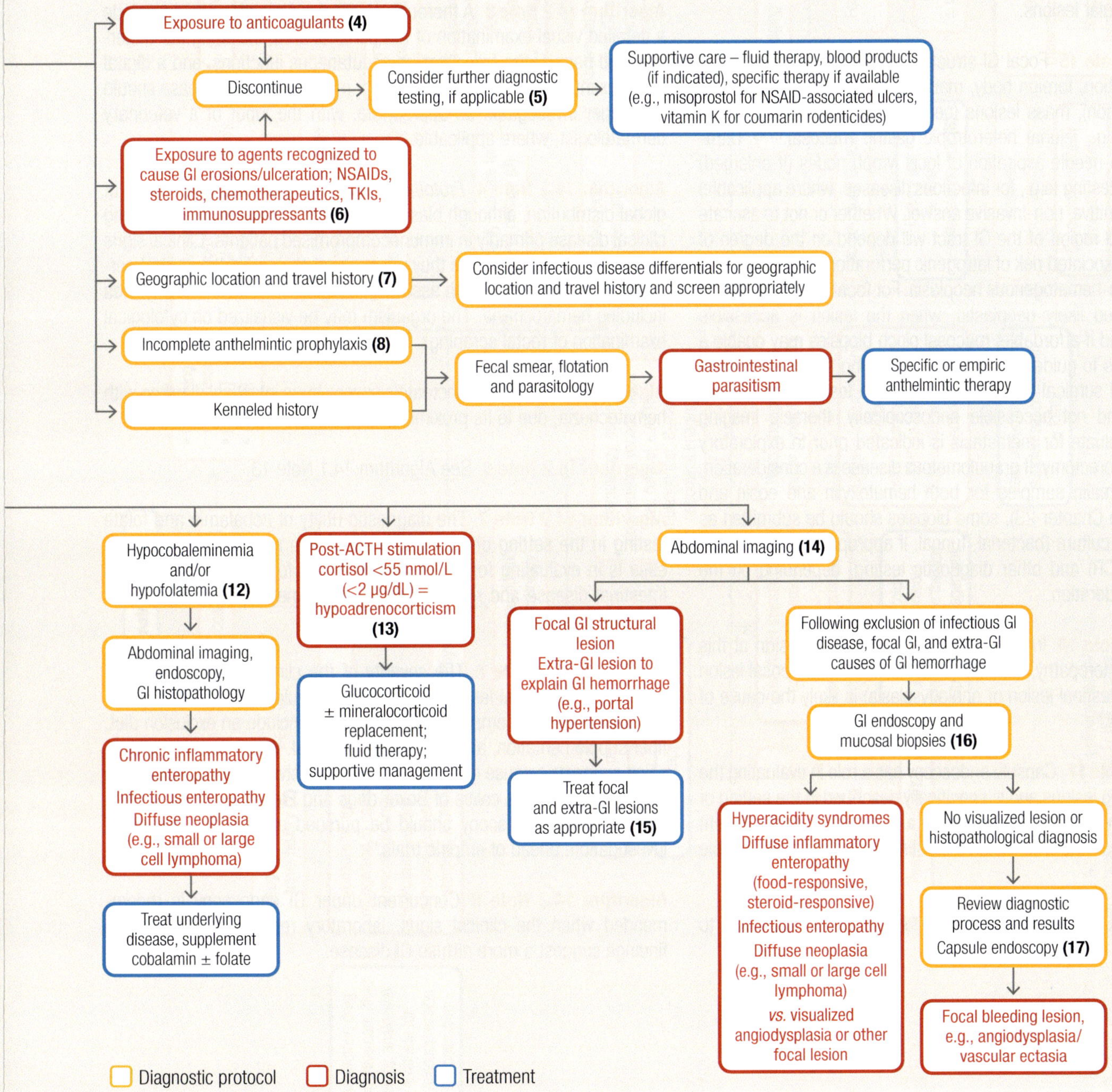
Exposure to anticoagulants (4)
Discontinue
Consider further diagnostic testing, if applicable (5)
Supportive care – fluid therapy, blood products (if indicated), specific therapy if available (e.g., misoprostol for NSAID-associated ulcers, vitamin K for coumarin rodenticides)
Exposure to agents recognized to cause GI erosions/ulceration; NSAIDs, steroids, chemotherapeutics, TKIs, immunosuppressants (6)
Geographic location and travel history (7)
Consider infectious disease differentials for geographic location and travel history and screen appropriately
Incomplete anthelmintic prophylaxis (8)
Kenneled history
Fecal smear, flotation and parasitology
Gastrointestinal parasitism
Specific or empiric anthelmintic therapy
Hypocobaleminemia and/or hypofolatemia (12)
Abdominal imaging, endoscopy, GI histopathology
Chronic inflammatory enteropathy
Infectious enteropathy
Diffuse neoplasia (e.g., small or large cell lymphoma)
Treat underlying disease, supplement cobalamin ± folate
Post-ACTH stimulation cortisol <55 nmol/L (<2 μg/dL) = hypoadrenocorticism (13)
Glucocorticoid ± mineralocorticoid replacement; fluid therapy; supportive management
Abdominal imaging (14)
Focal GI structural lesion
Extra-GI lesion to explain GI hemorrhage (e.g., portal hypertension)
Treat focal and extra-GI lesions as appropriate (15)
Following exclusion of infectious GI disease, focal GI, and extra-GI causes of GI hemorrhage
GI endoscopy and mucosal biopsies (16)
Hyperacidity syndromes
Diffuse inflammatory enteropathy (food-responsive, steroid-responsive)
Infectious enteropathy
Diffuse neoplasia (e.g., small or large cell lymphoma)
vs. visualized angiodysplasia or other focal lesion
No visualized lesion or histopathological diagnosis
Review diagnostic process and results
Capsule endoscopy (17)
Focal bleeding lesion, e.g., angiodysplasia/ vascular ectasia
Diagnostic protocol
Diagnosis
Treatment

dry and hard that the dog is no longer able to defecate, or just a small amount of liquid may be expelled past the impacted feces. Moreover, some dogs eat stones, bones, or gravel, and this can be responsible for a painful passage of feces through the colon; in these cases, supportive treatment (e.g., fluids, analgesics, laxatives) is needed according to the patient's condition. Obstipation should always be promptly investigated and managed medically to avoid a permanent loss of colonic function and motility, which would result in the development of megacolon.

Diagnostic approach

Algorithm 15.1 shows the diagnostic approach to dogs with fecal tenesmus.

Algorithm 15.1 Note When presented with a dog with tenesmus, it is fundamental to determine whether feces are being evacuated. Generally, the absence of defecation is indicative of constipation or obstipation and will require hospitalization of the patient for initiation of supportive therapy and colonic fecal evacuation. The presence of concurrent clinical signs (e.g., anorexia, weight loss, vomiting) should be assessed, as they are common consequences of the prolonged inability to defecate. It is equally important to determine fecal consistency and water content, the number of evacuations, and the presence or absence of mucus, fresh blood, or foreign material, as this will aid in understanding the disease pathophysiology and localizing the problem within the large intestine.

Algorithm 15.1 Note 2 The age of the patient should be considered in order to prioritize the cause of constipation: younger dogs are at a higher risk for foreign body ingestion, whereas older patients are more likely to present with concurrent conditions leading to constipation (e.g., polyuria/polydipsia associated with chronic kidney disease or with hypercalcemia, predisposing to dehydration) or to be treated with drugs interfering with gastrointestinal (GI) motility. For this reason, while taking the history, the owner should be questioned about the presence of clinical signs related to other diseases, any administered drugs, and diet composition to identify any possible cause of constipation (e.g., lack of dietary fiber, ingestion of raw bones). In addition, during the physical examination, the presence of abnormalities or clinical signs predisposing to evacuation difficulties (e.g., reluctance to move because of chronic pain or recent trauma, dehydration secondary to polyuria, sanguineous urethral discharge related to prostatic disease) should be identified. Thorough digital rectal palpation and visual inspection of the perianal region, any lesion or neoformation should be detected (e.g., perineal hernia, anal furunculosis, anal sac tumor, prostatic enlargement). Abdominal radiographs can confirm colonic distension, evaluate if fecal consistency is altered, and identify masses or lymph node enlargement responsible for extraluminal obstruction of the colon.

Algorithm 15.1 Note 3 A distal colonic or rectal mass deforming the feces should be investigated in these cases through imaging and, when possible, sampled during a colonoscopy to obtain diagnostic biopsies. Depending on the neoplasm, excision or adjunctive chemotherapy or radiation therapy may be appropriate.

Algorithm 15.1 Note 4 The presence of dyschezia associated with fecal tenesmus is highly indicative of anorectal or perianal disease. Therefore, visual inspection of the anal and perineal regions must be performed together with careful digital exploration of the rectum in the conscious or sedated/anesthetized patient (see Chapter 17).

Algorithm 15.1 Note 5 The etiopathogenesis of anal furunculosis is unclear. An immune-mediated basis is suspected, and breed predisposition is confirmed in German Shepherd Dogs, representing ~85% of affected patients. This supports the need for a complete physical examination in this breed in case of dyschezia and/or constipation. It has been hypothesized that the number and the specific characteristics of the apocrine sweat glands in the anal area in German Shepherd Dogs could represent a predisposing factor. Colitis can also often be associated with this condition. Male dogs seem to be more predisposed than females, and the median age of presentation is 5 years old. Because several conditions can be related to the development of ulcerative lesions, it is mandatory to rule out differentials such perianal adenoma, anal sac tumor, and mucocutaneous lupus.

Algorithm 15.1 Note 6 Adherent and invasive strains of *Escherichia coli* (AIEC) are causally associated with granulomatous colitis, most commonly in Boxers and French Bulldogs. Histopathologically, this syndrome is characterized by colonic mucosal erosions/ulcerations and periodic acid–Schiff positive macrophagic inflammation. Clinical signs vary based on the duration and severity of the disease but almost inevitably include increased frequency of defecation, tenesmus, hematochezia, and large bowel diarrhea. The age of onset is 1–2 years. Fluorescence *in situ* hybridization (FISH) on colonic tissue is required to confirm the presence of AIEC within the granulomatous infiltrate. See Chapter 48.

The overuse of enrofloxacin in dogs with suspected granulomatous colitis has led to widespread antimicrobial-resistant AIEC strains and increases in refractory cases of granulomatous colitis. For this reason, culture and antimicrobial susceptibility testing of representative colonic biopsies is strongly recommended before fluoroquinolone therapy.

Algorithm 15.1 Note 7 Mild constipation may occur with acquired primary hypothyroidism due to decreased intestinal motility. Congenital hypothyroidism is a rarer cause of chronic constipation, seen in young dogs. Constipation is associated with other clinical signs, such as lethargy, dullness, skeletal developmental abnormalities (e.g., small disproportionate size), and hair coat abnormalities, and with laboratory alterations (e.g., azotemia, hypercholesterolemia). Affected puppies may appear normal at birth but usually develop clinical signs by 1–2 months of age. Causes of the central form include thyroid-stimulating hormone (TSH) deficiency and TSH unresponsiveness, while thyroid dysgenesis, dyshormonogenesis, and iodine deficiency are causes of the primary form.

Algorithm 15.1 Note 8 One of the most important functions of intracellular potassium is the generation of normal resting membrane potential; this can explain the development of clinical signs such muscle weakness, arrhythmia, or decreased GI motility when serum potassium concentrations are below 3.5 mmol/L. Three main mechanisms can be considered in dogs to explain hypokalemia: decreased intake and increased loss of potassium through the GI tract (via vomiting or diarrhea), increased loss of potassium through the kidneys (impaired tubular potassium absorption as a consequence of a primary renal disease or drugs, such as diuretics affecting potassium reabsorption), and translocation from extracellular fluid to intracellular fluid caused by insulin or glucose-containing fluid administration. In addition to potassium supplementation, identification of the underlying cause of hypokalemia is necessary to stabilize the patient and prevent recurrence.

An increased concentration of calcium ions can reduce neuromuscular excitability and causes atonia of the GI tract. In dogs, the most common cause of hypercalcemia is neoplasia, followed by primary hyperparathyroidism and chronic kidney disease. Measurement of parathyroid hormone (PTH) concentrations can be useful to confirm the presence of primary hyperparathyroidism (increased plasma PTH and low or low–normal serum phosphorus) or malignancy-related hypercalcemia (increased PTH-related protein, low or low–normal PTH, and low or low–normal serum phosphorus). Among malignancies associated with hypercalcemia, anal sac apocrine gland adenocarcinoma is one of the most commonly reported and must be ruled out in dogs with constipation, tenesmus, and/or dyschezia.

Algorithm 15.1 Note 9 Abdominal and pelvic cavity ultrasound examination can identify primary GI diseases (e.g., neoplasia, chronic inflammation) but also extraintestinal lesions responsible for extraluminal compression (e.g., prostatic disease). Generally, in a constipated dog, the presence of abundant fecal material can decrease the quality of the ultrasound examination. For this reason, this procedure should be performed after fecal removal, in all cases in which the cause of constipation/dyschezia cannot be identified through clinical examination or abdominal radiographs. If a mass/neoplasm is detected, excision or adjunctive chemotherapy or radiation therapy may be appropriate.

Algorithm 15.1 Note 10 Orthogonal abdominal radiographs should be performed in case of severe constipation or obstipation to assess the degree and extent of any colonic fecal impaction and/or dilation, evaluate the presence of caudal abdominal organomegaly or masses, rule out pelvic bone fractures, and evaluate lumbosacral or coccygeal vertebral abnormalities. The diameter of the canine colon should be less than the length of the vertebral body of L7; a colonic diameter surpassing that value should raise suspicion for disease or injury.

Algorithm 15.1 Note 11 When presented with a severely constipated or obstipated dog, fecal evacuation of the colon must be ensured to avoid permanent loss of colonic function and motility. Prior to colonic evacuation, the patient must be adequately rehydrated with intravenous isotonic fluids and any electrolyte imbalances need to be corrected. For evacuation, large volumes (10 mL/kg) of warm isotonic crystalloid or polyethylene glycol solutions are instilled in the colon via a soft 12 Fr rubber catheter. To facilitate evacuation, the fecal mass is gently broken down with both hands and massaged out of the colon and rectum.

Algorithm 15.1 Note 12 Immunosuppressant/immunomodulatory treatment is the mainstay therapy for anal furunculosis. Half of affected dogs treated with topical tacrolimus experience clinical resolution within 16 weeks, whereas oral treatment with ciclosporin showed a higher (85%) success rate. Treatment cannot be completely discontinued in approximately 50% of dogs with anal furunculosis; in these cases, it should be given as maintenance therapy to avoid recurrence.

Algorithm 15.1 Note 13 Anal sac adenocarcinoma can be associated with malignant hypercalcemia. In case of metastatic disease, there is evidence that surgical removal of sublumbar lymph nodes is beneficial.

Algorithm 15.1 Note 14 Initially, in mildly constipated cases or following colonic evacuation of previously severely constipated or obstipated dogs, dietary modification is recommended alone or in conjunction with oral laxatives and/or prokinetics. Dietary modification is ensured either by feeding a commercial fiber-enriched diet or by adding a fiber supplement to the existing diet. Fiber exerts its beneficial effects by bulk formation, increasing fecal water content, reducing colonic transit time, and increasing the frequency of defecation. For fiber supplementation of an existing diet, psyllium (1–4 teaspoons) or pumpkin (1–4 tablespoons) can be added per meal, titrating to effect.

Algorithm 15.1 Note 15 Oral laxatives promote colonic evacuation by stimulating water and electrolyte transport and/or colonic propulsive motility. They include emollient laxatives (e.g., dioctyl sodium sulfosuccinate), lubricant laxatives (e.g., mineral oil), osmotic laxatives (e.g., polyethylene glycol, lactulose at 0.5 mL/kg PO every 8–12 h), and stimulant laxatives (e.g., bisacodyl 5–20 mg PO every 12–24 h). Laxatives can be used in conjunction with dietary modification and prokinetics. See Chapter 48.

Algorithm 15.1 Note 16 Subtotal colectomy is a salvage procedure in dogs and is much more likely to result in diarrhea and fecal incontinence than in cats. For this reason, this therapeutic option is not recommended.

ALGORITHM 15.1

Approach to the dog with fecal tenesmus.

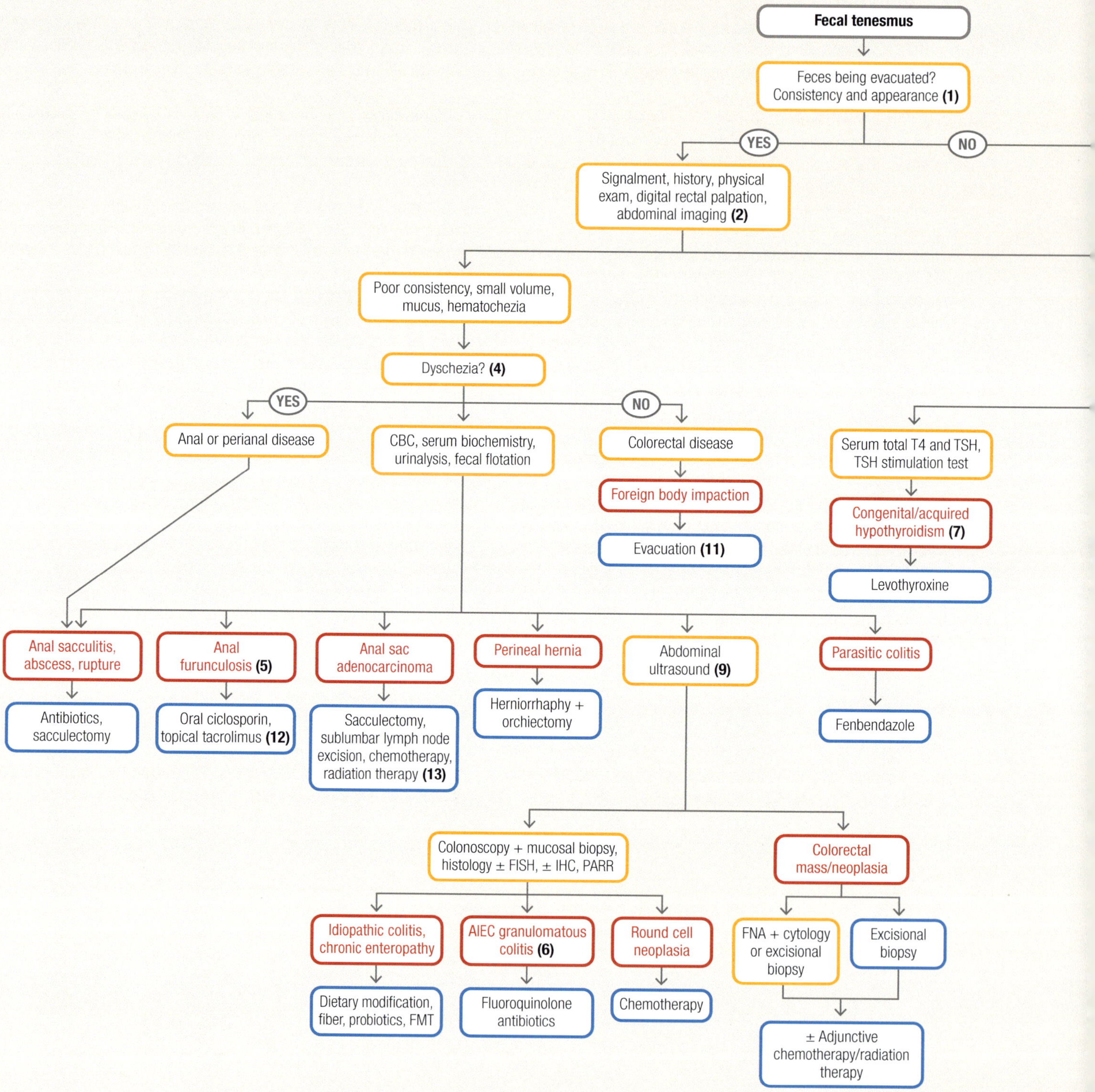

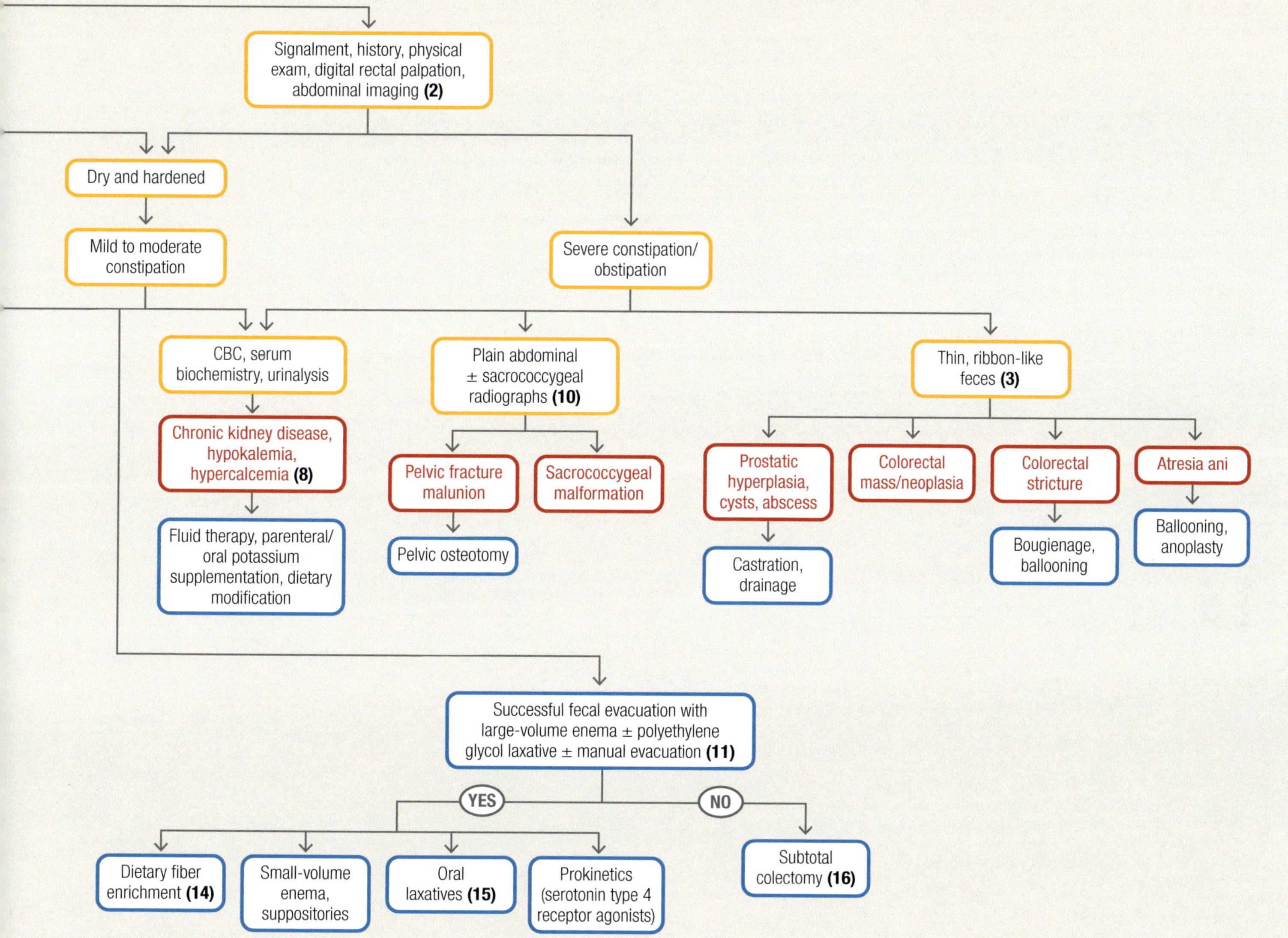

AIEC, adherent and invasive *Escherichia coli*; CBC, complete blood count;
FISH, fluorescence *in situ* hybridization; FMT, fecal microbiota transplantation;
FNA, fine needle aspiration; IHC, immunohistochemistry;
PARR, polymerase chain reaction for antigen receptor rearrangement
T_4, thyroxine; TSH, thyroid-stimulating hormone.

References

1. Jergens AE. Dyschezia and tenesmus. In: Washabau RJ, Day MJ (eds.). *Canine and Feline Gastroenterology.* Saunders; 2013, pp. 109–113.
2. Unterer S, Werner M. Diseases of the large intestine. In: Côté E, Ettinger SJ, Feldman EC (eds.). *Ettinger's Textbook of Veterinary Internal Medicine*, 9th ed. Elsevier; 2024, pp. 1729–1753.
3. Washabau RJ. Constipation. In: Washabau RJ, Day MJ (eds.). *Canine and Feline Gastroenterology.* Saunders; 2013, pp. 93–98.

CHAPTER 16

Flatulence

Beatrice Ruggerone
DVM, PhD, DECVIM-CA

Fabio Procoli
DVM, MVetMed,
DACVIM (SAIM),
DECVIM-CA, MRCVS

Flatulence refers to the expulsion of gas (flatus) originating from the gastrointestinal (GI) tract through the anus. Although infrequent or mild episodes of flatulence generally do not raise concern among pet owners, the concurrent presence of malodor and other clinical signs and/or a high frequency of flatulence can prompt owners to seek veterinary attention for their dog.[1] In the event of chronically recurrent or severe episodes, the occurrence of flatulence warrants careful attention and a structured diagnostic approach. Persistent flatulence may indicate underlying chronic GI disorders, especially when accompanied by other clinical signs such as diarrhea, vomiting, abdominal pain, hyporexia, or weight loss. Additionally, certain organic conditions, such as hiatal hernia, gastroesophageal reflux disease, upper airway obstruction, and peptic ulcer disease, can predispose dogs to aerophagia, which, in turn, contributes to excessive gas production and flatulence.

Pathophysiology

The primary sources of GI gas can be summarized as 1) swallowed air (aerophagia), particularly during rapid consumption of food or drink, as observed in voracious eaters or in brachycephalic dogs with upper airway obstruction; 2) carbon dioxide generated by chemical reactions between food components and gastric acid, bicarbonate, or alkaline secretions; 3) gas produced by bacterial fermentation of undigested food, especially in the colon; and 4) diffusion of gases from the bloodstream into the GI lumen. Under normal conditions, this gas is expelled via eructation or flatulence, metabolized by the resident intestinal bacterial flora, or absorbed into the bloodstream. More than 99% of GI gas consists of five odorless gases, carbon dioxide, hydrogen, methane, nitrogen, and oxygen, in varying proportions. The remaining 1% comprises sulfur-based compounds, which are responsible for the characteristic odor. Bacterial fermentation of dietary residues in both the small and large intestines is considered the primary source of gas production, of which 75% is represented by hydrogen, methane, and carbon dioxide. Nitrogen and oxygen mainly originate from aerophagia, often caused by rapid ingestion of food or water or by panting.

Breath analysis is used in human medicine as an indirect method to measure intestinal gas production. This approach is based on the diffusion of gases from the gut lumen into the bloodstream, which are subsequently exhaled through the lungs. Among intestinal gases, hydrogen and methane are uniquely produced by gut microbiota activity and demonstrate a strong correlation with their concentrations in breath. Due to this correlation, hydrogen- and methane-based breath tests are routinely employed in the diagnosis of conditions such as carbohydrate maldigestion syndromes and small intestinal bacterial overgrowth. However, the reproducibility and reliability of breath tests for other intestinal gases remain limited. This limitation arises either from their low concentrations in exhaled breath or from the inability to definitively attribute their origin to intestinal activity alone.[2]

Gas homeostasis in the GI tract is the result of a dynamic equilibrium governed by intestinal microbiota metabolism and the permeability and function of gas-absorptive intestinal pathways. Common factors contributing to excessive flatus include poor quality and digestibility of the diet with subsequent fermentation of excess carbohydrate residues, structural and inflammatory intestinal diseases with subsequent carbohydrate maldigestion and malabsorption, GI motility disorders, and exocrine pancreatic insufficiency. All of these can lead to abnormal composition and function of the intestinal microbiota, referred to as *dysbiosis*. Furthermore, excessive aerophagia due to ravenous food ingestion or associated with upper airway obstructive disease can lead to flatulence independently from bacterial production.

The type of diet significantly affects bacterial activity, gas volume, and flatulence frequency. Diets high in fiber (especially highly soluble and fermentable fibers) markedly increase flatus, whereas fiber-free diets nearly eliminate it, highlighting the pivotal role of dietary fiber. Fiber influences the GI tract through two main mechanisms: 1) producing fermentation by-products, such as short-chain fatty acids, which impact both the intestinal microbiota and the neuroendocrine regulation of the GI system, and 2) increasing fecal bulk and mechanically stimulating the colonic mucosa, thereby modulating secretion and peristalsis.

Dietary fiber is categorized based on its physical and chemical properties into soluble or insoluble, fermentable or nonfermentable, and as short- or long-chain carbohydrates. Soluble fiber is further classified as viscous or nonviscous. These distinctions are essential in understanding how different fiber types influence the volume and frequency of gas production, which is often a key factor in cases of flatulence. Fermentable carbohydrates, such as oligosaccharides, galactooligosaccharides, disaccharides, monosaccharides, and polyols (sugar alcohols), are poorly absorbed in the small intestine. This poor absorption increases intestinal osmolality, leading to greater gas production and larger volumes of fluid entering the colon. Similarly, fiber supplements such as psyllium or other bulk-forming agents may contribute to gaseous distension. In contrast, dietary fibers that are long chain, intermediately viscous, soluble, and moderately fermentable typically result in lower gas production, offering a potential dietary approach to minimize excessive flatulence.

Diagnostic approach

Algorithm 16.1 shows the diagnostic approach to dogs with flatulence. The first step in the evaluation of a dog with chronic flatulence is to identify any underlying organic disorder through a detailed history, physical examination, and relevant tests. The therapeutic approach involves determining which of the intrinsic variables of flatulence is most problematic: the volume of gas, the unpleasant odor, or both. This differentiation can guide subsequent management strategies.

Algorithm 16.1 Note 1 The signalment should be considered when a dog is presented for chronic flatulence. A brachycephalic conformation can represent a risk factor for excessive aerophagia as well as the tendency to eat voraciously of some breeds (e.g., retrievers).

Algorithm 16.1 Note 2 A comprehensive dietary history should be obtained for patients presenting with excessive flatulence, including details about the types and composition of food, treats, and table scraps provided. Diets containing mono/di/oligosaccharides (e.g., wheat, leeks, and zucchini), dairy products containing lactose, fruits (e.g., pears, apples, and apricots are rich in monosaccharides and polyols), and legumes (containing galactooligosaccharides) should be avoided. Any medications or supplements being administered also should be documented and withdrawn (when possible) to evaluate the clinical course, considering that multiple drugs can interfere with microbiota composition and health (e.g., antimicrobials and proton pump inhibitors). Owners should be questioned regarding the duration and frequency of the clinical signs as well as any potential correlation with the diet or recent dietary changes. Excessive flatulence is frequently reported alongside other clinical signs such as borborygmi, bloating or abdominal distension, weight loss, vomiting, diarrhea, and/or constipation.

Algorithm 16.1 Note 3 Despite these signs, the physical examination of a dog with excessive flatulence may appear largely unremarkable. Nonetheless, a thorough clinical evaluation, including abdominal palpation and a rectal examination, is essential to identify any underlying abnormalities.

Algorithm 16.1 Note 4 Because flatulence is most often reported in conjunction with other GI clinical signs, initial diagnostic testing should include a minimum database of a complete blood count, serum biochemistry panel, urinalysis, and fecal parasite screening. Thoracic and abdominal radiographs, abdominal ultrasound, and/or additional blood work to measure serum cobalamin, folate, trypsin-like immunoreactivity, and pancreatic lipase immunoreactivity levels also may be warranted based on initial physical examination findings and diagnostic test results. Although gastroduodenoscopy and colonoscopy are rarely indicated in dogs and cats presenting solely for flatulence, they may be recommended as part of diagnostic investigations if there is concurrent weight loss, vomiting, or diarrhea.

Algorithm 16.1 Note 5 Dogs are classified as aerophagic if they meet at least one of the following criteria: More than one third of the bolus volume contains air in more than 50% of swallows or air ingestion results in gastric distension exceeding one third of the final gastric volume, as determined by gross visual assessment by radiography. Reported factors contributing to aerophagia include a voracious appetite or being a brachycephalic breed exhibiting both GI and respiratory signs or having upper airway obstruction.[3]

Algorithm 16.1 Note 6 Plain abdominal radiography can help detect an excessive accumulation of gas in the stomach. However, videofluoroscopic swallow studies are considered a more precise method for diagnosing aerophagia in dogs, particularly when evaluating potential predisposing factors such as hiatal hernia (see Chapter 45).

Algorithm 16.1 Note 7 When aerophagia is suspected in dogs with a tendency to eat voraciously, implementing strategies to slow their food intake may be beneficial. Owners can be advised to use antigorging bowls designed to encourage slower eating or to add water to the dog's food to further reduce the speed of consumption. The administration of smaller meals several times per day or the mixing of dry and canned food also can be helpful. Another option is to consider a low-residue diet. In this case, most of the food is digested and absorbed before reaching the colon, where most of the gas would be produced.

Algorithm 16.1 Note 8 In cases where flatulence persists despite the discontinuation of drugs or inappropriate foods and after addressing concurrent GI diseases, the use of specific products may be beneficial. Given the critical role of the microbiota in regulating gas production in the GI tract, efforts to normalize its composition and maintain a healthy microbial balance may yield positive effects. Probiotics have been investigated for their efficacy in reducing flatulence and improving fecal consistency, but results remain inconsistent. Their potential benefits are attributed to their ability, when properly administered, to restore a healthy microbiome composition. Prebiotics, in contrast, serve as substrates selectively used by beneficial microorganisms for growth and activity. For example, the use of galactooligosaccharides promoting bifidobacteria has shown promising results in controlling flatulence and bloating in humans after two weeks of supplementation. Activated charcoal is another option, known for its capacity to bind sulfur-containing gases and reduce odor, although it does not lower the overall volume of gas produced.

Charcoal-based treats for dogs are available commercially, but their efficacy in mitigating flatulence remains unproven. Some supplements can be useful in controlling flatulence. For example, *Yucca shidigera* can bind ammonia and decrease fecal odor without reducing the amount of the excreted flatus, whereas zinc acetate can bind sulfhydryl compounds, serving to deodorize the gas. Simethicone, an antifoaming agent, works by reducing the surface tension and elasticity of mucus-coated gas

ALGORITHM 16.1

Approach to the canine patient with flatulence.

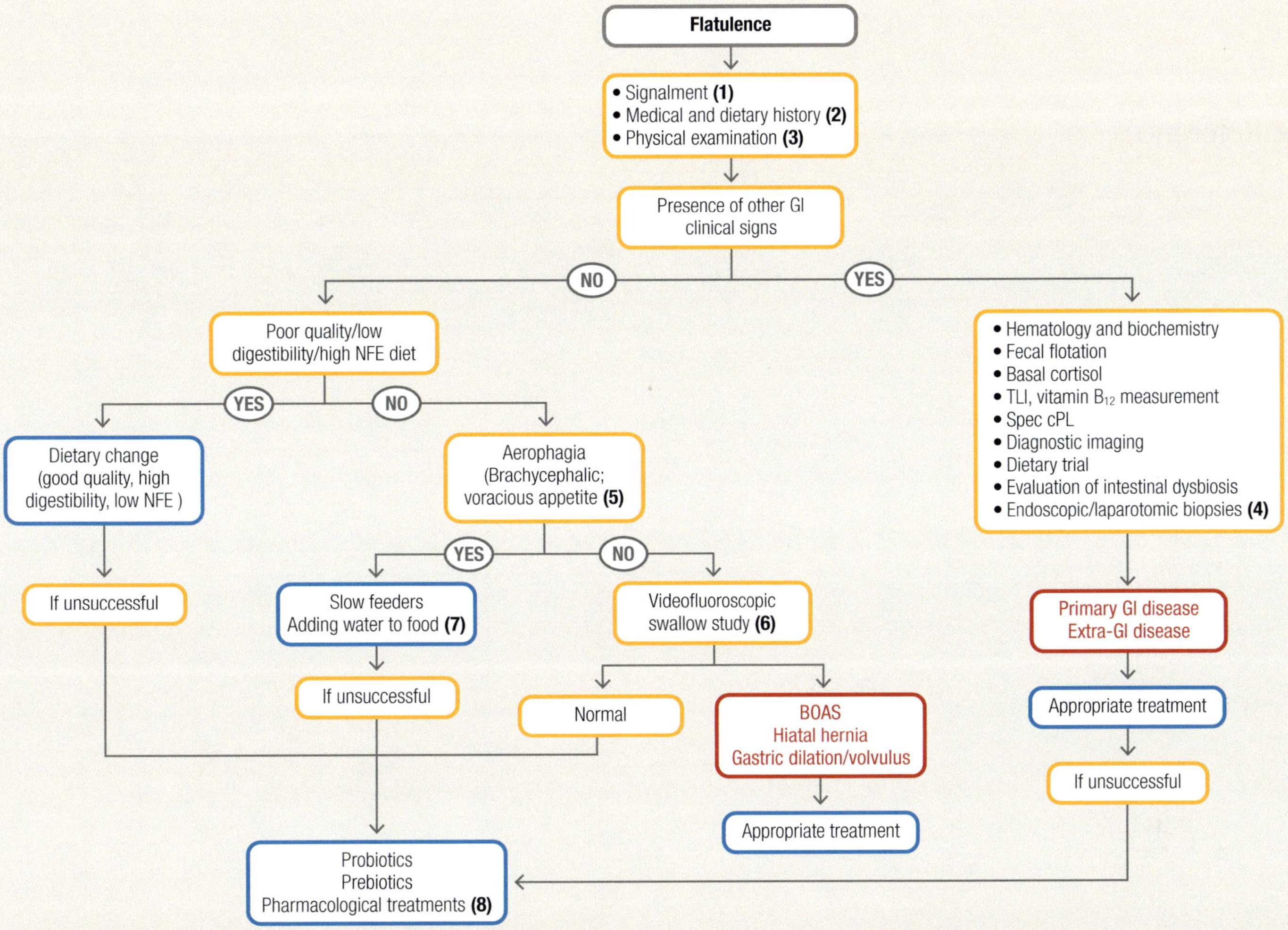

GI, gastrointestinal; TLI, trypsin-like immunoreactivity; Spec cPL, canine pancreas-specific lipase; NFE, nitrogen-free extract; BOAS, Brachycephalic obstructive airway syndrome

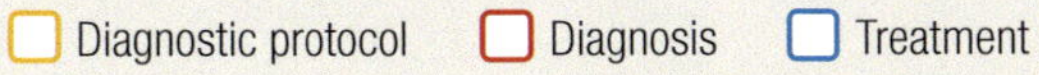

bubbles, causing smaller bubbles to merge into larger ones that are easier to expel. Although this could be helpful for managing flatulence, no specific studies have evaluated its effectiveness in this context. In humans, the main effect is to reduce flatulence without controlling the odor. The recommended dosage for dogs is 20–200 mg administered orally every 6 hours. Lastly, the use of antimicrobials to control flatulence is no longer recommended, considering the negative impact of these drugs on microbiota composition and health and the widespread diffusion of antibiotic resistance.

References

1. Mak G. Flatulence. In: Côté E, Ettinger SJ, Feldman EC (eds.). *Ettinger's Textbook of Veterinary Internal Medicine*. 9th ed. Elsevier; 2024. pp. 247–249.
2. Freire R, Mego M, Oliveira LF, et al. Quantitative GC-TCD measurements of major flatus components: a preliminary analysis of the diet effect. *Sensors (Basel)*. 2022;22(3):838.
3. Grobman N, Reinero C, Lee-Fawler T, Lever TE. Incidence and characterization of aerophagia in dogs using videofluoroscopic swallow studies. *J Vet Intern Med*. 2024;38(3):1449–1457.

Physical examination

Sarah O'Shaughnessy
BVetMed(Hons), PGCert (HPE), PGDip (clinical practice), FHEA, MRCVS

Effective physical examination of the canine patient with gastrointestinal (GI) disease helps to form the foundations for successful clinical reasoning. By facilitating the expansion and refinement of the patient's problem list, a physical examination will aid in identifying problems that need addressing to help maintain patient health and welfare (for example, the presence of pain should prompt the veterinarian to prescribe analgesia), formulating and prioritizing the patient's list of differential diagnoses, and selecting further diagnostic investigations.

As clinical signs that are commonly associated with the GI system may, in fact, be the result of "extra-GI disease" (e.g., vomiting in a patient with pyometra), a full physical examination should always be performed. A systematic (e.g., nose-to-tail) approach will help to ensure that significant findings are not overlooked. Otherwise, direct physical examination of the GI system is limited to:

- Oral examination.
- Palpation of the ventral neck.
- Abdominal palpation.
- Rectal examination.

A sound understanding of normal canine anatomy is essential and can be consolidated by practicing examination techniques on healthy patients and through experiences gained during dissections, diagnostic imaging, surgery, and postmortem examinations.

Oral examination and palpation of the ventral neck

If it is safe to do so, the lips should be lifted to allow examination of the buccal surfaces of the teeth and the mucosae of the gums and lips. The color and moistness of the mucous membranes should be noted. Capillary refill time is ideally performed on the buccal mucosa, away from gingival inflammation that could confound the results. Opening the mouth will allow examination of the lingual and occlusal surfaces of the teeth, the tongue, and the hard and soft palate. Table 17.1 reveals possible findings upon oral examination and their significance in patients with GI disease.

In dogs presenting with dysphagia or regurgitation, palpation of the cervical esophagus may provide further clues.[1] The normal esophagus is not palpable, but masses in this region may be intramural (e.g., diverticulum or esophageal foreign bodies), mural (e.g., esophageal carcinomas), or extramural (e.g., thyroid carcinomas). Gaseous distension may be evident in patients with advanced megaesophagus.[2]

A history of regurgitation should also prompt the veterinarian to look for evidence of aspiration pneumonia, such as dyspnea, pyrexia, and crackles upon auscultation of the cranioventral and/or craniomiddle lung fields.

TABLE 17.1 Possible findings upon oral examination and their significance in patients with gastrointestinal disease.

Examples of abnormal findings upon oral examination	Significance in the patient with gastrointestinal disease
Frequent lip licking and damp hair around the muzzle	Signs may be associated with nausea, oral pain, or anxiety.
Changes in mucous membrane color	Pale mucous membranes may indicate poor peripheral perfusion or anemia. Jaundiced mucous membranes may be associated with hepatic dysfunction or cholestatic disease.
Tacky or dry mucous membranes	Indicative of dehydration, a common consequence of excessive fluid loss or inadequate fluid intake. Hypersalivation in nauseous patients can make the oral mucosae of even markedly dehydrated patients moist. Thus, it is important to assess multiple indicators of hydration status, e.g., delays in the return of skin tenting.
Periodontal disease, fractured teeth, or other painful oral lesions	Painful lesions in the oral cavity may provide an alternative explanation for anorexia or inappetence.

Abdominal palpation

Despite being a valuable tool in the assessment of patients with GI disease, abdominal palpation is a challenging technique to teach and learn.[3,4] It should be acknowledged that not all normal abdominal organs are palpable, and, as a diagnostic tool, palpation has poor sensitivity, specificity, and accuracy.[5,6] Factors such as obesity, the tensing of the abdominal musculature, and the presence of significant volumes of free fluid will limit examination. Thus, this examination technique can rarely be used to make a definitive diagnosis and more commonly informs the selection of further diagnostic testing.

The approach to abdominal palpation can be observed in Video 17.1. The examination begins with distance observations of the patient's behavior and abdominal contour. Distension may be associated with organomegaly, pregnancy, or a large volume of free fluid. If the latter is suspected, the detection of a "fluid thrill" upon ballottement (Video 17.2) will further support the clinician's suspicion. A "tucked" appearance may be associated with pain, weight loss, or an empty GI tract. Adoption of a "prayer posture" may be associated with cranial abdominal pain.

A rough or abrupt approach to palpation is unpleasant for the patient and will cause sudden tensing of the abdominal wall (also known as "splinting"), which will limit the findings and/or be confused for abdominal pain. Time should be taken to alleviate patient anxiety and to gradually increase the amount of pressure that is being applied. The approach to abdominal palpation should be two-handed, using the flats of the fingers to apply rotational pressure contralaterally and systematically to the different abdomen regions. A single-handed approach may be useful in small dogs or for palpation of the caudoventral abdominal contents, e.g., the bladder.

Video 17.1

A systematic approach to abdominal palpation. Note the significant amount of time dedicated to acclimating the patient to being touched before embarking upon a systematic examination.

Video 17.2

Abdominal ballottement. The palm of one hand is placed upon the abdominal wall of the patient, and the fingers of the opposing hand are used to sharply tap the contralateral side. With large volumes of free fluid, a fluid "thrill" may be palpable (a vibrating sensation as the percussive force is transmitted through the free abdominal fluid).

A systematic approach to abdominal palpation will make it less likely that any abnormal findings are overlooked. One technique is to palpate the "four quadrants" of the abdomen in turn (Table 17.2). For each quadrant, the clinician may find it helpful to visualize the normal anatomy of the contents contained within this area (Fig. 17.1).[7] Raising the patient's forequarters may assist in palpation of the cranial abdominal organs (Fig. 17.2).[8] As structures are felt, their number, size, shape, position, mobility, margination, and compliance can be assessed. The patient's behavior should be observed throughout to detect any signs that may be indicative of pain. This may be as subtle as lip licking, sudden onset panting, arching of the back, tensing of the abdominal musculature, or turning of the head or ears.

TABLE 17.2 The four-quadrant approach to canine abdominal palpation with examples of possible findings in patients with gastrointestinal signs.

Quadrant	Organ	Palpable findings in normal dogs and possible findings in patients with gastrointestinal signs
Cranioventral	Liver	The normal liver is not readily palpable. Hepatomegaly may be suspected when firm, flat lobes of the liver extend caudally beyond the costal arch.
	Stomach	The normal stomach is rarely palpable. Ingestion of a very large meal may result in a "doughy" stomach being palpable upon the left side of the patient. Gastric dilatation-volvulus can result in profound abdominal distension, pain upon palpation, and resonance upon percussion.[9]
	Spleen	In most patients, palpation of the normal spleen is limited to the tail. Its flat, firm, and smooth structure may be appreciable, wrapping dorsoventrally from left to right. The body of the spleen may be more readily palpable when it is displaced by a distended stomach or with splenomegaly.[9] Space-occupying lesions in the cranioventral region may be difficult to accurately localize and may be associated with the liver, stomach, spleen, or pancreas.
	Pancreas	The normal pancreas is not palpable. Acute pancreatitis may be associated with detectable cranial abdominal pain.[10] Palpable masses in this region may be neoplastic (e.g., pancreatic adenocarcinoma) or non-neoplastic (e.g., chronic fibrosing pancreatitis).[11]
	Small intestine	The mobile and smooth loops of the jejunum will form most of the examination. The compliance of small intestinal loops is challenging to interpret and is likely to be affected by many factors, e.g., the contents, the degree of filling, as well as the thickness, tone, and health of the intestinal wall. Small intestinal masses can be highly mobile. Differential diagnoses include small intestinal foreign bodies, intussusception, and neoplasia.
Craniodorsal	Kidneys	The smooth and firm caudal pole of the left kidney may be palpable in healthy patients. Alterations in size, shape, consistency, and the presence of pain may be appreciated in patients with renal disease.[12]
Caudodorsal	Descending colon	Success in palpating the normal descending colon will be dependent upon its filling. With obstipation, the descending colon can distend to become a large, firm yet compressible tubular structure coursing craniocaudally. Colonic and other soft tissue masses will not yield upon pressure.
Caudoventral	Bladder	Success in palpating the normal bladder will depend upon its filling. The normal bladder is smooth, soft, and fluctuant. The prostate of male dogs is more likely to be palpated intra-abdominally when prostatomegaly is present.

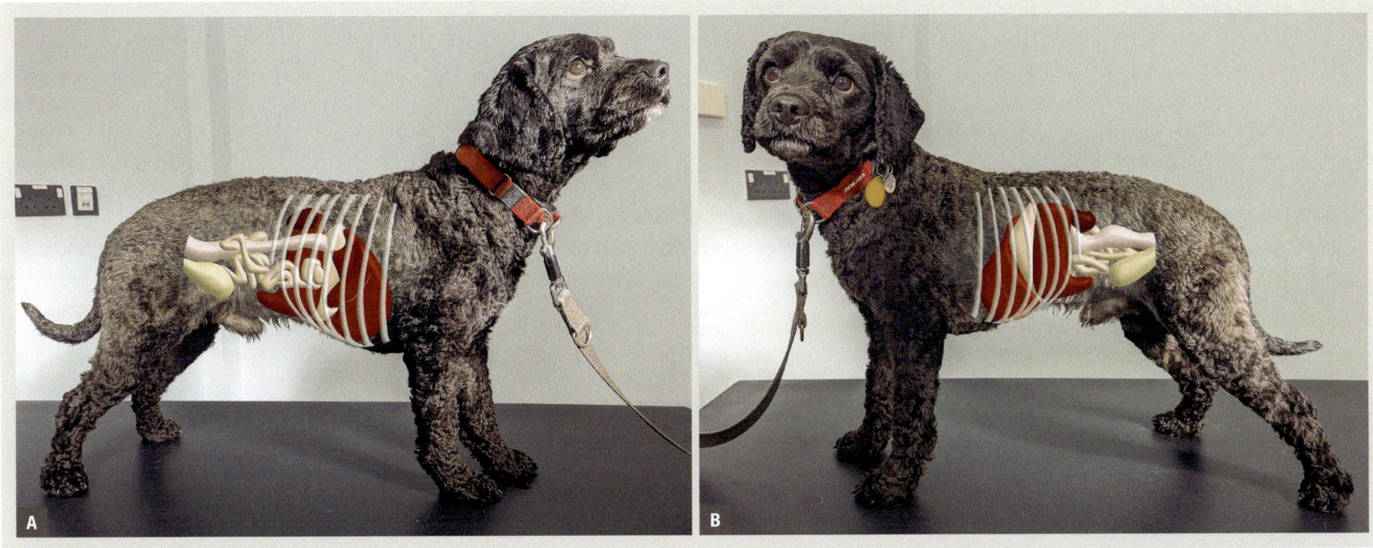

FIG. 17.1 Illustrations revealing the dog's internal abdominal anatomy from (**A**) the right and (**B**) left lateral aspects, respectively. Visualizing the topographical anatomy of the canine patient can assist in the interpretation of abdominal palpation. It is important to note that the liver, stomach, the right kidney, and most of the spleen are not routinely palpable, as these organs are housed within the rib cage. Illustrated photographs with courtesy to Oliver Robbins.

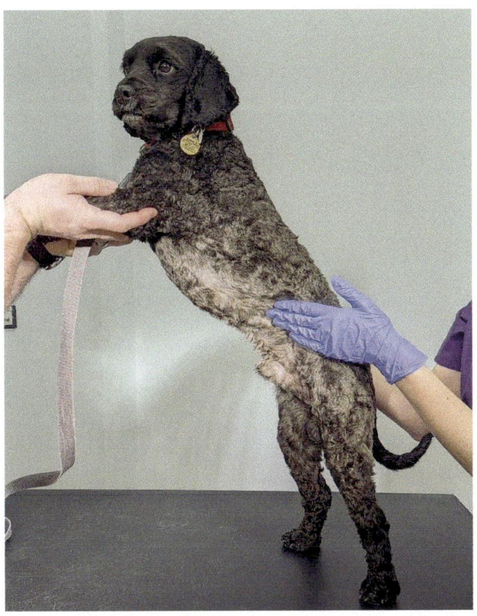

FIG. 17.2 Raising the patient's forequarters may assist in palpation of the cranial abdominal organs.

Comparing the behavioral response to abdominal palpation to that of the spine may help differentiate abdominal pain from back pain.

Rectal examination

The GI system can be examined by external examination of the perineum and a digital rectal examination. The perineum should be inspected for fecal staining. Bulging of the perineum may be seen with perianal herniation. The tone of the anal orifice can be assessed, and the anus should be inspected for evidence of anal prolapse or asymmetry. Measures to ensure patient comfort (e.g., lubrication and analgesia) and personnel safety (e.g., muzzling and chemical restraint) should be considered before embarking upon internal examination. A systematic rectal examination will facilitate assessment of the rectal wall (for strictures, diverticula, and masses) and the anal sacs (for impactions, abscesses or masses). The prostate may be palpable cranioventrally per rectum in male dogs. Once complete, the gloved finger can be inspected for abnormalities such as melena, hematochezia, and mucus.

KEY POINTS

- Effective clinical examination of the canine patient with GI disease forms the foundations for successful clinical reasoning.
- As clinical signs that are commonly associated with the GI system may, in fact, be the result of "extra-GI" disease, a full physical examination should always be performed.
- Examination of the GI system includes oral examination, palpation of the ventral neck, abdominal palpation, and rectal examination.
- A rough or abrupt approach to palpation will cause sudden tensing of the abdominal wall, which will limit the findings and/or cause abdominal pain. Time should be taken to alleviate patient anxiety and to gradually increase the amount of pressure that is being applied.

References

1. Ullal TV, Marks SL, Belafsky PC, et al. A comparative assessment of the diagnosis of swallowing impairment and gastroesophageal reflux in canines and humans. *Front Vet Sci* 9, 2022.
2. Neiger R. Megaesophagus and other problems causing regurgitation. *Proceedings of the NAVC Conference*, North American Veterinary Conference, Gainesville, pp. 550–552, 2010.
3. Esteves JE, Spence C. Developing competence in diagnostic palpation: perspectives from neuroscience and education. *Int J Osteopath Med* 17:52-60, 2014.
4. Hodges B, Regehr G, Martin D. Difficulties in recognizing one's own incompetence: novice physicians who are unskilled and unaware of it. *Acad Med* 76:S87–S89, 2001.
5. Abdellatif A, Kramer M, Failing K, Von Pückler K. Correlation between preoperative ultrasonographic findings and clinical, intraoperative, cytopathological, and histopathological diagnosis of acute abdomen syndrome in 50 dogs and cats. *Vet Sci* 4:39, 2017.
6. Allen WE, Meredith MJ. Detection of pregnancy in the bitch: a study of abdominal palpation, A-mode ultrasound, and Doppler ultrasound techniques. *J Small Anim Pract* 22:609–622, 1981.
7. Mario K, Besse JP. The role of mental imagery in osteopathic palpation: a qualitative study. *Eur J Osteopath Res* 1:17–27, 2019.
8. Elwood C. Investigation and differential diagnosis of vomiting in the dog. *In Practice* 25:374–386, 2003.
9. Monnet E. Gastric dilatation-volvulus syndrome in dogs. *Vet Clin North Am Small Anim Pract* 33: 987–1005, 2003.
10. Cridge H, Twedt DC, Marolf AJ, et al. Advances in the diagnosis of acute pancreatitis in dogs. *J Vet Intern Med* 35:2572–2587, 2021.
11. Watson PJ, Archer J, Roulois AJ, et al. Observational study of 14 cases of chronic pancreatitis in dogs. *Vet Rec* 167:968–976, 2010.
12. Kirk C, Bartges J. Abnormal renal palpation. Nephrol Urol Small Anim 422–424, 2011.

CHAPTER 18

Minimum database

Sonia Sanchez-Redondo
LdaVet, MSc, CSAVP (Internal Medicine), DACVP (Clinical Pathology), MRCVS

Kostas Papasouliotis
DVM, PhD, DECVCP, MRCVS

The routine laboratory database plays an important role in the diagnostic pathway in canine gastroenterology, but it should be recognized that clinicopathological findings are often nonspecific for gastrointestinal (GI) disorders. Nonetheless, these findings are indispensable in guiding the investigations and excluding other potential causes for the presenting clinical signs.

This chapter aims to describe and interpret the most common laboratory test abnormalities that could be found in dogs with GI signs. The minimum laboratory database includes routine hematology, serum biochemistry, urinalysis, basal cortisol levels, and the ACTH stimulation test.

Routine hematology

Erythrocytes

Erythrocytosis is found in diseases that induce dehydration and hypovolemia, such as those involving vomiting or diarrhea. This is frequently associated with mildly increased serum proteins, a pattern commonly observed in acute hemorrhagic diarrhea syndrome.

Regenerative anemia can be seen in cases of GI hemorrhage. Regeneration occurs 3-5 days following the onset of blood loss. Hence, in acute cases, signs of regeneration may not yet be apparent, i.e., preregenerative.

Nonregenerative anemia can be found secondary to chronic disease or due to iron deficiency (such as chronic GI bleeding). Iron deficiency anemia is typically microcytic (decreased mean corpuscular volume [MCV]) normochromic in mild or early stages, progressing to microcytic hypochromic (decreased mean corpuscular hemoglobin concentration [MCHC]) in more severe or advanced stages. The MCV and MCHC offer an overall estimate of red blood cell size and hemoglobin concentration, but these numeric parameters are generated by the hematology analyzer and can be affected by a suboptimal blood sample quality. For this reason, the presence of microcytosis and hypochromasia should be confirmed with a blood smear examination (Fig. 18.1).

It is also important to consider the patient's age when interpreting hematology results; dogs younger than 4 months old have lower numbers of erythrocytes, hemoglobin concentration, and hematocrit than adult dogs. So, puppies with suspected parvovirosis or acute gastroenteritis may be incorrectly considered anemic when reference intervals for adult dogs rather than for puppies are used.

Reticulocyte hemoglobin concentration can be an early indicator of iron-limited erythropoiesis, although it is not able to distinguish the underlying mechanism (i.e., true vs. functional iron deficiency).[1,2] This parameter is offered by some reference laboratories but can also be obtained from certain in-house hematology analyzers.[3]

Leukocytes

Mature neutrophilia can indicate inflammation but can also be seen as part of an epinephrine/norepinephrine (fight or flight) response or glucocorticoid (stress) induced leukogram. The former may be accompanied by lymphocytosis and the latter by lymphopenia, monocytosis, and eosinopenia.

Left-shift neutrophilia alongside toxic changes can be present in many but not all inflammatory conditions. Increased C-reactive protein (CRP) can confirm active inflammation in patients without hematological abnormalities; CRP can also be useful for evaluating disease progression and response to treatment.[4]

Overwhelming inflammation or bone marrow damage can lead to neutropenia as can be seen with parvovirosis or salmonellosis.

The neutrophil-to-lymphocyte ratio (NLR) can be a useful clinical marker.

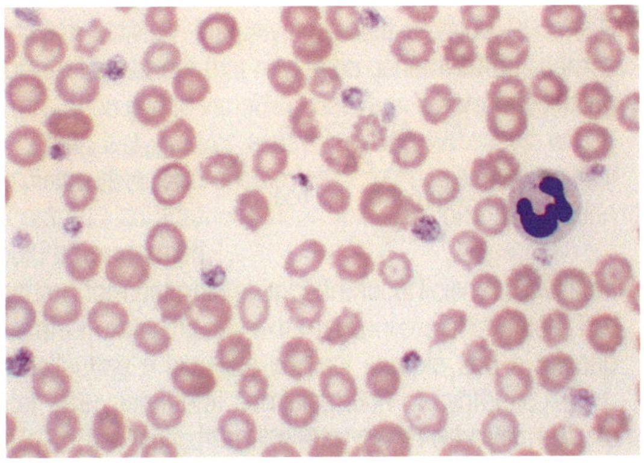

FIG. 18.1 Microcytic hypochromic anemia.

KEY POINTS

- The routine laboratory database is crucial in guiding the diagnostic pathway of canine gastrointestinal disease and excluding other potential causes for the presenting clinical signs.
- Minimum database components include hematology, serum biochemistry, urinalysis, basal cortisol, and ACTH stimulation test.
- Gastrointestinal disease can present with erythrocytosis due to dehydration or with anemia due to chronic disease or blood loss.
- Hypoalbuminemia is commonly associated with protein-losing enteropathy, which can serve as a diagnostic indicator and prognostic factor in dogs with chronic enteropathies.
- The lack of glucocorticoids can negatively impact GI health; thus, hypoadrenocorticism can lead to GI disease.
- Excluding hypoadrenocorticism should be part of the initial investigations in any dog with chronic GI signs.

References

1. Radakovich LB, Santangelo KS, Olver CS. Reticulocyte hemoglobin content does not differentiate true from functional iron deficiency in dogs. *Vet Clin Pathol* 44(4):511–518, 2015.
2. Fuchs J, Moritz A, Grußendorf E, Lechner J, Neuerer F, Nickel R, et al. Canine reticulocyte hemoglobin content (RET-He) in different types of iron-deficient erythropoiesis. *Vet Clin Pathol* 46(3):422–429, 2017.
3. Fuchs J, Moritz A, Grußendorf E, Lechner J, Neuerer F, Nickel R, et al. Evaluation of reticulocyte hemoglobin content (RET-He) in the diagnosis of iron-deficient erythropoiesis in dogs. *Vet Clin Pathol* 46(4):558–568, 2017.
4. Covin MA, Steiner JM. Measurement and clinical applications of C-reactive protein in gastrointestinal diseases of dogs. *Vet Clin Pathol* 50(S1):29–36, 2022.
5. Becher A, Suchodolski JS, Steiner JM, Heilmann RM. Blood neutrophil-to-lymphocyte ratio (NLR) as a diagnostic marker in dogs with chronic enteropathy. *J Vet Diagnostic Investig* 33(3):516–527, 2021.
6. Dinler AC. Neutrophil to lymphocyte ratio as a prognostic biomarker in puppies with acute diarrhea. *J Vet Emerg Crit Care* 32(1):83–89, 2022.
7. Guija-de-Arespacochaga A, Kremer L, Künzel F, Schwendenwein I. Peripheral blood eosinophilia in dogs: prevalence and associated diseases. *Vet Med Sci* 8(4):1458–1465, 2022.
8. Craven M, Simpson JW, Ridyard AE, Chandler ML. Canine inflammatory bowel disease: retrospective analysis of diagnosis and outcome in 80 cases (1995-2002). *J Small Anim Pract* 45(7):336–342, 2004.
9. Marchetti V, Lubas G, Lombardo A, Corazza M, Guidi G, Cardini G. Evaluation of erythrocytes, platelets, and serum iron profile in dogs with chronic enteropathy. *Vet Med Int* 28:2010:716040, 2010.
10. González-Domínguez A, Cristobal-Verdejo JI, López-Espinar C, Fontela-González S, Vázquez S, Justo-Domínguez J, et al. Retrospective evaluation of hematological ratios in canine parvovirosis: 401 cases. *J Vet Intern Med* 38(1):161–166, 2023.
11. Pierini A, Esposito G, Gori E, Benvenuti E, Ruggiero P, Lubas G, et al. Platelet abnormalities and platelet-to-lymphocyte ratios in canine immunosuppressant-responsive and non-responsive enteropathy: A retrospective study in 41 dogs. *J Vet Med Sci* 83(2):248–253, 2021.
12. Allenspach K, Wieland B, Gröne A, Gaschen F. Chronic enteropathies in dogs: evaluation of risk factors for negative outcome. *J Vet Intern Med* 21(4):700-708, 2007.
13. Pena-Ramos J, Barker L, Saiz R, Walker DJ, Tappin S, Hare CHZ, et al. Resting and postprandial serum bile acid concentrations in dogs with liver disease. *J Vet Intern Med* 35(3):1333–1341, 2021.
14. Lyngby JG, Sellon RK. Hypoadrenocorticism mimicking protein-losing enteropathy in 4 dogs. *Can Vet J* 57(7):757–760, 2016.
15. Venco L, Valenti V, Genchi M, Grandi G. A dog with pseudo-Addison disease associated with *Trichuris vulpis* infection. *J Parasitol Res* 2011(Figure 1): 6–8, 2011.
16. Gow AG, Gow DJ, Bell R, Simpson JW, Chandler ML, Evans H, et al. Calcium metabolism in eight dogs with hypoadrenocorticism. *J Small Anim Pract* 50(8):426–430, 2009.
17. Kimmel SE, Waddell LS, Michel KE. Hypomagnesemia and hypocalcemia associated with protein-losing enteropathy in Yorkshire Terriers: five cases (1992–1998). *J Am Vet Med Assoc* 217(5):703–706, 2000.
18. Hauck C, Schmitz SS, Burgener IA, Wehner A, Neiger R, Kohn B, et al. Prevalence and characterization of hypoadrenocorticism in dogs with signs of chronic gastrointestinal disease: A multicenter study. *J Vet Intern Med* 34(4):1399–1405, 2020.
19. Gallego AF, Gow AG, Boag AM. Evaluation of resting cortisol concentration testing in dogs with chronic gastrointestinal signs. *J Vet Intern Med* 36(2):525–531, 2022.
20. Gold AJ, Langlois DK, Refsal KR. Evaluation of basal serum or plasma cortisol concentrations for the diagnosis of hypoadrenocorticism in dogs. *J Vet Intern Med* 30(6):1798–1805, 2016.

CHAPTER 19

Fecal examination

Marta Costa
DVM, MSc, FRCPath, DECVCP, MRCVS

Although macroscopic evaluation of feces can provide information regarding the presence of hematochezia, melena, steatorrhea, mucus, or changes in coloration and consistency (see Section I Diagnostic approach), microscopic or laboratory fecal examination is often more useful in identifying possible underlying causes for gastrointestinal (GI) pathology. Nonetheless, the clinical information and macroscopic appearance of the fecal matter should help narrow down differential diagnoses and guide toward appropriate testing.

A wide variety of pathogens that can cause pathology of the GI tract can be detected on fecal examination. These include parasitic, viral, and bacterial pathogens as well as dysregulation of normal flora or opportunistic growth (dysbiosis). Detection/presence of some of these organisms may be incidental because they may be recovered from asymptomatic animals, and their absence or change in quantity does not always exclude pathology because intermittent excretion, diluted fecal matter in acute profuse diarrheic feces, and excess mucus may lead to false-negative results.

Occasionally, fecal examination is performed to identify the presence of zoonotic agents to assess for a possible source of clinical cases or assess risk for humans. Clinical signs are variable and may not be present, whereas the transmission of pathogens still may occur. This can depend on the site of infection, the underlying etiology, and the immunocompetence of the host, making selection of appropriate testing dependent on presentation and clinical question, and the result may require stepwise or multiple fecal examinations. Fecal examination also may include evaluation of fecal biomarkers, although these are used less commonly in practice and their utility may vary.

Parasitology

Detection of fecal parasites can be made by a variety of techniques, including direct visualization or detection of parasite molecules such as parasite antigens via immunoassays or genetic material using polymerase chain reaction (PCR) tests. It is important to recognize that the detection of antigen or DNA does not provide information regarding viability of the parasite, and these assays can be positive in the face of nonviable pathogens (e.g., immediately after treatment). These assays may be more sensitive in the detection of infection in prepatent infections (i.e. before egg excretion). False-positive results also may occur due to coprophagia or predation. Equally, intermittent excretion, incorrect sample collection and handling, and limitations inherent to each diagnostic technique may lead to false-negative results.

Sampling recommendations

Fecal samples should be collected from the rectum or swiftly after voluntary deposition to prevent contamination from the environment which may contain living nematodes. Samples should not be stored long (and should be stored at 4°C) for traditional fecal parasitology testing, as some eggs and larvae may continue to develop and change their diagnostic characteristics. Older fecal samples also may lead to loss of viability of lungworm and *Strongyloides* larvae for detection by the Baermann technique. Also some *Strongyloides* spp. eggs may hatch and lead to false-negative results. Repeat sampling (e.g., from 3 consecutive days) will increase the sensitivity of coproscopical assays due to intermittent excretion and increasing chances of detection in low-infestation cases. In cases of dilute diarrheic samples, a combined sedimentation–flotation method may increase sensitivity. If evaluation of macroscopic parasites collected from feces, vomit, or other secretions is required, specimens should be preserved in saline solution for short-term storage or in 70% ethanol.

Direct fecal smear

Macroscopic examination for excreted helminths (e.g., roundworms and tapeworm proglottids) should be done in collected fecal specimens. Although of relatively low sensitivity, a fresh direct fecal smear can provide quick and useful information. Unstained wet mounts can allow for identification of parasitic larvae and identify protozoal trophozoites such as *Giardia* spp. and some trichomonads. The type of movement can help differentiate between these ("falling leaves" for *Giardia* spp. vs direct straight movement for trichomonads).

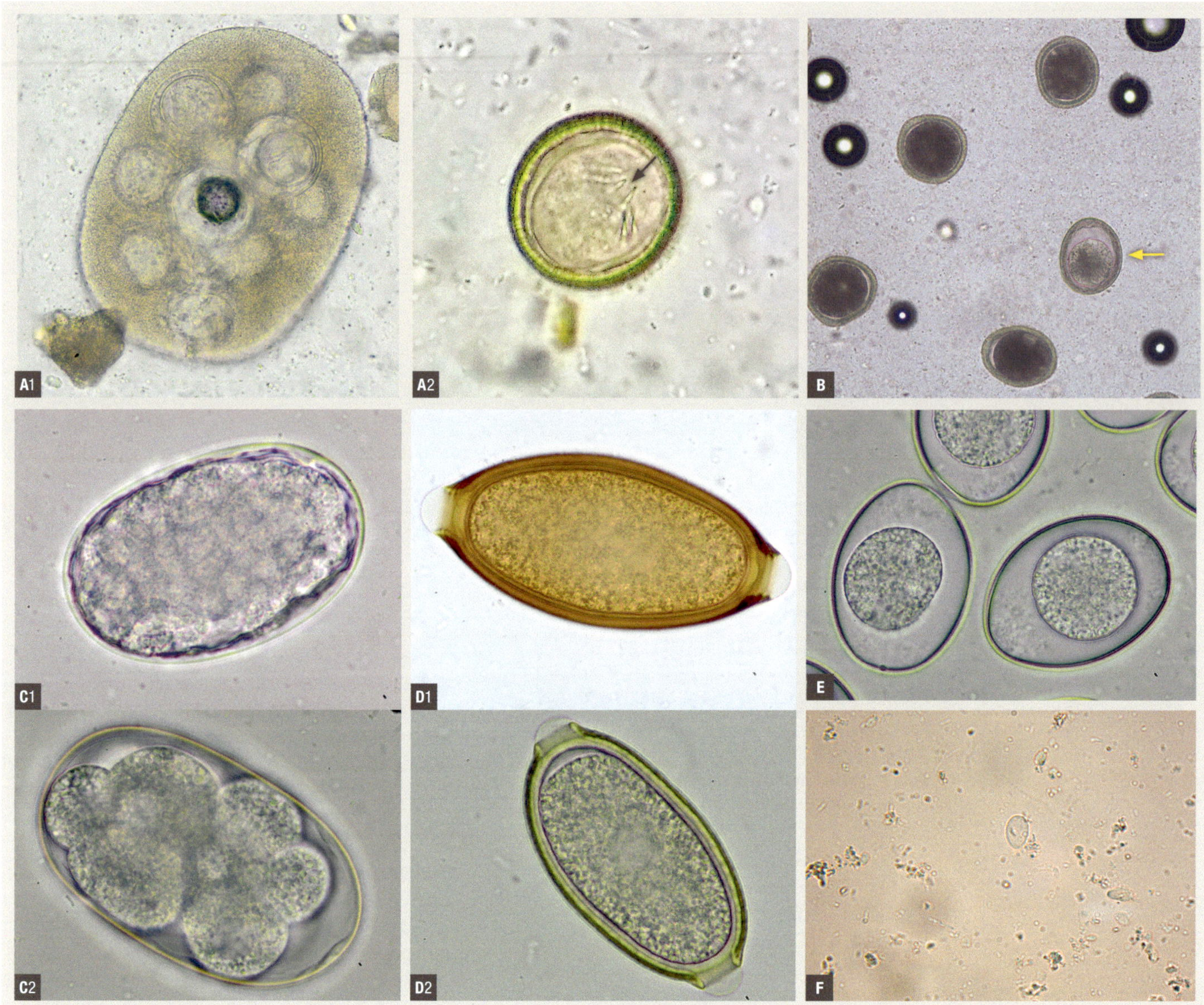

FIG. 19.1 (**A**) Tapeworm (×40): (**A**1) *Dipylidium caninum* egg capsule. Capsules are ~100–300 µm in size with 3–30 eggs; individual eggs are round, ~30–65 µm in diameter, and have a embryophore (shell) containing a hexacanth (six-hooked) embryo. (**A**2) Taeniid eggs are passed individually, measure ~25–40 µm in size, have a thick, radially striated embryophore surrounding an embryo with three pairs of hooks (arrow). *Taenia* spp. and *Echinococcus* spp. are morphologically indistinguishable.

(**B**) Roundworm eggs (×20) from *Toxocara canis* are ~75–90 µm in size, slightly oval, with a rough pitted outer shell wall. *Toxocara catis* also can be found in dogs feces (associated with coprophagia). These are similar to *T. canis* but smaller, ~65–75 µm (size is the main characteristic used for differentiation) with less space between the shell and embryo. *Toxascaris leonina* eggs (arrow) are ~70–80 µm in size with a smooth outer shell, and the embryo takes up less space within the egg.

(**C**) Hookworm eggs (×100), including *Ancylostoma* spp. and *Uncinaria* spp eggs, are ellipsoidal and thin shelled. (**C**1) *Ancylostoma* eggs are ~50–75 µm long and 30–50 µm wide, with (**C**2) *Uncinaria* eggs being larger (up to 90 µm in length). They have a smooth, clear shell and show an embryo in the morula stage with a variable number of divisions.

(**D**) Whipworm eggs (×100) such as (**D**1) *Trichuris* spp. are lemon shaped, ~70–90 µm in length, and 30–40 µm wide, with bipolar plugs. Each egg contains one cell. Capillarids such as *Eucoleus* spp. eggs (**D**2) are similar to *Trichuris* eggs but slightly asymmetrical and smaller in size.

(**E**) *Cystoisospora* spp. (formerly *Isospora*) oocysts (×100) are ovoid, ~30–40 µm in length, and have a thin, double-layered outer wall surrounding a small amount of clear cytoplasm and a single or occasionally double cell (sporont). The sizes of the oocysts range among species, with the larger ones ~40–50 µm long and ~25–35 µm wide, and the smaller coccidia ~15–25 µm × 15–25 µm. If the sporulated oocyst contains four cells, it represents *Eimeria* spp. (which is associated with coprophagia and predation, nonpathogenic for the dog).

(**F**) *Giardia* spp. cysts (×63) are small, ~7 × 10–15 µm in size, with a smooth wall and clear with one to four small, indistinct nuclei and an axostyle (flagella complex) that sometimes can be seen as a line through the length of the cyst.

Images (**A–E**) courtesy of Dr. Simone Manzocchi.

Fecal smears stained with Ziehl–Neelsen, Heine, or safranin stain can facilitate the identification of *Cryptosporidium* spp. oocysts. Immunofluorescent staining methods also increase the sensitivity of detection of *Giardia* and *Cryptosporidium* in fecal smears.

Concentration methods

Several concentrations methods have been described that increase the sensitivity of detection of parasitic worms and eggs. These include a combination of sedimentation and flotation techniques (including centrifugation followed by flotation), combined sedimentation and flotation methods, the Baermann technique, and a number of specific methods (e.g., Flotation Technique for Accurate Cyst Analysis [FLOTAC]). Several salt and sugar solutions can be used for the flotation methods, and although parasite eggs and oocysts can be detected by all methods, some methods may be preferred for specific parasites because they have greater sensitivity. For specific methodologies, readers are referred to the European Scientific Counsel Companion Animal Parasites website[1] and respective manufacturers' instructions. Figure 19.1 shows examples of the most common parasites recovered from dogs. Recently, in-house automated methods of scanning and evaluating coproscopical smears have been assessed and have shown similar sensitivity and specificity to evaluation by specialists.[2–4]

Immunoassays or coproantigen tests

The detection of parasite antigen in feces is of high sensitivity. Different methodologies include a variety of in-house and reference laboratory tests, such as immunofluorescence assays, enzyme-linked immunosorbent assays, or enzyme-based immunoassays and immunochromatographic tests. Because sensitivity is high when compared with coproscopical methods, these assays can detect patients with low parasite burden and single-sex infections, patients with prepatent infection, and patients that are asymptomatic carriers. Recently, antigen tests have become available for roundworms, whipworms, hookworms, flea tapeworms (*Dipylidium* spp.), and *Cystoisospora* spp.[5–7] Many immunoassays have been routinely available for a number of years for veterinary use for the detection of *Giardia* spp. and *Cryptosporidium* spp.

PCR

Molecular techniques are also used in fecal samples for the detection of parasitic infections with high sensitivity. For better sensitivity, fresh feces should be collected, and PCR methods are particularly helpful for the detection of organisms present in low numbers.

Virology

Several tests can be used to detect viral pathogens, including viral culture and electron microscopy. In practice, though, antigenic testing and PCR are the common tests employed. It is important to realize that modified live vaccines can interfere and lead to false-positive results with both modalities, with PCR being affected from days to weeks after vaccination. Most viral enteritis cases are acute and self-limited, but some can be life threatening, particularly in young or immunocompromised patients. The most common viruses tested in feces include parvovirus and coronavirus. Rotavirus is also offered as part of diagnostic panels by many laboratories (see also Chapter 36).

Sensitivity of diagnosis of viral infections (irrespective of method) is highly influenced by the time of sample collection, with false-negative results occurring in both pre- and post-shedding stages. False-negative results also may occur due to the presence of PCR inhibitors in feces. Equally with antigenic assays, in later stages of the infection, antibodies may bind to the viral antigen in feces and block detection in the assay.

Bacteriology

Bacteria are part of the normal fecal flora. Many of the genera and species that are associated with pathology also can be recovered from healthy and asymptomatic animals. Therefore, the significance of these bacteria when isolated is unclear and may be incidental or coinfections. Although many of these organisms may present a zoonotic risk for immunocompromised humans, attempts to eradicate them may not be advisable and can induce chronic carrier states and promote antimicrobial resistance.

Traditionally, evaluations for *Salmonella* spp., *Campylobacter* spp., *Escherichia coli*, *Clostridium perfringens*, *Clostridioides difficile*, and *Yersinia* spp. have been performed on fecal samples. Currently, there are no specific indications for when these bacterial pathogens should be considered significant or incidental. This is particularly more pertinent with PCR evaluation, which is more sensitive than culture. Isolation may be more relevant in patients with acute hemorrhagic diarrhea (particularly if there is evidence of sepsis), if more than one pet is affected, or if immunocompromised humans are at risk (see also Chapter 37).

Salmonella spp.

Salmonella is usually recovered from feces through a combination of enrichment and culture on selective media. Several serotypes can be recovered from canine patients, both in healthy asymptomatic patients and in patients with diarrhea. Dogs fed a raw-meat diet may be at increased risk of *Salmonella* carriage.[8–10] Although there is a zoonotic risk, most human cases of salmonellosis are associated with handling or consumption of contaminated food products.

Campylobacter spp.

There are more than 30 species and subspecies of *Campylobacter* that can be recovered from animal feces, but most are considered nonpathogenic. Several culture methods and sample collections can affect the likelihood of recovering different *Campylobacter* spp. Culture allows for identification up to the genus level, with speciation requiring PCR for some species. Matrix-assisted laser desorption ionization time-of-flight mass spectrometry (MALDI-TOF MS) can identify many *Campylobacter* spp., including *Campylobacter jejuni*, *Campylobacter coli*, and *Campylobacter upsaliensis*. These are the species most frequently recovered from dogs.[11,12]

Because *Campylobacter* spp. can be recovered from both healthy and diarrheic patients, a positive culture may not require antimicrobial treatment (see Chapter 29).

Escherichia coli

E. coli is part of the normal enteric flora and can be recovered by culture from most fecal samples. Some strains carry enteropathogenic virulence factors and can be associated with diarrhea, but these strains have been recovered from patients with and without diarrhea, and their role is poorly defined. Routine culturing of feces for *E. coli* therefore is not recommended.

E. coli have been recovered from tissue biopsies of some patients with granulomatous (histiocytic ulcerative) colitis, especially in Boxers and French bulldogs.[13,14] Evaluation for this should be done with colonic tissue culture, not fecal culture, and followed up by antibacterial sensitivity testing before any treatment (see Chapter 48).

Clostridium perfringens and *Clostridioides difficile*

Clostridia are part of the normal enteric flora from dogs and cats, but certain species may be pathogenic if overgrown or producing toxins. *C. perfringens* and *C. difficile* both have been implicated as pathogenic but also can be recovered from healthy asymptomatic patients. The detection of toxin production by these organisms is a better indication of pathogenic potential. This can be done by enzyme-linked immunosorbent assay detection of the respective toxins or PCR detection of the toxin genes for *C. perfringens* cases, although detection of the toxins does not necessarily correlate with disease.

Yersinia spp.

Yersinia pseudotuberculosis and *Yersinia enterocolitica* are enteropathogenic bacteria with worldwide distribution, and they have zoonotic potential. Dogs often can shed these organisms in feces with no clinical signs. There are occasional case reports of systemic disease in dogs. Culture for *Yersinia* spp. is offered as part of some diagnostic panels but may be of limited use for the diagnosis of chronic diarrhea in dogs.

Dysbiosis index

Dysbiosis refers to an imbalance or disruption in the normal intestinal microbiome that comprises a vast number of microorganisms. An imbalance in the intestinal microbiome has been putatively associated with a variety of conditions in dogs. Assessing this microbiome with culture-based methods is not possible because many of the organisms cannot be cultured, and next-generation sequencing of the whole microbiome is not directly applicable to individual patients.

As a surrogate marker of the microbiome, the *dysbiosis index* (DI) is based on a quantitative PCR-based assay that measures the abundance of seven bacterial taxa (*Fecalibacterium* spp., *Turicibacter* spp., *E. coli*, *Streptococcus* spp., *Blautia* spp., *Fusobacterium* spp., and *Clostridium hiranonis* [now *Peptacetobacter hiranonis*]) that have been demonstrated to be altered in a variety of enteropathies and after broad-spectrum antibiotic use.[15,16] Changes in the DI of bacterial groups are a result of changes in the intestinal environment. The DI calculates a single number that expresses the extent of intestinal dysbiosis present: A negative score is considered healthy, and a DI of ≥ 2 indicates dysbiosis.[15] A higher DI correlates with lower microbial diversity of the evaluated groups.

Causes of dysbiosis include chronic enteropathy, exocrine pancreatic insufficiency, and recent oral antibiotic or proton pump inhibitor (PPI) use. Dysbiosis has been associated with clinical entities that respond to antimicrobial agents, including small intestinal bacterial overgrowth and antibiotic-responsive diarrhea. Idiopathic chronic inflammatory enteropathies also may be associated with dysbiosis, but it is unclear whether this is a cause or a consequence of the changes in the intestine. The DI test is presently only available at a single reference laboratory. This lab currently recommends that the sample should reach the lab cold and fresh, with ~1 g of feces required. Patients should be off treatment with PPIs (for 1–2 weeks) and/or broad-spectrum oral antibiotics such as metronidazole or tylosin (for 2–4 weeks) because these agents have been demonstrated to at least transiently change the DI.[17,18] It is suggested that in addition to screening for dysbiosis, the DI can be used for screening of donors for fecal microbiota transplantation, if the latter is being considered[19] (see Chapter 27). The expanding literature and research into intestinal dysbiosis and DI may provide additional applications for these assays in the future.

Other fecal examination assays

Historically, tests such as quantification of fecal fat and proteolytic activity were used in the diagnosis of GI pathology, but many of these tests are unhelpful or unsuitable for practice. Newer fecal diagnostic tests have been developed, and a number of fecal biomarkers have become available, most of limited clinical use currently. Although not all are widely available, a number of biomarkers have been evaluated in fecal samples and may become useful in the diagnosis and monitoring of GI pathology, particularly chronic canine enteropathies[20,21] (see Chapter 20).

Fecal immunoglobulin A

Fecal immunoglobulin A (IgA) has been evaluated as a presumed reflection of the level of synthesis and secretion from the intestinal mucosa as either a cause or a consequence of GI pathology. Although decreased fecal IgA concentrations may be present in patients with GI pathology, the currently published literature does not lend enough support for the routine diagnostic use of fecal IgA concentrations in dogs.[20]

Fecal α_1-proteinase inhibitor

The presence of α_1-proteinase inhibitor in feces has been shown to be a marker for GI protein loss in the adult dog (>1 year old). It appears to be more sensitive than serum albumin concentration for early disease. Testing of at least three voluntarily evacuated fecal samples within a 48-hour period has been recommended to improve diagnostic accuracy. Abrasion of the colonic wall may lead to false increases of α_1-proteinase inhibitor. If there is hemorrhage into the GI tract, it invalidates the use of this test. This immunoassay is currently only available from a single laboratory in the United States.

Fecal calprotectin

Fecal calprotectin is a noninvasive biomarker for intestinal inflammation that has been evaluated in dogs with intestinal inflammatory diseases. In dogs, increased fecal calprotectin appears to be a useful biomarker of intestinal inflammation and has been associated with disease subclassification in chronic enteropathies, histological changes, and severity of endoscopic lesions. Fecal calprotectin appears to be stable to fecal bacterial degradation and has been shown to have stable concentrations for up to 1 week at room temperature.

Fecal calgranulin

Calgranulin C, a protein complex (S100A12), is stable in feces, and increased fecal concentrations of calgranulin C appear to correlate with clinical signs and endoscopic findings in some intestinal conditions. However, a definitive link to histological findings has not been established. It also may be helpful for monitoring treatment and assessing disease severity in animals with intestinal issues. However, the potential impact of GI neoplasia on fecal calgranulin C levels has not been studied. Fecal calgranulin may be more specific for inflammation than fecal calprotectin, but it is not currently routinely available for testing.[21]

Fecal elastase

Fecal elastase has been used to evaluate for exocrine pancreatic insufficiency, and an assay has been validated for use in dogs. However, it has been shown to have a high rate of false-positive results that limit the clinical utility of this assay.[22]

Fecal occult blood

Fecal occult blood testing is more sensitive than visual evaluation for the presence of blood, particularly in cases of upper GI hemorrhage. In veterinary medicine, most fecal occult blood assays are peroxidase-based guaiac tests. These are most useful in cases of iron-deficiency anemia (anemia with microcytosis and hypochromasia) because chronic GI hemorrhage (due to a variety of underlying causes) is a common cause for iron deficiency in adult animals. These assays are very sensitive[23] but nonspecific. They will detect any heme that is present in the sample, including that derived from diet and muscle. Equally, because they are based on peroxidase activity, they will test positive if the animal ingests or has a diet that is rich in plants with high endogenous peroxidase (e.g., beets, cantaloupe, broccoli, and cauliflower).[24] Hydrolyzed or meat-free diets have been recommended for at least 72 hours before sample collection to prevent false-positive results.[23] Intermittent bleeding may lead to false-negative results.

KEY POINTS

- Fecal examination allows for the detection of parasitic, bacterial, and viral pathogens, as well as assessment of dysbiosis.
- Pathogen significance depends on the clinical presentation, co-infections, and zoonotic risk. Both false negatives and incidental findings may occur. Knowledge of limitations of different techniques helps with interpretation.
- Recovery of some organisms from both healthy controls and patients with diarrhea may challenge their significance.
- Dysbiosis, an imbalance in gut microbiota, can be assessed using the Dysbiosis Index.
- Fecal biomarkers such as calprotectin, α_1-protease inhibitor, and occult blood tests may help evaluate inflammation, protein loss, and GI bleeding.

References

1. European Scientific Counsel Companion Animal Parasites (ESCCAP). Guidelines. GL4: Parasitological diagnosis in cats, dogs and equines [Internet]. 2025 [cited 2025 Feb 18]. Available from: https://www.esccap.org/guidelines/gl4/
2. Kanski S, Busch K, Hailmann R, Weber K. Performance of the Vetscan Imagyst in point-of-care detection of *Giardia duodenalis* in canine fecal samples. *J Vet Diagn Invest.* 37(1):63–70, 2025.
3. Nagamori Y, Scimeca R, Hall-Sedlak R, et al. Multicenter evaluation of the Vetscan Imagyst system using Ocus 40 and EasyScan One scanners to detect gastrointestinal parasites in feces of dogs and cats. *J Vet Diagn Invest.* 36(1):32–40, 2024.
4. Nagamori Y, Sedlak RH, DeRosa A, et al. Further evaluation and validation of the VETSCAN IMAGYST: in-clinic feline and canine fecal parasite detection system integrated with a deep learning algorithm. *Parasit Vectors.* 14(1):89, 2021.
5. Elsemore D, Bezold T, Geng J, et al. Immunoassay for detection of *Dipylidium caninum* coproantigen in dogs and cats. *J Vet Diagn Invest.* 35(6):671–678, 2023.
6. Little SE, Barrett AW, Beall MJ, et al. Coproantigen detection augments diagnosis of common nematode infections in dogs. *Top Companion Anim Med.* 35:42–46, 2019.
7. Little S, Braff J, Duncan K, et al. Diagnosis of canine intestinal parasites: improved detection of *Dipylidium caninum* infection through coproantigen testing. *Vet Parasitol.* 324:110073, 2023.
8. Groat EF, Williams NJ, Pinchbeck G, et al. UK dogs eating raw meat diets have higher risk of *Salmonella* and antimicrobial-resistant *Escherichia coli* faecal carriage. *J Small Anim Pract.* 63(6):435–441, 2022.
9. Joffe DJ, Schlesinger DP. Preliminary assessment of the risk of *Salmonella* infection in dogs fed raw chicken diets. *Can Vet J.* 43(6):441–442, 2002.
10. Solís D, Toro M, Navarrete P, et al. Microbiological quality and presence of foodborne pathogens in raw and extruded canine diets and canine fecal samples. *Front Vet Sci.* 9:799710, 2022.
11. Lemos ML, Nunes A, Ancora M, et al. *Campylobacter jejuni* in different canine populations: characteristics and zoonotic potential. *Microorganisms.* 9(11):2231, 2021.
12. Bessède E, Solecki O, Sifré E, et al. Identification of *Campylobacter* species and related organisms by matrix assisted laser desorption ionization–time

of flight (MALDI-TOF) mass spectrometry. *Clin Microbiol Infect.* 17(11):1735–1739, 2011.

13. Simpson KW, Dogan B, Rishniw M, et al. Adherent and invasive *Escherichia coli* is associated with granulomatous colitis in boxer dogs. *Infect Immun.* 74(8):4778–4792, 2006.
14. Sims CS, Nagle J, Tolbert MK, et al. Correlation of cytology to histology in a case of canine granulomatous colitis in a boxer dog. *Vet Clin Pathol.* 50(suppl 1):83–87, 2022.
15. AlShawaqfeh M, Wajid B, Minamoto Y, et al. A dysbiosis index to assess microbial changes in fecal samples of dogs with chronic inflammatory enteropathy. *FEMS Microbiol Ecol.* 93(11):fix136, 2017.
16. Suchodolski JS. Diagnosis and interpretation of intestinal dysbiosis in dogs and cats. *Vet J.* 215:30–37, 2016.
17. Garcia-Mazcorro JF, Suchodolski JS, Jones KR, et al. Effect of the proton pump inhibitor omeprazole on the gastrointestinal bacterial microbiota of healthy dogs. *FEMS Microbiol Ecol.* 80(3): 624–636, 2012.
18. Pilla R, Gaschen FP, Barr JW, et al. Effects of metronidazole on the fecal microbiome and metabolome in healthy dogs. *J Vet Intern Med.* 34(5):1853–1866, 2020.
19. Toresson L, Spillmann T, Pilla R, et al. Clinical effects of faecal microbiota transplantation as adjunctive therapy in dogs with chronic enteropathies—a retrospective case series of 41 dogs. *Vet Sci.* 10(4):271, 2023.
20. Heilmann RM, Steiner JM. Clinical utility of currently available biomarkers in inflammatory enteropathies of dogs. *J Vet Intern Med.* 32(5):1495–1508, 2018
21. Jergens AE, Heilmann RM. Canine chronic enteropathy—current state-of-the-art and emerging concepts. *Front Vet Sci.* 9:923013, 2022.
22. Steiner JM, Rehfeld JF, Pantchev N. Evaluation of fecal elastase and serum cholecystokinin in dogs with a false positive fecal elastase test: fecal elastase concentration. *J Vet Intern Med.* 24(3):643–646, 2010.
23. Pierini A, Bartoletti F, Lubas G, et al. The guaiac-based fecal occult blood test in healthy dogs: evaluation of the effects of diet, and the ability of the test to detect fecal occult blood. *Vet Clin Pathol.* 49(1):71–77, 2020.
24. Cook AK, Gilson SD, Fischer WD, Kass PH. Effect of diet on results obtained by use of two commercial test kits for detection of occult blood in feces of dogs. *Am J Vet Res.* 53(10):1749–1751, 1992.

CHAPTER 20

Biomarkers

Linda Toresson
DVM, Swedish Spec. Small Anim. Intern Med, PhD

Edward Hall
MA, VetMB, PhD, DECVIM-CA, FRCVS

Functional biomarkers

Linda Toresson

A *biomarker* is a naturally occurring molecule, enzyme, or gene found in blood, other bodily fluids, or tissue that can be measured objectively as an indicator of a pathogenic process or normality. Currently, in canine gastrointestinal (GI) disease, in addition to the minimum database (see Chapter 18), the biomarkers that are most useful clinically and readily available to practitioners are the functional biomarkers serum cobalamin and folate because they not only identify intestinal dysfunction, but any deficiencies also indicate the need for supplementation.

Cobalamin

Cobalamin (vitamin B_{12}) is a water-soluble vitamin that all cells in the mammalian body require for cell metabolism (Fig. 20.1). Long-standing GI disorders can lead to malabsorption and cobalamin deficiency, which can be associated with several clinical and metabolic consequences. Assessment of cobalamin status is an essential part of the investigation and treatment of dogs with chronic GI diseases.

Transport and metabolism in health

Cobalamin is ingested bound to dietary protein. In the stomach, the cobalamin is released from the dietary protein by pepsinogen and gastric acid. Cobalamin is then bound to haptocorrin (also named *R protein*), from which it is released in the duodenum when it binds to intrinsic factor (IF). IF is produced by the exocrine pancreas and the gastric mucosa in dogs. The cobalamin–IF complex is transported to the ileum, where specific cubam receptors are located. These receptors recognize the cobalamin–IF complex, which is absorbed via endocytosis.

In people, an alternative absorptive pathway exists where ~1% of dietary cobalamin is absorbed via passive diffusion across the small intestinal mucosa independent of IF.[1] This mechanism likely occurs in dogs too, which could explain why oral cobalamin is effective in treating cobalamin deficiency in dogs with chronic enteropathy (CE) and exocrine pancreatic insufficiency (EPI). After ileal absorption, cobalamin is bound to transcobalamin (TC) I and II in the circulation. Only cobalamin bound to TC II is available for uptake by body tissues. The major storage site for cobalamin is the liver, and its half-life in healthy dogs is 4 months.

When cobalamin enters the cells, conversion to adenosylcobalamin and methylcobalamin occurs. Adenosylcobalamin is required as a cofactor for methylmalonyl-CoA mutase within the mitochondrion, converting l-methylmalonyl-CoA to succinyl-CoA (Fig. 20.1). When intracellular cobalamin deficiency occurs, methylmalonyl-CoA accumulates within the mitochondrion and is converted to methylmalonic acid (MMA). An increased serum MMA concentration thus is a marker for intracellular cobalamin deficiency. Methylcobalamin is required for conversion of homocysteine to methionine within the cytoplasm. Thus, in cobalamin deficiency, homocysteine can accumulate.

Cobalamin deficiency in GI disorders

The most common GI disorders associated with cobalamin deficiency in dogs are CE and EPI. The reported prevalence of cobalamin deficiency is 19–38% in CE and 74–83% in EPI.[2] Cobalamin deficiency also has been reported in dogs with other GI disorders (Table 20.1). Suggested mechanisms behind cobalamin deficiency in canine CE include malabsorption secondary to decreased expression of ileal mucosal receptors, receptor dysfunction, increased tissue demand for cobalamin in CE, decreased half-life of cobalamin in CE, and/or dysbiosis, but the exact mechanisms are still unknown. The previous belief of decreased expression of cubam receptors in CE has been challenged in a very recent study in which the authors found an increased expression of cubam receptors in dogs with chronic inflammatory enteropathy (CIE) compared with healthy dogs.[3]

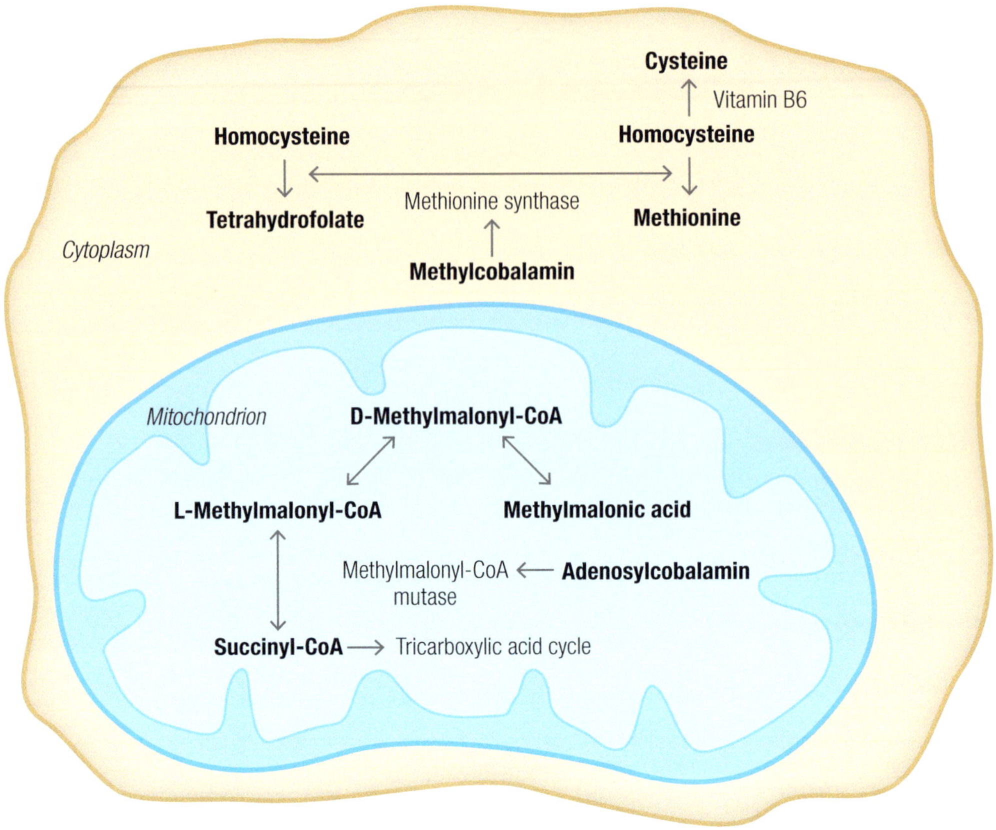

FIG. 20.1 Role of cobalamin in intracellular metabolic pathways.

Dysbiosis could contribute to hypocobalaminemia by bacterial competition for cobalamin, leaving less cobalamin available for absorption by the host, because several bacterial taxa also require cobalamin. Studies investigating the association between small intestinal bacterial overgrowth, based on culture of bacterial juice, and cobalamin deficiency have provided mixed results, showing everything from a good to no correlation between small intestinal bacterial overgrowth and cobalamin deficiency.[4–6] Because most bacterial species in the canine intestinal microbiota are anaerobes and very difficult to culture, studies based on bacterial culture are not optimal to assess intestinal dysbiosis. In a recent study using 16S rRNA sequencing, the intestinal microbiota were compared among dogs with CE and cobalamin deficiency versus dogs with CE and normocobalaminenia and healthy dogs.[7] Dogs with cobalamin deficiency were also analyzed after oral or parenteral cobalamin supplementation. Dogs with CE and cobalamin deficiency had significant dysbiosis compared with both dogs with CE and normocobalaminemia and healthy dogs. After 3 months of cobalamin supplementation, the microbiome changes between the groups were unaltered, suggesting that cobalamin deficiency may not have been the underlying cause for dysbiosis.

In exocrine pancreatic insufficiency, the pancreatic synthesis of IF is reduced or absent, contributing to cobalamin deficiency. Several other mechanisms are suggested to contribute, including decreased synthesis of digestive enzymes, potentially causing diminished release of cobalamin from haptocorrin and insufficient amounts of cobalamin available for binding to IF; dysbiosis; altered pH due to decreased release of bicarbonate from the exocrine pancreas; and mucosal damage due to malabsorption and altered luminal content.

In alimentary and multicentric lymphoma with presumed intestinal involvement, the proposed mechanism behind cobalamin deficiency is neoplastic infiltration of the ileal mucosa, impairing the receptor-mediated absorption of cobalamin.[8]

Congenital cobalamin malabsorption has been associated with mutations of the genes encoding the cubilin or amnionless subunits of the cubam receptors in Australian Shepherds, Beagles, Border Collies, Giant Schnauzers, and Komondors, resembling Imerslund–Gräsbeck syndrome in people.[2] In affected dogs, signs typically presents during the first year of life and include lethargy, failure to thrive, anorexia, poor body condition score (BCS), vomiting, diarrhea, and sometimes seizures and hyperammonemic encephalopathy. Familial cobalamin deficiency also has been described in Chinese shar peis, with a genetic defect localized to chromosome 13.[2] Affected shar peis show

TABLE 20.1 Diseases associated with cobalamin deficiency.

Gastrointestinal	Non-gastrointestinal
■ Exocrine pancreatic insufficiency ■ Chronic enteropathy ■ Alimentary lymphoma ■ Intestinal dysbiosis ■ Intestinal parasites ■ Short-bowel syndrome	■ Dietary deficiency* ■ Multicentric lymphoma ■ Congenital selective cobalamin malabsorption (Imerslund–Gräsbeck syndrome)

* No naturally occurring cases in dogs have been published.

clinical signs of CE and have a later onset of the disease than in the above-mentioned breeds.

Recent studies have shown decreased serum cobalamin concentrations in some dogs with acute gastroenteritis including parvovirosis. However, MMA concentrations were not different from those in healthy dogs, suggesting that intracellular cobalamin deficiency did not exist.[9]

Indications for cobalamin assessment

- Dogs with a history of chronic GI disease or pancreatic insufficiency.
- Young dogs of breeds known for congenital cobalamin deficiency with compatible clinical signs.

Diagnosing cobalamin deficiency

In people, there is no single perfect test to diagnose cobalamin deficiency. Consequently, diagnosis requires findings of subnormal serum concentrations and alterations in one additional biomarker of cobalamin deficiency, such as homocysteine (HCY), MMA, or holotranscobalamin. The latter measures cobalamin bound to TC II, which represents the biologically active form of cobalamin available in the circulation.

Several studies have been published on MMA and HCY in cobalamin deficiency in dogs. However, it is very likely that, as in human medicine, there is no single perfect test to diagnose cobalamin deficiency in veterinary medicine.

Serum cobalamin analysis

Serum cobalamin concentration is the standard initial routine diagnostic test to diagnose cobalamin deficiency in dogs because of the low cost, wide availability, and excellent stability of stored samples. The routinely used method is an automated chemiluminescence-based immunoassay.[2] The major disadvantage is that serum cobalamin concentrations do not assess intracellular cobalamin status and do not necessarily correlate with intracellular markers of cobalamin deficiency, such as MMA or HCY. Furthermore, serum cobalamin concentrations represent the total pool of cobalamin in the circulation, both the biologically available cobalamin bound to TC II and the unavailable cobalamin bound to TC I.

Serum cobalamin concentrations can be false negative or false positive in people and dogs. In one study, 12% of dogs with normal serum cobalamin concentrations had increased MMA concentrations, suggesting that these dogs may have intracellular cobalamin deficiency despite normal cobalamin concentrations.[10] When only dogs in the low end of the reference interval (RI), that is, 185–258 pmol/L, were studied, 19% had supranormal serum MMA concentrations. Of the dogs with serum cobalamin concentrations below the RI, 46% had serum MMA concentrations above the reference range. Consequently, 54% of dogs with serum cobalamin concentrations below the RI did not have evidence of intracellular cobalamin deficiency.

MMA analysis

In people, serum or urinary MMA above the RI is considered a more specific test for cobalamin deficiency than serum cobalamin or HCY concentrations. False-positive MMA results can occur in patients with renal disease, hemoconcentration, or intestinal dysbiosis. Even subclinical renal disease can cause a false increase in MMA, which stresses the importance of analyzing serum creatinine concentrations in all patients subject to MMA analysis. MMA is analyzed with gas chromatography–mass spectrometry or liquid chromatography–tandem mass spectrometry assay, and serum or urinary MMA analyses are currently only available in research settings. Increased serum MMA concentrations have been reported in 25–52% of dogs with CE and serum cobalamin concentrations below the RI.

If cobalamin deficiency can neither be excluded nor confirmed in people, a significant decrease in serum MMA concentration after cobalamin supplementation indicates preclinical deficiency. This is sometimes the only method to diagnose cobalamin deficiency. Similar observations have been made in a study in dogs with serum cobalamin concentrations at the end of or below the RI. At baseline, 75% of the dogs had serum MMA concentrations within the RI, but a significant decrease in serum MMA was found after 1 month of cobalamin supplementation.[11] The decrease in MMA suggests early cobalamin deficiency. MMA is a fairly stable compound, with accurate concentrations remaining in samples left unprocessed at room temperature for 24 hours and in serum samples left at room temperature for 8 days.

HCY analysis

Cobalamin is required as a cofactor for methionine synthase, which catalyzes the conversion of HCY to methionine in the cytosol (Fig. 20.1). If intracellular cobalamin deficiency occurs, this conversion may not take place, and HCY can accumulate. Supranormal HCY concentrations have direct toxic effects on neurons and endothelial cells in people and have been linked to, *inter alia*, thrombotic and vascular disease. Increased HCY concentrations are regarded as less specific for cobalamin deficiency than MMA because HCY also increases in response to deficiencies of folate (B_9), riboflavin (B_2), and pyridoxine (B_6). False-positive HCY results can occur in people with renal disease or hypothyroidism. Because HCY is mostly bound to albumin in the circulation, false-negative results can occur in conditions associated with hypoalbuminemia. HCY is very sensitive to delayed separation of blood cells from serum, causing false-positive results.

HCY, analyzed with the gas chromatography–mass spectrometry method in dogs, is mainly available in research settings. Increased HCY concentrations have been shown to correlate strongly with subnormal serum cobalamin concentrations in dogs with congenital cobalamin deficiencies. The biomarker appears less useful in dogs with CE. Only four of 35 dogs with CE and low serum cobalamin concentrations had increased HCY concentrations in one study.[11] In another study, HCY concentrations were similar in healthy greyhounds and greyhounds with cobalamin deficiency.[2] Homocysteine thus is regarded as a less useful marker in canine CE.

Interpretation of test results

- *Hypercobalaminemia* is defined as cobalamin concentrations above the RI. It has been associated with malignancies and renal and hepatic disorders in people and cats. The finding is less common in dogs.[2] Of the dogs with hypercobalaminemia, most had GI disorders. However, the most common reason to analyze serum cobalamin concentration is clinical signs of GI disorders, which may have resulted in a skewed population. In a recent retrospective case-control study, dogs with hypercobalaminemia were not more likely to have concurrent neoplastic disorders at baseline versus the control group or to develop neoplastic disorders over time.[12] Pancreatitis and hyperproteinemia were more common in hypercobalaminemic dogs. Chronic inflammatory disorders with increased protein synthesis potentially could result in increased production of cobalamin carrier proteins. MMA or HCY has not been analyzed in dogs with hypercobalaminemia.

- *Normocobalaminemia* is defined as serum cobalamin, MMA, and HCY concentrations within the RI. Cobalamin supplementation is generally not required in dogs when results are within the RI. However, in two studies, some dogs with serum cobalamin concentrations within the low end of the RI had increased serum MMA concentrations and/or serum MMA concentrations within the RI that significantly decreased over time after cobalamin supplementation.[10,11] This likely represents early cobalamin deficiency, resembling preclinical cobalamin deficiency in people, and supports supplementation of cobalamin in dogs at the low end of the RI. Different recommendations on when to start cobalamin supplementation are available, but the cutoff when supplementation should be started has not been defined. The author typically starts supplementation when the serum cobalamin concentration is within the lowest 10–15% of the RI.
- *Hypocobalaminemia* is defined as serum cobalamin concentrations below the RI but still measurable. MMA and HCY can be within or above the RI. This group of dogs should be supplemented with cobalamin.
- *Cobalamin deficiency* is defined as an undetectable serum cobalamin concentration. Serum MMA concentrations should be increased, and serum HCY concentrations should be within or above the RI. Urgent cobalamin supplementation is required in this group of dogs.

Clinical implications

In all dogs with hypocobalaminemia or cobalamin deficiency, serum trypsin-like immunoreactivity (TLI) should be measured. It can be impossible to differentiate clinical signs of CE from EPI, so it must be ruled out to facilitate the appropriate treatment of these dogs.

In dogs with congenital cobalamin malabsorption, as well as clinical signs already described, clinicopathological findings include normocytic nonregenerative anemia, neutropenia, hypoglycemia, hyperammonemia, hypoproteinemia, methylmalonic aciduria, and mild proteinuria. All changes are reversible with cobalamin supplementation except proteinuria.

Clinical signs of cobalamin deficiency in older dogs are often difficult to distinguish from the underlying disorder causing cobalamin deficiency. Inadequate response to concurrent treatment for CE has been suggested in dogs with cobalamin deficiency. The author's clinical impression is that mild lethargy, poor coat quality, and suboptimal BCS are often found in dogs with cobalamin deficiency despite treatment for the underlying condition. In cobalamin-deficient cats, improved appetite, BCS and decreased GI disease activity have been proven after cobalamin supplementation. Similar studies have not been performed in dogs.

Prognostic value

Cobalamin deficiency has been associated with a negative prognosis in dogs with CE, EPI, and multicentric lymphoma.[2,8]

Folate

Folate (vitamin B_9) is an essential water-soluble vitamin that is involved in numerous intracellular reactions as a cofactor, including DNA and RNA synthesis and protein metabolism. *Folate* is a generic term for naturally occurring folates in food, dietary supplements, and fortified foods including folic acid, which is the synthetic form. A wide variety of foods naturally contain folate, but it is especially abundant in raw green leafy vegetables, fruits (in particular citrus), and legumes. Clinical signs of folate deficiency in people include megaloblastic anemia, fetal neural tube defects, fatigue, oral ulcerations, and neurological signs. In dogs, the clinical effects of folate deficiency are poorly described.

Transport and metabolism in health

Folate is mainly available as tetrahydrofolate (THF) in the diet. Absorption of folate mainly takes place in the proximal small intestine, but there is also evidence of ileal absorption in dogs.[13] Folate is mainly absorbed as folate monoglutamate via the proton-coupled folate transporter on the brush border membrane. An alternative transport system via passive diffusion also occurs when high luminal concentrations of folate are present. A minor amount of folate can be absorbed in the colon in several mammals, including humans and possibly also dogs.[14] Within the epithelial cells, folate monoglutamate is metabolized to THF and further converted to methyl THF or formyl THF. Then THF enters the bloodstream. Folate is transported predominantly within the red blood cells. Unlike cobalamin, folate can enter and exit cells via several different transporters. Additionally, many bacterial species of the intestinal microbiota can synthesize folate, which also can be absorbed and used by the host.

Folate in GI disorders

Both serum folate concentrations above and below the RI have been reported in canine GI disorders. The proposed mechanism of hypofolatemia is malabsorption due to small intestinal inflammation, impairing the absorptive capacity. The reported prevalence of hypofolatemia in dogs with CE has varied from 1% to 14%. In one recent study, hypofolatemia was actually more common in 95 non-CE dogs than 99 CE dogs (20 and 8 %, respectively).[15] Multiple studies have shown a higher prevalence of hypocobalaminemia than hypofolatemia in CE.

Hyperfolatemia has been reported in dogs with CE and EPI. Increased serum folate concentrations also have been shown in dogs with small intestinal bacterial overgrowth diagnosed with bacterial culture of duodenal juice, but the sensitivity and specificity have been variable.

In cobalamin deficiency, serum folate concentrations can be falsely increased due to the *folate trap*. Cobalamin deficiency can cause decreased enzymatic conversion of 5-methylhydrofolate to THF because methionine synthase needs cobalamin as a cofactor (Fig. 20.1). Serum concentrations of folate then may be normal or high, but this is mostly 5-methylhydrofolate and not biologically active THF. In situations such as the folate trap and parallel folate malabsorption, folate deficiency may not be apparent until cobalamin has been supplemented, allowing trapped folate to be converted and used.

In EPI, most dogs have increased serum folate concentrations. Dysbiosis is very prevalent in dogs with EPI, which may explain the hyperfolatemia.

Methodology

The most common diagnostic tool for folate assessment is the serum folate concentration by automated chemiluminescence assays. Folate is sensitive to preanalytical errors such as delayed separation of whole blood or prolonged storage at room temperature. Hemolysis is associated with falsely increased serum folate concentrations in people but not in a very recent study in dogs.[15]

Interpretation of test results

- *Hypofolatemia* can be found in some dogs with malabsorption as well as in samples exposed to prolonged storage at room temperature. Treatment studies of hypofolatemia in dogs are lacking. According to personal (unpublished) experience, mildly decreased serum folate concentrations can normalize by treatment of the underlying condition, such as successful dietary trials in many dogs. The author recommends supplementation with folate in moderate to severe deficiency.
- *Hyperfolatemia* is indicative of CE with dysbiosis, EPI, vitamin supplementation, or the folate trap. Older recommendations to treat hyperfolatemic dogs with antibiotics for small intestinal bacterial overgrowth are not valid for several reasons, including lack of randomized, controlled trials, to maintain good antimicrobial stewardship and to avoid the negative impact of antibiotics on the intestinal microbiome.

Clinical implications and prognostic value

Studies on the clinical effects of folate deficiency are lacking in dogs. Megaloblastic anemia is a well-described sequela to folate deficiency in people but not in dogs.[16] Nonregenerative anemia is a well-known consequence of cobalamin or folate deficiencies in humans but is not recognized in hypocobalaminemic or hypofolatemic dogs. Establishment of relationships between hypocobalaminemia or hypofolatemia and hematologic disease would encourage vitamin B testing, and potentially supplementation, in anemic dogs.

Neither hypofolatemia nor hyperfolatemia has been associated with a negative prognosis in dogs with CE or EPI. In summary, folate is a marker of GI disease but less specific and apparently less important than cobalamin.

Indirect biomarkers

Edward Hall, Linda Toresson

Many indirect biomarkers are being developed and validated. They are generally considered research tools, although some are now available commercially.[17]

Genomic biomarkers

Genetic tests

Whole-genome sequencing is a research tool for identifying mutations associated with specific diseases that can lead to development of a DNA test for a specific disease. Genetic tests for inherited cobalamin deficiency (Imerslund–Gräsbeck syndrome; see above) and congenital megaesophagus in German shepherds, a sex-differentiated trait due to a mutation in the melanin-concentrating hormone receptor 2 gene, are available.[18]

Identification of single-nucleotide polymorphisms can help to explain differences in susceptibility or resistance to disease among individual dogs. For example, single-nucleotide polymorphisms in the genes for the toll-like receptors TLR4 and TLR5 have been demonstrated in dogs with CIE.[19]

MicroRNA (miR)

Transcriptomics is the study of the expression, structure, function, and regulation of all RNA molecules in a cell or organism. It is a research tool, but analysis of the expression of a subset of RNA molecules, miRs, may be useful clinically. They are small, highly conserved noncoding RNA molecules involved in the regulation of gene expression and are abundant and stable in body fluids including feces.[20] Alterations in the pattern of their expression may be markers of disease.[21] For example, canine intestinal T-cell lymphoma biopsies show downregulation of miR-192, -194, -141, and -203, whereas miR20b, -18b, and -363 are upregulated. Circulating miR-20b is a potential biomarker for distinguishing GI cancer from CIE in dogs.[22]

Damage biomarkers

Serum pepsinogen A

Pepsinogens are proenzymes secreted by the gastric mucosa. Their serum concentrations in people reflect gastric damage. Increased concentrations have been demonstrated in dogs with gastric dilatation–volvulus.[23]

Alpha-1 proteinase inhibitor (α_1PI)

Measurement of radioactivity in feces after intravenous administration of $^{51}CrCl_3$ to label serum albumin was used historically to identify protein-losing enteropathies (PLEs). Because this test involves radioactivity and is not a true biomarker, it has been abandoned, although it is still the "gold standard" test for PLEs by which the α_1PI test has been validated. Formerly known as alpha-1 antitrypsin, α_1PI is a serum antiproteinase that, when found in feces, is indicative of a PLE.[24] Low serum concentrations also have been described in PLEs, but fecal concentrations were superior for diagnostic purposes and reflected the severity of intestinal crypt abscessation or lacteal dilation.[25]

This biomarker has the same molecular size as albumin and is estimated to be lost into the feces at the same rate as albumin in PLEs. However, because it is an antiproteinase, it resists digestion and is passed whole, whereas albumin is digested and can only be measured indirectly using a radiolabel tracer.

However, fecal α_1PI is not very helpful when the diagnosis of a PLE is obvious because clinical signs (e.g., ascites and diarrhea) and severe hypoalbuminemia are already present. The serum-fecal canine α_1PI ratio has an improved accuracy in hypoalbuminemic dogs.

The fecal test alone is more useful in detecting a PLE during early, subclinical disease, particularly when screening breeds at risk of PLE, such as Norwegian Lundehunds, and for monitoring response to treatment. However, the test requires three spontaneously passed fecal samples, which must not contain any blood. Samples must not be obtained by digital rectal evacuation because any rectal trauma and bleeding will result in a false-positive test. Currently, the test is only available in North America.

Metabolic markers

Metabolomics and proteomics

Metabolomics is the comprehensive measurement of all metabolites and low-molecular-weight molecules in mammalian and microbial specimens. *Proteomics* is the study of the structure and function of all the proteins, the proteome, in biological systems, including their actions and interactions. They are research tools that are helping to elucidate the interaction of the microbiome, intestine, and whole body and have been applied to dogs with intestinal diseases and their microbiomes. For example, decreased plasma tryptophan is a marker in PLEs.[26] Measurements of specific metabolites, such as MMA and HCY, related to cobalamin deficiency were discussed earlier.

Vitamin D

Hypovitaminosis D is a fairly common finding in canine chronic enteropathies and may be part of the reason for ionized hypocalcemia in some PLEs.[27,28] What is not clear is whether vitamin D deficiency is a risk factor for chronic enteropathies, perhaps because it affects immunocompetency, or whether it is merely a marker of malabsorption. Nevertheless, hypovitaminosis D has been shown to be a negative prognostic factor in PLEs.[29]

Microbiome biomarkers

Microbiome analysis

Next-generation sequencing and bioinformatic analysis of bacterial 16S rRNA have allowed characterization of the diversity and relative abundance of bacterial populations, and when applied to feces, they provide some indication of intestinal health. This methodology has been used in dogs as a research tool, but testing is becoming available commercially, although how results should be interpreted is not clear because the lack of standardization and high interassay variability are associated with low reproducibility.

Dysbiosis index

Intestinal dysbiosis is defined as an unhealthy change in the normal microbial ecology of the intestine and includes decreases in microbial richness and diversity, loss of beneficial bacterial groups, blooms of intestinal pathogens, and alterations in the metabolic functions and end products of the microbiota. Alterations in the microbiome probably occur in most intestinal diseases In CIEs there tends to be a decrease of Faecalibacterium and *Peptacetobacter hiranonis* (formerly *Clostridium hiranonis*), an increase of Enterobacteriaceae, and a loss of diversity.

The dysbiosis index (DI) is a validated method, now available commercially, that assesses the relative abundance of nine key fecal bacteria (total fecal bacteria, *Turicibacter* spp., *Blautia* spp., *Fusobacterium* spp., *Bifidobacterium* spp., *Bacteroides* spp., *Peptacetobacter hiranonis*, *Streptococcus* spp., and *Escherchia coli*) in canine fecal samples, giving a numerical score for the degree of dysbiosis.[30] *Peptacetobacter hiranonis* appears to be a critical component of a healthy intestinal microbiome, being responsible for the conversion of primary to secondary bile acids.[31]

Healthy animals typically have a negative DI score, whereas DI numbers >2 are indicative of dysbiosis. Proton pump inhibitors have been shown to induce a dysbiosis, with an increased DI score, but the score generally normalizes within 2–4 weeks of stopping treatment.[32] Antibacterials, especially metronidazole, may produce either a temporary or permanent dysbiosis[33] (see Chapter 29). Recent research suggests that a high DI score is associated with a less favorable response to treatment with probiotics or fecal microbiota transplantation (see Chapters 26 and 27). Current research suggests that a persistently high DI score and low *P. hiranonis* abundance may be associated with bile acid diarrhea.

Urinary nitrosonaphthol

This rarely used test measures the urinary excretion of 4-hydroxyphenylacetic acid and related compounds as a marker of bacterial metabolism in the intestine.[34]

Inflammatory biomarkers

C-reactive protein

This is an acute-phase protein produced by the liver in response to inflammation of any kind. Finding an increased serum C-reactive protein (CRP) concentration is a sensitive but nonspecific marker of inflammation. It may suggest intestinal inflammation if it is increased in conjunction with intestinal signs, but it does not indicate the cause or type of inflammation. The Canine Inflammatory Bowel Disease Activity Index has been shown to be correlated with serum CRP concentrations.[35] However, results may not be reliable if the dog has a PLE because CRP may be lost in feces. Fecal CRP can be measured, but there are better fecal markers of inflammation.

Fecal calprotectin

Calprotectin is a protein dimer (S100A8/A9) from the S100 calcium- and zinc-binding protein family. It is expressed mainly by neutrophils but also by activated macrophages and epithelial cells. It presents a ligand for TLR4 in inflammation and is classed as a damage-associated molecular pattern molecule. Calprotectin expression has been shown to be increased in inflamed canine intestinal biopsies.[36] Serum calprotectin concentrations are also increased in CIEs.[37]

The presence of calprotectin in feces is a consequence of neutrophil migration into intestinal tissue and is a biomarker for intestinal inflammation. It is resistant to pancreatic enzymes, intestinal proteases, and bacterial degradation; distributes homogeneously within stool; and is stable for up to 1 week at room temperature.

Measurement of fecal calprotectin has been validated in dogs as a marker of intestinal inflammation correlating with the Canine Chronic Enteropathy Clinical Activity Index score and histologic severity.[38,39] A validated assay is available commercially in several countries.

Fecal calgranulin C

Calgranulin C (S100A12) is another molecule in the S100 protein family. It is released primarily from activated neutrophils and binds to several innate immune receptors, including RAGE, the receptor for advanced glycation end products, having a role in innate and acquired immune responses. Again, measurement of fecal calgranulin C is a marker of intestinal inflammation.[40] It may be superior to the fecal calprotectin assay because it is not affected by corticosteroid treatment and may distinguish dogs with nonresponsive or immunosuppressant-responsive enteropathy from those with food-responsive enteropathy.

Neutrophil–lymphocyte ratio

A change in the neutrophil–lymphocyte ratio is a totally nonspecific indicator of disease. It may be altered in inflammatory enteropathies and may have use as a prognostic marker and method of monitoring the response to treatment.[41–43] However, one study indicated that the monocyte–lymphocyte ratio may be a better discriminator of CIEs than the neutrophil–lymphocyte ratio.[44]

N-Methylhistamine

A metabolite of histamine and serum, both urinary and fecal *N*-methylhistamines have been proposed as markers for mast cell activation in intestinal inflammation.[45] However, results did not correlate with histologic findings nor disease activity indices.[46]

3-Bromotyrosine

A stable by-product of eosinophil peroxidase activity, 3-bromotyrosine in serum or urine may be a marker of eosinophilic disease, including eosinophilic enteritis.[47]

Immunologic biomarkers

Measurements of cytokines and chemokines, including soluble RAGE molecules, and their underlying messenger RNA expression are research tools that have helped elucidate the mechanism of intestinal inflammation but are not used clinically.

Immunoglobulin A

Secretory immunoglobulin A (IgA) is the main mucosal protective antibody in the GI tract, and IgA deficiency has been incriminated in some canine enteropathies. While absolute IgA deficiency in people predisposes them to intestinal (and other) infections, absolute IgA deficiency has not been proven in dogs. Studies have indicated a relative deficiency of serum IgA in German shepherds with enteropathies.[48] Yet, serum concentrations do not necessarily correlate with mucosal IgA secretion, and measurement of fecal IgA has not shown absolute IgA deficiency.[49] German shepherds do express a specific allotype of IgA, but this does not correlate with intestinal disease.[50]

Anti-gliadin antibodies

Human celiac patients express antibodies to tissue transglutaminase that crossreact with gliadin, which is the immunogenic component of wheat gluten. There are now commercially available assays for tissue transglutaminase and IgA autoantibodies to gliadin as markers of gluten sensitivity, as demonstrated in gluten-sensitive paroxysmal dyskinesia of Border Terriers. However, no studies have yet shown that dogs with CIE that are antibody positive necessarily respond to a gluten-free diet.

Perinuclear anti-neutrophilic cytoplasmic antibodies

This marker is an autoantibody that stains material around the nucleus of a neutrophil and is found in some CIEs and other immune-mediated diseases in dogs. A survey of Soft Coated Wheaten Terriers in the United Kingdom found that ~21% were positive for perinuclear anti-neutrophilic cytoplasmic antibodies, with a significant association with dogs suffering a PLE.[51] A sensitivity of 0.34 and a specificity of 0.86 have been reported for dogs with CIE.[52] A commercially available anti-neutrophilic cytoplasmic antibody assay for humans has been validated in dogs.[53]

Biomarker panels

Combining a series of independent tests of biomarkers in a panel may increase testing specificity. Estruch et al. initially reported that the combined detection of IgA autoantibodies to polymorphonuclear leukocytes (APMNA), calprotectin (ACNA), gliadins (AGA), the microbial outer membrane porin C (ACA), and flagellins (AFA) differentiated dogs with inflammatory bowel disease from non–inflammatory bowel disease and healthy dogs. However, this publication was withdrawn after criticism, and a study that measured serum concentrations of ACA, ACNA, and AGA showed poor specificity and was not recommended.[54] Estruch et al.[55] have subsequently published a prospective study to detect APMNA, ACNA, AGA, ACA, and AFA. Dogs with histological evidence of a CIE displayed a 39–76% prevalence of seropositivity against selected serological markers, whereas any seropositivity was <13% in non-CIE and healthy dogs.

KEY POINTS

- Serum cobalamin is the most useful biomarker because it indicates intestinal dysfunction and a need to supplement.
- Hypocobalaminemia has metabolic consequences that cause clinical signs and worsen preexisting intestinal disease.
- Cobalamin can be supplemented either by periodic parenteral injections or by daily oral dosing.
- Folate deficiency can be a marker of intestinal dysfunction, but its clinical significance is less clear.
- Assays of many other biomarkers are only research tools.

References

1. Berlin H, Berlin R, Brante G. Oral treatment of pernicious anemia with high doses of vitamin B_{12} without intrinsic factor. *Acta Med Scand.* 184(4):247–258, 1968.
2. Kather S, Grützner N, Kook PH, et al. Review of cobalamin status and disorders of cobalamin metabolism in dogs. *J Vet Intern Med.* 34(1):13–28, 2020.
3. Kather S, Kacza J, Pfannkuche H, et al. Expression of the cobalamin transporters cubam and MRP1 in the canine ileum-upregulation in chronic inflammatory enteropathy. *PLoS One.* 19(1):e0296024, 2024.
4. Batt RM, Needham JR, Carter MW. Bacterial overgrowth associated with a naturally occurring enteropathy in the German shepherd dog. *Res Vet Sci.* 35(1):42–46, 1983.
5. Rutgers HC, Batt RM, Elwood CM, Lamport A. Small intestinal bacterial overgrowth in dogs with chronic intestinal disease. *J Am Vet Med Assoc.* 206(2):187–193, 1995.
6. German AJ, Day MJ, Ruaux CG, et al. Comparison of direct and indirect tests for small intestinal bacterial overgrowth and antibiotic-responsive diarrhea in dogs. *J Vet Intern Med.* 17(1):33–43, 2003.
7. Toresson L, Suchodolski JS, Spillmann T, et al. The intestinal microbiome in dogs with chronic enteropathies and cobalamin deficiency or normocobalaminemia—a comparative study. *Animals (Basel).* 13(8):1378, 2023.
8. Cook AK, Wright ZM, Suchodolski JS, et al. Prevalence and prognostic impact of hypocobalaminemia in dogs with lymphoma. *J Am Vet Med Assoc.* 235(12):1437–1441, 2009.
9. Hung M, Heinz J, Steiner JM, et al. Serum cobalamin and methylmalonic acid concentrations in juvenile dogs with parvoviral enteritis or other acute enteropathies. *J Vet Intern Med.* 37(4):1368–1375, 2023.
10. Berghoff N, Suchodolski JS, Steiner JM. Association between serum cobalamin and methylmalonic acid concentrations in dogs. *Vet J.* 191(3):306–311, 2012.
11. Toresson L, Steiner JM, Spodsberg E, et al. Effects of oral versus parenteral cobalamin supplementation on methylmalonic acid and homocysteine concentrations in dogs with chronic enteropathies and low cobalamin concentrations. *Vet J.* 243:8–14, 2019.
12. Henry PMN, Williams TL. Prevalence of neoplasia and concurrent diseases in dogs and cats with hypercobalaminemia: a retrospective case-control study. *Vet Clin Pathol.* 52(4):613–620, 2023.
13. Beiler HA, Steinorth J, Witt A, et al. Absorption of D(+)-xylose, cobalamin, and folic acid after autologic-allotopic ileum mucosa transplantation in beagles. *J Pediatr Surg.* 39(9):1362–1367, 2004.
14. Alpers DH. Absorption and blood/cellular transport of folate and cobalamin: pharmacokinetic and physiological considerations. *Biochimie.* 126:52–56, 2016.
15. Ullal TV, Marks SL, Huebner SN, et al. Association of folate concentrations with clinical signs and laboratory markers of chronic enteropathy in dogs. *J Vet Intern Med.* 37(2):455–464, 2023.
16. Stanley E, Appleman E, Schlag A, Siegel A. Relationship between cobalamin and folate deficiencies and anemia in dogs. *J Vet Intern Med.* 33(1):106–113, 2019.
17. Chantawong P. Clinical applications of current biomarkers in canine chronic enteropathies. *Vet Integr Sci.* 22(3):713–717, 2024.
18. Bell SM, Evans JM, Evans KM, et al. Congenital idiopathic megaesophagus in the German shepherd dog is a sex-differentiated trait and is associated with an intronic variable number tandem repeat in melanin-concentrating hormone receptor 2. *PloS Genet.* 18(3):e1010044, 2022.
19. Kathrani A, House A, Catchpole B, et al. Polymorphisms in the TLR4 and TLR5 gene are significantly associated with inflammatory bowel disease in German Shepherd dogs. *PLoS One.* 5(12):e15740, 2010.
20. Cirera S, Willumsen LM, Johansen TT, Nielsen LN. Evaluation of microRNA stability in feces from healthy dogs. *Vet Clin Pathol.* 47(1):115–121, 2018.
21. Varvil MS, dos Santos AP. A review on microRNA detection and expression studies in dogs. *Front Vet Sci.* 10:1261085, 2023.
22. Irving JR, Hiron TK, Davison LJ, et al. Characterization of canine intestinal microRNA expression in inflammatory bowel disease and T-cell lymphoma. *J Comp Pathol.* 204:23–29, 2023.
23. Israeli I, Steiner J, Segev G, et al. Serum pepsinogen-A, canine pancreatic lipase immunoreactivity, and C-reactive protein as prognostic markers in dogs with gastric dilatation–volvulus. *J Vet Intern Med.* 26(4):920–928, 2012.
24. Melgarejo T, Williams DA, Asem EK. Enzyme-linked immunosorbent assay for canine alpha(1)-protease inhibitor. *Am J Vet Res.* 59(2):127–130, 1998.
25. Heilmann RM, Parnell NK, Grützner N, et al. Serum and fecal canine α_1-proteinase inhibitor concentrations reflect the severity of intestinal crypt abscesses and/or lacteal dilation in dogs. *Vet J.* 207:131–139, 2016.
26. Kathrani A, Allenspach K, Fascetti AJ, et al. Alterations in serum amino acid concentrations in dogs with protein-losing enteropathy. *J Vet Intern Med.* 32(3):1026–1032, 2018.
27. Gow AG, Else R, Evans H, et al. Hypovitaminosis D in dogs with inflammatory bowel disease and hypoalbuminaemia. *J Small Anim Pract.* 52(8):410–417, 2011.
28. Serafini F, Maxwell KM, Zhu XJ, Lennon EM. Dysregulated serum concentrations of fat-soluble vitamins in dogs with chronic enteropathy. *J Vet Intern Med.* 38(5):2612–2619, 2024.
29. Allenspach K, Rizzo J, Jergens AE, Chang YM. Hypovitaminosis D is associated with negative outcome in dogs with protein losing enteropathy: a retrospective study of 43 cases. *BMC Vet Res.* 13(1):96, 2017.
30. AlShawaqfeh MK, Wajid B, Minamoto Y, et al. A dysbiosis index to assess microbial changes in fecal samples of dogs with chronic inflammatory enteropathy. *FEMS Microbiol Ecol.* 93(11):fix136, 2017.
31. Lopes BC, Chen CC, Sung CH, et al. Correlation between *Peptacetobacter hiranonis*, the *baiCD* gene, and secondary bile acids in dogs. *Animals (Basel).* 14(2):216, 2024.
32. Burrows CF, Jezyk PF. Nitrosonapthol test for screening of small intestinal diarrheal disease in the dog. *J Am Vet Med Assoc.* 183(3):318–322, 1983.
33. Garcia-Mazcorro JF, Suchodolski JS, Jones KR, et al. Effect of the proton pump inhibitor omeprazole on the gastrointestinal bacterial microbiota of healthy dogs. *FEMS Microbiol Ecol.* 80(3):624–636, 2012.
34. Pilla R, Gaschen FP, Barr JW, et al. Effects of metronidazole on the fecal microbiome and metabolome in healthy dogs. *J Vet Intern Med.* 34(5):1853–1866, 2020.
35. Jergens AE, Schreiner CA, Frank DE, et al. A scoring index for disease activity in canine inflammatory bowel disease. *J Vet Intern Med.* 17(3):291–297, 2003.
36. Heilmann RM, Nestler J, Schwarz J, et al. Mucosal expression of S100A12 (calgranulin C) and S100A8/A9 (calprotectin) and correlation with serum and fecal concentrations in dogs with chronic inflammatory enteropathy. *Vet Immunol Immunopathol.* 211:64–74, 2019.
37. Heilmann RM, Jergens AE, Ackermann MR, et al. Serum calprotectin concentrations in dogs with idiopathic inflammatory bowel disease. *Am J Vet Res.* 73(12):1900–1907, 2012.
38. Heilmann RM, Berghoff N, Mansell J, et al. Association of fecal calprotectin concentrations with disease severity, response to treatment, and other biomarkers in dogs with chronic inflammatory enteropathies. *J Vet Intern Med.* 32(2):679–692, 2018.
39. Nestler J, Syrjä P, Kilpinen S, et al. Duodenal and colonic mucosal S100A8/A9 (calprotectin) expression is increased and correlates with the severity of select histologic lesions in dogs with chronic inflammatory enteropathy. *BMC Vet Res.* 20(1):393, 2024.
40. Heilmann RM, Grellet A, Allenspach K, et al. Association between fecal S100A12 concentration and histologic, endoscopic, and clinical disease severity in dogs with idiopathic inflammatory bowel disease. *Vet Immunol Immunopathol.* 158(3–4):156–166, 2014.
41. Becher A, Suchodolski JS, Steiner JM, Heilmann RM. Blood neutrophil-to-lymphocyte ratio (NLR) as a diagnostic marker in dogs with chronic enteropathy. *J Vet Diagn Invest.* 33(3):516–527, 2021.

42. Benvenuti E, Pierini A, Gori E, et al. Neutrophil-to-lymphocyte ratio (NLR) in canine inflammatory bowel disease (IBD). *Vet Sci.* 7(3):141, 2020.
43. Cagnasso F, Borrelli A, Bottero E, et al. Comparative evaluation of peripheral blood neutrophil to lymphocyte ratio, serum albumin to globulin ratio and serum c-reactive protein to albumin ratio in dogs with inflammatory protein-losing enteropathy and healthy dogs. *Animals (Basel).* 13(3):484, 2023.
44. Marchesi MC, Maggi G, Cremonini V, et al. Monocytes count, NLR, MLR and PLR in canine inflammatory bowel disease. *Animals (Basel).* 14(6):837, 2024.
45. Berghoff N, Hill S, Parnell NK, et al. Fecal and urinary N-methylhistamine concentrations in dogs with chronic gastrointestinal disease. *Vet J.* 201(3):289–294, 2014.
46. Anfinsen KP, Berghoff N, Priestnall SL, et al. Urinary and faecal N-methylhistamine concentrations do not serve as markers for mast cell activation or clinical disease activity in dogs with chronic enteropathies. *Acta Vet Scand.* 56(1):90, 2014.
47. Sattasathuchana P, Thengchaisri N, Minamoto Y, et al. Serum and fecal 3-bromotyrosine concentrations in dogs with chronic inflammatory enteropathy: clinical parameters and histopathological changes. *Animals (Basel).* 13(17):2804, 2023.
48. Grützner N, Heilmann RM, Tress U, et al. Genomic association and further characterisation of faecal immunoglobulin A deficiency in German shepherd dogs. *Vet Med Sci.* 7(6):2144–2155, 2021.
49. Peters IR, Calvert EL, Hall EJ, Day AJ. Measurement of immunoglobulin concentrations in the feces of healthy dogs. *Clin Diagn Lab Immunol.* 11(5):841–848, 2004.
50. Peters IR, Helps CR, Calvert EL, et al. Identification of four allelic variants of the dog IGHA gene. *Immunogenetics.* 56(4):254–260, 2004.
51. Wieland B, Summers JF, Haesler B, et al. Prevalence of perinuclear antineutrophilic cytoplasmic autoantibodies in serum of healthy soft coated Wheaten terriers in the United Kingdom. *Am J Vet Res.* 73(3):404–408, 2012.
52. Mancho C, Sainz A, García-Sancho M, et al. Detection of perinuclear antineutrophil cytoplasmic antibodies and antinuclear antibodies in the diagnosis of canine inflammatory bowel disease. *J Vet Diagn Invest.* 22(4):553–558, 2010.
53. Florey J, Viall A, Streu S, et al. Use of a granulocyte immunofluorescence assay designed for humans for detection of antineutrophil cytoplasmic antibodies in dogs with chronic enteropathies. *J Vet Intern Med.* Jul;31(4):1062–1066, 2017.
54. Langlois DK, Pritchard JC, Tolbert MK, et al. Clinical utility of an immunoglobulin A-based serological panel for the diagnosis of chronic enteropathy in dogs. *J Vet Intern Med.* 37(2):446–454, 2023.
55. Estruch JJ, Barken D, Bennett N, et al. Evaluation of novel serological markers and autoantibodies in dogs with inflammatory bowel disease. *J Vet Intern Med.* 34(3):1177–1786, 2020.

results obtained with ultrasonography.[3] Computed tomography has shown promising results in the diagnosis and staging of GI tumors[4] and can be used for the diagnosis of mechanical obstruction.[5] Examples of GI pathology on CT are shown in Figure 21.1.

Magnetic resonance imaging has the advantage of not using ionizing radiation and provides exquisite soft tissue differentiation. It is the most advanced technique used in people.[6] Magnetic resonance imaging of the GI tract suffers from movement-related artefacts from normal gut peristalsis and lack of adequate luminal filling, which can cause erroneous diagnoses in human patients. Although the advances in MRI sequences have reduced motion artefacts, this modality is not widely used in GI investigations in canine patients, with reported lesions of the GI tract often found during imaging of other body systems. There are no comprehensive veterinary studies characterizing the appearance of the GI tract on MRI at this stage.

Magnetic resonance imaging and CT are modalities that are both used in the investigation of rectal and anal sac lesions as this region does not suffer from physiological movement blur or require gating techniques for image acquisition. Magnetic resonance imaging and CT have higher sensitivity than ultrasonography to detect sacral lymphadenopathy from anal sac adenocarcinomas[7,8] and can be considered in cases where an additional metastatic site would affect the treatment plan. Few MRI descriptions of normal GI and abdominal lymph nodes exist in the veterinary literature.

Contrast agents

Barium sulfate is used as the contrast medium for upper GI tract studies and can be obtained as suspensions or pastes. Barium mixed with food of increasing levels of solidity (from liquid to kibble) usually provides the best diagnostic results. Administration of barium sulfate is contraindicated when perforation of the GI tract is suspected, in patients with known hypersensitivity to barium sulfate preparations, and in cases of fistulae. If a perforation is suspected and an esophagram is considered rather than endoscopy, the best choice of contrast medium is a nonionic iodinated contrast medium such as iohexol or iopamidol, although these agents have an unpleasant taste, making patients reluctant to ingest them.

Intravascular administration of water-soluble, nonionic, low-osmolality iodinated contrast agents such as iohexol and iopamidol is used for contrast CT studies. These contrast agents are contraindicated in patients with renal disease, liver disease, dehydration, and a known history of hypersensitivity reactions to iodinated contrast media.

Radiation safety

Care must be taken with regard to radiation safety for the personnel and the patient during all studies involving ionizing radiation (radiography, fluoroscopy, and CT). Hand holding of patients even with lead glove protection during radiographic and fluoroscopic examinations constitutes unsafe radiation safety practice and should never be performed, although it has not yet been banned in all countries. Gloved or ungloved hands should never be included in the primary beam. Computed tomographic examinations should be performed with adequate sedation or anesthesia so that all personnel can leave the room during image acquisition. All procedures should follow the ALARA (As Low As Reasonably Achievable) principles to reduce radiation dose to personnel by increasing distance, using appropriate shielding, minimizing exposure time, and limiting exposure factors.

Imaging technique and patient preparation

Obtaining images of diagnostic quality is paramount for complete evaluation of the GI tract in all modalities. Patients should ideally be fasted for 6–12 hours prior to imaging in all modalities. This is particularly important in ultrasonography. However, the results of fasting can be inconsistent, particularly with regard to stomach emptying. Access to water prior to ultrasound examination can be helpful to improve visibility of the walls, in particular of the stomach. Sedation or anesthesia greatly improves image quality and acquisition.

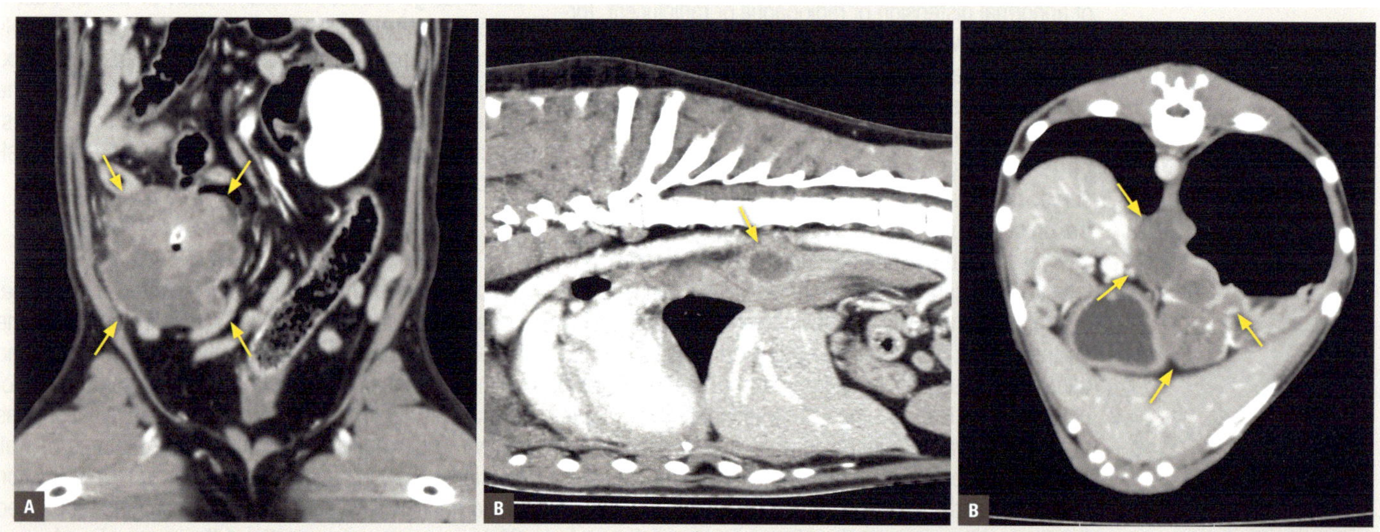

FIG. 21.1 Computed tomography images of gastrointestinal pathologies. (A) Gastrointestinal stromal tumor surrounding the cecum. (B) Paraesophageal abscess. (C) Stomach mass.

Radiography

A complete survey radiographic study of the abdomen should include four views: right lateral, left lateral, ventrodorsal, and dorsoventral; these should include the entire region between the diaphragm and the pelvis. This is to obtain a complete picture of the location, distribution, and amount of fluid and gas in the GI tract. In practice, however, time constraints usually limit the acquisition to three views: right lateral, left lateral, and either ventrodorsal or dorsoventral views. The radiographic technique employed for the abdomen should be tailored to the patient via previously established exposure charts. In general, a low Kvp, high mAs technique is required to enhance the inherently poor abdominal detail. Acquisition at peak expiration is preferred. A grid and bucky are used, except for very small dogs. Conversely, radiography of the thorax to assess the esophagus requires a high Kvp, low mAs technique, with acquisition timed with peak inspiration.

Contrast radiographic studies should always include precontrast survey views. This allows evaluation of normal anatomical structures and the diagnosis of any condition that would preclude the requirement for a contrast study to be performed. It also enhances the visibility of strongly radiopaque structures, may reveal contraindications to a contrast study, and ensures the radiographic acquisition parameters are accurate prior to starting the contrast study.

Fluoroscopy

Following the acquisition of a survey image, boluses of food mixed with a barium sulfate preparation are ingested by the conscious, standing patient. Frame rates must be set between 30 and 60 frames per second to obtain enough detail for frame-by-frame analysis. Liquid barium is offered to the patient, followed by soft food and finally kibble (both mixed with barium). The prehension, formation of the bolus, passage of the bolus through the upper esophageal sphincter, esophagus, and lower esophageal sphincter are sequentially imaged by tracking boluses of food as the patient eats. This allows the evaluation of the oral, cricopharyngeal, pharyngeal, and esophageal phases of swallowing. If a sliding hiatal hernia or regurgitation is suspected, focusing the screening on the caudal esophageal sphincter and stomach once the stomach is full offers a higher chance of witnessing an event. Elevating the caudal half of the patient and ensuring complete stomach filling can sometimes enhance the chances of seeing a regurgitation event.

Ultrasonography

Patients can be scanned in dorsal or lateral recumbency or in standing position. High-frequency probes are used (5–8 MHz or higher), with the smallest patients requiring the highest frequency probes (7–18 MHz) and larger patients requiring lower frequency probes (3.5–5 MHz) to examine the deepest portions of the abdomen. Curvilinear or linear transducers or a combination of both are used to scan the GI tract. In some patients, the wall layering is best visualized with a linear probe. The shape of the curvilinear probes allows assessment of the stomach and proximal duodenum, which are located under the patient's ribs. Transverse and longitudinal views of the structures should be obtained for a complete evaluation. Measurements of the wall thickness of each segment are obtained from the inner mucosal surface to the outer part of the serosa.

Ultrasonography can be challenging in very large patients[7] (i.e., large breeds and/or obese patients) and in patients with significant amounts of gas in the GI tract. Computed tomography can be considered in these patients.

Point-of-care ultrasound can be performed as a noninvasive, quick, reliable patient-side technique even by less experienced ultrasonographers in patients with GI disease when free fluid accumulation is suspected.[9,10] This involves looking for free fluid by scanning the patient in four locations: caudal to the xyphoid process (diaphragmatico-hepatic window), caudal to the ribs on the left flank (splenorenal window), caudal to the ribs on the right flank (hepatorenal window), and midline over the urinary bladder (cystocolic window). Abdominocentesis can then be performed for fluid collection and analysis and for detecting immediate life-threatening conditions such as a septic peritonitis from bowel perforation.

Advanced imaging: MRI and CT

Protocols for CT of the GI tract[11] include the acquisition of a pre- and postcontrast series of images extending from the cranial abdomen to the caudal pelvis. Low to medium kernel frequency is used to obtain images in soft tissue reconstruction, with the usual window level being around +45/50 HU with a window width of 300–400 HU. Tube voltage should be between 120–140 kVp, tube current between 100 and 250 mA depending on the size of the patient, and slice thickness 1–1.25 mm, with a collimator pitch of 1–1.5 and reconstruction interval one half of the slice width to allow for good quality multiplanar reconstructions. These parameters are general and should be tailored for each individual machine with the help of the equipment manufacturer and engineers for optimal results. Fluid or air can be added as contrast medium to increase the visibility of the hollow organ walls. Intravenous injection of iodinated contrast medium is required to highlight some aspects of layering of the GI tract and to improve visualization of disease processes.

A protocol for pneumocolonography established in normal dogs determined the optimum insufflation pressure for maintaining pneumocolon to be 20 mmHg.[12]

There is little information in the veterinary literature concerning MRI protocols for the canine GI tract. One study looking at MRI at 1.0 T of the canine abdomen as a whole suggested that the sequence with the best diagnostic quality score was a dorsal T2 turbo spin echo with fat saturation and breath holding and the sequence with the highest signal to noise ratio was the sagittal T1 spin echo sequence, although smaller structures suffered from volume averaging.[13] Another study in low field MRI showed good visual correlation between MRI and ultrasound using transverse, sagittal, and dorsal T1- and T2-weighted spine echo pulse sequences.[14]

Imaging of the pharynx and esophagus

Normal appearance

Anatomy

The oropharynx and laryngopharynx are the spaces cranial to the esophagus and caudal to the mouth and nasal cavity; they are involved in the digestive function of the pharynx. The function of the pharynx is to carry food to the esophagus and air to the larynx. On plain radiography, the pharynx is located at the caudal aspect of the oral and nasal cavities and is of gas opacity. The oropharynx is delineated by the ventral aspect of the soft palate and the base of the tongue. The laryngopharynx is located just caudal to the nasopharynx, just distal to the tip of the soft palate, and cranial to the larynx. The epiglottis serves as a moving barrier between these two pharyngeal structures, directing food into the esophagus and air in the trachea. These spaces are gas-filled on CT. The pharynx cannot be evaluated on ultrasound images due to the presence of air.

The esophagus starts cranially at the cricopharyngeal sphincter. This structure is visible on radiographs when a small amount of gas is present in the esophagus as a thickening of the walls of the cranial esophagus just dorsal to the laryngeal cartilages and corresponding narrowing of the width of the esophageal lumen.

The esophagus then courses in the neck slightly to the left and in the thorax to the left and dorsal to the trachea; it then joins the diaphragm at the level of the esophageal hiatus.

The portion of the esophagus located in the thoracic cavity cannot be examined via ultrasonography due to gas in the lungs. Functional studies are best obtained using fluoroscopy and contrast medium such as barium sulfate, although plain radiography with contrast can also be considered to obtain some diagnostic information.

Radiography

On radiographic examinations, the esophagus is usually empty and silhouetting with the mediastinal structures, and it is therefore not readily visible. Small accumulations of gas are normal and may highlight portions of the esophagus, particularly dorsal to the carina, for example. On the left thoracic radiograph, a small amount of fluid is commonly seen accumulating in the caudal esophagus, forming a faint tube of soft tissue opacity between the heart base and the diaphragm. General anesthesia, heavy sedation, and marked aerophagia may result in artefactual dilation of the esophagus.

Ultrasonography

The cervical esophageal wall is constituted of four layers visible with ultrasonography: a hypoechoic mucosa, a hyperechoic submucosa, a hypoechoic muscularis, and a faint hyperechoic fibrous adventitia layer. These layers are not distinguishable on CT. The esophageal mucosa has multiple longitudinal folds and the esophageal muscularis is composed of striated muscle in dogs.

Computed tomography

On CT examinations, the esophagus is closely related to the trachea, longus colli and longus capitis muscle, left common carotid artery, internal jugular vein, and vagosympathetic trunk. It can be followed along its entire length as an ellipsoid-shaped soft tissue density structure in the neck and cranial mediastinum, before becoming slightly more triangular in the caudal mediastinum. Fluid and air variably distend its lumen.

Fluoroscopy

In dynamic fluoroscopic contrast studies, food boluses of increased levels of solidity are offered to the patient. The contrast medium highlights the bolus as it passes through the pharynx and esophagus. The food bolus should form by accumulation at the caudal aspect of the mouth before being pushed towards the oro- and laryngopharynx by a combination of tongue, hyoid, and pharyngeal muscle contractions. The epiglottis forms a vertical barrier obstructing the larynx, thus preventing the food bolus from entering the airways. The cricopharyngeal sphincter should then open in a synchronous fashion to the bolus being presented at the caudal aspect of the pharynx for progression into the esophagus. The bolus can then be followed along the length of the esophagus. Primary and then secondary waves of esophageal contractions should propel the bolus along the esophagus up to the level of the cardia prior to entry into the stomach. A very small amount of regurgitation of contrast material at the cardia immediately after the bolus passes this sphincter is normal. During the examination, most of the esophageal lumen should remain empty aside from the area occupied by the bolus. Thin streaks of contrast medium along the esophageal longitudinal folds can persist for a small amount of time in the esophagus, particularly if the thicker barium formulations are used. Timings of all the phases of swallowing have been documented in the literature but are beyond the scope of this chapter.[15]

Pharyngeal, cricopharyngeal, and esophageal dysphagia

Dysphagia can be functional or result from trauma, foreign bodies, pharyngeal masses, and occasionally regional lymph node enlargement. Survey radiography is indicated to rule out radiopaque foreign material. Ultrasonography can be used to assess the surrounding tissues and identify radiolucent foreign objects. Fluoroscopic contrast studies are required to assess any functional disorder as survey radiographs are often normal. The study is examined for pharyngeal and tongue movements, propulsion of the food bolus through the pharynx, and finally, for cricopharyngeal sphincter opening and closure timings and function.

In a normal examination, following the oral phase, the bolus enters the laryngopharynx, where craniodorsal movement of the hyoid due to pharyngeal contraction is visualized. This pushes the bolus against the tongue towards the pharyngeal region. The tongue stops the to-and-fro motion that formed the bolus. The epiglottis closes the entrance to the trachea. This constitutes the pharyngeal phase. The cricopharyngeal phase is characterized by the relaxation and opening of the cricopharyngeal sphincter to allow the formed bolus to enter the proximal aspect of the esophagus. The esophageal phase starts at the closure of the cricopharyngeal sphincter. Primary and then secondary waves propel the bolus towards the stomach.

Pharyngeal dysphagia in isolation is rare. This condition is difficult to diagnose as the signs often overlap with cricopharyngeal dysphagia and many patients have combined disease. Myomectomy or myotomy can result in clinical improvement for patients with disorders of the upper esophageal sphincter, but it will result in deterioration in patients with pharyngeal contraction disorders. Careful examination of the fluoroscopic studies and classification of the disease are therefore very important.[15] Normal timings of each phase of the swallowing process are available in the literature to aid distinction between the different origins of dysphagia.[15]

In pharyngal dysphagia, the timing of the opening of the cricopharyngeal sphincter remains normal; however, the pharyngeal contraction is weak, the formation of the bolus is abnormal or delayed, or the bolus is not propelled aborally. Calculation of the pharyngeal constriction ratio is used to identify this condition.[16] Pharyngeal dysphagias can be caused by neuromuscular diseases, inflammatory myopathies, or trauma but may be idiopathic or congenital.

Cricopharyngeal dysphagias can be classified into three groups: achalasia, which is characterized by incomplete or absence of opening of the cricopharyngeal sphincter; asynchrony, which is characterized by a mismatch between the timing of the opening of the upper esophageal sphincter relative to bolus presentation; and chalasia, which is rare and can be seen in cases of myasthenia gravis, and occurs when the sphincter remains open following the passage of the bolus. Gas in the sphincter and cranial esophagus can be seen in these cases.

Esophageal dysmotility can present with segmental or generalized distension of the esophagus on survey radiography. On dynamic contrast studies, the bolus is either transported more slowly through the esophagus, can remain stagnant in parts of the esophagus after two subsequent swallows, or is seen to be sent in an oral direction during regurgitation events.

Structural malformations

Esophageal diverticula or redundancies

Esophageal diverticula or redundancies, which are segmental sacculations of the esophageal wall, are common as a congenital malformation in brachycephalic breeds but can also be acquired.

They are most readily identifiable on CT examinations or contrast radiography. Small dilations can be missed on plain radiography if no air or food is filling the dilation. These lesions, which are not visible on ultrasound due to their intrathoracic nature, appear on CT and radiography as a focal dilation of the esophagus that is usually found in the cranial mediastinum. Fluid or gas can be found in the resulting pouch or U-shaped distension, which is usually orientated ventrally or laterally (Fig. 21.2A). The lung fields should be examined for signs of secondary aspiration pneumonia.

Hiatal malformations

Sliding hiatal hernia, paraesophageal hernias, gastroesophageal intussusception, and gastroesophageal reflux all constitute abnormalities of the esophageal hiatus.

Hiatal hernias and paraesophageal hernias can be transient and therefore missed on plain radiography, CT, and even fluoroscopy. They are characterized by a soft tissue opacity visible adjacent or in line with the esophageal sphincter, cranial to the diaphragm between the aorta and caudal vena cava. This opacity is broad-based, caudally silhouettes with the diaphragm, and has a rounded cranial shape (Fig. 21.2B). Rugal folds can occasionally be seen on radiographs but are more easily identified on CT examination; they are particularly evident with the administration of intravenous contrast material.

Gastroesophageal reflux events are mostly diagnosed with the aid of contrast fluoroscopy when an event is witnessed during the study, as both static and fluoroscopic contrast esophagrams are usually normal unless secondary ulceration that has led to retention of contrast along the mucosal folds is present in the esophageal mucosa.

Cases of gastroesophageal intussusception are a surgical emergency with a poor prognosis. These are readily diagnosed on plain film radiographs, which show a large, rounded structure of mixed opacity (air, fluid, ingesta), sometimes with evident rugal folds, within the lumen of the distended esophagus. The stomach is absent from the abdominal cavity, and the structure creates a semilunar-shaped, sharply delineated gas interface with the dilated esophageal lumen cranially. Other organs such as the spleen can also enter the esophagus in severe cases.

Megaesophagus

Megaesophagus is defined as an abnormal and persistent dilation of part or the entirety of the esophagus and can be congenital in origin or acquired secondary to neuromuscular disease, intoxication (e.g., lead, organophosphates), esophageal obstruction, stricture, or various vascular ring anomalies.

This is readily identifiable on plain radiographs, which reveal a generalized or focal dilation filled with gas/ingesta (Fig. 21.3). This is often accompanied by a tracheal stripe sign, which is seen as an increased soft tissue density thickness of the dorsal wall of the trachea due to the draping of the ventral esophageal wall over the dorsal tracheal wall. The dorsal and ventral walls of the esophagus are often seen in the caudodorsal lung fields on lateral views, with a hyperlucent tubular area between these walls. Thin, converging, V-shaped stripes of soft tissue opacity can be seen converging at the esophageal hiatus caudally on dorsoventral/ventrodorsal views and correspond to the caudal esophagus connecting with the caudal sphincter.

Contrast radiography allows further characterization of the degree of esophageal distension, esophageal function, and any structural abnormalities of the esophagus. This approach must be weighed against the risk of aspiration pneumonia and barium aspiration. Computed tomography can be used to identify structural causes but is often not required in cases of megaesophagus.

The lung fields should be examined for signs of secondary aspiration pneumonia.

Vascular ring anomalies

Secondary dilation of the esophagus following entrapment by vascular ring anomalies can be identified on radiographs or CT images. The most common type of vascular ring anomaly causing esophageal entrapment is the persistence of the right fourth aortic arch, which results in segmental dilation of the esophagus cranial to the heart base and ventral and rightward deviation of the trachea (Fig. 21.4).[17] However, a double aortic arch, a left aortic arch with a persistent right ligamentum arteriosum and/or right subclavian arteries, or the presence of an aberrant right subclavian

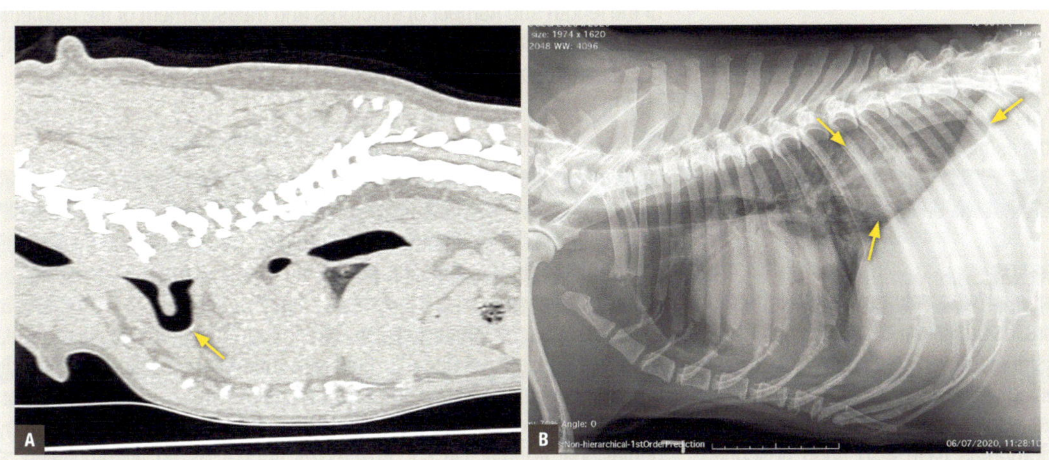

FIG. 21.2 (A) U-shaped gas-filled esophageal diverticulum or redundancy in the cranial thorax. (B) Lateral radiographic view. Soft tissue and gas opacity with a rounded cranial border just cranial to the cardia, consistent with hiatal herniation including of part of the stomach fundus.

Ultrasonography

All segments of the GI tract present distinct wall layering on ultrasonography, correlating with the histological layers that make up the walls of these organs. Five layers are distinguished in all segments: hyperechoic mucosal interface with the lumen, hypoechoic to anechoic mucosa, hyperechoic submucosa, hypoechoic to anechoic muscularis, and hyperechoic serosa (Fig. 21.6). The thickest layers are the mucosa and muscularis in all segments except the colon, where all the layers are equivalent in size. With high frequency probes, it may be possible to identify:

1. Dual echogenicity of the mucosa attributable to the differentiation between the mildly echogenic intestinal villi and hypoechoic lamina propria and lacteal dilation.
2. A hyperechoic mucosal line parallel to the submucosa corresponding to enlarged Peyer's patches in the ileum.
3. A fine hyperechoic line in the muscularis corresponding to the interface between the inner and outer layers of the muscularis. It is present in all intestinal segments (Fig. 21.7).[19]

All segments should be evaluated for motility, wall thickness, integrity, and character of the wall layering and luminal contents. Wall thickness and relative motility of all segments of the GI tract are presented in Table 21.2.

Prominent rugal folds are readily visualized on ultrasonography of the stomach, and measurements should be obtained in the inter-rugal fold area but should be interpreted in the context of the degree of distension of the stomach. The duodenum is characterized by a greater overall thickness than the remainder of the small intestine, a thicker mucosal layer, and the presence of the duodenal papilla. Peyer's patches, which appear as rectangular invaginations of the duodenal mucosa on the antimesenteric border of the duodenum, are normal and should not be confused with ulceration. The ileum has a characteristic cartwheel appearance when viewed transversely. The colonic wall is markedly thinner than the remainder of the segments of the GI tract, and the luminal contents are highly echogenic causing dirty distal acoustic shadowing due to the gas present in the feces. Peristaltic waves are not often seen in the colon.

Advanced imaging: MRI and CT

All GI segments are visible on CT examinations, with the gross anatomy as described above. The layering that is visible on CT examination does not correspond to histological layers and is not present in all segments. Gastric rugal folds readily contrast enhance and are visible on CT examination.

There are no comprehensive studies showing the appearance of the GI tract on MRI.[26]

Gastric and intestinal pathology

In all cases of GI pathology, interpretation of the imaging findings must be performed in light of the patient's history, clinical signs, and laboratory findings, as many imaging features significantly overlap between disease processes.

Gastric dilation vs. gastric dilatation-volvulus

Distinguishing between gastric dilation and gastric dilatation-volvulus (GDV) is important to decide between medical and surgical treatment. Both diseases are best diagnosed on radiographs and/or CT images.

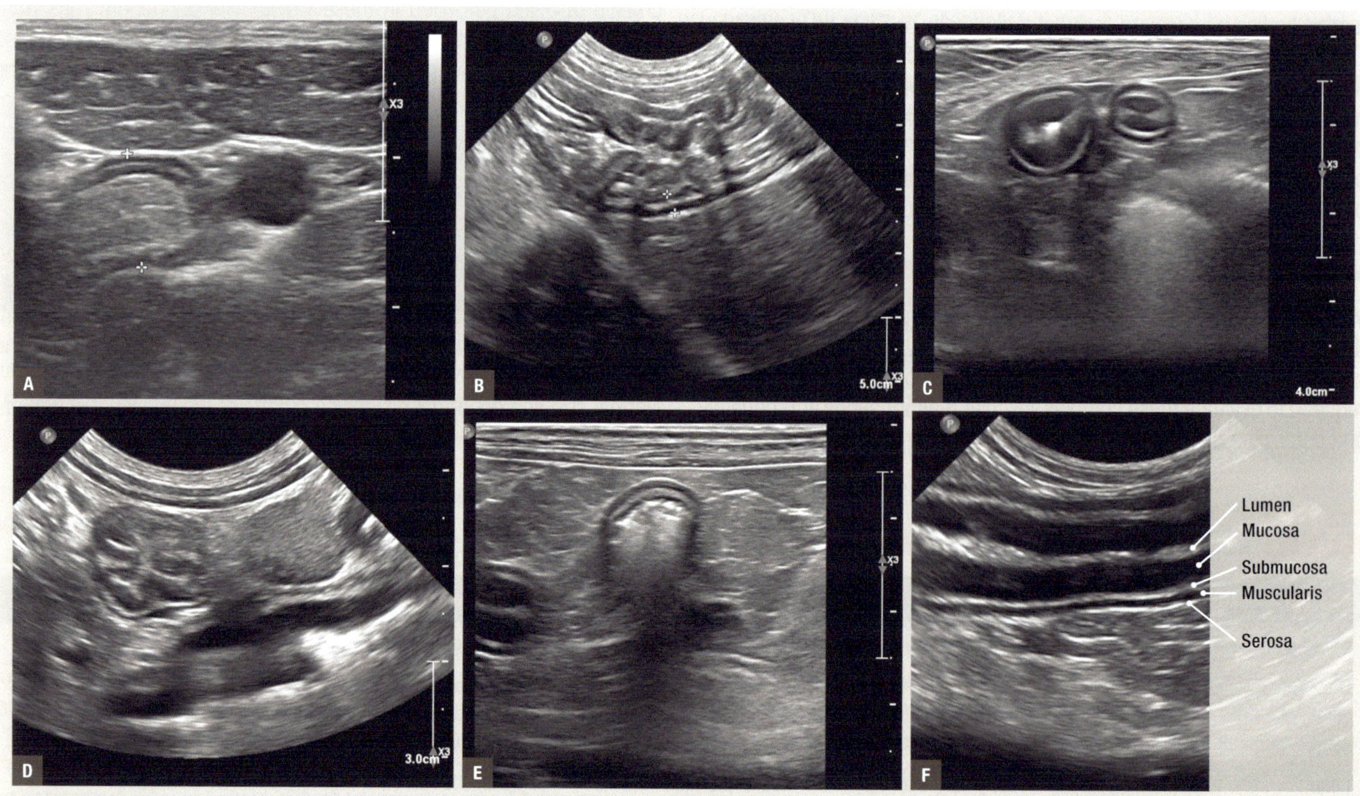

FIG. 21.6 Ultrasonographic appearance of the normal gastrointestinal tract. (A) Esophagus. (B) Stomach. (C) Duodenum (left loop), and jejunum (right loop). (D) Ileum. (E) Colon. (F) Normal wall layering, illustrated in the duodenum.

Gastric dilatation is characterized by severe enlargement of the stomach, with variable contents (gas vs. ingesta most commonly) and preservation of the anatomical location of the segments of the stomach (Figs. 21.8A and B). Gastric dilation-volvulus is characterized by mispositioning of the pylorus, which shifts to the left, dorsally, and cranially, and of the fundus and body, which shift to the right. Compartmentalization of the stomach, visible as soft tissue bands overlying the stomach, often occurs as a result of the volvulus (Figs. 21.8C and D). The spleen is also found to have followed the greater curvature of the stomach. The presence of gas in the stomach wall indicates a poorer prognosis as it is due to gastric wall necrosis. Obtaining two lateral views is helpful to identify the location of the pylorus in these patients. Cases of 360-degree rotation are more difficult to identify as the anatomical position of the stomach is maintained.

In both dilation and GDV, distension of the esophagus and aspiration pneumonia may be present concurrently.

Ileus

Ileus can affect all segments of the GI tract and is classified as mechanical or functional (see Chapter 43). Mechanical ileus may be secondary to foreign body ingestion, intussusception, the presence of a mass (neoplastic or benign), adhesions, mesenteric or colonic torsion, strangulation, and areas of stenosis such as pyloric stenosis or chronic hypertrophic pyloric gastropathy. Functional ileus may be observed postlaparotomy or after opioid administration, and in cases of severe gastroenteritis, peritonitis, volvulus without strangulation of the vascular supply, electrolyte imbalances, dysautonomia and visceral myopathy, certain toxicities, peritonitis, and pancreatitis. General principles apply to distinguish between mechanical and functional ileus on radiographic examination (Fig 21.9). In mechanical obstructions, the bowel is usually more distended than in functional ileus, some segments of the GI tract are usually normal in size, and the dilation usually involves a combination of gas and fluid. Conversely, in functional ileus, the dilation is often mostly gaseous and generalized throughout the tract. Measurements have been suggested to distinguish normal from pathological dilation of bowel segments (Table 21.1); however, the usefulness of these absolute measurements has been questioned, and radiographic interpretation experience and subjective assessment remain very important.[27] The diagnostic criteria overlap, and therefore, the combination of ultrasonography and radiography are seen as complementary techniques to distinguish between mechanical and functional ileus. Ultrasonography may identify the cause of the ileus if it is not apparent on radiographs. Serial radiographs over time following medical management may also help diagnosis if the first series of radiographs acquired is equivocal.

In cases of chronic longstanding GI tract obstructions, accumulations of small, mineralized debris oral to the site of obstruction can create a gravel sign visible on radiographs.

Gastrointestinal foreign bodies

Foreign bodies show a great variation in size, shape, radiopacity, and echogenicity. Abnormal distension of the segments of the intestine oral to the foreign material is sought on all modalities. On ultrasonography, the presence of a luminal structure with a strongly hyperechoic interface and marked distal acoustic shadowing is strongly suggestive of foreign material. Linear foreign bodies can sometimes be identified as a hyperechoic line spanning multiple loops of intestine. Plication of

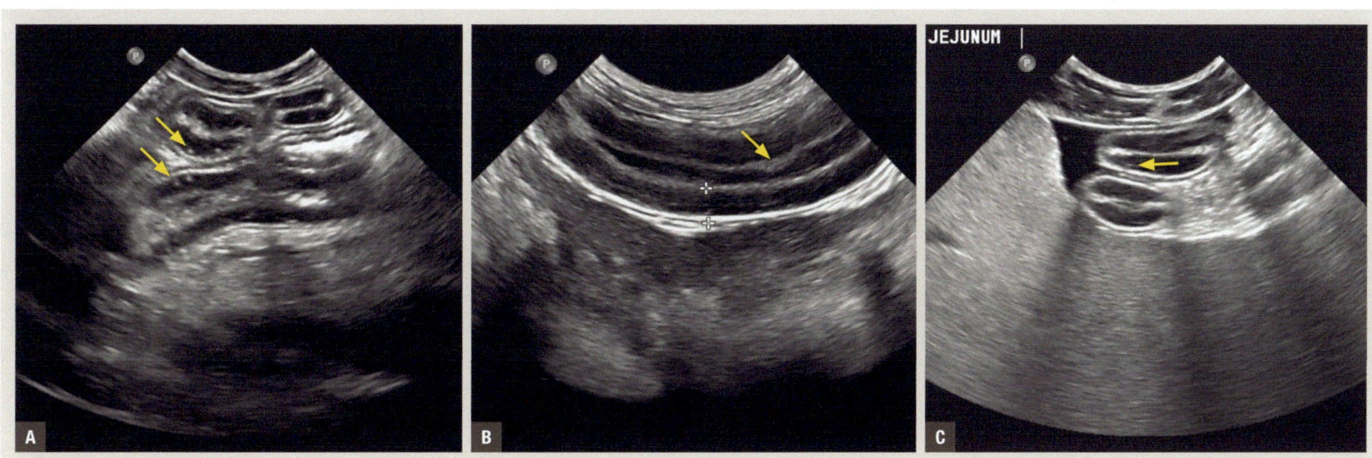

FIG. 21.7 Nonpathological ultrasonographic mucosal changes. (A) Hyperechoic speckles in the mucosal layer of the intestine. (B) Hyperechoic mucosal surface in a duodenal segment postprandium. (C) Fine hyperechoic line at the base of the jejunal mucosa. A small amount of anechoic free fluid is present adjacent to the loops of jejunum.

TABLE 21.2 Mean normal wall thickness and relative motility of the gastrointestinal tract segments.[21-24]

Anatomical segment	Wall thickness, adult dogs (mm)		Wall thickness, puppies (mm)[21]	Motility[22,23]
Stomach	3–5		2.7 ± 0.4	4–5 contractions per minute
Duodenum	Up to 30 kg: ≤5.3	Over 30 kg: ≤6	3.8 ± 0.5	4–5 contractions per minute
Jejunum	Up to 30 kg: ≤4.4[24]	Over 30 kg: ≤4.7	2.5 ± 0.5	1–3 contractions per minute
Ileum	3–4		Data not available	1–3 contractions per minute
Colon	1.2–2.5		1.3 ± 0.3	1 to 4 per minute

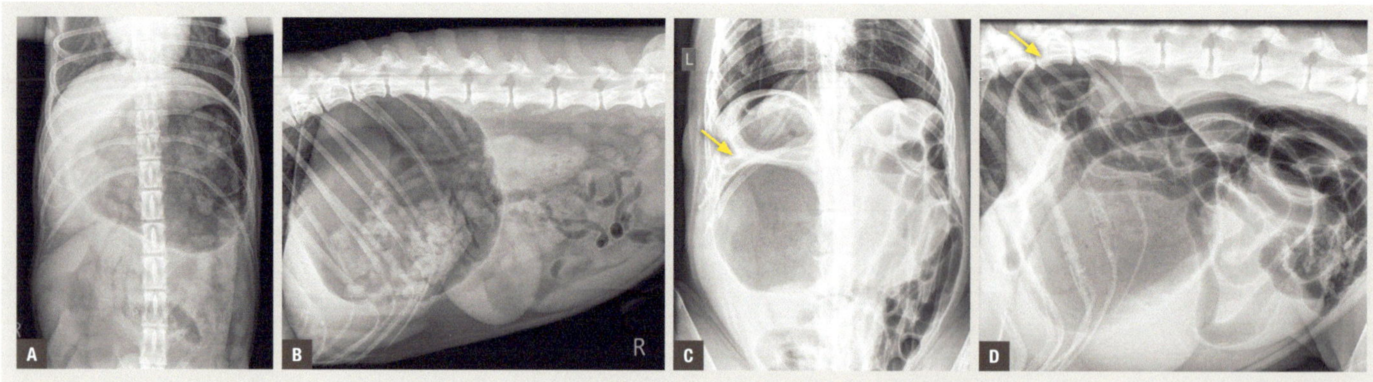

FIG. 21.8 (**A, B**) Ventrodorsal and lateral views of a gastric dilation with foreign material. (**C, D**) Ventrodorsal and lateral radiographic views of a gastric dilation-volvulus with compartmentalization of the gas in the stomach and abnormal positioning of the pylorus on the left side and dorsal aspect of the abdomen.

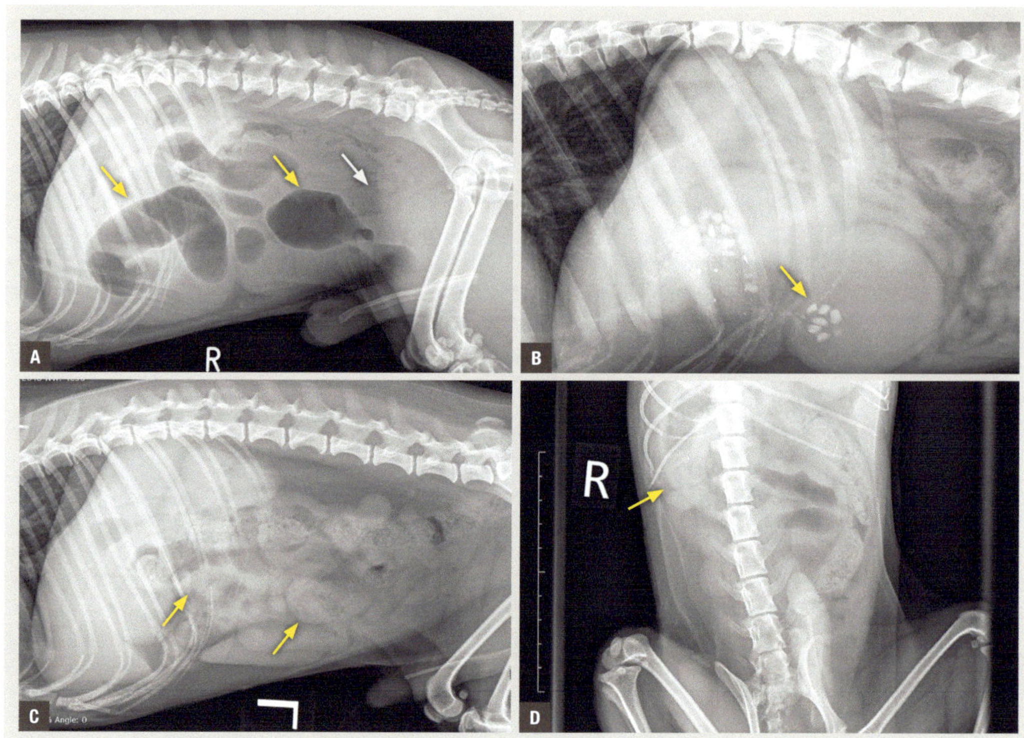

FIG. 21.9 (**A**) Mechanical ileus due to obstruction from a corn on the cob (white arrow). Note the severely gas-distended loops of small intestine (yellow arrows). (**B**) Gravel sign following chronic obstruction (arrow). (**C, D**) Linear foreign body. Note the abnormal gas pattern distribution in the small intestine (**C**) and the plication of the duodenum (**D**).

the small intestine over this hyperechoic line is strongly suggestive of an obstructive linear foreign body. On radiography, if the material is of soft tissue opacity and therefore not readily visible, abnormal fluid and gas distension of the intestinal segments, two populations of bowel, stacking of the small intestine, and distension of GI segments beyond the boundaries presented in Table 21.2 are suggestive or a mechanical obstruction due to foreign material ingestion. Linear foreign bodies can present with a lesser degree of distension of the GI segments. Radiographic signs of linear foreign body include focal loss of serosal detail and paisley-, crescent- or geometric-shaped gas bubbles overlying ill-defined loops of intestine. In all cases, careful inspection of the imaging studies for the presence of free gas and free fluid indicative of perforation should be performed.

Intussusception

Although occasionally visible radiographically, particularly in cases of ileocolic intussusception, cecal inversions and colonocolic intussusceptions, ultrasonography is the method of choice for the diagnosis of intussusceptions (Fig. 21.10). The characteristic appearance of this disease in transverse view on ultrasonography is a very distended loop of bowel with hypoechoic, thickened, edematous walls (intussuscipiens), which contains one or more loops of bowel within its lumen (intussusceptum). This gives the appearance of a multilayered wall. The lumen is also usually filled with strongly echogenic mesenteric fat that has been invaginated at the same time as the intussusceptum. The mesenteric vasculature and lymph nodes can also be identified within the intussusception in some cases, depending on the length of the intussusception.

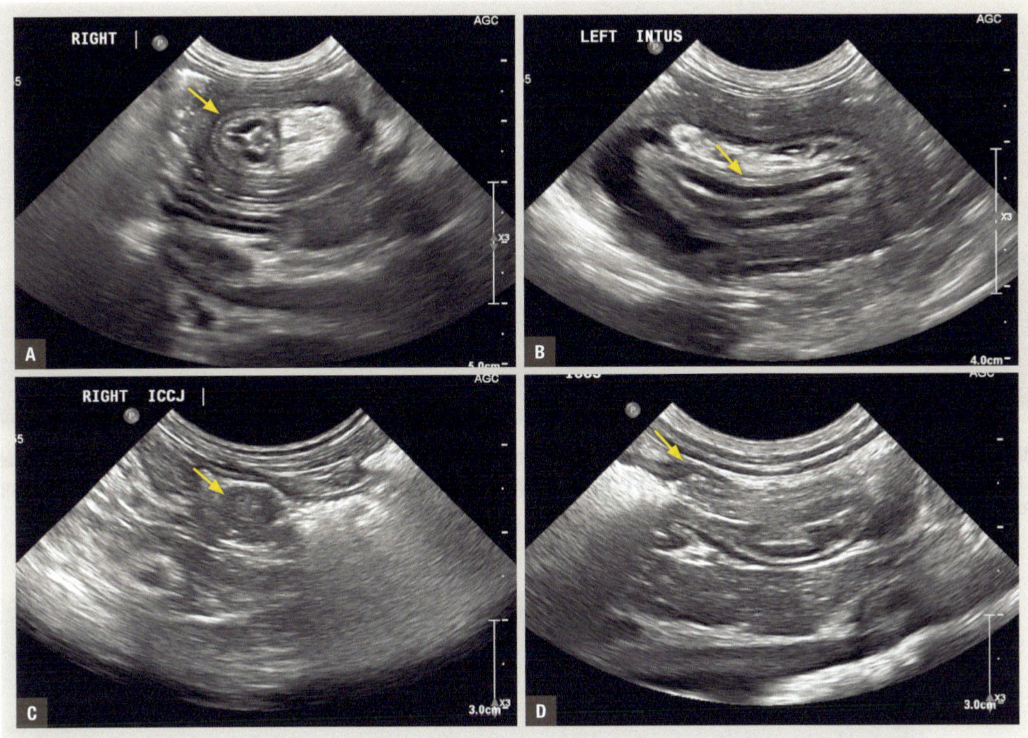

FIG. 21.10 (A, B) Transverse and longitudinal section of an intussusception. Note the jejunal loop with normal layering encircled by another jejunal loop with thickened walls and loss of layering. The hyperechoic material around the inner loop corresponds to hyperechoic mesentery. (C, D) Transverse and longitudinal sections of the ileocecocolic junction. Note the normal thin layering in all segments and the absence of invagination in the longitudinal view. The hyperechoic material represents colonic content causing dirty acoustic shadowing consistent with feces and gas.

Pyloric stenosis

This disease can be identified on ultrasonography and contrast radiography (or endoscopy). On ultrasound images, this disease appears as concentric hypertrophy of the pyloric walls, in particular of the muscularis layer. Observation of the sphincter may reveal lack of passage of gastric contents despite active contraction.

Focal wall changes

Malignant masses

The most common malignant masses found in the GI tract are adenocarcinoma, carcinoma, leiomyosarcoma, histiocytic sarcoma, fibrosarcoma, lymphoma, mast cell neoplasia, and GI stromal tumor. GI stromal tumors range from malignant to benign in classification.

Although some lesions are visible on radiographs as intraluminal or concentric soft tissue masses that can contain areas of mineralization, ultrasonography is the method of choice for detection and characterization of these lesions. CT can also be used for surgical planning if required, particularly in cases of very large masses.

Common ultrasonographic features of neoplasia include thickening of the GI walls, alteration of the normal wall layering, presence of pseudolayering and altered motility and echogenicity of the segments affected. Pseudolayering is characterized by the replacement of the normal five layers of the walls by two hypoechoic layers surrounding one more echogenic layer; it is strongly suggestive of gastric carcinoma. This is thought to be due to the uneven distribution of tumor cells within the lesion. The thickening of the walls can vary from a few millimeters to several centimeters. Neoplastic lesions tend to present with a larger degree of thickening than inflammatory lesions. Mast cell neoplasia can be seen as focal asymmetric eccentric strongly hypoechoic masses with loss of layering. This has been described as a feature in cats, but now also in two dogs.[28] Gastrointestinal stromal tumors are usually heterogenous and very large, making their anatomical localization difficult. These masses are often associated with the cecum; however, their appearance mimics smooth muscle tumors.

There is overlap in the imaging features between neoplasia and inflammatory disease. Therefore, interpretation should always be considered in light of the patient's history, clinical signs, and laboratory and cytology findings. The type of tumor is also difficult to establish based on imaging studies, and cytology and/or histopathology are often required for a definitive diagnosis. Regional lymph nodes should be evaluated, and sampling may help provide further diagnostic information.

Benign masses

Non-neoplastic masses of the GI tract include granulomas, leiomyomas, polyps, adenomatous hyperplasia, or adenomas (Fig. 21.11). These may have a benign or a more aggressive biological behavior.

Polyps appear as pedunculated rounded lesions that project into the lumen. Vascularization of the pedicle and polyp can be observed with Doppler ultrasonography. Hyperplasia of the mucosal or muscular layers is difficult to differentiate from large polypoid lesions based on appearance alone. Smooth muscle tumors are most often large in size (over 3 cm) at the time of diagnosis, hypoechoic, and growing eccentrically from the serosal layer or extraluminally. Granulomatous lesions have features that significantly overlap with neoplastic lesions in appearance.

Diffuse wall changes

Corrugation

Corrugation is a nonspecific sign associated with many different pathological processes such as enteritis, peritonitis, renal disease, neoplasia, bowel ischemia, protein-losing enteropathy, and pancreatitis.[29] The

- Dilation of the lower esophageal sphincter (Video 22.6).
- Luminal stenosis (Video 22.7).
- Intussusception (Videos 22.8 and 22.9).
- Masses, such as varices (Video 22.10), parasitic nodules (e.g., *Spirocerca lupi*),[5] polyps (Video 22.11), focal lipogranulomatous lymphangitis,[6] and neoplasia (Video 22.12).

The main ancillary procedures that can be performed via endoscopy include the following:

- Biopsy or fine-needle aspiration of the GI wall (Video 22.13).
- Foreign body retrieval, directly by means of the endoscope (Video 22.14), by passing rigid forceps alongside the endoscope (Video 22.15), or assisted by laparotomy (Video 22.16).[7]
- Treatment of esophageal or rectal strictures.[8]
- Injection of drugs using a per-endoscopic needle (Video 22.17).
- Temporary complete endotracheal tube obstruction to increase the transdiaphragmatic pressure gradient, and to highlight a hiatal hernia.[9]
- Electrosurgical ablation of polyps (Fig. 22.2; Video 22.18).
- Electrocoagulation of non-neoplastic ulcerations (Video 22.19).
- Placement of percutaneous gastric or jejunal feeding tubes.[10]

Since endoscopic examination of the digestive system is always performed with the patient under anesthesia, the main contraindications for endoscopic examination of the GI tract are primarily anesthesia-related risk factors (e.g., cardiorespiratory disorders, moderate/severe anemia) as well as coagulopathy, metabolic disturbances, kidney/liver failure, immunodeficiency, and intestinal perforation.

It must not be forgotten that, for the most part, endoscopy is an inspection procedure, and similar morphological appearances can correspond to different diseases. Therefore, histological confirmation is always necessary before a final diagnosis can be reached (Fig. 22.3). In addition, since endoscopic biopsy specimens rarely include the submucosa, the etiology of pathological changes involving deeper layers of the GI wall will likely not be identified via this procedure.

Video 22.1

Jejunoscopy in a dog with intestinal lymphangiectasia. Note the white spots at the tips of the villi, representing severe cystic lacteal dilation.

Video 22.2

Endoscopy in a dog with chronic gastritis. Note the thickening of the fundic and antral mucosa, and the cobblestone appearance of the antral mucosa.

Video 22.3

Colonoscopy in a dog with a flare-up of chronic colitis. Note the diffuse mucosal thickening with loss of visualization of the submucosal vascular pattern, and the numerous bleeding erosions.

Video 22.4

Esophagoscopy in an English Bulldog with brachycephalic syndrome. Note the salmon-pink tongues of mucosal tissue at the distal esophagus, proximal to the gastroesophageal junction, which corresponds to mucosal metaplasia (Barrett's esophagus) in response to damage caused by chronic gastroesophageal reflux. The change from a normal squamous epithelium into a columnar epithelium with goblet cells is a premalignant condition that can lead to the development of an esophageal adenocarcinoma.

Video 22.5

Endoscopy showing three benign gastric ulcers with slightly thickened margins, one in the fundus/body, one at the lesser curvature, and one in the body/pyloric antrum region.

Video 22.6

Forward and backward views of the esophagus with the endoscope in the esophagus and cardia, respectively. The lower esophageal sphincter is dilated, and there is severe hiatal dilatation. Note the hyperemic and erosive lesions of the mucosa at the terminal portion of the esophagus.

Video 22.7

Endoscopy showing esophageal stenosis at the heart base due to a persistent right aortic arch. Note the esophageal diverticulum cranial to the heart base, and the severe distal compression due to the vascular ring.

Video 22.8

Esophagoscopy suggestive of occlusion of the lower esophageal sphincter by gastric mucosa due to gastroesophageal intussusception (retrograde invagination of a part of the stomach into the caudal part of the thoracic esophagus without the displacement of the gastroesophageal junction).

Video 22.9

Colonoscopy showing narrowing of the proximal colon due to a pseudopolypoid mass consisting of the cecum invaginated into the colon (i.e., cecal inversion or cecocolic intussusception).

Video 22.10

Endoscopy showing swollen veins in the lining of the esophagus. These are esophageal varices, defined as veins of the esophagus that are abnormally dilated due to increased vascular resistance in the portal venous system or in the cranial vena cava, or due to arteriovenous fistulae formation from the pulmonary arteries, or from the aorta.

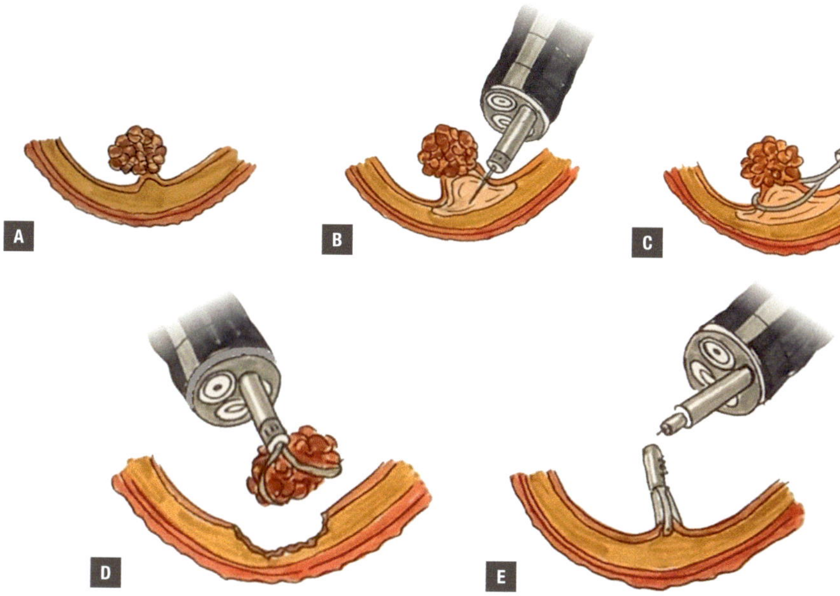

FIG. 22.2 Schematic representation of endoscopic polyp removal via electrocoagulation and electrosection using a generator providing electrical current flow. A dispersive grounding pad must be placed on the patient's shaved decubitus side, ensuring good skin contact, wet with saline solution and not with alcohol. (A) Polyp before removal. (B) Saline solution and epinephrine (1:10,000 epinephrine in 0.9% saline) are injected submucosally to form a cushion and lift the mucosa from the underlying layers. If possible, two injections should be made: first proximal and then distal to the polyp. (C) A snare loop is positioned around the base of the polyp. Electrocoagulation is activated followed by electrosection. (D) The polyp is removed with a basket/forceps. (E) A hemostatic clip is placed on the mucosa. Original drawn by Dr. Alessandra Ghelli, with permission.

Equipment needed for upper and lower gastrointestinal endoscopy

The canine species is characterized by a wide range of somatic variability between individuals of different breeds, ranging from animals weighing just 1 kg (e.g., Chihuahua, Yorkshire Terrier) up to the 80–90 kg of giant breeds (e.g., Great Dane). This influences the choice of instruments to be used in GI endoscopy. If it is not possible, for economic reasons, to have a wide range of endoscopes of different diameters and lengths, an endoscope with a working length of 140 cm, a tip diameter of 7–8 mm, and at least a 2.8 mm working channel will be suitable for most small and all giant dog breeds. It will also be possible to insert biopsy forceps and most endoscopic ancillary instruments, which, in general, have a diameter of 2.3 mm. Importantly, four-way tip deflection with complete retroflexion (≥180°) in one direction must be available to examine the gastric cardia, enable passage through the pylorus, and make ileal intubation easier.

Use of videoendoscopes is recommended. The image is acquired by a video chip (charge-coupled device [CCD] or complementary metal-oxide-semiconductor chip [CMOS]) at the tip of the instrument and transmitted as electrical signals to the processor. Modern videoscopes offer high-definition quality imaging. In contrast, fiberscopes transmit images by means of optical fibers, resulting in a lower-quality, pixelated image. The necessary instrumentation also includes a light source (a 100–300 W xenon or a LED light source are preferred to a tungsten-halogen bulb), an image processor to reconstruct the electrical signals received by the video chip, a pump/insufflator, a monitor, and devices for photo and video documentation.

Numerous accessories and ancillary instruments with diagnostic and therapeutic capabilities can be added to the basic endoscope system. These include sheaths and instruments for biopsy, grasping, cytological sampling, aspiration/fluid infusion, electrosurgery, and laser surgery. In addition, the following are useful and often necessary: baskets and loop snares for foreign body retrieval, polypectomy snares, endoscopic needles for injection/aspiration, suction traps to collect fluid specimens, and hydrostatic balloon dilators and bougies (or bougie caps[11]) to treat esophageal stenosis. To prevent damage to the lower esophageal

Video 22.11

Endoscopy of the descending colon showing the presence of polyps covered by normal mucosa.

Video 22.12

Colonoscopy using water immersion showing a single mass in the midrectum with a cauliflower-like appearance (rectal adenocarcinoma).

Video 22.13

Endoscopy showing a malignant ulcer at the lesser curvature of the stomach (gastric adenocarcinoma). Repeated biopsy on the margin and endoscopic needle aspiration were performed.

Video 22.14

Endoscopic removal of a gastric foreign body (cork) using basket forceps.

Video 22.15

Removal of an esophageal foreign body (bone) using a flexible endoscope and a rigid foreign body retrieval forceps, designed for passage alongside the endoscope. Note the ulcerated and hemorrhagic appearance of the terminal esophageal mucosa after foreign body removal.

Video 22.16

Combination of exploratory laparotomy and endoscopy to remove a linear foreign body. One part of the foreign body was in the stomach, and the remaining portion through the pylorus into the duodenum and jejunum. The foreign body should not be pulled retrogradely until the surgeon has released it from the intestinal loop. Therefore, the intestinal part of the foreign body was gently milked by hand into the stomach to allow its safe removal by endoscopy, thus avoiding the need for enterotomy.

Video 22.17

Preventive treatment of stenosis recurrence, after balloon dilation of an esophageal stenosis, by means of submucosal injection of slow-release methylprednisolone using a per-endoscopic needle. Performing intralesional injections around the entire circumference of the esophagus is recommended. Published studies also recommend injecting before dilating the stricture and using triamcinolone.

Video 22.18

Electrosurgical ablation of a sessile lesion (rectal polyp) using a monopolar endoscopic snare. After debulking, a clip is placed endoscopically, with positioning confirmed by radiographic examination.

Video 22.19

Endoscopic treatment of proximal duodenal ulceration using a monopolar electrocoagulation technique. The strong thermal effect produces coagulation and hemostasis in the intestinal wall, resulting in clot formation in the submucosal vessels and bleeding arrest.

sphincter during removal of sharp gastric foreign bodies, a rubber cap can be mounted on the endoscope tip; during withdrawal of the endoscope through the lower esophageal sphincter, the bell portion is reversed so that the hood flips back to its original shape, thereby protecting the esophagus and pharynx from the pointed/cutting edges of the foreign body.[12] It should be remembered that most endoscopic accessories are intended for use in human medicine. Although the application of these products in dogs is usually satisfactory, there are some exceptions. Anatomically, the space between the greater horns of the hyoid bone in humans is smaller than in many dogs; therefore, compared to humans, dogs can ingest significantly larger foreign bodies. For this reason, accessories designed specifically for veterinary use (e.g., foreign body basket forceps with a 14 × 10 cm opening) may be required. In fact, these are mandatory in the case of large foreign bodies that need to be removed from the esophagus or stomach.

After endoscopic examination, the procedure must be completed by taking proper care of the instruments to avoid transmission of pathogens from one patient to the next. Meticulous cleaning, of both the outside and the internal channels using a brush and an enzymatic cleaner to remove biological material, must precede high-level disinfection/sterilization. Disinfection can be carried out with an approved disinfectant. Sterilization can be achieved utilizing ethylene oxide, glutaraldehyde, or peracetic acid, after appropriate risk assessment for use of these potentially toxic sterilants. Table 22.1 summarizes the steps to follow for completing the procedure, according to the Centers for Disease Control and Prevention.[13]

Patient preparation

A scheduled endoscopic examination of the GI tract involves the assessment of the clinical and laboratory findings justifying the procedure (see above) and a 12-hour fast, leaving water available up to 3 hours before the examination. Upper GI endoscopy is performed first when lower GI endoscopy is also required.

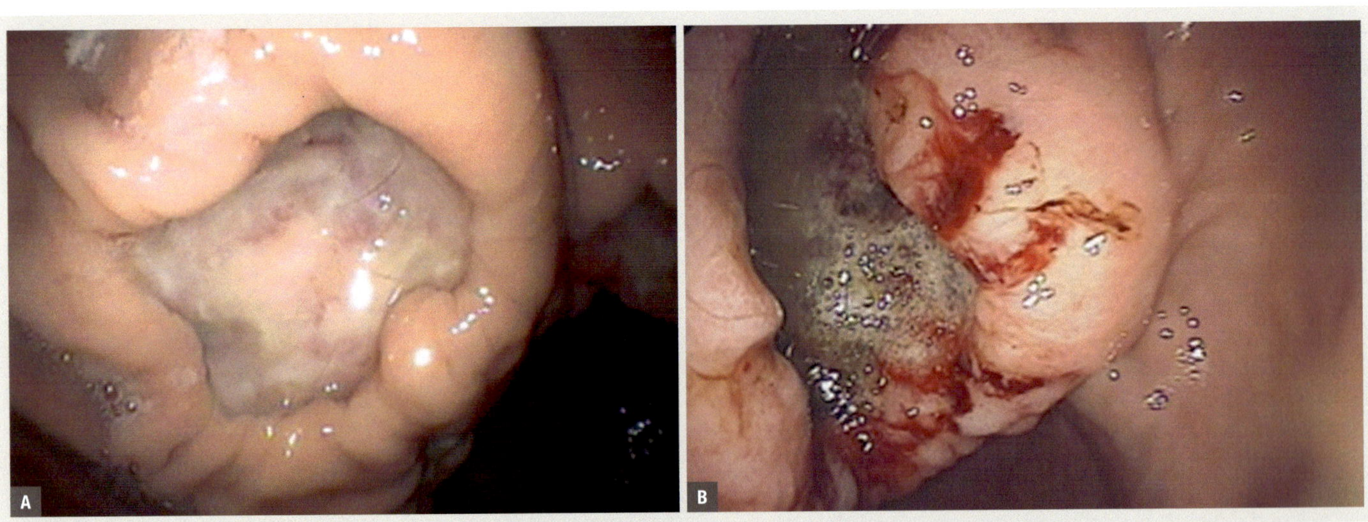

FIG. 22.3 (A) Benign vs. (B) malignant gastric ulcer (carcinoma). Macroscopic appearance does not always allow differentiation between the two forms, in the same way that biopsy is not always diagnostic (if too superficial or if only necrotic tissue is collected).

TABLE 22.1 Guidelines for flexible endoscope reprocessing.

1	Educate all personnel about the biological, chemical, and environmental hazards associated with the procedures which require disinfectants.
2	Make protective equipment available (e.g., gloves, gowns, eyewear, face mask or shields, respiratory protection devices) and use these items appropriately to protect workers from exposure to both chemicals and microorganisms.
3	Before the procedure, attach the cap designed to protect the electrical connections, and test the endoscope for leaks using a pressure tester. Ensure that all pressure is removed prior to disconnecting the leak tester.
4	Disconnect and disassemble the endoscopic components (suction valves and biopsy channel cap), and completely immerse all components in the enzymatic cleaner.
5	Meticulously clean the internal and external surfaces of the components. Brush the internal channels passing the brush in a single direction, avoiding a back-and-forth scrubbing motion; alternatively, push and pull a double-ended brush through the channels.
6	Flush the external surface and each internal channel with water and an enzymatic cleaner that is compatible with the endoscope.
7	Immerse the endoscope in an approved high-level disinfectant or sterilant (e.g., ethylene oxide, glutaraldehyde, or peracetic acid) and perfuse the disinfectant into all accessible channels, such as the suction/biopsy channel and air/water channel. Use the disinfectant manufacturers' recommended exposure conditions.
8	Rinse the endoscope and all channels with tap water.
9	Rinse the insertion tube and inner channels with alcohol, and dry with forced air.
10	Store the endoscope, hanging it vertically, not in its travel suitcase.
Remember to follow the manufacturer's warnings for your specific endoscope.	

The anesthetic protocol for GI endoscopy should include drugs that avoid spasm of the sphincters in order to allow easier access through the pylorus and, if lower GI tract examination is to be performed as well, through the ileal papilla. The safest anesthetic protocol is the one the anesthetist is familiar with and is confident in. A suitable anesthetic protocol is as follows:

1. After placement of a catheter into the cephalic vein, the patient is administered butorphanol (0.4 mg/kg intramuscular [IM]) and dexmedetomidine (7–15 µg/kg IM) as premedication.
2. After 20 minutes, general anesthesia is induced with propofol or alfaxalone administered intravenously and titrated to effect in order to achieve endotracheal intubation with a cuffed tube.[14]
3. The dog is placed in left lateral recumbency and connected to a multiparameter monitor to evaluate heart rate, mean arterial pressure, SpO_2, respiratory rate, and end-tidal CO_2 and/or isoflurane concentration.
4. General anesthesia is maintained with isoflurane or sevoflurane vaporized in 100% oxygen delivered through an appropriate breathing system.[15]

In case of reduced visibility of the lower esophagus or stomach due to excessive foaming produced by swallowed saliva, it is recommended to spray a simethicone syrup (25 mg for small dogs, up to 200 mg for large dogs) and/or acetylcysteine through the working channel.[16] It should be remembered that the use of simethicone in dogs, although common, is empirical, and studies regarding safety and adverse effects in dogs have not yet been published.

During endoscopic GI examination, the dilation medium utilized to distend the bowel is usually air or, less frequently, carbon dioxide. However, improvement in visualization can also be achieved by the instillation of warm (~37°C) water, instead of air, through the working channel (Fig. 22.4); part of this water is aspirated at the end of the examination and the rest spontaneously absorbed.[17] The water volume introduced should be enough to fill the duodenal lumen completely and varies from 40 to 100 mL, depending on the size of the dog (Video 22.20).[17]

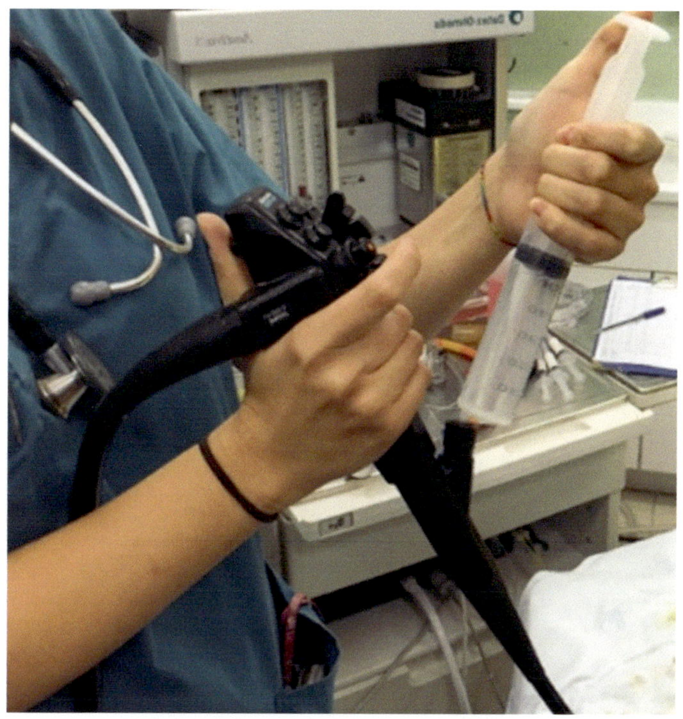

FIG. 22.4 Inoculation of warm water through the endoscope working channel to distend the intestinal lumen and improve visualization of the mucosal surface during an upper gastrointestinal endoscopy.

Video 22.20

Endoscopic view of the duodenum using air insufflation vs. water infusion. Note the better visualization of the mucosal surface and villous pattern under water immersion as compared to the examination carried out with air insufflation.

Preparing the lower GI tract for endoscopy is more complex and time-consuming than preparation of the upper GI tract for examination, since removal of the feces from the colon is essential to allow visualization of the wall and reduce the execution time of the procedure.

If there are no contraindications (e.g., food-responsive enteropathy), administering a low-fiber diet (chicken or white fish) for 4–5 days before a colonoscopy is recommended. Food, but not water, should be withheld for 24 hours prior to general anesthesia, excluding dogs with protein-losing enteropathy, which should only be fasted for 8 hours before the examination. The literature recommends the administration of a bowel-cleansing agent (e.g., macrogol [PEG 3350] with or without isotonic electrolytes at 25–30 mL/kg[18,19]) 18 and 12 hours before the endoscopy. This is not easy for owners to carry out, as few dogs will drink the agent voluntarily, even if dissolved in a meat-flavored solution. The large volume of cleansing fluid often requires nasogastric or orogastric intubation, which is not without risk and increases the hospitalization period and the cost of the procedure.[20]

A reasonable degree of colon cleansing can be achieved by administering a significantly smaller volume of bowel-cleansing fluid (e.g., 50 mL of macrogol for dogs weighing less than 10 kg, 100 mL for dogs weighing 11–25 kg, and 150 mL for dogs weighing more, plus sodium and potassium salts, administered orally) 18 and 16 hours before general anesthesia. This should be followed by enemas (30–50 mL/kg) using warm water without soap, at least three times 1 hour apart, in the 6 hours before anesthesia, until the liquid emitted is clean.

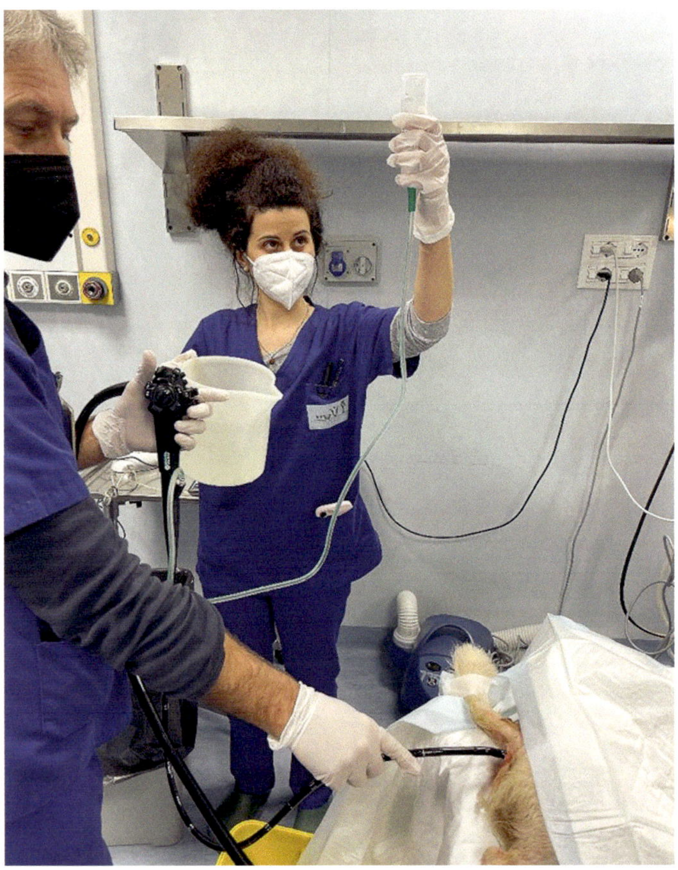

FIG. 22.5 Continued inoculation of warm water through the endoscope working channel during a colonoscopy to optimize colon cleansing, distend the lumen, and improve visualization of the mucosal surface.

The colonoscopic procedure begins with the animal under anesthesia, positioned in left lateral recumbency, with the table slightly lowered, so as to keep the caudal portion of the body lower. Intraprocedural cleaning allows the elimination of any remaining fecal material which, despite performing enemas, always remains in the colon, significantly improving the visualization of the mucosa. The working channel of the endoscope can be connected, by means of a modified Levin tube with the end cut off, to a funnel which is continuously filled with warm (~37 °C) water at a low pressure (Fig. 22.5, Video 22.21). This water (which should be allowed to flow and not injected to avoid barotrauma) will be released from the endoscope tip, washing the mucosa as the instrument is passed proximally. A peristaltic flushing pump can also be attached via a channel adapter. The liquid flows freely out of the anus and is collected in a specially positioned container, avoiding any increase in intra-abdominal pressure. At the end of the examination, before the endoscope is removed, any remaining liquid should be aspirated.

The use of prophylactic antibiotic treatment for digestive endoscopy in dogs should be avoided. Whilst bacteremia resulting from endoscopic procedures has been reported in a small percentage of animals,[21] the risks linked to the development of antibiotic resistance, from a One Health perspective, clearly negate the utilization of antibiotic prophylaxis except in immunosuppressed dogs.

Advantages and disadvantages

When compared to biopsy via laparotomy, endoscopic biopsy is faster, cheaper, less invasive, and less painful for the patient on recovery. It also allows direct visualization of any lesion within reach, which is not always possible when using a surgical approach. Moreover, it can be performed even in hypoproteinemic dogs.

While the number of surgical biopsies is limited to 3–4, they are relatively large and full thickness. With endoscopic examination, multiple samples can be taken from sites that are distant from each other, with a reduced recovery time. Collecting a minimum of six good-quality specimens from each part of the GI tract is recommended;[22] 10–15 from each sector is ideal. However, compared to biopsy by laparotomy (or laparoscopy), endoscopic biopsy has limitations, namely the aforementioned inability to completely examine and sample the whole jejunal tract and other abdominal organs (lymph nodes, spleen, and liver), the small size of the samples, and the impossibility of performing full-thickness sampling. Therefore, it may not allow identification of conditions that affect the entire gastric or enteric wall, or of diseases in the layers deeper than the muscularis mucosae. Furthermore, even if rare, there are cases (e.g., carcinoma with extensive stromal desmoplasia) in which the hardness of the tissue does not allow it to be sampled with endoscopic forceps; in this situation, surgery is necessary.

Video 22.21

Endoscopic cecal examination using water as the dilation medium.

Biopsy collection techniques

The acquisition of biopsies is usually mandatory in the course of diagnostic endoscopic procedures, since a simple inspection of the mucosal surface is unlikely to indicate the specific disease. In contrast, in therapeutic endoscopy (e.g., foreign body removal) biopsy findings may be irrelevant; it is very often impossible to determine whether the presence of an inflammatory histological picture is due to the foreign body or to an underlying condition.

Acquiring good-quality biopsies depends upon numerous factors, the first being the choice of biopsy forceps, which must have the largest biopsy cup that will fit down the biopsy channel. Oval or ellipsoid cups will provide larger biopsies than round cups. Of note, the presence of a spike or other features in the cups (alligator vs. smooth edge, fenestrated vs. nonfenestrated) does not significantly influence the diagnostic value of the histological examination.[23] Biopsy forceps can be disposable or reusable; however, it is essential to check that the blade is sharp and does not tear the sample. To ensure that a satisfactory biopsy sample is obtained, the forceps must be positioned perpendicularly against the mucosa avoiding advancing the forceps too far from the endoscope tip to maintain greater pressure on the mucosa, and then suction should be applied to make the mucosa collapse into the biopsy cups before closing them.

In order to reduce intubation time, it is possible to perform a double-bite technique instead of a single bite: two successive bites of the mucosa are taken to collect two samples each time the forceps are withdrawn.[24]

In ulcers, biopsy specimens should be taken from the rim of all four quadrants, and not from the central portion of the lesion, which often consists of necrotic material. In the case of submucosal masses with normal overlying mucosa (e.g., leiomyoma, leiomyosarcoma), it may be necessary to attempt needle aspiration (Video 22.22) or repeat biopsies from the same site ("well-excavation biopsy") in order to introduce the forceps under the mucosa and sample the underlying muscular layer (Video 22.23). Samples obtained by endoscopic biopsy can be used for histological/immunohistochemical examination, clonality testing, and bacteriological examination.

In general, care must be taken when extracting the biopsy from the forceps; the use of tweezers should be avoided. The sample should be gently removed from the cup with the tip of a micropipette or a needle and placed onto a cellulose acetate filter in order to maintain correct orientation (i.e., mucosal surface up and muscularis mucosae side down).

Video 22.22

Per-endoscopic fine-needle aspiration for cytological sampling of a submucosal mass (gastric cardia leiomyoma).

Video 22.23

Well-excavation biopsy of a submucosal mass (leiomyoma) at the level of the cardia. To collect samples of the tissue beneath the mucosal layer, repeated biopsies are performed in the same area until closed forceps can be introduced beneath the mucosa. The forceps are then opened to obtain neoplastic smooth muscle tissue.

Each strip containing specimens from the same organ is deposited into a test tube with 10% buffered formalin. Alternatively, biopsies may be placed directly into formalin or onto a foam insert within a tissue cassette that is then immersed in formalin.[25]

For bacteriological testing—e.g., necessary for checking the sensitivity of antibiotics against *Escherichia coli* in granulomatous (histiocytic ulcerative) colitis—it is essential to use a disinfected endoscope and new, sterile forceps. After cleaning the colonic surface with 0.9% sterile saline solution and taking the biopsy, the tissue is placed on a sterile surface and washed with 0.9% sterile saline to reduce surface contamination. The sample is then stored in a test tube with 0.9% sterile saline and sent to a microbiology laboratory, which will take material for culture and susceptibility testing after homogenizing the tissue.

New endoscopy methods

New techniques, routinely used in human medicine, have been introduced into the veterinary field in recent years. Capsule videoendoscopy is commonly used in people with chronic GI hemorrhage to explore sections of the intestinal tract that cannot be reached with a flexible endoscope. In veterinary medicine, this technique can be used in patients with a systemic illness that makes them unsuitable for general anesthesia and traditional flexible endoscopy, if the pet owners declined endoscopy due to cost/invasiveness, or especially in cases of chronic intestinal bleeding of unknown origin.

The capsule is administered orally and records the mucosal appearance of the GI tract while it is propelled by peristalsis. There are various types of commercially available endoscopic capsules capable of recording images of the GI tract, differing in size and system (lateral- vs. axial-viewing). They contain a camera with high magnification, a light source, a transmitter, and a battery. Some are connected wirelessly to a recording device and computer and collect video in real-time. There is a veterinary-specific system that stores multiple images on an internal flash drive, and images can be downloaded after retrieval of the capsule from the feces.

The main advantages of capsule videoendoscopy over conventional endoscopy are visualization of the entire small intestine and lower risks and costs, since anesthesia is not necessary. However, incomplete recording of the GI tract is the most common complication, due to gastric or intestinal retention of the capsule, encountered in approximately 38% of cases.[26,27] Biopsies cannot be obtained by this device, which limits the procedure to simple observation.

In addition to imaging, endoscopy capsules can be used as wireless sensors to measure pH, temperature, peristaltic pressure, and transit time simultaneously within the GI tract.[28] Also, the possibility of endoscopically fixing a radiotelemetric pH-monitoring capsule in the distal esophagus, using vacuum suction and a lock and pin mechanism, allows continuous recording of the pH in this sector. This is useful for a precise diagnosis of gastroesophageal reflux, even in patients without apparent esophageal mucosal lesions.[29]

Another new technique that could be useful in endoscopy in the coming years is narrow-band imaging, which is based on removing red light from the illumination. This highlights the submucosal vascular bed and aids in assessing the degree of tissue inflammation or the presence of dysplasia or neoplasia. It should be emphasized, however, that at the time of writing of this chapter, the information provided by narrow-band imaging is not comparable to that obtained by histological examination of biopsies.[30]

In white light endoscopy, mucosal visualization can be improved by spraying dyes (5 mL of dye in an air-filled 20–30 mL container) onto the mucosal surface (a technique called "chromoendoscopy"), either using a syringe inserted into the rubber biopsy valve of the scope or via a wash tube passed down the working channel. Based on their staining properties, dyes can be classified into three groups:

- Vital stains (e.g., Lugol's iodine, methylene blue, crystal violet, acetic acid) are absorbed by specific cells, delineating dysplastic or neoplastic areas.
- Nonabsorptive stains (e.g., indigo carmine) fix themselves to irregularities of the mucosa, highlighting the detailed contour of the mucosal surface. Currently, the use of chromoendoscopy in veterinary medicine to detect subtle changes suggesting preneoplastic processes or malignancies, followed by targeted biopsies for histology, is limited to indigo carmine.[31]
- Reactive stains (e.g., Congo red, phenol red) change color due to chemical reactions with cellular components.[32]

KEY POINTS

- Like other ancillary techniques, endoscopy is only part of the diagnostic process.
- With the exception of therapeutic endoscopy (e.g., foreign body removal, polypectomy), endoscopic examination of the gastrointestinal tract should include all sectors: esophagus, stomach, duodenum, jejunum, ileum, and colon.
- It is preferable to use a videoendoscope with four-way tip deflection, 140 cm of working length, a tip diameter of 7–8 mm, and a working channel diameter that allows the use of 2.3 mm ancillary instruments.
- In case of reduced visibility of the lower esophagus or stomach due to excessive foaming produced by swallowed saliva, spraying a simethicone syrup is recommended.
- Visualization of the intestinal mucosal surface is improved by instillation of warm water instead of air or carbon dioxide insufflation.
- Collecting a minimum of six biopsy specimens from each region of the gastrointestinal tract is recommended.

References

1. Irom S, Sherding R, Johnson S, Stromberg P. Gastrointestinal perforation associated with endoscopy in cats and dogs. *J Am Anim Hosp Assoc* 50(5):322–329, 2014.
2. Procoli F, Mõtsküla PF, Keyte SV, et al. Comparison of histopathologic findings in duodenal and ileal endoscopic biopsies in dogs with chronic small intestinal enteropathies. *J Vet Intern Med* 27(2):268–274, 2013.
3. Sarria R, López Albors O, Soria F, et al. Characterization of oral double balloon endoscopy in the dog. *Vet J* 195(3):331–336, 2013.
4. Sarriá R, López Albors O, Soria F, et al. Characterization of anal double balloon endoscopy in the dog. *Vet J* 197(3):886–888, 2013.
5. Aroch I, Markovics A, Mazaki-Tovi M, et al. Spirocercosis in dogs in Israel: A retrospective case-control study (2004–2009). *Vet Parasitol* 211(3–4):234–240, 2015.
6. Lecoindre A, Lecoindre P, Cadoré JL, et al. Focal intestinal lipogranulomatous lymphangitis in 10 dogs. *J Small Anim Pract* 57(9):465–471, 2016.
7. Demars C, Boland L, Minier K. Surgical removal of intestinal foreign bodies using a laparotomy-assisted endoscopic approach in dogs and cats and comparison with enterotomy. *J Small Anim Pract* 64(1):43–50, 2023.
8. Da Riz F, Béguin J, Manassero M, et al. Outcome of dogs and cats with benign oesophageal strictures after balloon dilatation or stenting: 27 cases (2002–2019). *J Small Anim Pract* 62(10):886–894, 2021.
9. Freiche V, German AJ. Digestive diseases in brachycephalic dogs. *Vet Clin North Am Small Anim Pract* 51(1):61–78, 2021.
10. Hinden SE, Schweighauser A, Francey T. Evaluation of a novel non-surgical post-pyloric feeding technique in dogs with severe acute kidney injury. *J Vet Emerg Crit Care (San Antonio)* 30(4):384–395, 2020.
11. Cortez-Pinto J, Mão de Ferro S, Dias Pereira A. Use of the novel BougieCap in the treatment of esophageal peptic stricture. *Endoscopy* 51(9):E251–E252, 2019.
12. Wood AN, Gallagher AE. Survey of instruments and techniques for endoscopic retrieval of esophageal and gastric foreign bodies in cats and dogs. *Top Companion Anim Med* 45:100555, 2021.
13. Rutala WA, Weber DJ. Guideline for Disinfection and Sterilization in Healthcare Facilities, 2008 [Internet]. Available from: https://www.cdc.gov/infection-control/hcp/disinfection-and-sterilization/.
14. Grubb T, Sager J, Gaynor JS, et al. 2020 AAHA anesthesia and monitoring guidelines for dogs and cats. *J Am Anim Hosp Assoc* 56(2):59–82, 2020.
15. McFadzean WJ, Hall EJ, van Oostrom H. Effect of premedication with butorphanol or methadone on ease of endoscopic duodenal intubation in dogs. *Vet Anaesth Analg* 44(6):1296–1302, 2017.
16. Basford PJ, Brown J, Gadeke L, et al. A randomized controlled trial of pre-procedure simethicone and N-acetylcysteine to improve mucosal visibility during gastroscopy – NICEVIS. *Endosc Int Open* 4(11):E1197–E1202, 2016.
17. Galiazzo G, Costantino F, Foglia A, et al. Water immersion vs. air insufflation in canine duodenal endoscopy: is the future underwater? *Pol J Vet Sci* 23(4):581–588, 2020.
18. Rychlik A, Nowicki M, Kander M, Szweda M. The effect of macrogol administration on the quality of macroscopic images and transit time in canine capsule endoscopy. *Pol J Vet Sci* 17(4):673–679, 2014.
19. Richter KP, Cleveland MB. Comparison of an orally administered gastrointestinal lavage solution with

traditional enema administration as preparation for colonoscopy in dogs. *J Am Vet Med Assoc* 195(12):1727–1731, 1989.

20. Leib MS, Baechtel MS, Monroe WE. Complications associated with 355 flexible colonoscopic procedures in dogs. *J Vet Intern Med* 18(5):642–646, 2004.
21. Gaspardo A, Sabetti MC, Zanoni RG, et al. Incidence of bacteremia consequent to different endoscopic procedures in dogs: a preliminary study. *Animals (Basel)* 10(12):2265, 2020.
22. Day MJ, Bilzer T, Mansell J, et al. Histopathological standards for the diagnosis of gastrointestinal inflammation in endoscopic biopsy samples from the dog and cat: a report from the World Small Animal Veterinary Association Gastrointestinal Standardization Group. *J Comp Pathol* 138 Suppl 1:S1–43, 2008.
23. Goutal-Landry CM, Mansell J, Ryan KA, Gaschen FP. Effect of endoscopic forceps on quality of duodenal mucosal biopsy in healthy dogs. *J Vet Intern Med* 27(3):456–461, 2013.
24. Muhammad H, Burch N, Gordon V, et al. One bite or two? A comparison of single bite and double bite biopsy techniques in gastrointestinal endoscopy (BITES). *Scand J Gastroenterol* 58(6):680–683, 2023.
25. Ruiz GC, Reyes-Gomez E, Hall EJ, Freiche V. Comparison of 3 handling techniques for endoscopically obtained gastric and duodenal biopsy specimens: a prospective study in dogs and cats. *J Vet Intern Med* 30(4):1014–1021, 2016.
26. Davignon DL, Lee AC, Johnston AN, et al. Evaluation of capsule endoscopy to detect mucosal lesions associated with gastrointestinal bleeding in dogs. *J Small Anim Pract* 57(3):148–158, 2016.
27. Stiller J, Defarges AM, Brisson BA, et al. Feasibility, complications, and quality of visualization using video capsule endoscopy in 40 dogs with overt or questionable gastrointestinal bleeding. *J Vet Intern Med* 35(4):1743–1753, 2021.
28. Warrit K, Boscan P, Ferguson LE, et al. Effect of hospitalization on gastrointestinal motility and pH in dogs. *J Am Vet Med Assoc* 251(1):65–70, 2017.
29. Kook PH, Kempf J, Ruetten M, Reusch CE. Wireless ambulatory esophageal pH monitoring in dogs with clinical signs interpreted as gastroesophageal reflux. *J Vet Intern Med* 28(6):1716–1723, 2014.
30. Salavati M, Pérez-Accino J, Tan YL, et al. Correlation of minimally invasive imaging techniques to assess intestinal mucosal perfusion with established markers of chronic inflammatory enteropathy in dogs. *J Vet Intern Med* 35(1):162–171, 2021.
31. Candido MV, Syrjä P, Kilpinen S, et al. Can chromoendoscopy improve the early diagnosis of gastric carcinoma in dogs? *Animals (Basel)* 12(17):2253, 2022.
32. Singh R, Chiam KH, Leiria F, et al. Chromoendoscopy: role in modern endoscopic imaging. *Transl Gastroenterol Hepatol* 5:39, 2020.

CHAPTER 23

Intestinal biopsy

Simon L. Priestnall
BSc(Hons), BVSc, PhD, PGC(VetEd), FHEA, FRSB, DACVP, FRCPath, FRCVS

Alejandro Suárez-Bonnet
DVM, MVetMed (Distinction), PhD(Hons), DipRCPath, DACVP, MRCVS

Histopathological examination of the gastrointestinal (GI) tract is generally still considered to offer the potential for a "gold standard" diagnosis of many diseases and lesions within this body system. However, it must be stressed that the accuracy and specificity of this diagnosis is, perhaps more than in any other location, highly dependent on the quality and number of samples examined by the pathologist. It is also important to consider that, even within one species, establishing what is considered histologically "normal" across a range of breeds, ages, diets, etc., is largely based on experience, and thus examination and reporting of GI biopsies should ideally be performed by specialized or experienced pathologists.

The sample

Most upper and lower GI samples are obtained endoscopically using forceps. The quality and number of samples (as a rule of thumb, the more the better) are paramount, both in terms of actual sampling (see Chapter 22) and then handling. This chapter will focus on handling and submission to the laboratory.

The best sample is generally the one handled the least, but some handling will be unavoidable. Not only are the samples very small and delicate, but they also have an inherent tendency to curl up when placed into formalin. Although various techniques have been devised to aid sample handling and avoid crushing, such as mounting on filter paper or even dehydrated cucumber slices, good results are usually obtained when samples are submitted between two synthetic formalin-soaked sponges and then sealed within a plastic histological cassette (Fig. 23.1).[1] This protects the samples physically and ensures that no samples are lost in the formalin pot when reaching the laboratory. If sponges or histological cassettes are not available, samples can be submitted free-floating in formalin.

Ten percent neutral buffered formalin should be used and is widely commercially available. Formalin does have a shelf life, so ensuring that it is in date (still neutral pH) is important, as is adequate storage at room temperature.

For surgical (full-thickness) samples of the stomach or intestine where surgical margins might be important, such as tumor resections, inking of surgeon-cut margins is crucial, as samples can become markedly distorted following fixation. Alternatively, sutures can be used to indicate oral and aboral margins. These samples must be fixed adequately, which is best achieved by very gently removing any content (e.g., by very gentle rinsing) and then ideally by making a single longitudinal incision to open the lumen and allow adequate formalin penetration. If this is performed, it should be indicated on the submission form, so the laboratory staff are aware when undertaking further dissection and trimming for histological processing. Fixation generally takes place at a rate of 1 mm/hour (of each surface in contact with formalin, i.e., both serosal and luminal); therefore, most stomach or intestinal samples will be fixed and suitable for trimming within 24 hours. In samples with a larger "mass", such as a tumor, one or two incisions partway into the lesion will greatly aid fixation.

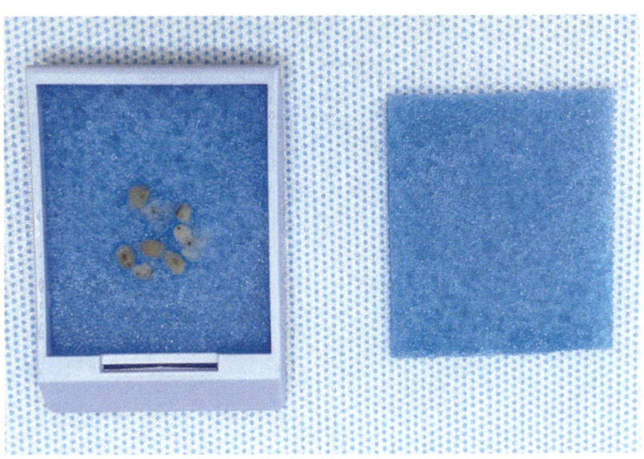

FIG. 23.1 Endoscopically retrieved stomach biopsies placed between two formalin-soaked sponges within a histological cassette. Use of sponges reduces the handling of the tissues with forceps and increases the chance that all samples will be processed at the laboratory.

Sample submission to the laboratory

Samples should ideally be submitted with a relevant and concise clinical history—ideally, a short description of the gross (endoscopic or intraoperative) appearance of the tissue and any interpretation provided by the endoscopist/surgeon. It is also helpful to provide any specific working differential diagnosis or questions that the pathologist should address. Samples can be accompanied by images from the endoscopy to provide additional (and very helpful) context to the pathologist.

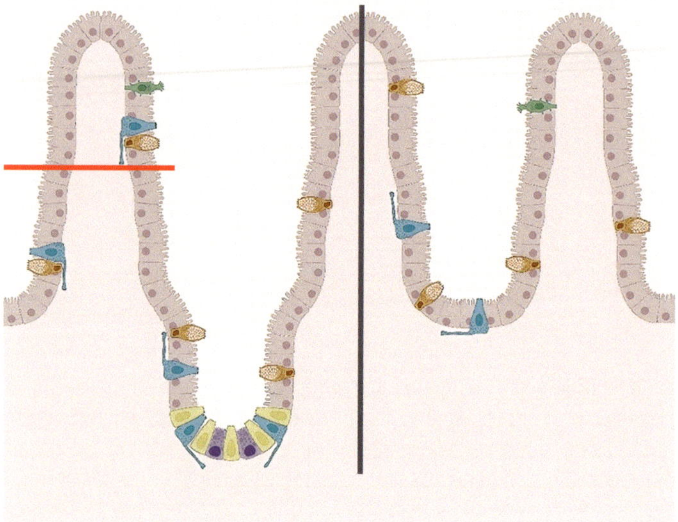

FIG. 23.2 Correct sectioning orientation (black line) for a full villus and crypt profile. If villi are sectioned transversely (red line) due to poor tissue orientation during embedding, assessment for evidence of atrophy will be virtually impossible.

Once received within the laboratory, samples should be processed as quickly as possible. Endoscopic specimens will almost always be fully fixed by the time they are received, so extended periods of fixation (longer than 48–72 hours) should be avoided if subsequent immunohistochemical labeling is to be optimally performed.

Ideally, a histology laboratory that is familiar with handling and processing of GI samples is preferred, as they will be familiar with sample orientation during embedding within molten paraffin wax to ensure that the sections are cut such that villi and crypts can be viewed longitudinally and not transversely through the middle of the villus (Fig. 23.2).

Histopathological evaluation

As mentioned earlier, GI tissues (particularly the small intestine) pose a challenge in interpretation of what is considered normal. Assessment and interpretation of both morphological (structural) and inflammatory changes therefore requires experience in order to calibrate one's own "baseline" with careful evaluation of all samples at low and high magnification. Poor sample orientation (as discussed above) can have a marked influence on the interpretation of villous and cryptal length, and villi of normal length can appear artefactually atrophic when sectioned tangentially. Additionally, there is a resident population of lymphocytes and plasma cells within the GI tract that are present most notably in the small intestine, particularly the ileum. Numbers of cells within the mucosa can fluctuate with age, immune status, concurrent non-GI disease, diet, and medical therapy, amongst others, and thus the presence of inflammatory cells (within the mucosa) does not on its own constitute a diagnosis of "-itis".

The WSAVA histopathological standards for the diagnosis of GI inflammation in endoscopic biopsy samples published in 2008 provided the first, and still most comprehensive, guide for the pathologist in assessing the severity of microscopic changes in the stomach, duodenum, and colon.[2] Although these standards act as a reference to try to standardize reporting between pathologists, they still require considerable experience to put into practice.

When hematoxylin and eosin (H&E)–stained sections are examined, a range of morphological and inflammatory parameters are assessed and, in most cases, graded from 0 to 3 (Table 23.1). Morphological parameters include surface epithelium (e.g., evidence of erosion or ulceration), villous length and width, lacteal dilation (e.g., physiological, lymphangiectasia), and presence of mucosal fibrosis. Inflammatory parameters include the quantification of numbers of lymphocytes, plasma cells, eosinophils, neutrophils, and histiocytes. The standards were originally established for endoscopic biopsies of the stomach (antrum and fundus), duodenum, and colon, and thus relate specifically

TABLE 23.1 Example of a histopathology report of a gastrointestinal mucosal biopsy.

Feature		Stomach fundus	Stomach antrum	Duodenum	Ileum	Colon
Morphological	Surface epithelium	0	0	0	0	2
	Gastric pit epithelium	1	1	–	–	–
	Villus stunting	–	–	1–2	1	–
	Crypt dilation/distortion	–	–	1	0–1	1
	Lacteal dilation	–	–	1	0	–
	Colonic goblet cells	–	–	–	–	Dec1
	Mucosal fibrosis	0	0	0	0	1
Inflammatory	Intraepithelial lymphocytes	1	1	1	0	0
	LP lymphocytes and plasma cells	2	1	2–3	0	1–2
	LP eosinophils	0	0	1	0	0
	LP neutrophils	1	1–2	0–1	1	2
	LP macrophages	0	0	0	0	0
	Gastric lymphoid follicular hyperplasia	0	1	–	–	–

Modified from the Texas A&M University GI Lab (https://vetmed.tamu.edu/gilab/service/assays/histopathology-service/).
LP, lamina propria; 0, normal; 1, mild; 2, moderate; 3, marked; Dec1, mild decrease.

to the mucosa (and not deeper levels *per se*). Modified versions of the original standards have been published that include the ileum and additional parameters such as numbers of colonic goblet cells, which can be altered in various conditions.[3] The histopathological scores were envisaged to represent a single ("mean") value per parameter and tissue site, but the degree often varies across the samples examined. There is no standardized approach to this by pathologists, with some giving the number corresponding to the greatest severity found, whereas others might use a range (e.g., 0–1 or 2–3) to indicate heterogeneity of the change across the multiple samples assessed.

Apart from grading the histopathological changes, each tissue submitted should be accompanied by a histopathological description of the changes. Additionally, and somewhat unusually, microscopic descriptions of the GI tract usually include mention of the number and quality of the samples and thus how representative they may be of the organ sampled. The pathologist describes what is present and to some degree what is not present, since exclusion of certain changes (e.g., lymphangiectasia, neoplasia) may be sufficient for clinical decision-making.

Neutrophils are one of the most informative cell types, as they are not present in the normal canine GI mucosa. Thus, their presence usually does suggest a lesion, but often not much more than that. For example, gastric foreign bodies can result in an influx of neutrophils within the upper small intestinal mucosa, despite there not being an actual lesion at that level.

Evaluation can be limited by tissue orientation, as previously discussed, with sometimes just tips of villi available for assessment. However, this can often be remedied by reorientation of the sample by the histologist (Fig. 23.3). Crushed samples are harder to rectify, and in endoscopic specimens it tends to be the inflammatory cell population (the mucosal lymphocytes in particular) that suffers most, which can lead to very challenging evaluation and interpretation, especially if there is a concern for lymphoma (Fig. 23.4).

Obviously, endoscopically retrieved samples can only ever give an indication of possible mucosal lesions, and, even then, they may miss focal changes (e.g., gastric carcinoma) if these are not sampled. If deep mucosal lesions are suspected, full-thickness specimens are preferable.

Microscopic diagnosis and comment

Description and scoring are followed by a microscopic diagnosis, which effectively is the pathologist's interpretation of the changes present. A comment in which the microscopic changes, or their absence, can be related back to the clinical history or clinician's specific questions is also paramount.

As mentioned above, the intestine (particularly the small intestine) contains a resident population of lymphocytes and plasma cells (as well as lesser populations of eosinophils and mast cells) that can vary with age, breed, diet, and potentially other iatrogenic factors such as concurrent or prior antimicrobial or anti-inflammatory therapies. Thus, the presence of lymphocytes and plasma cells on its own does not constitute an -itis (in contrast to most other tissues in the body)—a common pitfall for many inexperienced pathologists and trainees. Alterations in cellular numbers and in particular the relative proportions of lymphocytes to plasma cells as well as their distribution (especially high numbers of intraepithelial lymphocytes) are more useful, and -itis (e.g., duodenitis) should be reserved for cases with both inflammatory and morphological changes.

An additional area of controversy surrounds the pathologist's diagnosis of "inflammatory bowel disease". This is mostly due to a lack of consensus on what the histopathological criteria are to make this diagnosis, which is largely a diagnosis of exclusion by the clinician. When a pathologist does make this diagnosis, what they usually mean is that there is lymphoplasmacytic (usually) enteritis without a specific etiology identified. Other causes of similar histopathological changes including food- or antibiotic-responsive enteropathies should be excluded by the clinician first.

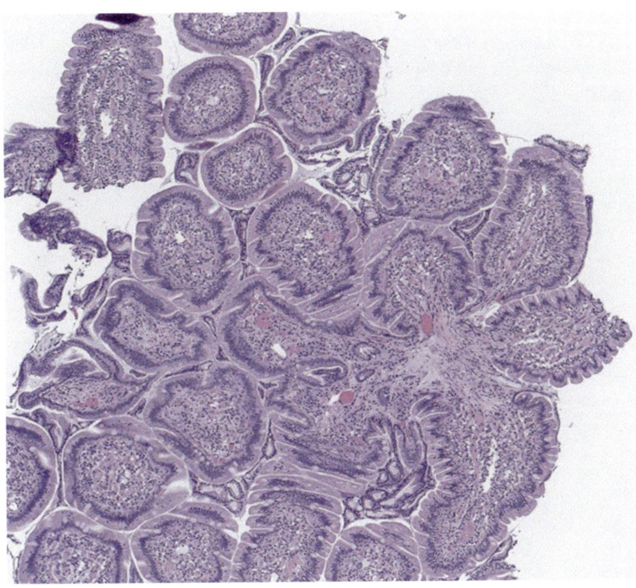

FIG. 23.3 When sectioned transversely, villus (and therefore presence of atrophy) and crypt length cannot be accurately assessed. Also, evaluation of mucosal inflammation is only based on the villous lamina propria, so this sample is potentially unrepresentative of the wider mucosa.

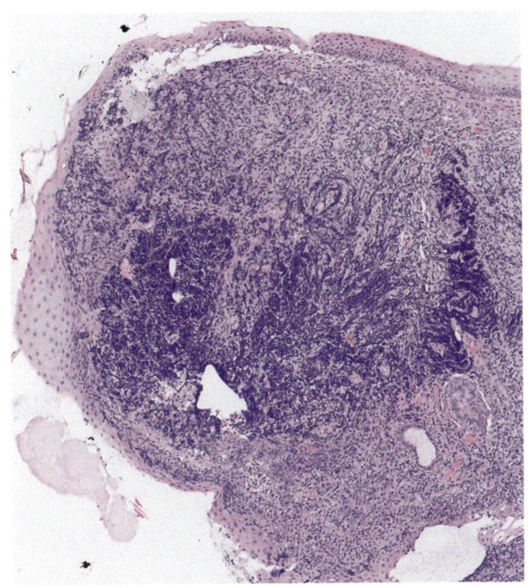

FIG. 23.4 Crushed samples are very hard to interpret and cannot be rectified. Crush artefact, for example by forceps, tends to disproportionately affect the inflammatory cell population in the mucosa (especially lymphocytes), which can make differentiating lymphocytic inflammation from lymphoma very challenging.

Use of special stains

Special histochemical stains are essentially any stain other than H&E. Those most frequently used for GI biopsies are listed in Table 23.2. They are most often employed to either identify or confirm the presence of microorganisms (e.g., fungi, protozoa, algae) or, conversely, to exclude the presence of organisms such as mycobacteria in granulomatous inflammation. They may also be used to identify cell types (e.g., toluidine blue to highlight the cytoplasmic metachromatic granules in a duodenal mast cell tumor; Fig. 23.5) or to help identify and potentially quantify normal features (e.g., goblet cell numbers; Fig. 23.6).

In most cases, the pathologist has a very strong suspicion of the presence and likely type of infectious agent from the H&E evaluation based on the size and shape of the microorganism and on the clinical information provided (e.g., geographic location of the animal). Indeed, certain infectious agents (e.g., *Prototheca* sp., *Histoplasma capsulatum*, *Pythium insidiosum*) are strongly associated with specific geographic locations, and when faced with histiocytic/granulomatous or pyogranulomatous inflammation in the intestine, the pathologist should be mindful of these agents, although it should be borne in mind that these agents could occur outside their more typical endemic areas. Special stains are then used to either confirm or exclude a particular agent.

Special stains can be helpful in the diagnosis of certain conditions, such as granulomatous (histiocytic ulcerative) colitis, in which periodic acid–Schiff positive histiocytes can usually be found within the mucosa. However, more specific assays, in particular fluorescence *in situ* hybridization (FISH) using specific, fluorescent, antibacterial nucleic acid probes, are now considered more sensitive and specific. FISH may be helpful when there is a concern for enteroinvasive bacteria such as *Escherichia coli* or *Salmonella* spp. (e.g., when an animal is fed a raw diet).

TABLE 23.2 Common histochemical stains used in gastrointestinal tract biopsy interpretation.

Stain	Use	Color
Alcian blue	Mucopolysaccharides (acid mucins)	■ Blue
Alcian blue–PAS	Mucins (acid and neutral)	■ Blue (acid mucins) ■ Magenta (neutral mucins)
Congo red	Amyloid, elastic fibers, and eosinophil granules	■ Red (apple-green birefringence under polarized light)
Giemsa	Protozoa, eosinophils, and mast cell granules	■ Dark blue
Gram	Bacteria	■ Blue-purple (gram-positive organisms) ■ Pink-red (gram-negative organisms)
Grocott (Gomori methenamine silver)	Fungi	■ Black
Masson's trichrome	Collagen (fibrosis)	■ Blue
Periodic acid–Schiff (PAS)	Carbohydrates (e.g., goblet cells, fungi)	■ Magenta
Toluidine blue	Mast cell granules	■ Dark blue-purple
Warthin-Starry (Young's)	Spirochetes (*Leptospira* spp., *Helicobacter* spp.)	■ Black

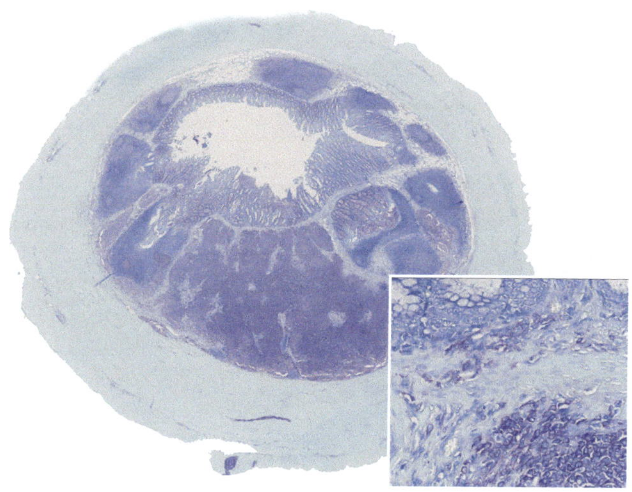

FIG. 23.5 Histological image of a canine duodenum with a mast cell tumor. Toluidine blue stain highlights the deep blue-purple (metachromatic) granules within the cell cytoplasm.

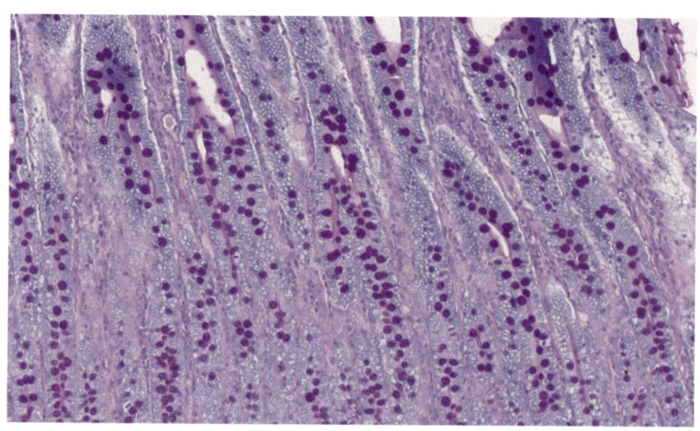

FIG. 23.6 Histological image of goblet cells stained with periodic acid–Schiff. This stain dyes carbohydrates within the mucus of goblet cells a magenta color and can be helpful if quantification is required. It also stains carbohydrates in the cell walls of fungi.

Immunohistochemistry and PARR

The use of antibodies to aid in identification of neoplastic cell types within biopsies is becoming increasingly popular as more diagnostic laboratories either acquire or gain access to automated immunostainers. Although these ancillary tests significantly add to the cost, they can transform a diagnosis from a possible "round cell malignancy" to a "small cell epitheliotropic T-cell lymphoma" (Fig. 23.7). Immunohistochemistry (IHC) can be performed on the same formalin-fixed paraffin-embedded tissue originally submitted to the laboratory; this is optimum indeed, since the comparison of the IHC-labeled tissue to the cells of interest in the H&E-stained section is essential. A non-comprehensive list of some of the most frequently utilized antibodies in GI biopsies is given in Table 23.3. The most commonly used antibodies are those to differentiate T- and B-cell lymphomas (see Chapter 42).

Regarding the limitations of IHC, antibodies tend to bind nonspecifically around the edges of tissues on a slide; small samples (e.g., endoscopic biopsies) disproportionately suffer from this "edge effect". Additionally, inadequately, or more likely overfixed, tissues can have a weaker signal due to formation of protein cross-links with target antigens and can thus sometimes appear falsely negative. Crushed samples or those with excessive hemorrhage or necrosis are also poor candidates for IHC, so it is always best to be guided by the pathologist on the suitability for IHC testing. PARR (polymerase chain reaction for antigen receptor rearrangement) is essentially a test of clonality of a cellular infiltrate and, again, is most often used to aid in the diagnosis of lymphoma. While the use of PARR is on the increase, it is still quite a specialized test and not that widely available. The value of PARR is in the ability to differentiate an inflammatory lymphocytic infiltrate from a neoplastic infiltrate. However, PARR should only be used following IHC to determine if the infiltrate is predominantly T cell, B cell, or mixed. If either of the former two, then PARR may be helpful, but in the latter case it would not be warranted.

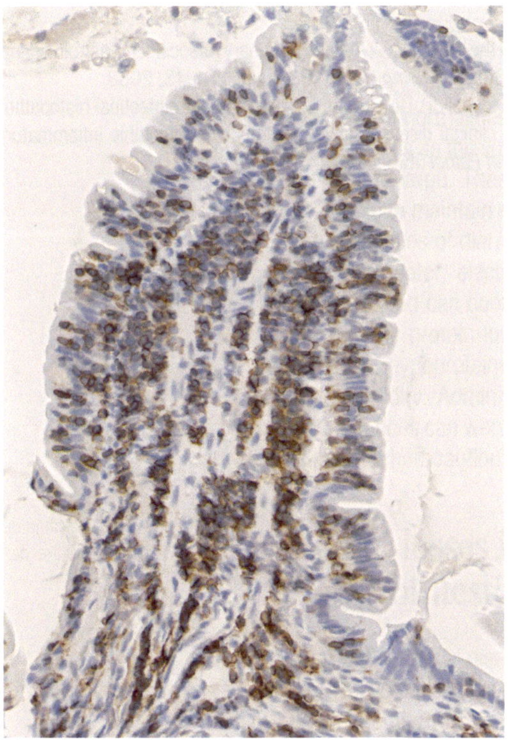

FIG. 23.7 Immunohistochemical image of a small cell epitheliotropic T-cell lymphoma. CD3 immunohistochemistry labels neoplastic T cells, which can be seen expanding the villous lamina propria and infiltrating the villous enterocytes.

TABLE 23.3 Main cell markers used in gastrointestinal immunohistochemistry.

Antigen	Details	Use
Alpha-smooth muscle actin	Contractile microfilament of smooth muscle	Smooth muscle tumors
AE1/AE3 (multikeratin)	Antibody "cocktail" of keratins	Carcinomas and adenocarcinomas
Chromogranin A	Neurosecretory granules of neuroendocrine cells	Neuroendocrine tumors
CD3	High specificity to confirm T-cell origin of lymphomas	T-cell lymphomas
CD79α	High specificity to confirm B-cell origin of lymphomas Can aberrantly label smooth muscle fibers	B-cell lymphomas
CD20	Transmembrane protein expressed in immature and mature B cells, and in lymphomas	B-cell lymphomas
CD31	Transmembrane glycoprotein present in endothelial cells, megakaryocytes, and platelets	Endothelial tumors (e.g., hemangiosarcoma)
Carcinoembryonic antigen (CEA)	Carbohydrate-rich glycoprotein	Stomach, pancreas, and cholangiocellular carcinomas
CD117 (C-Kit)	Transmembrane receptor for the stem cell factor	Mast cell tumors and gastrointestinal stromal tumors
Iba1	Ionized calcium-binding adapter molecule 1	Histiocytic sarcomas
MUM-1	Transcription factor involved in regulation of cell growth and immune response	Plasma cell neoplasms
Vimentin	Intermediate filament	Mesenchymal neoplasms (sarcomas)

Clinicopathological evaluation

A clinicopathological evaluation is indicated in dogs presenting with fluid disturbances as a result of acute GI signs, as this may influence fluid choices or management. A minimum database should include packed cell volume and refractometric TP, electrolytes, blood glucose, creatinine ± urea, and lactate. Many point-of-care blood gas analyzers will provide most of these results from a single sample. Blood gas analysis may provide additional information but is not essential, as many abnormalities will be effectively treated through appropriate fluid resuscitation and correction of electrolytes.

Electrolyte and blood gas abnormalities in acute gastrointestinal disease

Electrolyte abnormalities are relatively common in dogs with acute onset vomiting and diarrhea. The most common abnormality is hypokalemia. Potassium can be lost both with vomiting and diarrhea.[2] This coupled with inappetence can result in significant hypokalemia. Some diseases associated with GI signs are associated with specific electrolyte abnormalities, such as hyponatremia and hyperkalemia in hypoadrenocorticism. Loss of intravascular volume associated with hypoperfusion can result in a metabolic acidosis as a result of hyperlactatemia.

Upper gastrointestinal obstruction

Vomiting of gastric contents is thought to result in the loss of hydrogen ions, chloride, and potassium. Excessive losses of these can result in hypochloremic metabolic alkalosis, and this is reported in up to 45% percent of cases,[3] although more recent studies have suggested this is less common than previously described, with only about 10% of cases presenting with metabolic alkalosis.[4] However, upper GI obstruction remains an important cause of metabolic alkalosis and so should prompt investigation for this if identified.[5] Mild to moderate hyponatremia, hypochloremia, and hypokalemia are common in upper GI obstruction.[4] If metabolic alkalosis is identified and associated with hypochloremia, treatment with 0.9% saline is indicated in order to replace the chloride ions. Resolution of alkalosis requires adequate provision of both chloride and volume in order to promote chloride and sodium retention by the kidney.

Fluid therapy

Fluid therapy is the mainstay of treatment of hypovolemia and dehydration as well as the electrolyte and acid–base abnormalities associated with acute GI signs. Dogs without significant cardiovascular compromise may be managed on an outpatient basis. This has been described as effective, even in dogs with severe causes for their signs such as parvovirosis.[6] Dogs that are hypoperfused should be hospitalized until they are considered well enough to be discharged to home care. This will be dependent on individual client expectations and abilities.

The value of nutritional support, when tolerated, in the management of mild dehydration and electrolyte abnormalities should not be underestimated.

Management of hypovolemia

Hypovolemia should be treated as a priority. Recommendations for first-line management of hypovolemia with fluid therapy are to use a balanced isotonic crystalloid fluid at a dose of 10–20 mL/kg given intravenously over 10–20 minutes, with reassessment at the end of this initial dose. This dose can be repeated at least twice. If there is no response after three doses, the dog should be carefully reassessed to ensure that there is no other cause for the clinical signs, for example, sepsis or cardiac insufficiency. It is not unusual to have to give a total of 60–80 mL/kg in dogs with very severe signs, such as those presenting with acute hemorrhagic diarrhea syndrome.

The use of natural and artificial colloids in the management of hypovolemia has been described. These types of fluids are usually used when dogs have failed to show a good response to isotonic crystalloid fluids. There is a lack of good supportive evidence for the use of these fluids, but there are some anecdotal reports of their effectiveness. In human medicine, there is a lack of evidence of benefit and a demonstration of harm associated with artificial colloids, and it is therefore difficult to recommend these. The author would use natural colloids such as plasma in preference, but still does so rarely. In most cases, crystalloid fluids provide adequate resuscitation. Natural colloids may benefit as they do not have the diluting effect that crystalloid fluids do, but they are expensive, and large doses are required to have any effect on protein concentrations, so this effect should not be expected. As most dogs with hypovolemia due to GI disease are dehydrated, hypertonic saline is of limited use in this population.

Management of dehydration

In stable dogs with mild dehydration that are able to eat and drink, oral fluid intake is recommended and should be attempted. Many owners will be familiar with oral rehydration therapy, which has the benefit of being safe and economic. In its simplest form, water can be administered, but a variety of solutions are available. Large volumes can be administered in this way, either via the oral route or via feeding tubes.

In dogs that are unstable, vomiting, unwilling to drink, or losing large volumes of diarrhea, intravenous fluid replacement is recommended. The simplest way to achieve this is through the use of isotonic crystalloid fluids. The estimation of the degree of dehydration is used to calculate the total fluid deficit, and this volume is added to the dog's usual fluid requirements and administered over a 12- to 24-hour period. Reassessment after 6 hours should demonstrate improvement in clinical signs. If the animal deteriorates or passes larger than expected volumes of diarrhea during this time, the fluid plan will need adjustment. Fluid therapy is dynamic, and adequate planning is required to ensure that the dog is appropriately managed. Overadministration of fluids results in polyuria, peripheral edema, chemosis, and pleural effusion.

Example:

10% dehydration in a 7-kg dog

$$10/100 \times 7 \times 1000 = 700 \text{ mL deficit}$$

Normal fluid requirement for 12 hours: $7 \times 12 \times 2 = 168$ mL

The total to be administered is 868 mL, which is a rate of 72 mL/h.

Clinicians should be prepared to readjust the fluid rate if large volumes of diarrhea are passed.

Management of electrolyte abnormalities

Severe electrolyte abnormalities are uncommon. If hypokalemia is present, this should be managed through potassium supplementation in the

TABLE 24.1 Supplementation with potassium for management of hypokalemia.

Serum potassium (mmol/L)	Amount of KCl needed per liter (mmol)	Maximum rate to avoid exceeding 0.5 mmol/kg/h
<2,0	80	6
2.1–2.5	60	8
2.6–3.0	40	12
3.1–3.5	28	18
3.6–5.0	20	25

Fluid bags should be well shaken after addition of potassium chloride to ensure adequate mixing. Fluids containing high concentrations of potassium (e.g. >40 mmol/L) should not be flushed into fluid lines as this can be associated with cardiac arrhythmias or arrest.

Adapted from AAHA/AAFP, 2013.[7]

replacement fluids (Table 24.1) or orally. Chloride should be supplemented aggressively if there is concurrent metabolic alkalosis. The use of a balanced electrolyte solution is typically associated with a resolution of most other electrolyte abnormalities. Nutritional support will also assist with the management of these, typically quite quickly.

Management of hypoproteinemia

Fluid therapy for management of hypoproteinemia/oncotic support is unlikely to have long-term efficacy. Artificial and natural colloids such as plasma will have less of a diluting effect on colloid osmotic pressure than isotonic crystalloids, but their effects are short term, particularly if there is chronic hypoproteinemia. Dogs with hypoproteinemia as a result of protein-losing enteropathy may require general anesthesia to allow GI biopsy. Endoscopic biopsies are usually preferred as there is an increased risk of breakdown associated with full-thickness biopsy. As any albumin infused through plasma administration is short-lived, it is unlikely to mitigate this risk; however, hypotension during anesthesia may be more appropriately managed with colloid solutions. The author's preference in these situations is to use a natural colloid. However, artificial colloids are more readily available and may provide the short-term volume support required during anesthesia, with fewer side effects than isotonic crystalloid fluids.

Fresh frozen plasma is usually available, although expensive. Additionally, large volumes of plasma are required, although there is controversy over the appropriateness of published calculations. Based on the various calculations, 10–20 mL/kg of fresh frozen plasma is a reasonable starting point[8] if this is selected and used to manage hypoproteinemia, but even these doses may have a limited effect on hypoalbuminemia.[9] The use of cryosupernatant in dogs with hypoalbuminemia has been described and can be considered, particularly as it is typically cheaper than fresh frozen or frozen plasma. It also has a slightly higher concentration of albumin compared with frozen plasma.[10]

Until 2013, the most frequently used artificial colloids were the starches. One of the main proposed benefits of starches is that, due to their high colloid osmotic pressure, lower volumes are required for stabilization. This has not been studied in clinical veterinary medicine; however, in a randomized trial of human septic patients, equal volumes of colloid and crystalloid were used over the first 24 hours. As starches are not readily available, they are no longer commonly used. Gelatins are more easily available, and some clinicians use these when there is a need for acute volume resuscitation. However, there is limited evidence base to support their use.

Human serum albumin has also been described for management of hypoproteinemia in dogs, but it can be associated with both type 2 and 3 hypersensitivity reactions.[8] Human serum albumin is costly and not readily available and so should only be used with caution and appropriate informed client consent. The routine use of albumin for management of hypoproteinemia in people is not recommended as it is commonly ineffective or associated with significant side effects.

KEY POINTS

- Fluid therapy is essential in the management of severe acute gastrointestinal signs.
- Management of hypovolemia is a priority and may require infusion of large quantities of fluids.
- Isotonic crystalloids are the first-line choice for management of both hypovolemia and dehydration.
- Mild to moderate dehydration can be managed with oral fluid administration, and outpatient management should be considered with financial limitations.
- Electrolyte abnormalities, particularly hypokalemia, are common, especially when dogs are hyporexic.
- Nutritional management should be considered once vomiting is controlled, as it will help manage fluid, electrolyte, and protein losses.
- Management of hypoproteinemia with fluid therapy is often ineffective. Avoiding complications of excessive administration of crystalloid fluids through careful administration and monitoring prevents morbidity associated with fluid therapy.
- Although commonly used, there is limited evidence base to support the use of either natural or artificial colloids in the management of hypoproteinemia or severe hypovolemia.
- Administration of human serum albumin to dogs is not recommended.

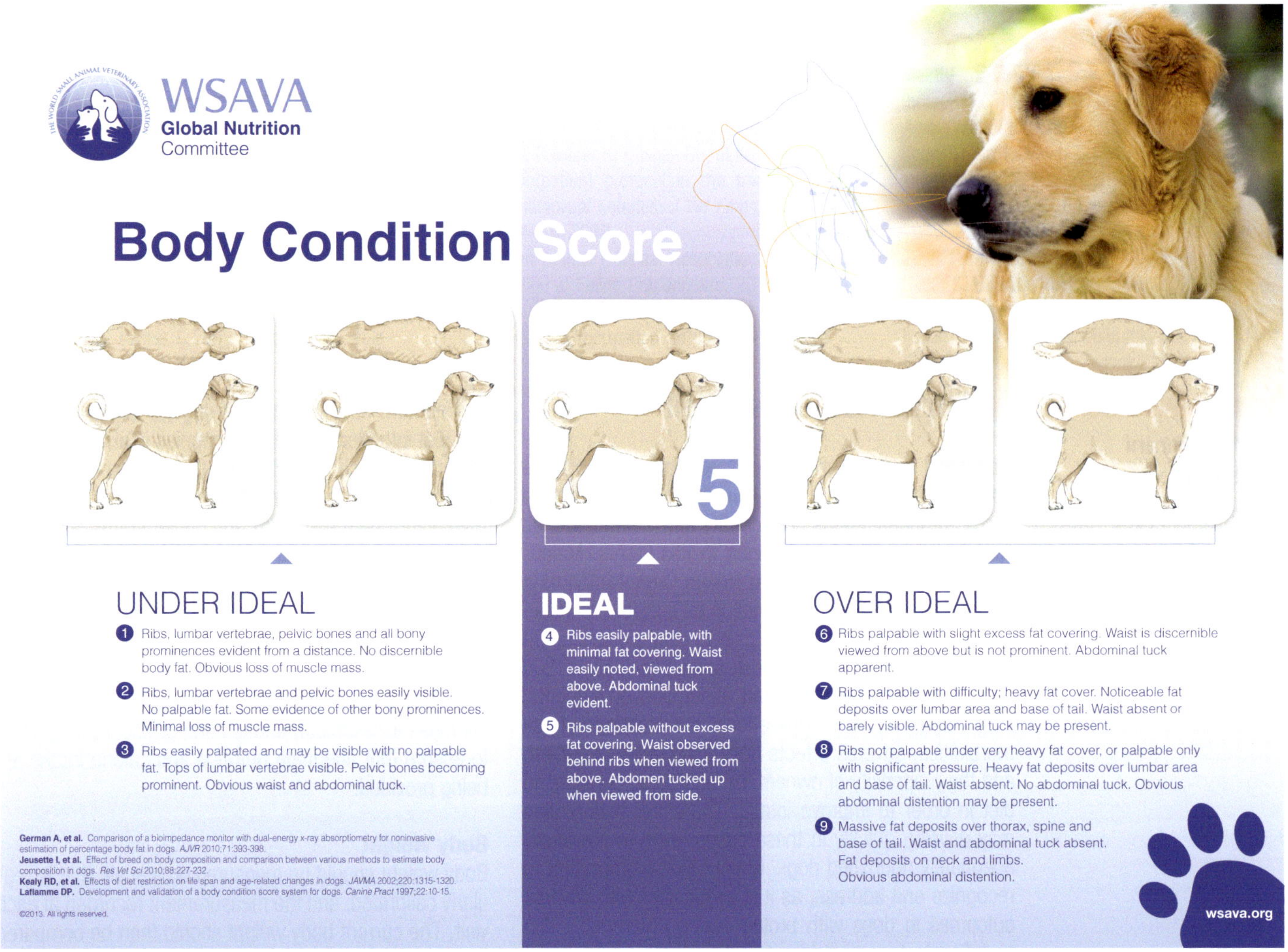
WSAVA
Global Nutrition
Committee
Body Condition Score
5
UNDER IDEAL
1 Ribs, lumbar vertebrae, pelvic bones and all bony prominences evident from a distance. No discernible body fat. Obvious loss of muscle mass.
2 Ribs, lumbar vertebrae and pelvic bones easily visible. No palpable fat. Some evidence of other bony prominences. Minimal loss of muscle mass.
3 Ribs easily palpated and may be visible with no palpable fat. Tops of lumbar vertebrae visible. Pelvic bones becoming prominent. Obvious waist and abdominal tuck.
IDEAL
4 Ribs easily palpable, with minimal fat covering. Waist easily noted, viewed from above. Abdominal tuck evident.
5 Ribs palpable without excess fat covering. Waist observed behind ribs when viewed from above. Abdomen tucked up when viewed from side.
OVER IDEAL
6 Ribs palpable with slight excess fat covering. Waist is discernible viewed from above but is not prominent. Abdominal tuck apparent.
7 Ribs palpable with difficulty; heavy fat cover. Noticeable fat deposits over lumbar area and base of tail. Waist absent or barely visible. Abdominal tuck may be present.
8 Ribs not palpable under very heavy fat cover, or palpable only with significant pressure. Heavy fat deposits over lumbar area and base of tail. Waist absent. No abdominal tuck. Obvious abdominal distention may be present.
9 Massive fat deposits over thorax, spine and base of tail. Waist and abdominal tuck absent. Fat deposits on neck and limbs. Obvious abdominal distention.
German A, et al. Comparison of a bioimpedance monitor with dual-energy x-ray absorptiometry for noninvasive estimation of percentage body fat in dogs. AJVR 2010;71:393-398.
Jeusette I, et al. Effect of breed on body composition and comparison between various methods to estimate body composition in dogs. Res Vet Sci 2010;88:227-232.
Kealy RD, et al. Effects of diet restriction on life span and age-related changes in dogs. JAVMA 2002;220:1315-1320.
Laflamme DP. Development and validation of a body condition score system for dogs. Canine Pract 1997;22:10-15.
©2013. All rights reserved.
wsava.org

FIG. 25.1 World Small Animal Veterinary Association nine-point body condition scoring system for dogs (with permission).

will then be able to assess this regularly at home. It is important to note that BCS is informative of peripheral fat status and does not take into account intra-abdominal fat, muscle condition, or bone density, all of which can be affected by malnutrition and are therefore likely important in nutrition assessment.

Muscle condition

Inadequate nutrition, cachexia, or sarcopenia can lead to reduced muscle condition. Cachexia is a complex metabolic syndrome associated with an underlying illness resulting in loss of muscle with or without loss of fat mass. Although sarcopenia also refers to the loss of muscle mass, it differs from cachexia in that sarcopenia can be an age-related condition not necessarily associated with disease. Sarcopenia is characterized by low muscle mass, muscle strength, and physical performance.

Assessment of muscle condition is important to identify malnutrition, cachexia, and sarcopenia. However, there is currently no standardized scoring system for muscle mass in dogs. Therefore, assessment of muscle condition can be performed subjectively by using the four-point scale recommended by the WSAVA Global Nutrition Committee (Fig. 25.2) or by assessing the muscle mass as adequate or atrophied (mild, moderate, or severe) together with characterization of the symmetry and distribution of this loss. Muscle mass should be evaluated both by visual assessment and palpation of the head, scapulae, epaxial muscles over the thoracic and lumbar vertebrae, and pelvic bones (Fig. 25.3). In order to ensure accuracy for both BCS and muscle condition, it is important that they be assessed not just visually but also by palpation, especially in dogs with medium- or long-haired coats.

Clinicopathological tests

At the time of writing this chapter, there are no clinicopathological tests available that can definitively assess a dog's nutritional status. Although the packed cell volume, serum albumin, and electrolytes can be an indication of the nutritional status, these are poor markers as they can also be influenced by additional factors such as the disease process itself, reduced intake, or increased losses. Similarly, as serum vitamin B_{12} and folate concentrations can also be influenced by GI disease, they are unreliable markers of malnutrition in dogs with these conditions.

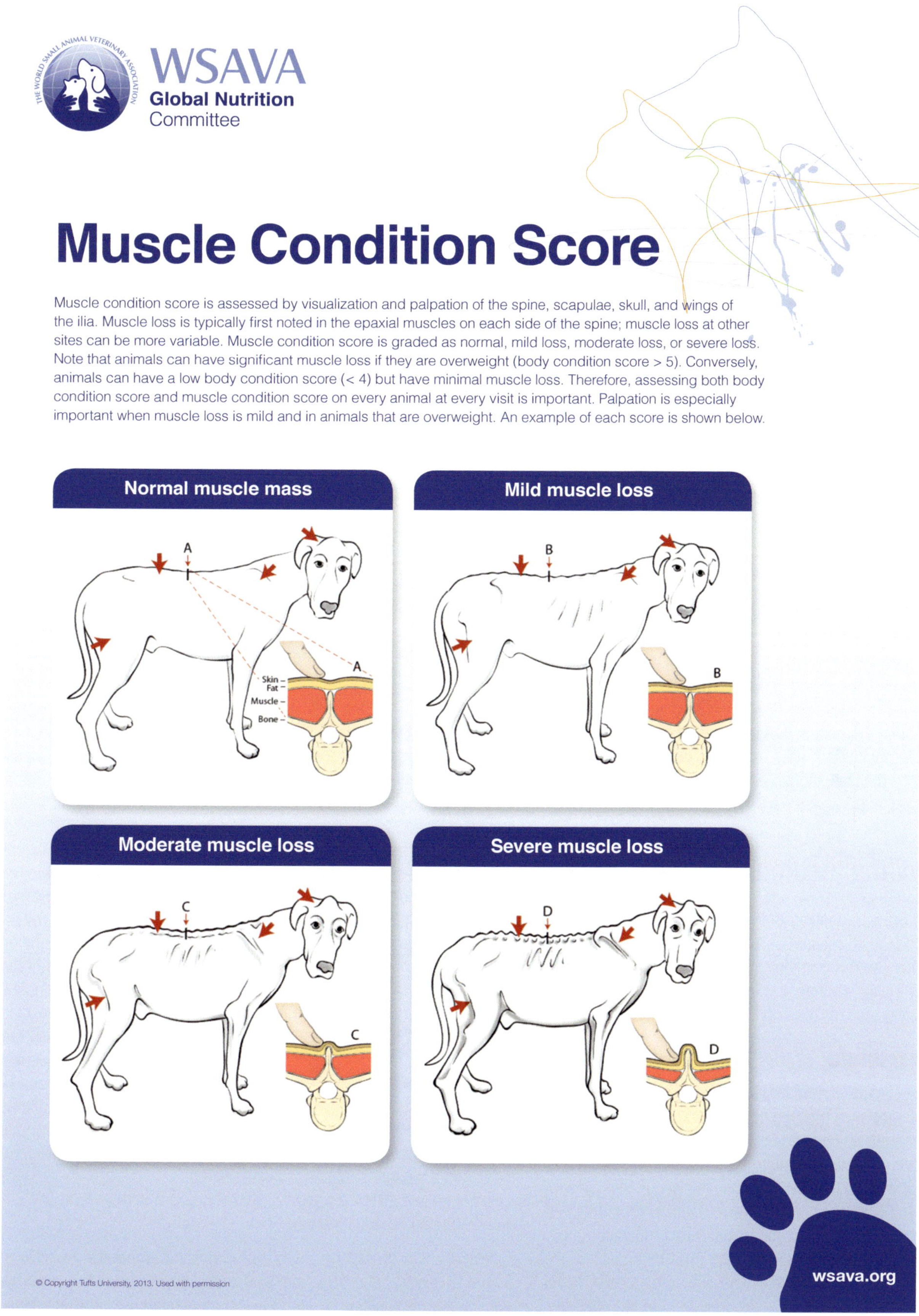

FIG. 25.2 World Small Animal Veterinary Association muscle condition score chart for dogs (with permission).

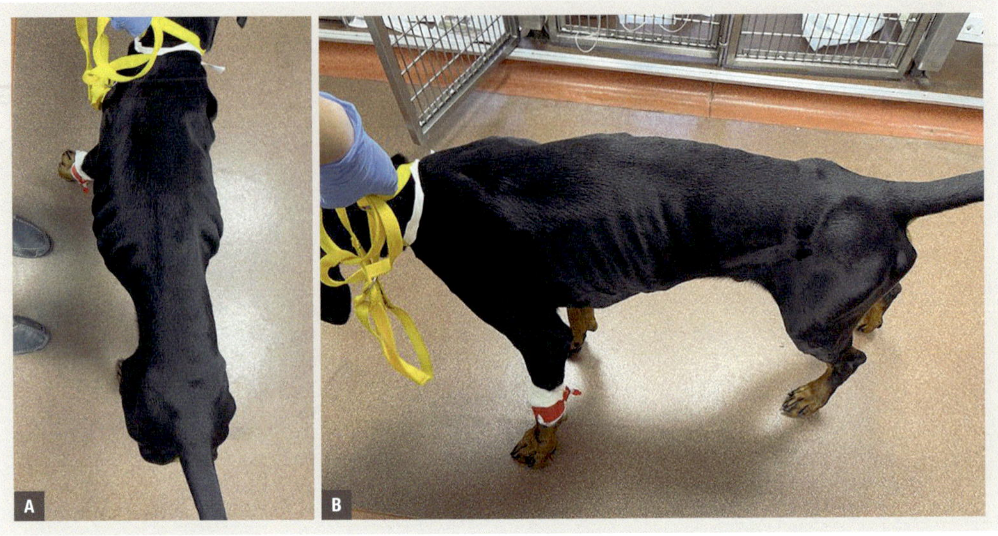

FIG. 25.3 Malnourished neutered male Doberman with reduced body and muscle conditions. Note the prominence of the ribs and pelvic bones in both views. Images courtesy of Dr. Sarah Tayler.

Assessment of the diet

A complete and thorough diet history is paramount in determining whether nutrient intake is sufficient or immediate nutritional intervention is needed. Collection of the diet history should encompass all foods that the dog is eating, including commercial pet food, commercial treats, human food, dietary supplements, and foods used to administer medications, with specification of the manufacturer, formula (dry or tinned) and flavor where applicable. The ability to scavenge and the access to additional food from friends and family members should also be ascertained. Correlation of historical GI signs with dietary ingredients and fat and fiber content will help in the prioritization of specific dietary strategies to trial in dogs with GI disease. A thorough diet history will also enable compilation of a detailed antigen exposure list, which can help to determine which ingredients would be truly novel for the dog.

Assisted feeding methods

For those dogs that are not meeting their daily energy and nutrient requirements, assisted feeding methods are indicated to try to correct or prevent any malnutrition and its adverse consequences. Assisted feeding can take the form of trying to enhance voluntary oral intake, utilizing an assisted enteral feeding tube, or resorting to parenteral nutrition (PN).

Voluntary oral intake

Measures to increase voluntary oral intake center around adjustments to the environment and food offered and optimization of appetite, nausea, and pain through medical intervention. Environmental adjustments are focused on providing a quiet and stress-free place to eat, utilizing bowls with the same material as those the dog is familiar with at home if feeding in hospital or utilizing novel feeding receptacles if feeding at home, and encouraging owner visits during hospitalization. With regard to the food offered, warming the food or adding warm water may help to increase acceptance. The use of diets with novel proteins, if the underlying disease permits, may help to increase appetite. Similarly, the use of unbalanced foods, such as low-fat cottage cheese or skinless, boneless chicken breast with cooked white rice for a few days may help to improve intake while the animal is recovering. Appetite stimulants, such as mirtazapine or capromorelin, can be used to improve appetite. Palatant enhancers, such as probiotics with animal digest, may also help to improve intake. Optimization of nausea and pain management through the use of anti-nausea medication and analgesics (see Chapters 28 and 32), respectively, may also help to improve voluntary oral intake.

Assisted enteral feeding tubes

For those dogs that have been anorexic for at least 3 days and in which the above strategies to increase voluntary oral intake have not helped, assisted enteral feeding may be required. Placement of an enteral feeding tube should be pursued to help prevent or treat malnutrition, provide nutrition to the enterocytes, and support gut health. The most common assisted enteral feeding tubes are nasoenteral, esophagostomy, and gastrostomy tubes. The decision to place one over the other depends on many factors, including the ability of the dog to undergo general anesthesia, clinical signs and location of GI disease, anticipated length of assisted feeding, and financial considerations. Once an enteral feeding tube is in place, feeds should be started at 25% of the resting energy requirement (RER). Feeds can be via bolus or continuous administration, with the recommendation to administer no more than 5–10 mL/kg of slurry per feed initially. Feeding should be increased by 25% of RER increments daily if the dog's tolerance is adequate. Feeding above 100% of RER is not recommended in critically ill hospitalized GI patients due to complications associated with overfeeding. The animal should be monitored closely for any signs of intolerance, and the rate of enteral feeds should be decreased or the caloric density of the diet increased if volume intolerance is suspected.

Parenteral nutrition

Enteral feeding should be prioritized and used whenever possible to ensure GI health, but enteral nutrition is not always feasible (e.g., animals with intractable vomiting or diarrhea, dull mentation, or coagulopathy). In such cases, PN may be indicated to help address or prevent malnutrition.

However, PN should only be used until the dog can tolerate feeding tube placement or is eating voluntarily. More dogs and cats have been reported to survive when PN was administered with some enteral nutrition compared to animals receiving no concurrent enteral nutrition.[2] Therefore, PN should be complemented with enteral feeding whenever possible, even if the latter makes up no more than 10% of the daily RER. Administration of PN is achieved via central or peripheral venous access, depending on the osmolality of the formulation. Parenteral formulations consist of three main components: amino acid, lipid, and dextrose solutions. PN is not typically used long term, as it does not meet all of the dog's daily nutrient requirements. Three-in-one PN solutions are commercially available, or they can be compounded. Ideally, 100% of RER should be attained over 2–3 days when administered centrally. PN should be administered through a dedicated previously unused line and in-line filter via a continuous rate infusion using an infusion pump, and the patient should be hospitalized in the intensive care unit for close monitoring. Each bag of PN solution should not be used for more than 24–48 hours, and the line should not be disconnected, even for walks or diagnostic investigations. Once the animal is eating voluntarily or until a more permanent enteral feeding tube can be placed, the animal can be slowly weaned off PN (it should not be stopped abruptly).

Diets for acute gastrointestinal disease

Although research defining the ideal dietary composition for dogs with acute GI disease is lacking, some studies have shown beneficial responses to increased digestibility or dietary fiber in dogs with colitis. It is important to note that as the etiology of acute GI disease in dogs is heterogenous, different nutritional strategies may need to be trialed before a beneficial response is seen in an individual dog. Fortunately, a range of commercial therapeutic GI diets utilizing different strategies that may be beneficial in acute GI disease (e.g., high digestibility with moderate or low fat, or high dietary fiber) and containing commonly fed ingredients, such as chicken or pork, is available.

Therapeutic gastrointestinal diets with high digestibility

Digestibility, usually expressed as a percentage, refers to the extent to which food or macronutrients present in food are digested and absorbed by the GI tract. Many factors influence digestibility and therefore, this value is not constant (Table 25.2). Although there are currently no standard criteria for the definition of a highly digestible diet, diets with a total digestibility of at least 80% and a digestibility of macronutrients of at least 90% are considered to meet this definition. Commercial therapeutic GI diets that are not fiber enriched are generally classified as highly digestible and are often used for nutritional management of acute GI disease in dogs. As acute GI disease may compromise the digestion and absorption of nutrients, diets with high digestibility can be advantageous in these cases. Additionally, diets with high digestibility produce fewer residues in the GI tract, which can help to prevent overloading of the gut and alleviate any osmotic diarrhea if present.

TABLE 25.2 Example of ingredient- and dog-related factors that may affect the digestibility of a diet.

Ingredient-related factors	Dog-related factors
Processing of the diet (e.g., heat processing generally increases the digestibility of starch but decreases the digestibility of protein)	Breed, as the size of the dog has been shown to have an effect on digestion (larger-breed dogs typically display lower food digestibility compared to smaller-breed dogs)[25]

Therapeutic gastrointestinal diets with low fat

Diets high in fat may have detrimental effects on the GI tract, including delayed gastric emptying. Animal models of GI disease have also shown adverse effects of high-fat diets on the intestinal microbiota, GI permeability, and the mucosal immune response in susceptible animals. As a reduction in dietary fat may help to hasten gastric transit, this strategy may be beneficial in dogs with nausea, regurgitation, or vomiting associated with acute GI disease. In addition, some dogs with acute GI disease may experience reduced fat digestion and absorption resulting in excess dietary fat passing into the colon, which may cause dysbiosis and secretory diarrhea. Therefore, reducing the dietary fat in these dogs may help to decrease or alleviate these effects. Consequently, a low-fat diet should be considered in those dogs with clinical signs of acute GI disease that are likely to benefit from this strategy.

Therapeutic gastrointestinal diets with high fiber

Dietary fiber is defined as carbohydrates derived from plants, which cannot be digested by host enzymes or absorbed in the upper GI tract of mammals. This fiber has many beneficial effects in the GI tract, including modification of gastric emptying, normalization of intestinal motility, optimization of the intestinal mucosal barrier function, anti-inflammatory effects via generation of short-chain fatty acids, buffering of toxins, binding of excess water, promotion of beneficial bacterial growth, and alteration of the viscosity of the ingesta. Diets high in fiber may be beneficial for dogs with predominantly or exclusively large intestinal signs associated with acute GI disease. However, not all dogs with these signs will respond to a high-fiber strategy. Therefore, trial and error with this approach is needed and should be prioritized for those dogs with large intestinal signs that do not respond to a highly digestible diet, and especially before considering the use of empirical antimicrobials. It is important to note that a randomized controlled clinical trial showed that, for dogs with noninfectious acute colitis, dietary management with an easily digestible diet with or without the soluble, nonfermentable fiber psyllium proved to be a superior treatment strategy versus metronidazole.[3]

Diets for chronic gastrointestinal disease

Chronic enteropathy (CE) is the most common chronic GI disease in dogs. Food-responsive enteropathy (FRE) is a subclassification of CE and includes a group of diseases resulting in chronic GI signs that are responsive to dietary management alone. Therefore, the diagnosis of FRE is made retrospectively, based on the dog's response to a therapeutic diet trial. It has been demonstrated that FRE encompasses approximately two-thirds of dogs presenting with CE in a secondary or tertiary referral population.[4,5] The exact etiology of CE and FRE is unknown. Therefore, dogs with FRE may respond to different dietary strategies, necessitating trials with multiple therapeutic diets before this condition can be ruled out. Indeed, a study showed that trials with up to three different therapeutic diets may be needed before a response is seen in dogs.[6] Nutritional management should therefore be individualized in dogs with CE to ensure that the most effective dietary strategy that will allow control of the clinical signs is used.

The diet history of the dog can help to determine if certain ingredients and nutritional strategies (e.g., low fat, high digestibility, high fiber) have been used previously and whether they helped, as the information can then be used to prioritize the specific formula within a selected category of diets. However, despite this information, dietary management may remain trial and error in dogs with CE to determine which strategy is most effective. Although owners may find it frustrating to trial different dietary strategies, studies have demonstrated that most dogs with CE that respond to dietary therapy alone respond quickly, usually within 1–2 weeks, suggesting that these diets do not need to be fed long-term to determine clinical response.[4,7,8]

Diets that are most commonly trialed in dogs with CE include either commercial therapeutic GI diets, hydrolyzed diets, limited-ingredient novel protein diets, fiber-enriched diets, low-fat diets, or therapeutic complete and balanced home-prepared diets. To date, two studies have assessed a commercial therapeutic veterinary elemental diet and a human enteral diet that was formulated with additional ingredients to ensure it was complete and balanced for canine maintenance in dogs with CE and protein-losing enteropathy, respectively.[9,10] The first study showed that exclusive feeding of the diet improved clinical signs in 16 of 23 dogs with uncontrolled CE. The second study revealed that short-term in-hospital feeding of the diet via an esophagostomy feeding tube was well tolerated and resolved anorexia in all dogs and helped to improve selected biochemical parameters associated with protein-losing enteropathy in some dogs. Further studies will help to further determine the utility of these diets in dogs with GI disease.

Therapeutic gastrointestinal diets

Commercial therapeutic GI diets incorporate commonly fed ingredients, such as chicken or pork, and typically have higher digestibility. The high digestibility of these diets is likely the key feature for their proposed beneficial effect in dogs with CE. It may result in less protein being presented intact to the immune system, which may be dysregulated in CE, and less digestion may be required, which would be advantageous for the already compromised GI tract. However, for dogs with CE, diets with high digestibility alone may be unlikely to maintain remission, as a study showed that although a therapeutic GI diet was able to induce remission, these dogs were less likely to remain asymptomatic at subsequent rechecks when compared to dogs managed with a hydrolyzed protein diet.[11] Therefore, further studies comparing therapeutic GI diets with hydrolyzed protein diets are needed to help define the subset of dogs with CE that are likely to benefit the most from these diets.

Therapeutic hydrolyzed protein diets

Hydrolyzed diets have been used successfully in the management of CE in dogs,[5,7,11–13] with some studies reporting a response in two-thirds of affected animals.[11,12] Even though the exact mechanism for their effectiveness is unknown, the following could explain the beneficial effects of this category of diet in dogs with CE:

- The hydrolyzed protein strategy may help to dampen the immune response, which may be exaggerated in dogs with CE.
- The hydrolyzed protein strategy helps to increase digestibility, which may be beneficial.
- Some hydrolyzed protein diets have a lower fat content, which may be beneficial.
- Some hydrolyzed protein diets contain soy and/or omega-3 fatty acids, which are immunomodulatory.
- Some hydrolyzed protein diets are vegetarian, and a study in humans showed that a semivegetarian diet was highly effective for maintaining remission in patients with inflammatory bowel disease.[14]
- Some hydrolyzed protein diets are gluten free, and these diets have been shown to improve clinical symptoms in people with inflammatory bowel disease.[15]

Therapeutic limited-ingredient novel protein diet

The term *limited-ingredient novel protein* is preferred over *single novel protein*, as the carbohydrate source of the diet can also contain some protein to which the dog may be sensitive. A study showed that 60% of dogs with chronic GI signs responded to a novel protein diet.[16] Another study showed no difference in response rate between hydrolyzed protein and limited-ingredient novel protein diets for dogs with CE.[5] Some therapeutic limited-ingredient novel protein diets may have higher total dietary fiber and may therefore be beneficial in dogs with large intestinal signs, especially if a highly digestible diet failed to improve the GI signs. The presence of other common food antigens in over-the-counter novel protein diets has been reported, so these diets should be avoided for the management of CE.[17]

Therapeutic fiber-enriched diets

Fiber-enriched diets may be effective for dogs with large intestinal signs, as reported by a handful of studies. Overall, these studies showed that the prognosis for dogs with large intestinal signs was good, with a response rate ranging from 63 to 96%. They also determined that fiber-enriched diets were safe and well tolerated. Response to fiber-enriched diets was relatively quick, with improvement reported in a mean of 8.5 days in one study[18] and within 1 day in another.[19] Long-term use of fiber-enriched diets may be needed to ensure control of the clinical signs.[20] Overall, most of these studies were retrospective in design and used fiber-enriched diets, rather than fiber supplements. Additionally, no control group or no good comparison group was included and some studies lacked statistical power. Therefore, more studies are needed on the effects of dietary fiber in dogs with CE and, in particular, in dogs with small bowel or mixed bowel diarrhea.

Therapeutic low-fat diets

CE may reduce fat digestion and absorption in the small intestine, resulting in increased passage of undigested fat into the colon, dysbiosis, and secretory diarrhea. Trialing a low-fat diet may thus be beneficial in these cases. In addition, CE dogs with nausea, regurgitation, or vomiting may also benefit from a low-fat strategy, as this may increase the rate of gastric emptying. Low-fat diets should also be used in dogs with CE leading to secondary lymphangiectasia.[21–23]

Therapeutic complete and balanced home-prepared diets

Certain emulsifiers and preservatives have been shown to have negative effects on the intestinal microbiota and the GI mucosal immune system in rodent gene-knockout models of inflammatory bowel disease. Therefore, there may be a subset of dogs with CE that, because of the underlying pathogenesis, may not be able to tolerate commercial foods due to these additives and may need a home-prepared diet for resolution of their GI signs. Home-prepared diets incorporating novel ingredients, low fat, or high fiber can be used in these cases. However, these diets must be formulated using the guidance of a board-certified veterinary nutritionist to ensure that they are complete and balanced for long-term feeding. A study showed that a change to a low-fat home-prepared diet may be an alternative to further immunosuppression or anti-inflammatory strategies in some dogs with difficult-to-treat protein-losing enteropathy.[21]

Diet trials

Correctly performed diet trials are important to help rule in or out a FRE. The new diet should be fed exclusively, without any treats, additional food, supplements, or flavored medication or toothpaste, in order to allow accurate assessment of the chosen diet strategy. Providing detailed instructions to the owner, including the exact name of the diet, tinned or dry formula, amounts to feed, number of meals per day, and duration of the trial, will help to improve compliance. Transition to the new diet should be performed slowly over 7–10 days. Owners should be contacted after 2 weeks of exclusive feeding to check the response to the diet. At this time, if a positive response is seen, the diet should be continued for another 6 weeks. In case of a partial response, a further update should be obtained in another 2 weeks. If there is no response to the diet in 2 weeks and no more than a partial response is observed after 4–6 weeks of exclusive feeding, then a change in diet, addition of medication, or further diagnostic investigations, if not previously performed, should be considered.

Most dogs with CE can be transitioned back to their original diet without showing signs of relapse. A study reported that only 21% of dogs with GI signs relapsed following challenge.[4] In dogs with protein-losing enteropathy, however, a change away from the therapeutic diet was associated with relapse, so long-term feeding of the diet is recommended in these cases.[24] In addition, if a response is seen to a fiber-enriched diet, long-term feeding using this strategy may be indicated to prevent relapse of GI signs.

KEY POINTS

- The purpose of nutritional assessment is to determine the dog's nutritional status, identify malnutrition, and monitor any changes to this status.
- Nutritional assessment involves evaluation of the dog and all diets being fed.
- In dogs with GI disease, the severity and duration of disease, impaired digestion and absorption of nutrients, comorbidities, complications of disease, adverse effects from treatment, and an unbalanced diet are all risk factors for malnutrition.
- Nutritional management of acute GI disease in dogs includes consideration of the digestibility, fat, and fiber of the diet.
- Dietary management of chronic enteropathy in dogs involves trial and error to determine the most effective nutritional strategy. The types of diets commonly used include commercial therapeutic GI diets (e.g., low-fat or fiber-enriched diets), commercial therapeutic hydrolyzed protein diets, commercial therapeutic limited-ingredient novel protein diets, and complete and balanced home-prepared diets. Different amounts of dietary fat and fiber within these categories of diets can be trialed to determine the most effective for the individual dog.

References

1. Wootton FE, Hoey CSFK, Woods G, et al. An undernutrition screening score for dogs with protein-losing enteropathy: A prospective multicenter study. *J Vet Intern Med* 37(5):1821–1829, 2023.
2. Chan DL, Freeman LM, Labato MA, Rush JE. Retrospective evaluation of partial parenteral nutrition in dogs and cats. *J Vet Intern Med* 16(4):440–445, 2002.
3. Rudinsky AJ, Parker VJ, Winston J, et al. Randomized controlled trial demonstrates nutritional management is superior to metronidazole for treatment of acute colitis in dogs. *J Am Vet Med Assoc* 260(S3):S23–S32, 2022.
4. Allenspach K, Wieland B, Gröne A, Gaschen F. Chronic enteropathies in dogs: evaluation of risk factors for negative outcome. *J Vet Intern Med* 21(4):700–708, 2007.
5. Allenspach K, Culverwell C, Chan D. Long-term outcome in dogs with chronic enteropathies: 203 cases. *Vet Rec* 178(15):368, 2016.
6. Schramm A, Kook PH. A descriptive study on the extent of dietary information obtained during consultations at a veterinary teaching hospital. *Animals (Basel)* 12(5):661, 2022.
7. Walker D, Knuchel-Takano A, McCutchan A, et al. A comprehensive pathological survey of duodenal biopsies from dogs with diet-responsive chronic enteropathy. *J Vet Intern Med* 27(4):862–874, 2013.
8. Schmitz S, Glanemann B, Garden OA, et al. A prospective, randomized, blinded, placebo-controlled pilot study on the effect of *Enterococcus faecium* on clinical activity and intestinal gene expression in canine food-responsive chronic enteropathy. *J Vet Intern Med* 29(2):533–543, 2015.
9. Manchester AC, Dow S, Chow L, et al. Efficacy of an elemental diet in achieving clinical remission in dogs with chronic enteropathy. *J Vet Intern Med* 37(6):2322–2333, 2023.

10. Kathrani A, Parkes G. A preliminary study of Modulen IBD liquid diet in hospitalized dogs with protein-losing enteropathy. *Animals (Basel)* 12(12):1594, 2022.
11. Mandigers PJ, Biourge V, van den Ingh TS, et al. A randomized, open-label, positively-controlled field trial of a hydrolyzed protein diet in dogs with chronic small bowel enteropathy. *J Vet Intern Med* 24(6):1350–1357, 2010.
12. Marks SL, Laflamme DP, McAloose D. Dietary trial using a commercial hypoallergenic diet containing hydrolyzed protein for dogs with inflammatory bowel disease. *Vet Ther* 3(2):109–118, 2002.
13. Wang S, Martins R, Sullivan MC, et al. Diet-induced remission in chronic enteropathy is associated with altered microbial community structure and synthesis of secondary bile acids. *Microbiome* 7(1):126, 2019.
14. Chiba M, Abe T, Tsuda H, et al. Lifestyle-related disease in Crohn's disease: relapse prevention by a semi-vegetarian diet. *World J Gastroenterol* 16(20):2484–2495, 2010.
15. Herfarth HH, Martin CF, Sandler RS, et al. Prevalence of a gluten-free diet and improvement of clinical symptoms in patients with inflammatory bowel diseases. *Inflamm Bowel Dis* 20(7):1194–1197, 2014.
16. Luckschander N, Allenspach K, Hall J, et al. Perinuclear antineutrophilic cytoplasmic antibody and response to treatment in diarrheic dogs with food responsive disease or inflammatory bowel disease. *J Vet Intern Med* 20(2):221–227, 2006.
17. Raditic DM, Remillard RL, Tater KC. ELISA testing for common food antigens in four dry dog foods used in dietary elimination trials. *J Anim Physiol Anim Nutr (Berl)* 95(1):90–97, 2011.
18. Rossi G, Cerquetella M, Gavazza A, et al. Rapid resolution of large bowel diarrhea after the administration of a combination of a high-fiber diet and a probiotic mixture in 30 dogs. *Vet Sci* 7(1):21, 2020.
19. Fritsch DA, Wernimont SM, Jackson MI, et al. A prospective multicenter study of the efficacy of a fiber-supplemented dietary intervention in dogs with chronic large bowel diarrhea. *BMC Vet Res* 18(1):244, 2022.
20. Leib MS. Treatment of chronic idiopathic large-bowel diarrhea in dogs with a highly digestible diet and soluble fiber: a retrospective review of 37 cases. *J Vet Intern Med* 14(1):27–32, 2000.
21. Wennogle SA, Stockman J, Webb CB. Prospective evaluation of a change in dietary therapy in dogs with steroid-resistant protein-losing enteropathy. *J Small Anim Pract* 62(9):756–764, 2021.
22. Rudinsky AJ, Howard JP, Bishop MA, et al. Dietary management of presumptive protein-losing enteropathy in Yorkshire terriers. *J Small Anim Pract* 58(2):103–108, 2017.
23. Okanishi H, Yoshioka R, Kagawa Y, Watari T. The clinical efficacy of dietary fat restriction in treatment of dogs with intestinal lymphangiectasia. *J Vet Intern Med* 28(3):809–817, 2014.
24. Green J, Kathrani A. Incidence of relapse of inflammatory protein-losing enteropathy in dogs and associated risk factors. *J Vet Intern Med* 36(6):1981–1988, 2022.
25. Zentek J, Meyer H. Normal handling of diets—are all dogs created equal? *J Small Anim Pract* 36(8):354–359, 1995.

CHAPTER 26

Prebiotics, probiotics, and synbiotics

Silke Salavati Schmitz
Dr.med.vet., PhD, DECVIM-CA, FHEA, FRCVS

Over the past decades, it has become clear that dysbiosis, defined as perturbations of the intestinal microbiota (the community of microorganisms in the gut), is involved in the etiopathogenesis of many conditions, and more particularly chronic inflammatory processes such as canine chronic enteropathy. Based on this, attempts at preventing or treating dysbiosis or modifying immune and gut functions via manipulation of the microbiota is increasingly popular.

Pre-, pro- and, synbiotics (as defined in Box 26.1) have gained interest as a means of introducing or promoting microorganisms with transient or permanent beneficial effects on the intestinal microbiota.[1] As a result of the growing concern regarding indiscriminate antimicrobial use for clinical signs such as diarrhea, which has been shown to aggravate intestinal dysbiosis and to possibly contribute to the rise in global antimicrobial resistance, pre- or synbiotics are promoted as a valid alternative.

While prebiotics are well-defined substances, the word *fiber* does not have a single broadly accepted definition. Generally, dietary fibers (DFs) are carbohydrates that are found in plants and are naturally resistant to digestion by host enzymes. From a gut health perspective, DFs often function as prebiotics.[2]

The evidence base for the use of specific pre-, pro-, or synbiotics in dogs with gastrointestinal (GI) disease is increasing, but still patchy. This chapter will summarize concepts of pre- and probiotic actions and the available information on their specific use in canine GI conditions.

> **Box 26.1 Definition of pre-, pro-, syn-, and postbiotics.**
>
> - **Prebiotic.** Nondigestible food ingredients that beneficially affect the growth and/or activity of one or a limited number of bacterial species already established in the gastrointestinal tract.
> - **Probiotics.** Live microorganisms which, when administered in adequate amounts, confer a health benefit to the host.
> - **Synbiotics.** A mixture of probiotics and prebiotics that beneficially affect the host by improving the survival and implantation of live microbial dietary supplements.
> - **Postbiotics.** Inanimate microorganisms and/or their (metabolic) components that confer a health benefit on the host.

Mechanisms of action

Several mechanisms of action within the GI tract and the gut-associated immune system have been proposed for probiotics. These include displacement of intestinal pathogens, production of antimicrobial substances such as organic acids or defensins, enhancement of innate and adaptive immune responses, and upregulation of various nonspecific cellular defense mechanisms.[3] Many of these actions are strain-specific; even bacterial strains of the same species can alter cellular responses differently.[4]

Details on cellular interactions of specific probiotic strains have been summarized in several reviews,[1,3,4] but it is overall believed that key biological signaling pathways (e.g., transcription of cytokines, cell survival, and apoptosis) are common targets for probiotics or their products both *in vitro* and *in vivo*.[4] Probiotics particularly modulate signaling pathways in innate immune cells such as macrophages and intestinal epithelial cells, but they also regulate adaptive immunity by promoting T cell differentiation into regulatory T cells (Tregs) and subsequently generating a more tolerogenic environment, as well as by stimulating plasma cell class switching.[4]

For prebiotics and DFs, the main proposed mechanism of action is an increase in metabolic products (sometimes called postbiotics[5]) such as short-chain fatty acids, which are a primary energy source for colonocytes, hence promoting barrier function and repair. They also directly and indirectly modulate the mucosal immune response, colonic motility, and microbiota composition.[2]

Pre-, pro-, and synbiotics in gastrointestinal health

Effect of probiotics in healthy dogs

Enterococcus faecium (EF) is one of the most widely used probiotics in small animals, with some information stemming from administering EF to healthy dogs. For example, when EF 10415 SF68 was given to healthy puppies for a year, these had significantly higher total fecal and serum IgA concentrations compared to control animals.[6]

Other studies have investigated the safety and effect of other single-strain lactic acid bacteria (LAB) (e.g., lactobacilli, bifidobacteria) or LAB mixtures in healthy dogs, but they often assessed routine clinico-pathological parameters of minor clinical relevance alongside fecal scores, fecal pH, dry matter, and fermentation end products.[6]

Few studies have used next-generation sequencing methods to assess fecal microbiota composition changes with probiotic administration, and these changes were either as expected (increase in Lactobacillaceae when lactobacilli were administered as probiotics) or absent.[6]

Pre- and probiotics in acute gastrointestinal conditions

There is evidence supporting the use of DF in the management of acute GI signs in dogs. Fiber-enhanced diets have been shown to reduce the effect of antibiotics on fecal consistency. An easily digestible diet with or without psyllium supplementation improved time to clinical resolution in acute noninfectious colitis, but the number of dogs with recurrence of colitis was less for dogs receiving the fiber supplement.[2] In puppies with shelter-associated diarrhea, feeding a diet high in both crude fiber and soluble fiber resulted in faster resolution of clinical signs.[2]

Studies investigating *in vivo* use of pro- and synbiotics in the prevention or treatment of specific naturally occurring GI disease in dogs are scarce. For acute GI diseases these can be divided into infectious diseases, idiopathic or otherwise ill-defined gastroenteritis, and antibiotic-induced diarrhea (Table 26.1).[6]

In several studies of dogs with acute uncomplicated diarrhea of different origins, results of the benefit of probiotics are mixed. Overall, even reported significant differences are of unclear clinical relevance. A recent systematic review of the available literature concluded that the administration of probiotics did not show a clinically significant effect in shortening the duration of acute diarrhea, and that the available evidence was of very low to moderate quality.[7]

In canine parvoviral enteritis, one study reports a significant clinical improvement with a commercially available LAB mixture added to standard treatment compared to standard treatment alone. The mortality rate was reduced by probiotic administration, with 90% of dogs in the oral probiotic group surviving compared to 70% of the nonprobiotic group.

In acute hemorrhagic diarrhea syndrome, the "de Simone formulation" probiotic blend (Table 26.1) lowered clinical severity and increased fecal abundance of bacterial markers of gut health (e.g., *Faecalibacterium* sp.), while *Clostridium perfringens* abundance and enterotoxin levels were reduced.

In parasitic disease, pro- and synbiotics have limited to no effects. *Giardia* cyst shedding was not altered by the administration of EF, while subclinical *Ancylostoma* egg shedding was significantly, albeit only transiently, suppressed using a LAB mixture.

Antibiotic-induced diarrhea was only assessed in one experimental study, in which the duration of lincomycin-induced diarrhea was significantly shortened by the administration of *Saccharomyces boulardii* in comparison to placebo.

Pre- and probiotics in chronic gastrointestinal conditions

The potential benefits of pro- and synbiotics on chronic GI conditions in dogs have been assessed using both clinical trials (Table 26.2) and *ex vivo* stimulation of biopsies.[6] There are minimal or no effects observed in most of the studies of chronic GI disease. In food-responsive chronic enteropathy, the probiotics used (EF and a LAB mixture) seemed to show promising results in *ex vivo* experiments (i.e., shift of cytokines towards a more tolerogenic microenvironment) but failed to produce similar responses when assessed in clinical trials.

Lactobacillus acidophilus DSM13241 was used in dogs with unspecific dietary sensitivity in a very small study and improved their fecal consistency. In dogs with tylosin-responsive diarrhea, *Lacticaseibacillus rhamnosus* GG failed to prolong the asymptomatic period once clinical remission was achieved and tylosin administration discontinued.

In cases of chronic enteropathy refractory to dietary and antibiotic treatment trials, specific probiotics seem to be a promising adjunctive or even possibly sole treatment. One study administering the de Simone formulation mixture demonstrated that it was as good as the control treatment (consisting of metronidazole and prednisolone) in inducing clinical remission and reduction of inflammatory cells in duodenal biopsies.[8] This study also demonstrated an increase in tissue markers representative of a more tolerogenic intestinal microenvironment, which was significantly stronger in the probiotic-treated dogs.

In another study, a significant improvement in clinical signs and defecation frequency was achieved using *S. boulardii* as a probiotic in dogs with immunosuppressant-responsive chronic enteropathy with or without protein-losing enteropathy. In the latter cases, probiotic administration resulted in significant improvement of serum albumin concentrations; however, the number of dogs with protein-losing enteropathy was very small (see Table 26.2).

There is also evidence that probiotics modulate intestinal epithelial permeability by changing expression of tight junction proteins such as E-cadherin, occludin, and zonulin, which could be seen as beneficial in a number of chronic GI conditions.

Studies investigating the effect of DF on chronic diarrhea are mostly specific to animals with large bowel diarrhea termed "fiber-responsive colitis".[2] This is likely not a diagnosis in itself, but a heterogenous group of diseases with characteristics that overlap with canine chronic enteropathies. In a number of studies using both soluble and insoluble fiber in dogs with colitis, excellent short- and long-term clinical response rates (ranging between 63% and 96%) were reported.[2] When attempts at reducing or stopping fiber supplementation were made, clinical signs recurred in some animals, indicating the likely need for long-term supplementation in these cases.

TABLE 26.1 Pro- and synbiotics assessed for their effect in acute gastrointestinal conditions in dogs.

Pre-, pro-, synbiotic, or DF used (and trade name where appropriate)	Dose	Number of animals in study	Condition treated	Observed outcomes
Bifidobacterium animalis AHC7 (isolated from healthy dog)	1×10^{10} CFU every 12 h	31	Acute idiopathic diarrhea	■ Significantly shorter duration to resolution of diarrhea in probiotic group (3.9 ± 2.3 days) compared to placebo group (6.6 ± 2.7 days)
B. animalis AHC7 (isolated from healthy dog)	Either: 1×10^{7} CFU/day, 1×10^{8} CFU/day or 1×10^{9} CFU/day (or placebo)	121	Kennel stress–associated diarrhea	■ No difference between fecal scores at week 1–2 ■ Significantly better fecal score for all probiotic groups compared to placebo at week 3 ■ No difference in diarrhea occurrences between groups
EF DSM 10663 NCIMB 10415 4b/E1707 + fructo-oligosaccharides and gum arabic	2×10^{9} CFU/day	733 (399 treated, 374 placebo)	Shelter-associated diarrhea	■ On treatment, significant fewer dogs have diarrhea (2% vs. 3% with placebo) ■ On treatment, fewer dogs with >1 day of diarrhea (18.8% vs. 27.2% with placebo)
EF SF68 NCIMB 10415	2.1×10^{9} CFU/day	182 (102 treated, 80 placebo)	Shelter-associated diarrhea (some animals also positive for various parasites)	■ No difference in number of dogs having diarrhea (9.8% vs. 12.5% with placebo)
LAB mixture in sour milk: – *Lactobacillus fermentum* VET 9A, – *Lacticaseibacillus rhamnosus* VET 16A, – *Lactobacillus plantarum* VET 14A	4×10^{11} CFU/day	44 (25 treated, 19 placebo)	Acute or intermittent, mild to moderate diarrhea	■ Statistical difference in change in mean fecal score on day 7, but not day 1–6 or 28
LAB mixture: – *Lactobacillus acidophilus* ATCC 4536, – *Lactobacillus plantarum* ATCC 8014, – *Lactobacillus delbrueckii* UFV H2B20	1×10^{6} CFU/day	20 (10 treated, 10 placebo)	*Ancylostoma* egg shedding	■ At day 28 of treatment, eggs per gram of feces reduced by 88.8% in the probiotic group, compared to 11.8% with placebo ■ This was not sustained by day 42
LAB mixture: – *Lactobacillus acidophilus*, – *Pediococcus acidilactici*, – *Bacillus subtilis*, – *Bacillus licheniformis*, – *Lactobacillus farciminis*	n/a	36 (15 treated, 21 placebo)	Acute gastroenteritis	■ Treatment resulted in significantly shorter duration of diarrhea ■ Days to last abnormal feces shorter in probiotic group (1.3 d; range 0.5–2.1 d) compared to controls (2.2 d; range 1.3–3.1 d)
LAB mixture DSF: – *L. plantarum* DSM 24730, – *Streptococcus thermophilus* DSM 24731, – *Bifidobacterium breve* DSM 24732, – *Lactobacillus paracasei* DSM 24733, – *L. delbrueckii* subsp. *bulgaricus* DSM 24734, – *L. acidophilus* DSM 24735, – *Bifidobacterium longum* 120 DSM 24736, – *Bifidobacterium infantis* DSM 24737	4.5×10^{10} CFU/day	20 (10 standard treatment alone, 10 standard treatment and probiotics)	Parvoviral enteritis	■ Significant improvement in clinical scores in probiotic group
LAB mixture DSF	225×10^{9} CFU for 1–10 kg dogs; 450×10^{9} CFU for 10–20 kg dogs; 900×10^{9} CFU for 20–40 kg dogs	25 (13 treatment, 12 control)	Acute hemorrhagic diarrhea syndrome	■ Significantly lower clinical severity in probiotic group ■ Increased fecal abundance of *Turicibacter* spp. and *Faecalibacterium* spp. in probiotic group ■ Significantly lower abundance of *C. perfringens* counts and enterotoxin in probiotic group

CFU, colony-forming units; DSF, de Simone formulation; EF, *Enterococcus faecium*; LAB, lactic acid bacteria.

Adapted from Salminen et al.[5]

TABLE 26.2 Pro- and synbiotics assessed for their effect in chronic gastrointestinal conditions in dogs.

Pre-, pro-, synbiotic, or DF used (and trade name where appropriate)	Dose	Number of animals in study	Condition treated	Observed outcomes
EF SF68 NCIMB 10415	5×10^{8} CFU/day	20 (10 treatment, 10 placebo)	*Giardia* cyst shedding (subclinical natural infection)	■ No statistical difference in fecal score ■ All dogs remained subclinical
EF DSM 10663 NCIMB 10415 4b/E1707 + fructo-oligosaccharides and gum arabic	1×10^{9} CFU/day	12 (7 synbiotic, 5 placebo) + healthy controls	Food-responsive chronic enteropathy	■ Small increase in fecal microbiota diversity in dogs treated with synbiotic ■ No significant differences in microbial community composition before and after 6 weeks of treatment in either synbiotic or placebo group or healthy controls
L. acidophilus DSM13241	6×10^{6} CFU/g dry food Control period 1: 12 weeks control diet Probiotic period: 12 weeks probiotic diet Control period 2: 12 weeks control diet	6 German Shorthair Pointers	Nonspecific dietary sensitivity	■ Unacceptable fecal consistency/defecation rates observed in 50% of the samples/study days during control period 1, but was reduced during the probiotic period and persisted in control period 2 ■ Fecal dry matter was significantly higher in the probiotic period compared to both control periods ■ Culturable bacteria concentrations (*C. perfringens*, *E. coli*, *Lactobacillus* spp., *Bifidobacterium* spp.) were similar in each dietary period
L. rhamnosus GG	5×10^{9} CFU every 12 h	14	Tylosin-responsive diarrhea	■ When tylosin was discontinued (in 9/14 dogs), diarrhea reappeared in all 9 dogs after a median of 7 days (range 3–26 days)
LAB mixture: – *L. acidophilus* NCC2628, – *L. acidophilus* NCC2766, – *Lactobacillus johnsonii* NCC2767	1×10^{10} CFU/day	21 (10 novel protein diet and placebo, 11 novel protein diet and LAB)	Food-responsive chronic enteropathy	■ Similar reduction in clinical severity ■ No difference in cytokines assessed in both groups, numbers of culturable Enterobacteriaceae decreased
LAB mixture DSF	$112–225 \times 10^{9}$ CFU/10 kg BW/day	10 probiotic treatment, 10 control treatment (metronidazole and prednisolone), 10 healthy control	Inflammatory bowel disease	■ Clinical improvement in both groups ■ TGFβ expression higher in the probiotic group ■ Similar reduction in overall inflammatory cells ■ Treg cells increased in the probiotic group ■ *Faecalibacterium* spp. increased in probiotic group
LAB mixture DSF	$112–225 \times 10^{9}$ CFU/10 kg BW/day	14 standard treatment + probiotic, 12 standard treatment + placebo	Inflammatory bowel disease	■ No difference in clinical remission or histopathology score ■ Total number of mucosal bacteria assessed by FISH increased in probiotic group ■ Increased number of intestinal mucosal and fecal *Lactobacillus* spp. in probiotic group, but decreased *Bifidobacteria* spp. (FISH) ■ Intestinal tight junction proteins upregulated in the probiotic group ■ Increased bifidobacteria in probiotic group
Saccharomyces boulardii	1×10^{10} CFU/day	20 (13 finished trial: 6 treated, 7 placebo)	Inflammatory bowel disease with or without protein-losing enteropathy	■ CCECAI improved more in probiotic group ■ Stool frequency reduced in probiotic group ■ In dogs with protein-losing enteropathy, serum albumin was >2 g/dL in 3/3 dogs in the probiotic group and 2/3 dogs in the placebo group

BW, body weight; CCECAI, canine chronic enteropathy clinical activity index; CFU, colony-forming units; EF, *Enterococcus faecium*; DSF, de Simone formulation; FISH, fluorescent *in situ* hybridization; LAB, lactic acid bacteria; TGFβ, transforming growth factor beta; Treg cells, regulatory T cells.

Adapted from Salminen et al.[5]

Conclusions

DF and other prebiotics as well as pro- and synbiotics have a place in treating GI conditions in dogs. However, their use cannot be indiscriminate or interchangeable. The level and strength of evidence is variable across studies and diseases. The outcomes observed are most often clinical, while functional effects on the mucosal immune system and microbiota remain largely unexplored. Currently, the main advantage of these measures, even if given empirically, seems to be their potential to reduce antibiotic prescription in both acute and chronic GI diseases in dogs.

KEY POINTS

- While general beneficial effects of moderate to high dietary fiber (DF) intake to improve gastrointestinal (GI) health have been demonstrated, probiotic effects in studies in healthy dogs are mostly minor and transient.
- For acute GI signs, evidence supports the use of DF such as psyllium, but strong evidence for the use of pro- or synbiotics is lacking.
- In chronic GI signs, it seems that specific probiotic strains or blends are needed for defined clinical scenarios such as chronic enteropathy or protein-losing enteropathy, and some promising results regarding functional improvement of the microbiota and local immune response are emerging.
- Additional research is needed to document the effect of probiotics in canine "colitis" and related conditions, but response rates to both soluble and insoluble DF can be excellent.

References

1. Schmitz S, Suchodolski J. Understanding the canine intestinal microbiota and its modification by pro-, pre- and synbiotics - what is the evidence? *Vet Med Sci* 2(2):71–94, 2016.
2. Moreno AA, Parker VJ, Winston JA, Rudinsky AJ. Dietary fiber aids in the management of canine and feline gastrointestinal disease. *J Am Vet Med Assoc* 260(S3):S33–S45, 2022.
3. Oelschlaeger TA. Mechanisms of probiotic actions—A review. *Int J Med Microbiol* 300(1):57–62, 2010.
4. Thomas CM, Versalovic J. Probiotics-host communication: Modulation of signaling pathways in the intestine. *Gut Microbes* 1(3):148–163, 2010.
5. Salminen S, Collado MC, Endo A, et al. The International Scientific Association of Probiotics and Prebiotics (ISAPP) consensus statement on the definition and scope of postbiotics. *Nat Rev Gastroenterol Hepatol* 18(9):649–667, 2021.
6. Schmitz SS. Value of probiotics in canine and feline gastroenterology. *Vet Clin North Am Small Anim Pract* 51(1):171–217, 2021.
7. Scahill K, Jessen LR, Prior C, et al. Efficacy of antimicrobial and nutraceutical treatment for canine acute diarrhoea: A systematic review and meta-analysis for European Network for Optimization of Antimicrobial Therapy (ENOVAT) guidelines. *Vet J* 303:106054, 2024.
8. Rossi G, Pengo G, Caldin M, et al. Comparison of microbiological, histological, and immunomodulatory parameters in response to treatment with either combination therapy with prednisone and metronidazole or probiotic VSL#3 strains in dogs with idiopathic inflammatory bowel disease. *PLoS One* 9(4):e94699, 2014.

CHAPTER 27

Fecal microbiota transplantation

Linda Toresson
DVM, Swedish Spec. Small Anim. Intern Med, PhD

Fecal microbiota transplantation (FMT) is a technique used to transfer feces from a healthy donor to a recipient with a disease to restore their intestinal microbiota and metabolome and decrease disease activity. The treatment was mentioned in a Chinese textbook of emergency medicine by Ge Hong in 320 A.D. but had rarely been used in traditional medicine until the last two decades.

In people, FMT is superior to antibiotics in recurrent *Clostridioides difficile* (rCDI) infection.[1] There is also evidence from several randomized controlled trials (RCTs) that FMT is associated with decreased disease activity and induction of remission in people with inflammatory bowel disease (IBD).[1] It has been shown that both the microbial composition of the donor stool and that of the recipient are important for a successful outcome.[2] Patients responding to FMT had increased fecal microbial diversity both before and after FMT compared to nonresponders.

Gastrointestinal (GI) disorders are by far the most common reasons to perform FMT in people, but multiple research studies have been performed using FMT for other indications, including hepatic disorders, metabolic syndrome, treatment of antibiotic-resistant microbes, psychiatric disorders, obesity, and others.[3]

The transplant can be administered rectally as a retention enema, orally as lyophilized feces in capsules, or deposited in the duodenum or colon using an endoscope. The route of administration does not appear to affect the outcome in people. Likewise, fresh or thawed frozen feces are equally effective in people with rCDI.[4]

FMT in dogs with gastrointestinal disorders

Several case reports, case series, and studies have been published on the use of FMT in dogs. An RCT in puppies with parvovirosis showed a beneficial effect of FMT.[5] Sixty-six puppies with parvovirosis were treated with FMT and standard treatment or standard treatment alone. The puppies in the FMT group were treated with one FMT every other day until recovery, with a median of 1.8 FMTs. Puppies treated with FMT had a significantly reduced time to recovery and hospitalization time (median, 3 days in the FMT group versus 6 days in the control group). Survival was also higher in the FMT group (26/33, 79%) compared to the other group (21/33, 64%), although this difference was not statistically significant. In a study of 18 dogs with acute diarrhea, dogs were treated with one single FMT or metronidazole for a week.[6] At day 7, the fecal scores were similar in both groups. At day 28, the dogs treated with FMT had significantly improved fecal scores versus the metronidazole-treated group. Dogs treated with metronidazole had significant dysbiosis at day 28, compared to dogs treated with FMT and healthy dogs. In studies of dogs with acute hemorrhagic diarrhea syndrome (AHDS), FMT treatment has not been shown to be superior to placebo or probiotics. However, only a small number of dogs have been included in the published studies. Furthermore, these dogs were only treated with one single FMT. Since AHDS is an aggressive condition associated with necrotizing inflammation, it may be beneficial to use multiple FMTs, as in the study on parvovirosis.

In dogs with chronic enteropathy (CE) with clinical signs such as diarrhea, vomiting, weight loss, or lethargy, there is evidence from several case reports and case series that FMT can decrease disease activity. In one retrospective study of 41 dogs with poorly responsive CE, FMT was used as adjunctive treatment.[7] Multiple rectal FMTs (median, 3) were given as a series of treatments. Thirty-one of 41 dogs responded to FMT, of which the majority showed further improvement of the clinical signs after the second or third FMT treatment. This was manifested as a significant reduction in the canine IBD activity index after FMT. Repeated FMTs have also been beneficial in people with IBD.[8,9]

In the CE dogs responding to FMT, the maintenance dose of corticosteroids could be reduced to doses that had not been possible before in 10/31 dogs, and frequent use of antibiotics could be reduced or stopped in 3 dogs. The most common clinical response was increased activity level in 24/31 dogs, and fecal quality was also improved in 24/31 dogs.[7] Additional clinical improvement after FMT consisted in less frequent flare-ups or milder flare-ups, weight gain, and improved appetite.

Reduction of fatigue and improved quality of life have been shown in RCTs in people with IBD as well as irritable bowel syndrome (IBS) for up to 6 months post FMT. This effect may partially be explained by increased production of short-chain fatty acids (SCFAs) by beneficial microbes. SCFAs stimulate the enterochromaffin cells to synthesize and secrete serotonin, which is one of the most important modulators of the gut–brain axis. Additionally, several intestinal microbes can synthesize neurotransmitters, such as γ-amino butyric acid (GABA), glutamate, noradrenaline, and dopamine. These can have a local effect in the gut but also modulate the brain and behavior.

Donor screening, FMT dose, and preparation of feces

The fundamental principle of donor screening is to find a donor with lots of beneficial microbes and no potential fecal pathogens. Current recommendations for donor screening are listed in Table 27.1. It is recommended to retest donors every 6 months.

There is currently no consensus on the FMT dose in veterinary medicine. The amount of donor stool given for FMT in dogs varies between studies. At the author's clinic, 5 grams of donor feces per kg body weight (BW) of the recipient are used for dogs up to 25 kg BW, and 3 grams of feces per kg BW for dogs with a BW >25 kg. In dogs with CE, three FMTs are given with a 10- to 20-day interval as one set of treatment. If there is no clinical response to the first two FMT doses, a third treatment is not recommended, based on previous results.[7]

Fresh frozen feces without cryopreservatives are used by the author. Frozen feces are stored at -20 °C for a maximum of 1 month. Cryopreservatives, such as glycerol, increase the amount of viable bacteria in frozen feces. Several gastroenterologists make a fecal slurry and add 10% glycerol before freezing the feces. However, it is not known if adding cryopreservatives actually makes a clinical difference. In several published studies on FMT to date, frozen feces without cryopreservatives have been used with a good outcome.[5–7]

Frozen feces should be thawed overnight in a fridge or in a 37°C water bath on the day of the procedure. The volume of the transplant after blending with saline should not exceed 20 mL/kg BW of the recipient.[10]

TABLE 27.1 Donor requirements and screening for fecal microbiota transplantation.

Donor requirements	Fecal screening
■ 12 months–middle age ■ Body condition score of 4 to 6/9 ■ Healthy, no medication ■ Canine inflammatory bowel disease activity index (CIBDAI) ≤3 ■ No antibiotics for 6 months (minimum) ■ Not being fed a raw food diet ■ Normal hematology and serum biochemistry	Normal dysbiosis index Exclude: ■ *Salmonella* spp. ■ *Campylobacter jejuni* ■ *Giardia* and other intestinal parasites

Rectal FMT procedure

On the day of the procedure, food is withheld from the recipient for 4–6 hours prior to FMT, but water is allowed. The rationale behind withholding food is that a recent meal may initiate motility of the lower GI tract via the gastrocolic reflex. However, there are no studies comparing FMT retention in dogs that have been fasted prior to FMT versus those that have not been fasted. Just prior to the procedure, the recipient dog should be walked for 30–40 minutes in order to defecate. Prior bowel cleansing is not recommended.

The author uses a low dose of acepromazine (0.1 mg/kg) subcutaneously, given 15 minutes prior to the procedure, unless there are contraindications to premedication. Many clinicians do not use premedication or sedation prior to FMT, depending on the individual animal's temperament. However, premedication usually makes it easier for the dog to relax and rest after the procedure, which allows for a longer contact time between the transplant and the colonic mucosa. The stepwise procedure for FMT is available in Figure 27.1. FMT can be given with the dog in a standing position or sternal or lateral recumbency. It is easiest to insert the catheter if the dog is in a standing position or in sternal recumbency. For details of the full procedure, see Figure 27.1. The author uses 16-French flexible suction catheters with atraumatic, rounded

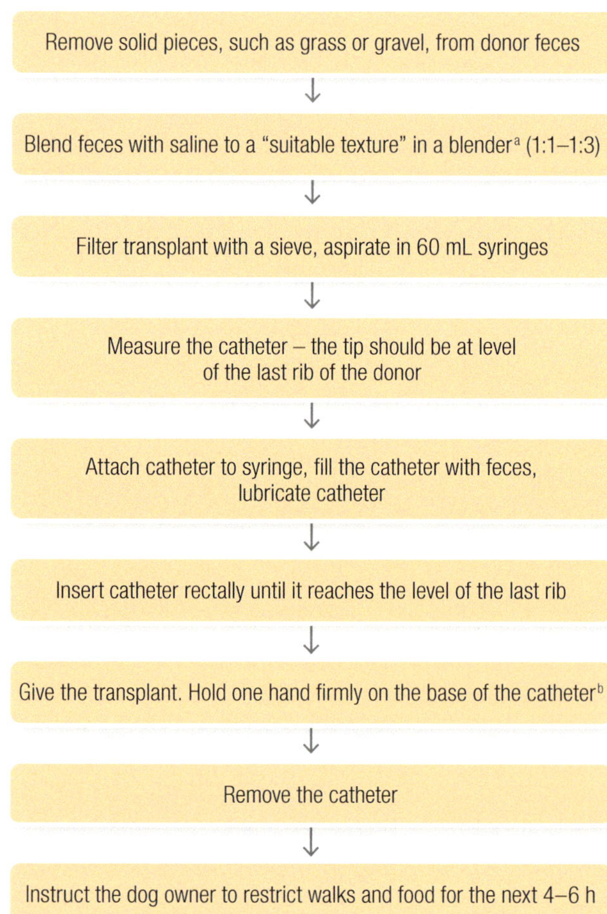

[a] Equivalent to a "thick smoothie" or purée.
[b] Holding a hand on the base of the catheter/syringe attachment prevents leakage and detachment.

FIG. 27.1 Stepwise procedure for fecal microbiota transplantation.

tips for most dogs, and 14-French catheters for toy breeds. Red rubber catheters or similar can also be used.

Adverse effects

Mild side effects have been described in 10/41 CE dogs and occurred in both responders and nonresponders.[7] The most prevalent was self-limiting diarrhea or worsening of diarrhea within 48 hours after FMT.

Lyophilized FMT capsules

Several studies have been published using lyophilized FMT capsules. This has been proven effective in people and dogs and is quick and convenient, since no special preparation of the dog is required.[11] However, it may not provide the same booster effect as rectal FMT, since it is difficult to give the equivalent amount of feces in capsules as one rectal FMT. Lyophilized capsules have been used by the author to extend the interval between rectal FMTs in a few dogs with poorly responsive CE requiring frequent rectal FMTs. If commercial lyophilized capsules are used, less information on the microbial composition of the donor stool is available compared to personally screened donors. The microbial composition of the donor stool has been associated with the outcome in ulcerative colitis in people.[2]

Gastrointestinal indications for FMT

Fecal microbiota transplantation can be used in both acute and chronic GI disorders. It has saved the life of several of the author's canine patients with nonresponsive or poorly responsive CE. In dogs with CE responding to FMT, FMT will not "cure" the dogs of CE, but the disease activity and maintenance doses of concurrent medication can often be decreased. However, the author has personal experience of a few young dogs with immunosuppressive-responsive enteropathy that could be weaned off corticosteroids after having been treated with three FMTs at a 10- to 20-day interval.

KEY POINTS

- Fecal microbiota transplantation (FMT) is used to restore the patient's intestinal microbiota and metabolome and decrease disease activity.
- Studies have shown that FMT led to a reduced time to recovery and hospitalization time in puppies with parvovirosis and can decrease disease activity in dogs with chronic enteropathy and signs such as diarrhea, vomiting, weight loss, or lethargy.
- Further research is needed to assess the potential beneficial effects of FMT treatment in dogs with acute hemorrhagic diarrhea syndrome.
- FMT can be used in both acute and chronic gastrointestinal disorders.
- There is currently no consensus on the FMT dose to be used in veterinary medicine.
- Fresh frozen feces with or without cryopreservatives may be used. Lyophilized FMT capsules are an option, but a booster effect may be more difficult to achieve, and less information about the microbial composition of the donor stool is available if commercial capsules are used.

References

1. Jaramillo AP, Awosusi BL, Ayyub J, et al. Effectiveness of fecal microbiota transplantation treatment in patients with recurrent Clostridium difficile infection, ulcerative colitis, and Crohn's disease: a systematic review. *Cureus* 15(7):e42120, 2023.
2. Paramsothy S, Nielsen S, Kamm MA, et al. Specific bacteria and metabolites associated with response to fecal microbiota transplantation in patients with ulcerative colitis. *Gastroenterology* 156(5):1440–1454.e2, 2019.
3. Green JE, Davis JA, Berk M, et al. Efficacy and safety of fecal microbiota transplantation for the treatment of diseases other than Clostridium difficile infection: a systematic review and meta-analysis. *Gut Microbes* 12(1):1–25, 2020.
4. Chapman BC, Moore HB, Overbey DM, et al. Fecal microbiota transplant in patients with Clostridium difficile infection: A systematic review. *J Trauma Acute Care Surg* 81(4):756–764, 2016.
5. Pereira GQ, Gomes LA, Santos IS, Alfieri AF, Weese JS, Costa MC. Fecal microbiota transplantation in puppies with canine parvovirus infection. *J Vet Intern Med* 32(2):707–711, 2018.
6. Chaitman J, Ziese AL, Pilla R, et al. Fecal microbial and metabolic profiles in dogs with acute diarrhea receiving either fecal microbiota transplantation or oral metronidazole. *Front Vet Sci* 7:192, 2020.
7. Toresson L, Spillmann T, Pilla R, et al. Clinical effects of faecal microbiota transplantation as adjunctive therapy in dogs with chronic enteropathies— a retrospective case series of 41 dogs. Veterinary Sciences. 2023;10(4):271.
8. He Z, Li P, Zhu J, et al. Multiple fresh fecal microbiota transplants induces and maintains clinical remission in Crohn's disease complicated with inflammatory mass. *Sci Rep*;7(1):4753, 2017.
9. Paramsothy S, Kamm MA, Kaakoush NO, et al. Multidonor intensive faecal microbiota transplantation for active ulcerative colitis: a randomised placebo-controlled trial. *Lancet* 389(10075):1218–1228, 2017.
10. Winston JA, Suchodolski JS, Gaschen F, et al. Clinical guidelines for fecal microbiota transplantation in companion animals. *Advances in Small Animal Care*. 2024;5(1):79-107. doi:10.1016/j.yasa.2024.06.006
11. Innocente G, Patuzzi I, Furlanello T, et al. Machine learning and canine chronic enteropathies: a new approach to investigate FMT effects. *Vet Sci* 9(9):502, 2022.

Analgesia

Jo Murrell
BVSc(Hons), PhD,
DECVAA, MRCVS

Visceral pain is generally difficult to localize and can be very severe. The pain scoring tools currently available have not been specifically developed to quantify visceral pain, thus making pain assessment and management of visceral pain with analgesia challenging. The reader can also refer to Chapter 6 for more information on abdominal pain.

Opioids form the backbone of analgesia protocols for the management of visceral pain. Nonsteroidal anti-inflammatory drugs (NSAIDs) must be used cautiously because of their gastrointestinal (GI) side effects. However, paracetamol (acetaminophen) can be used very safely in dogs. There is a limited evidence base for other classes of analgesic drugs for the management of visceral pain.

Principles of visceral pain management

As with any pain condition, there are two major principles that should be applied to the management of visceral pain, namely preventive analgesia and multimodal analgesia. Preventive analgesia has recently replaced the concept of preemptive analgesia (the administration of analgesic drugs before the onset of pain) because it is recognized that preemptive analgesia is not always practical and that pain is sustained by the afferent barrage of nociceptive input into the central nervous system (CNS).[1] Preventive analgesia encompasses the principles of giving analgesic drugs early and continuing them until this nociceptive barrage is over in order to prevent ongoing peripheral and central sensitization. This means getting analgesic drugs on board as soon as possible after the patient is presented to the clinic and maintaining analgesic drug administration until the pain has subsided, although there is little data available on how long analgesia should be administered in common visceral pain conditions. Therefore, this means combining analgesic drug administration with pain assessment and continuing analgesia until pain scores are below the threshold for intervention using validated pain assessment tools.

Multimodal analgesia is the concept of using different classes of analgesic drugs in combination to target pain more effectively. The pain pathway is very complex, with multiple neurotransmitters and receptors, and effective pain control can therefore rarely be achieved by the administration of a single class of analgesic drug. However, it is important to make a distinction between multimodal analgesia and uncontrolled polypharmacy. Analgesic drugs should ideally be chosen based on the underlying pain mechanisms (e.g., NSAIDs are most appropriate to treat pain of inflammatory origin; gabapentinoids are more appropriate to treat pain with a neuropathic component) so that there is a rationale for their selection. However, it is also true that many visceral pain conditions are of mixed etiology (e.g., ischemic and inflammatory pain), thus making the rational selection of analgesic drugs problematic. Due to the lack of consistent and effective pain models to mimic visceral pain, most analgesic drugs have a poor evidence base for the management of visceral pain, and in many cases, selection of an appropriate analgesic drug is based on trial and error combined with rigorous pain assessment.

Drug classes used to manage visceral pain

Opioids

Opioids form the backbone of most analgesic drug regimens in the USA and Europe in hospitalized patients, although it must be acknowledged that in many parts of the world (e.g., large parts of Asia) opioids are restricted and not available for use in veterinary patients. Many different opioid drugs are available, and they can be classified according to their effects at opioid receptors (Table 28.1). Opioids exert their analgesic action at multiple sites along the nociceptive pathway, with opioid receptors being ubiquitous in the dorsal horn of the spinal cord and higher brain centers. In the dorsal horn of the spinal cord, opioid drugs reduce the release of neurotransmitters, thereby reducing the transmission of information from the first-order primary afferent fibers to second-order dorsal horn neurons. They also play a pivotal role in the activation of descending inhibitory pathways and silence activity in nociceptive pathways in higher brain centers. Silent opioid receptors also exist in peripheral tissues

KEY POINTS

- The principles of multimodal and preventive analgesia should be used in the approach to visceral pain management.
- There is a paucity of data to support rational analgesic drug selection for visceral pain.
- Opioids (where available) form the mainstay of analgesic protocols.
- NSAIDs should be used cautiously, although paracetamol is an appropriate alternative in dogs.

References

1. Pogatzki-Zahn EM, Zahn PK. From preemptive to preventive analgesia. *Curr Opin Anaesthesiol* 19(5):551–555, 2006.
2. Columbano N, Secci F, Careddu GM, et al. Effects of lidocaine constant rate infusion on sevoflurane requirement, autonomic responses, and postoperative analgesia in dogs undergoing ovariectomy under opioid-based balanced anesthesia. *Vet J* 193(2):448–455, 2012.
3. Pypendop BH, Ilkiw JE. Assessment of the hemodynamic effects of lidocaine administered IV in isoflurane-anesthetized cats. *Am J Vet Res* 66(4):661–668, 2005.
4. Steagall PVM, Benito J, Monteiro B, et al. Intraperitoneal and incisional analgesia in small animals: simple, cost-effective techniques. *J Small Anim Pract* 61(1):19–23, 2020.
5. Slingsby LS, Waterman-Pearson AE. The post-operative analgesic effects of ketamine after canine ovariohysterectomy--a comparison between pre- or post-operative administration. *Res Vet Sci* 69(2):147–152, 2000 Oct.
6. Buisman M, Wagner MC, Hasiuk MM, et al. Effects of ketamine and alfaxalone on application of a feline pain assessment scale. *J Feline Med Surg* 18(8):643–651, 2016.
7. Boscan P, Monnet E, Mama K, et al. Effect of maropitant, a neurokinin 1 receptor antagonist, on anaesthetic requirements during noxious visceral stimulation of the ovary in dogs. *Am J Vet Res* 72(12):1576–1579, 2011.
8. Kinobe RT, Miyake Y. Evaluating the anti-inflammatory and analgesic properties of maropitant: A systematic review and meta-analysis. *Vet J* 259–260:105471, 2020.
9. Valtolina C, Robben JH, Uilenreef J, et al. Clinical evaluation of the efficacy and safety of a constant rate infusion of dexmedetomidine for postoperative pain management in dogs. *Vet Anaesth Analg* 36(4):369–383, 2009.

CHAPTER 29

Antibacterials

Fergus Allerton
BSc, BVSc, CertSAM, DECVIM-CA, FRCVS

Gastrointestinal (GI) disease represents the most common situation where antibacterials are prescribed in companion animal medicine. This is because diarrhea is a frequent reason for consultation and antibacterials are prescribed in a high proportion (28–70%) of diarrhea cases. Given the serious and growing threat posed to human and animal health by antimicrobial resistance, there is a pressing need to ensure that all antibacterial use is rational and supported by the best available evidence. Multiple antimicrobial stewardship guidelines from across Europe recommend against the use of antibacterials to manage cats and dogs with acute diarrhea.[1] However, adherence to these recommendations remains low, with veterinarians citing pet owner pressure, diagnostic uncertainty, and fear of disease progression as reasons for antibacterial use. More work is required to address these barriers and optimize antimicrobial stewardship.

Antimicrobial treatment of canine acute diarrhea

The European Network for Optimization of Veterinary Antimicrobial Treatment (ENOVAT) has recently developed antimicrobial use guidelines for treatment of canine acute diarrhea based on a systematic review of the available evidence.[2,8] According to these guidelines, dogs with acute diarrhea (duration <7 days, of any etiology) can be subdivided into three groups depending on their clinical severity (**Table 29.1**). These groupings mirror categorization from a study performed in primary care practice which found that the majority (84%) of dogs presenting for diarrhea have mild clinical signs, while 15% have moderate disease and only 1% are considered to be severe presentations.[3] The presence or absence of blood is specifically addressed in the recommendations, as this feature has previously been identified as a key driver in the decision to prescribe antibacterials. In fact, dogs presenting with hemorrhagic diarrhea are four times more likely to be prescribed an antibacterial than dogs presenting diarrhea without blood.[3]

The ENOVAT guideline panel made strong recommendations, with a high certainty of evidence, against antimicrobial treatment of dogs with mild or moderate acute diarrhea regardless of whether blood was present in the feces. These recommendations were based on outcome data from 232 dogs from six randomized controlled trials.[2] Among the studies included in the meta-analysis was a randomized, placebo-controlled trial that found no difference in morbidity or mortality in dogs with acute hemorrhagic diarrhea syndrome whether given systemic amoxicillin–clavulanate or a placebo.[4] A second randomized, double-blinded, placebo-controlled clinical trial found a small, but statistically significant, reduction in the duration (from 3.6 to 2.1 days) of acute diarrhea following treatment with metronidazole.[5] However, this benefit must be carefully weighed against the negative consequences of using this drug; the risk of neurotoxicity[6] and/or disruption of the GI microbiome[7] are important considerations for the individual animal. In addition, any antibacterial use can potentiate antimicrobial resistance. Metronidazole administration to healthy dogs caused a significant and sustained decrease in the richness and diversity of fecal microbial communities.[7] With the increasing availability of commercial assays to analyze the GI microbiome, the understanding of the dysbiotic impact of antibacterials will likely improve further in the coming years and should raise awareness of this adverse effect.

For dogs with acute diarrhea classed as severe disease, there was only low certainty evidence, as this group was not represented in any of the randomized controlled treatment trials. These animals represent a small minority of very sick dogs in which sepsis is a relevant clinical concern. In the absence of any supportive evidence, only a weak or conditional recommendation could be made. Antibacterial treatment with broad-spectrum coverage is suggested. Combination therapy using aminopenicillins or clindamycin (good gram-positive activity) alongside fluoroquinolones or aminoglycosides (for gram negatives) for a short period (<7 days) was proposed, adapted according to the clinical progression.[8] Alternative therapeutic strategies for dogs with severe disease may be considered, allowing for different drug availability (e.g., intravenous amoxicillin–clavulanate ± a fluoroquinolone).

Dogs presenting with parvovirus may require antibacterial therapy should severe neutropenia accompany the GI signs. Thresholds for prophylactic administration have not been established, but most authorities recommend

TABLE 29.1 Clinical categorization of dogs with acute diarrhea based on disease severity.

Clinical severity	Mild	Moderate	Severe
Management	■ May be treated on an outpatient basis	■ Hospitalization, warrants IVFT	■ Hospitalization, warrants IVFT
Mental status	■ Bright, alert, responsive	■ Mildly to moderately depressed	■ Moderately to severely depressed
Systemic response to disease	■ No clinical signs of dehydration or hypovolemia ■ Circulatory stable ■ Absence of fever	■ Clinically detectable dehydration or hypovolemia, but adequate improvement in response to appropriate IVFT ■ Absence of fever	■ Clinically detectable dehydration or hypovolemia, but no adequate improvement in response to appropriate IVFT ■ Severe circulatory compromise ■ Fever (>39.5°C)
Blood in feces	■ Nonhemorrhagic or hematochezia	■ Nonhemorrhagic or hemorrhagic (AHDS)	■ Nonhemorrhagic or hemorrhagic (AHDS)
Antibiotic use recommendation	■ No	■ No	■ Weak/conditional

AHDS, acute hemorrhagic diarrhea syndrome; IVFT, intravenous fluid therapy.

broad-spectrum antibacterial coverage when the neutrophil count drops below 1.0×10^9/L.

Metronidazole is consistently the antibacterial of choice to manage diarrhea in dogs and is often selected for putative nonantibacterial, anti-inflammatory, or immunomodulatory properties.[9] The scientific basis for this rationale is poorly established, but its widespread adoption may, in part, explain the continued popularity of metronidazole despite guidance to the contrary. Future stewardship resources may need to recognize and address this mechanistic belief to redirect prescribing behaviors away from this medication.

Historically, a therapeutic trial with metronidazole, tylosin, or oxytetracycline was considered a logical step in the approach to chronic enteropathy, as 15–35% of presentations were attributed to antibiotic-responsive diarrhea.[10] The category of antibiotic-responsive enteropathy was positioned just above food-responsive enteropathies in the pyramidal functional classification of inflammatory gut disease.[10] However, recent studies have proposed a new nomenclature that emphasizes more holistic means to modulate the microbiome and reduce the reliance on antibacterials. Revised terms including *idiopathic intestinal dysbiosis*[11] or *microbiota-related modulation-responsive enteropathy*[12] have been suggested to encourage clinicians to trial prebiotics, probiotics, postbiotics, synbiotics, fecal microbiota transplantation, or bile acid sequestrants in preference to antibacterials (hopefully supported by further robust evidence in the future). Furthermore, a group of eminent veterinary gastroenterologists advocated that antibiotics should only be introduced once all other etiologies have been excluded and other empirical treatments have been exhausted, or based on compatible histopathology from GI biopsies.[13] Enteropathies that may respond to antibacterial therapy include granulomatous (histiocytic ulcerative) colitis in Boxers and French Bulldogs, caused by a mucosally invasive *Escherichia coli* (see Chapter 49), and antibiotic-responsive diarrhea in young German Shepherd Dogs, potentially linked to altered expression of certain toll-like receptors.[14] A diagnosis of antibiotic-responsive enteropathy is contingent on a positive response to antibiotics after exclusion of other causes. Frustratingly, prolonged treatment courses are often required, as relapses are common following withdrawal of therapy.

Communication with pet owners

Adopting a nonantibacterial management strategy may meet objections from pet owners, so careful communication of the risks and benefits is necessary. To facilitate this conversation, a nonprescription form may be considered, with options developed by the British Small Animal Veterinary Association (BSAVA) and the Small Animal Medicine Society (SAMSoc),[15] and the American Veterinary Medical Association (AVMA). These forms reassure owners that the clinical decision not to prescribe antibacterials has been made based on careful balancing of risks and benefits, offer preferred options for management, and incorporate safety netting advice lest there is clinical deterioration. Similar tools have been effective in reducing antibiotic use without compromising patient outcome in people with respiratory disease.[16]

A short, animated educational film (Fig. 29.1) centered on a dog presenting to the veterinarian with acute diarrhea has recently been created for pet owners.[17] Viewing the animation can exert an important positive impact on pet owners' attitudes towards antimicrobial stewardship and could represent a low-cost aid that practices can host in their waiting rooms.

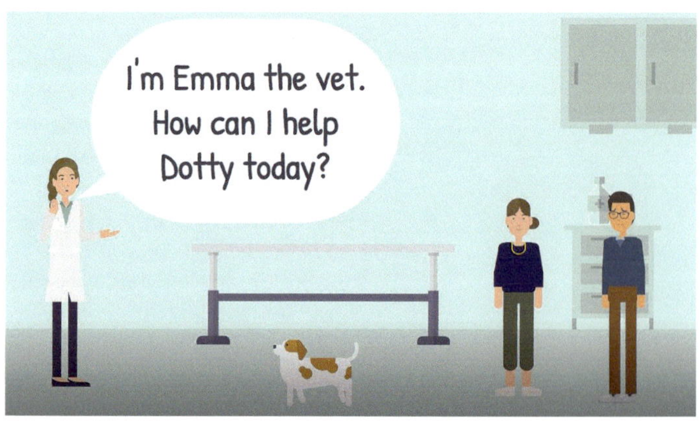

FIG. 29.1 Screenshot from the ENOVAT pet owner educational animation.[18]

Conclusion

GI disease offers few indications for justified antibacterial use. In summary, for pets with acute or chronic diarrhea with or without the presence of blood, or for pets presenting with acute vomiting, antibacterial treatment is not warranted unless the animal has concurrent systemic clinical signs consistent with sepsis. Important exceptions to this recommendation include dogs with parvovirus and severe neutropenia and dogs with histiocytic ulcerative colitis.

KEY POINTS

- Antibacterial therapy is not indicated in the vast majority of dogs presenting with gastrointestinal signs.
- Recommendations for antibiotic use in canine acute diarrhea have been developed based on a thorough appraisal of the available evidence.
- Antibacterials are only warranted in dogs and cats with gastrointestinal disease and severe systemic disease (suspicion of sepsis) or in specific disorders with a confirmed infectious etiology (e.g., granulomatous colitis).
- Resources such as the nonprescription form and pet owner educational animations may support veterinarians to avoid unnecessary antibiotic use.

References

1. Allerton F, Prior C, Bagcigil AF, et al. Overview and evaluation of existing guidelines for rational antimicrobial use in small-animal veterinary practice in Europe. *Antibiotics (Basel)* 10(4):409, 2021.
2. Scahill K, Jessen LR, Prior C, et al. Efficacy of antimicrobial and nutraceutical treatment for canine acute diarrhoea: A systematic review and meta-analysis for European Network for Optimization of Antimicrobial Therapy (ENOVAT) guidelines. *Vet J* 303:106054, 2024.
3. Singleton DA, Noble PJM, Sánchez-Vizcaíno F, et al. Pharmaceutical prescription in canine acute diarrhoea: A longitudinal electronic health record analysis of first opinion veterinary practices. *Front Vet Sci* 6:218, 2019.
4. Unterer S, Strohmeyer K, Kruse BD, et al. Treatment of aseptic dogs with hemorrhagic gastroenteritis with amoxicillin/clavulanic acid: a prospective blinded study. *J Vet Intern Med* 25(5):973–979, 2011.
5. Langlois DK, Koenigshof AM, Mani R. Metronidazole treatment of acute diarrhea in dogs: A randomized double blinded placebo-controlled clinical trial. *J Vet Intern Med* 34(1):98–104, 2020.
6. Tauro A, Beltran E, Cherubini GB, et al. Metronidazole-induced neurotoxicity in 26 dogs. *Aust Vet J* 96(12):495–501, 2018.
7. Pilla R, Gaschen FP, Barr JW, et al. Effects of metronidazole on the fecal microbiome and metabolome in healthy dogs. *J Vet Intern Med* 34(5): 1853–1866, 2020.
8. Jessen LR, Werner M, Singleton D, et al. European Network for Optimization of Veterinary Antimicrobial Therapy (ENOVAT) guidelines for antimicrobial use in canine acute diarrhoea. *Vet J* 307:106208, 2024.
9. Ellis C, Odunayo A, Tolbert MK. The use of metronidazole in acute diarrhea in dogs: a narrative review. *Top Companion Anim Med* 56–57:100824, 2023.
10. Dandrieux JR. Inflammatory bowel disease versus chronic enteropathy in dogs: are they one and the same? *J Small Anim Pract* 57(11):589-599, 2016.
11. Jergens AE, Heilmann RM. Canine chronic enteropathy—Current state-of-the-art and emerging concepts. *Front Vet Sci* 9:923013, 2022.
12. Dupouy-Manescau N, Méric T, Sénécat O, et al. Updating the classification of chronic inflammatory enteropathies in dogs. *Animals (Basel)* 14(5):681, 2024.
13. Cerquetella M, Rossi G, Suchodolski JS, et al. Proposal for rational antibacterial use in the diagnosis and treatment of dogs with chronic diarrhoea. *J Small Anim Pract* 61(4):211–215, 2020.
14. Allenspach K, House A, Smith K, et al. Evaluation of mucosal bacteria and histopathology, clinical disease activity and expression of Toll-like receptors in German shepherd dogs with chronic enteropathies. *Vet Microbiol* 146(3-4):326–335, 2010.
15. BSAVA, SAMSoc. *BSAVA/SAMSoc Guide to Responsible Use of Antibacterials: PROTECT ME.* 2018. https://www.bsavalibrary.com/content/chapter/10.22233/9781910443644.app15#-supplementary_data. Accessed June, 2025.
16. Spurling GK, Del Mar CB, Dooley L, et al. Delayed antibiotic prescriptions for respiratory infections. *Cochrane Database Syst Rev* 9(9):CD004417, 2017.
17. Wright E, Jessen LR, Tompson A, et al. Influencing attitudes towards antimicrobial use and resistance in companion animals—the impact on pet owners of a short animation in a randomized controlled trial. *JAC Antimicrob Resist* 6(3):dlae065, 2024.
18. ENOVAT videos on the rational use of antibiotics https://enovat.eu/search/?search=pet+owners Accessed June 2025

CHAPTER 30

Gastrointestinal parasiticides

Ian Wright
BVMS, BSc, MSc, MRCVS

A wide range of drugs are effective against different endo- and ectoparasites. In the case of gastrointestinal (GI) disease, these are anthelmintics and antiprotozoal drugs used in the treatment and prevention of disease and zoonotic risk caused by intestinal worms such as *Toxocara canis* (Fig. 30.1) and protozoa. When deciding whether a parasiticide is required in a particular case and which would be suitable, several factors need to be considered:

- **Is a product available that is licensed against the target parasite and safe for use in dogs?** Where possible, a product should be selected that has been licensed to be effective against target parasites but also has licensed safety profiles for the patient species. Even when using licensed products, drugs may cause side effects in certain situations, such as the use of macrocyclic lactones at incorrect dosages in Collie breeds or when cross reactions between drugs occur.
- **Is the aim to treat disease or eliminate infection?** Sometimes, a parasiticide will be selected to treat disease, but elimination of the causative organism is impractical or not desirable. For example, treatment of individual cases of giardiosis with parasiticides will often rapidly resolve the clinical signs, although the parasite can be extremely difficult to eliminate from the intestine. Prolonged attempts to treat subclinical infections may promote drug resistance and result in little clinical benefit. In some cases, however, such as for preventing the shedding of zoonotic parasitic life stages of *Toxocara* spp. or *Echinococcus* spp. into the environment, elimination of patent infection is essential.
- **Is a wide spectrum of activity required?** Some parasiticides treat both some internal and external parasites (endectocides) or a wide range of helminths. These are useful to improve owner compliance and restrict the number of drugs/products required when multiple parasites need treatment or prevention. If broad-spectrum activity is not required, however, selection of these products may have unintended effects, such as the promotion of drug resistance in nontarget parasites or impact on free-living invertebrates in the environment.
- **Is use warranted when weighed against potential drug resistance and environmental contamination concerns?** There is growing concern around drug resistance in companion animal parasites and potential environmental contamination with parasiticides. There is currently no evidence of environmental contamination with anthelmintics or antiprotozoals used in cats and dogs, but little research has been carried out in this area. There is also little or no surveillance of parasiticide drug resistance in many parts of the world, including Europe, making the extent of drug resistance largely unknown. Parasiticides should only be used when a significant positive impact on human and animal health can be demonstrated.

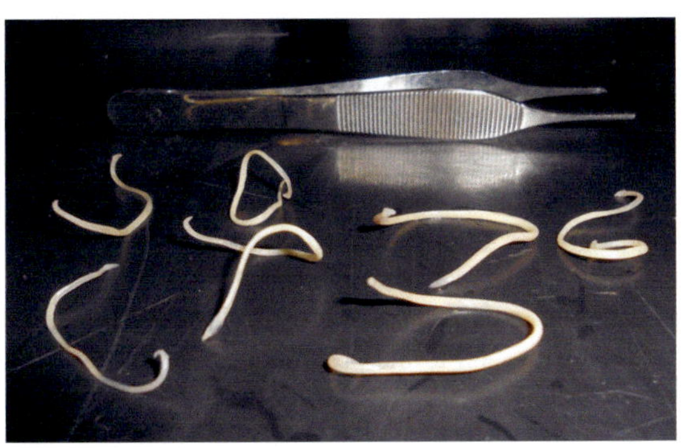

FIG. 30.1 Adult *Toxocara canis* worms.

Classes of parasiticide

Parasiticides targeted at GI parasites can be classed broadly as anthelmintics or antiprotozoals, although some compounds (e.g., fenbendazole) have activity against both. Endoparasiticides are compounds able to kill parasites living inside the animal, such as GI and cardiorespiratory parasites.

Anthelmintics

The anthelmintics commonly used to treat worms infecting companion animals fall into the drug classes described below. See also Chapter 39. A summary of the parasites each drug class is active against is summarized in Table 30.1.

KEY POINTS

- A wide range of drugs are effective against different helminths and protozoa of dogs.
- Benzimidazoles, macrocyclic lactones, and tetrahydropyrimidines are commonly used to treat intestinal nematode infections with a broad-spectrum of activity.
- Macrocyclic lactones are also used for essential heartworm prevention in dogs visiting or living in endemic countries.
- Ivermectin should not be used in breeds likely to carry the *MDR1* gene due to toxicity risks.
- Praziquantel has broad-spectrum activity against tapeworms and is an essential component in limiting zoonotic risk from exposure to *Echinococcus* spp. from infected dogs. Routine use is essential for dogs visiting or living in endemic countries with outdoor access.
- Anthelmintic resistance is becoming an increasing concern in dogs, with rapid spread of multiple drug-resistant hookworms in North America. There is little surveillance of anthelmintic resistance developing in helminths of dogs, and studies looking at potential environmental contamination from anthelmintics are still minimal.
- Increased surveillance is essential, and parasiticides should only be used if a significant positive impact on human and animal health can be demonstrated.
- Some antimicrobials have activity against intestinal protozoa, with fenbendazole and metronidazole being commonly used to treat *Giardia*, and sulfonamides and triazones being used to treat *Cystoisospora* species.
- The development of antibiotic resistance in some of these compounds and emerging drug resistance to fenbendazole in *Giardia* spp. mean that only clinical protozoal cases should be treated, unless the strategy is to reduce clinical disease in wider groups of animals.

References

1. Epe C, Kaminsky R. New advancement in anthelmintic drugs in veterinary medicine. *Trends Parasitol* 29:129–134, 2013.
2. Jimenez Castro PD, Venkatesan A, Redman E, et al. Multiple drug resistance in hookworms infecting greyhound dogs in the USA. *Int J Parasitol Drugs Drug Resist* 17:107–117, 2021.
3. Kopp SR, Kotze AC, McCarthy JS, Coleman GT. High-level pyrantel resistance in the hookworm *Ancylostoma caninum*. *Vet Parasitol* 143: 299–304, 2007.
4. Loftus JP, Acevedo A., Bowman DD, et al. Elimination of probable praziquantel-resistant *Dipylidium caninum* with nitroscanate in a mixed-breed dog: a case report. *Parasites Vectors* 15:438, 2022.

CHAPTER 31

Prokinetic drugs

Mark G. Papich
DVM, MS, DACVCP

Prokinetic drugs are medications that increase gastrointestinal (GI) motility—that is, more rapid stomach emptying and/or intestinal transit.[1] In people gastroparesis is a complication of diabetes, neuropathies, medications (opioids), and surgery. Much of the veterinary studies have focused on prokinetic drug use in horses, and not in dogs, but reviews of GI motility disorders in dogs provide additional information about the causes and clinical presentation of these cases.[2,3]

The GI tract is an abundant source of serotonin (5-HT), and several of the drugs discussed in this chapter affect 5-HT activity or 5-HT receptors. Motility of gastric and intestinal smooth muscle is influenced by at least six types of 5-HT receptors. Generally, 5-HT$_3$ receptors are inhibitory and 5-HT$_4$ receptors are stimulatory (Box 31.1).

Metoclopramide

Metoclopramide has multiple actions, but overall it is more effective as an antiemetic than as a motility modifying agent (see Chapter 32). It can increase gastric emptying, increase the tone of the lower esophageal sphincter, and stimulate motility of the duodenum, but these effects require high doses or a constant rate infusion, and it has much less effect on distal segments of the intestine.

Mechanism of action

Metoclopramide is a dopamine (D_2) antagonist, weak 5-HT$_4$ agonist, and 5-HT$_3$ antagonist, all of which can affect GI motility. The D_2 antagonist effects on the chemoreceptor trigger zone are responsible for the antiemetic action and may also antagonize its inhibitory action on GI motility. Among the additional proposed actions of metoclopramide is an increase in the release of acetylcholine in the GI tract, possibly via a prejunctional mechanism, or by increasing the sensitivity of the cholinergic response. At high doses it acts as a 5-HT$_4$ agonist to increase motility. In canine studies this required a constant rate infusion for a consistent effect.

Adverse effects of metoclopramide are mostly attributed to D_2 antagonism affecting the central nervous system and can include excitement (rarely observed in dogs), anxiety, and involuntary muscle movements. There are also endocrine effects including a transient increase in prolactin and aldosterone. Consequently, there has been some concern about the carcinogenicity of this drug in women, but these effects are unknown in dogs.

Clinical use

Metoclopramide is often used as an antiemetic in dogs, but other agents are more popular (see Chapter 32). The clinical dose is 0.25–0.5 mg/kg every 8–12 hours, but it can be increased to 1–2 mg/kg to produce a more consistent effect. Although it has been used to stimulate GI motility, it is probably less effective for this indication than previously thought. For example, it is of little benefit to increase stomach emptying in case of gastroparesis or chronic regurgitation. Metoclopramide stimulates upper GI motility following corrective surgery for gastric dilatation, but it does not promote gastric emptying in dogs with gastric dilatation–volvulus.[4] In another study, it reduced, but did not prevent, gastroesophageal reflux in anesthetized dogs at a dose of 1 mg/kg.[5]

Box 31.1 Significance of serotonin (5-HT) receptors.

- Over 90% of the 5-HT in the body is in the gastrointestinal tract
- There are several 5-HT receptor types:
  - 5-HT$_4$ agonists and 5-HT$_3$ antagonists stimulate gastrointestinal motility
  - 5-HT$_{1A}$ inhibits gastrointestinal motility
  - Stimulation of brainstem 5-HT$_3$ receptors induces vomiting
  - 5-HT$_3$ antagonists act as antiemetics

Cisapride

In July 2000, cisapride was removed from the human pharmaceutical market because of serious cardiac adverse events and some deaths in people due to cardiac arrhythmias. Despite discontinuation of the drug for people, there is continued interest among veterinarians, and it is still available via compounding pharmacists. Until new replacement drugs, such as prucalopride or tegaserod, become available and are shown to have utility in dogs, veterinarians must rely on compounded cisapride formulations.

Mechanism of action

The effect of cisapride on animals has been described in older reviews.[1,6–8] It has greater prokinetic effects in comparison to metoclopramide, being an agonist for 5-HT_4 receptors on myenteric neurons, stimulating cholinergic transmission. Cisapride may also be an antagonist for 5-HT_3 receptors, but it increases smooth muscle motility in the stomach, small intestine, and colon, primarily through 5-HT_4 receptors. It accelerates the transit of contents in the bowel, and because of the 5-HT_3 antagonist properties it also has some antiemetic effects.

Pharmacokinetics

Oral absorption of cisapride is variable, ranging from 30 to 60%, because of extensive metabolism. The elimination half-life is approximately 5 hours in dogs.

Clinical use

In dogs, cisapride at a dose of 0.1 mg/kg (range 0.08–1.25 mg/kg) orally stimulates the stomach, small intestine, and colon, with a duration of action of about 3 hours. Routine clinical doses can range from 0.1 to 0.5 mg/kg, and as high as 1 mg/kg every 8–12 hours.

It is used in dogs for treatment of gastroesophageal reflux, delayed gastric emptying, and small bowel motility disorders. Compared to metoclopramide, cisapride is more effective for increasing the lower esophageal sphincter tone, which is helpful for preventing reflux esophagitis.[9]

Although cisapride has been used for treatment of megaesophagus in dogs, the response is usually poor because the canine esophagus is largely composed of striated muscle.

Availability of formulations

The previously available 10 mg tablet is no longer on the market. Oral formulations have been prepared from the bulk powder administered in a capsule, via a suspension in a flavored vehicle or dissolved in an oil vehicle. Although cisapride is insoluble in most aqueous solutions, solubility is possible in acidic solutions.

Side effects and interactions

Adverse effects have not been reported in clinical cases; however, abdominal discomfort has been observed when dogs received high doses of cisapride. In safety studies, dogs have tolerated high doses (40 mg/kg) for prolonged periods without problems.

In people, high plasma concentrations have caused cardiac arrhythmias by prolonging the QT interval. This can lead to serious ventricular arrhythmias (e.g., torsade de pointes) and has been responsible for deaths in people. These reactions have not been reported in animals. Nevertheless, caution should be used when combining cisapride with drugs (e.g., itraconazole, ketoconazole) that may increase plasma concentrations by interfering with its metabolism.

Macrolide antibiotics: erythromycin and azithromycin

Erythromycin is a macrolide antibiotic ordinarily used to treat bacterial infections. It has been associated with vomiting and regurgitation in small animals as an adverse consequence of treatment. This effect is caused by stomach contraction and expulsion of gastric contents when high doses are administered. At doses below the antibacterial effects, it can produce a beneficial stimulation of GI motility and an increase in stomach emptying. However, responsible antibiotic stewardship raises significant concerns over the use of low doses of these antibiotics and the potential development of antibiotic resistance (see Chapter 29).

Although erythromycin may not be commonly used in small animal practice, azithromycin, an antibiotic with a similar spectrum, is used in some countries. It has a longer half-life and fewer adverse effects.[10] Azithromycin is typically administered for some infections, but it also has a promotility effect.[11] In people the effects are equivalent to those of erythromycin, with fewer adverse effects and drug interactions.[10] Not all macrolide antibiotics exhibit this property, because it requires a unique chemical structure that not all drugs in this class (e.g., tylosin) possess.

Mechanism of action

These macrolide antibiotics stimulate GI motility via activation of motilin receptors, either via release of endogenous motilin or via cholinergic mechanisms in the upper GI tract.[1,12,13] Motilin is a peptide released from endocrine cells of the duodenal mucosa. It increases the motor contractions (housekeeper waves) during the interdigestive period. Motility is initiated specifically in the pyloric antrum or the smooth muscle cells of the proximal small intestine.[14,15] The effective prokinetic dose of erythromycin is 1 mg/kg or less—much lower than the antibacterial dose. Because most of the motilin receptors are on the stomach and proximal small intestine, the response in the distal GI tract is weaker. In people, erythromycin has been utilized to promote gastric motility and increase stomach emptying in patients with diabetic gastroparesis and is used in conjunction with enteral feeding in critical care patients.[13] Azithromycin has similar effects to erythromycin, with fewer adverse reactions. In cats, azithromycin administered at 3.5 mg/kg once daily had similar prokinetic effects compared to erythromycin administered at 1 mg/kg three times daily.[11] These studies have not been performed in dogs, but a similar effect is anticipated.

Lidocaine

Lidocaine is a well-known local anesthetic, but intravenous infusion of lidocaine also improves intestinal motility in horses.[16] The mechanism for this effect is not understood but may be attributed to a lower pain response, decreased intestinal inflammation following surgery, or effects on the sympathetic nervous system. However, these effects have not been observed in dogs: lidocaine infusions produced a mild decrease in intestinal transit time but did not increase gastric emptying, and higher sedation and nausea scores were observed.[17] Because of the only mild intestinal motility effects and increased adverse effects, this use of lidocaine as a prokinetic drug in dogs is not recommended.

Opiate antagonists

Mechanism of action

Administration of opioid analgesics postoperatively[18,19] or increased levels of endogenous opioids (endorphins) stimulate μ-opioid receptors in the submucosal plexus, myenteric plexus, and longitudinal muscle of the ileum, decreasing propulsive motility and causing postoperative ileus and constipation.[20] Postoperative ileus may be treated by μ-opioid receptor blockers,[21] while agonists for these receptors (e.g., loperamide) can be useful in treating some forms of diarrhea.

Clinical use

Selective peripheral opiate antagonists have been used to reduce the effects of opioids on GI motility. These agents are considered peripheral opioid antagonists, rather than central opioid antagonists. They do not produce a central effect because they are unable to cross the blood-brain barrier. Such agents include alvimopan, methylnaltrexone, naldemedine, and naloxegol. These drugs are approved for use in people, but there has been very limited use in dogs, and they may not be safe in dogs with the MDR1 mutation. They restore GI motility while preserving opioid-mediated analgesia. Naloxone should not be used for this indication because it will cross the blood-brain barrier and diminish the analgesic effect of opioids.

Drugs for Chronic Constipation

The following drugs are used to treat chronic constipation in people but are not yet approved for clinical use in dogs:

- Prucalopride: High-affinity 5-HT_4 receptor agonist.
- Mosapride: Selective 5HT_4 agonist; its major active metabolite (M1) additionally acts as a 5-HT_3 antagonist.
- Tegaserod: 5-HT_4 receptor agonist.
- Linaclotide and plecanatide: Guanylate cyclase-C receptor agonists.
- Lubiprostone: Prostaglandin derivative that activates intestinal chloride channels.

Laxatives and cathartics

Laxatives and cathartics are drugs which increase bowel motility and change the character of the stool. These drugs promote the elimination of soft-formed stool or increase the water content of feces, which increases their bulk. Laxatives and cathartics can be divided into stimulants, hyperosmotic agents, and bulk-forming laxatives (see also Chapter 48). They may also be categorized by their onset of action: osmotic (saline) laxatives act in 1–3 hours, direct stimulants act in 6–8 hours, and "bulk laxatives" and surfactants act in 1–3 days.

Stimulant (irritant) laxatives

Stimulant (irritant) laxatives produce their action by inhibiting the Na^+/K^+-ATPase in the intestine and increasing electrolyte loss through intestinal tight junctions, followed by increased fluid loss. These drugs act within 6–8 hours of administration. They can have a potent stimulant effect on the GI tract. Excessive fluid and electrolyte loss can result from overdose. Adverse effects associated with damage to enterocytes can be caused by chronic use and abuse.

- Diphenylmethane: Use is not documented in veterinary medicine.
- Phenolphthalein: Once an ingredient found in over-the-counter laxative preparations, it is no longer available.
- Anthraquinone: Glycoside derivative found in bisacodyl, senna, and cascara sagrada.
- Castor oil: Hydrolyzed in the bowel to release ricinoleic acid, which causes increased secretion of water in the small intestine.

Hyperosmotic cathartics (saline cathartics)

Saline cathartics are nonabsorbed electrolytes that draw fluid into the bowel via osmosis. These are the most rapidly acting of the cathartics, with an onset of action in 1–3 hours. The fluid content of the stool increases, which causes intestinal distention and promotes increased peristalsis. They have been the most common cathartics used in veterinary medicine. Most often they are dissolved in an aqueous solution (water-based) and administered via gastric gavage. These drugs have been used to prepare animals for colonoscopy or for cathartic treatment of poisoning. They are relatively safe drugs, but overdose can cause dehydration in a patient. Examples of these drugs include:

- Sodium sulfate (Glauber's salt) solution is administered orally usually combined with magnesium or potassium sulfate. The sulfate anions produce an osmotic catharsis.
- Magnesium salts such as magnesium sulfate (Epsom salts), magnesium hydroxide, and magnesium citrate. Magnesium sulfate combined with psyllium is used to treat sand enteropathy in horses, but this has not been described in dogs.
- Nonabsorbed sugars: Lactulose, polyethylene glycol (PEG). Lactulose is used to treat hepatic encephalopathy, partly through its cathartic action, but macrogol (PEG 3350) is considered a more effective laxative.
- Combination products: Strong osmotic cathartics that are a combination of inorganic salts (e.g., sodium sulfate, potassium chloride, sodium chloride, sodium bicarbonate) and PEG 3350 (see Chapter 22).
- Low-volume sodium phosphate bowel preparation solutions used in people are highly concentrated, drawing water into the bowel to produce an osmotic catharsis. Other products are difficult to use in dogs: a tablet formulation requires 32 large tablets (with 1 cup of water per 4 tablets) for its effects. Nausea, vomiting, bloating, and abdominal discomfort can occur in dogs. They can also cause electrolyte imbalances and severe water loss, although this is less likely with the combination products.

Bulk laxatives (hydrophilic colloids)

Bulk laxatives are mostly natural products and dietary plant fibers. They are composed of nonabsorbed synthetic or natural polysaccharide and cellulose derivatives, are resistant to digestion, and attract water into the intestine. By imbibing water, they increase the mass of nondigestible material in the bowel, and motility is increased through the stimulation of mechanoreceptors. They are more slowly acting than other drugs, with an onset of action of up to 24 hours. They are relatively safe drugs with few side effects. Examples include methylcellulose, carboxymethylcellulose, psyllium, canned pumpkin, prunes, and wheat bran—and other proprietary attempts to increase "fiber" in the diet.

KEY POINTS

- Metoclopramide is a weak prokinetic and more effective antiemetic.
- Cisapride is a more effective prokinetic than metoclopramide.
- Low-dose erythromycin is prokinetic, but this use is not compliant with good antibiotic stewardship.
- Generally, 5-HT_3 receptors are inhibitory and 5-HT_4 receptors are stimulatory.
- Opioids can cause ileus and constipation, but use of μ-receptor blockers is not common practice.
- Laxatives and cathartics include stimulants, hyperosmotic agents, and bulk-forming agents.

References

1. Washabau RJ, Hall JA. Diagnosis and management of gastrointestinal motility disorders in dogs and cats. *Compend Contin Educ Pract Vet* 19(6):721–736, 1997.
2. Husnik R, Gaschen F. Gastric motility disorders in dogs and cats. *Vet Clin North Am Small Anim Pract* 51(1):43–59, 2021.
3. Whitehead K, Cortes Y, Eirmann L. Gastrointestinal dysmotility disorders in critically ill dogs and cats. *J Vet Emerg Crit Care (San Antonio)* 26(2): 234–253, 2016.
4. Hall JA, Solie TN, Seim HB 3rd, Twedt DC. Effect of metoclopramide on fed-state gastric myoelectric and motor activity in dogs. *Am J Vet Res* 57(11):1616–1622, 1996.
5. Wilson DV, Evans AT, Mauer WA. Influence of metoclopramide on gastroesophageal reflux in anesthetized dogs. *Am J Vet Res* 67(1):26–31, 2006.
6. Washabau RJ, Sammarco J. Effects of cisapride on feline colonic smooth muscle function. *Am J Vet Res* 57(4):541–546, 1996.
7. Van Nueten JM, Schuurkes JAJ. Development of a gastrointestinal prokinetic: pharmacology of cisapride. In: Scarpignato C (ed.). *Advances in Drug Therapy of Gastroesophageal Reflux Disease.* Frontiers of Gastrointestinal Research, vol. 20, pp. 54–63, 1992.
8. King JN, Gerring EL. Actions of the novel gastrointestinal prokinetic agent cisapride on equine bowel motility. *J Vet Pharmacol Ther* 11(4):314–321, 1988.
9. Kempf J, Lewis F, Reusch CE, Kook PH. High-resolution manometric evaluation of the effects of cisapride and metoclopramide hydrochloride administered orally on lower esophageal sphincter pressure in awake dogs. *Am J Vet Res* 75(4):361–366, 2014.
10. Potter TG, Snider KR. Azithromycin for the treatment of gastroparesis. *Ann Pharmacother* 47(3):411–415, 2013.
11. Rutherford S, Gaschen F, Husnik R, et al. Ultrasonographic evaluation of the effects of azithromycin on antral motility and gastric emptying in healthy cats. *J Vet Intern Med* 36(2):508–514, 2022.
12. Lester GD, Merritt AM, Neuwirth L, et al. Effect of erythromycin lactobionate on myoelectric activity of ileum, cecum, and right ventral colon, and cecal emptying of radiolabeled markers in clinically normal ponies. *Am J Vet Res* 59(3):328–334, 1998.
13. Hawkyard CV, Koerner RJ. The use of erythromycin as a gastrointestinal prokinetic agent in adult critical care: benefits versus risks. *J Antimicrob Chemother* 59(3):347–358, 2007.
14. Nouri M, Hajikolaee MR, Constable PD, Omidi A. Effect of erythromycin and gentamicin on abomasal emptying rate in suckling calves. *J Vet Intern Med* 22(1):196–201, 2008.
15. Nouri M, Constable PD. Effect of parenteral administration of erythromycin, tilmicosin, and tylosin on abomasal emptying rate in suckling calves. *Am J Vet Res* 68(12):1392–1398, 2007.
16. Torfs S, Delesalle C, Dewulf J, et al. Risk factors for equine postoperative ileus and effectiveness of prophylactic lidocaine. *J Vet Intern Med* 23(3):606–611, 2009.
17. Johnson RA, Kierski KR, Jones BG. Evaluation of gastric emptying time, gastrointestinal transit time, sedation score, and nausea score associated with intravenous constant rate infusion of lidocaine hydrochloride in clinically normal dogs. *Am J Vet Res* 78(5):550–557, 2017.
18. Boscan P, Van Hoogmoed LM, Pypendop BH, et al. Pharmacokinetics of the opioid antagonist N-methylnaltrexone and evaluation of its effects on gastrointestinal tract function in horses treated or not treated with morphine. *Am J Vet Res* 67(6):998–1004, 2006.
19. Sojka JE, Adams SB, Lamar CH, Eller LL. Effect of butorphanol, pentazocine, meperidine, or metoclopramide on intestinal motility in female ponies. *Am J Vet Res* 49(4):527–529, 1988.
20. DeHaven-Hudkins DL, DeHaven RN, Little PJ, Techner LM. The involvement of the mu-opioid receptor in gastrointestinal pathophysiology: therapeutic opportunities for antagonism at this receptor. *Pharmacol Ther* 117(1):162–187, 2008.
21. Hicks GA, DeHaven-Hudkins DL, Camilleri M. Opiates in the control of gastrointestinal tract function: current knowledge and new avenues for research. *Neurogastroenterol Motil* 16 Suppl 2:67–70, 2004.
22. Taguchi A, Sharma N, Saleem RM, et al. Selective postoperative inhibition of gastrointestinal opioid receptors. *N Engl J Med* 345(13):935–940, 2001.

CHAPTER 32

Antiemetic drugs

Mark G. Papich
DVM, MS, DACVCP

Vomiting in dogs can be due to a variety of etiologies (see Chapter 10), and the underlying cause must be addressed to provide long-lasting resolution. Antiemetic and anti-nausea medications can suppress clinical signs and reduce fluid and electrolyte loss and discomfort but will not address the underlying cause, so they only provide temporary relief of nausea and vomiting. Antiemetic drugs are directed at the various neurotransmitter receptors that stimulate vomiting and nausea. Table 32.1 provides a summary of antiemetic drugs and suggested dosages.

TABLE 32.1 Antiemetic drugs and doses.

Antiemetic		Doses
Antihistamines	Diphenhydramine	2–4 mg/kg IM or PO every 8–12 h
	Dimenhydrinate	4–8 mg/kg PO every 8–12 h
	Promethazine	0.2–0.4 mg/kg IM or PO every 8 h
Phenothiazines	Chlorpromazine	0.5 mg/kg IM or PO every 6–8 h
	Prochlorperazine	0.1–0.5 mg/kg IM every 6–8 h
	Acepromazine	0.1 mg/kg IM or PO every 12 h
	Triflupromazine	0.1–0.3 mg/kg IM or PO every 8–12 h
	Trifluperazine	0.03 mg/kg IM every 12 h
	Triethylperazine	0.13–0.2 mg/kg IM every 8–12 h
	Metoclopramide	0.1–0.3 mg/kg IM or PO every 12 h
Anticholinergic drugs	Atropine	0.02–0.04 mg/kg IM or SC every 8–12 h
	Methscopolamine	0.3–1.0 mg/kg PO every 8 h
	Isopropamide	0.2–1.0 mg/kg PO every 12 h
Antiserotoninergic drugs	Ondansetron	0.5–1.0 mg/kg IV or PO 30 minutes prior to administration of cancer drugs For vomiting from other causes: 0.1–0.2 mg/kg slow IV injection and repeated every 6–12 h
Neurokinin-1 receptor blockers	Maropitant	1 mg/kg SC every 24 h, 2 mg/kg PO every 24 h, or 8 mg/kg PO (for prevention of motion sickness)

IM, intramuscular; IV, intravenous; PO, per os; SC, subcutaneous.

Neurotransmitters involved in vomiting

A variety of inputs to the vomiting center can trigger the vomiting reflex (see Chapter 10). The neurotransmitters at these sites include dopamine, histamine, acetylcholine, neurokinin, and serotonin (Fig. 32.1). Successful antiemetic treatment involves blocking one or more of the receptors for these neurotransmitters. There are differences among dogs, cats, and people with respect to the relative importance of the various neurotransmitters. Dogs readily vomit in response to the administration of apomorphine or ropinirole, which are agonists for dopamine type 2 (D_2) receptors. Efferent stimuli from the emetic center then trigger the familiar sequence of events: nausea, abdominal and diaphragmatic contraction, and consequent ejection of gastric contents.

The variety of neurotransmitters and their origins and targets can have overlapping effects on nausea and vomiting. The properties of these neurotransmitters can be confusing, but there are some generalities:

- Afferents from the gastrointestinal (GI) tract: After injury to the GI mucosa by cisplatin and other anticancer drugs, GI diseases, or GI distension, serotonin is released by enterochromaffin cells in the mucosa to stimulate the vagal afferents leading to the vomiting center and chemoreceptor trigger zone (CRTZ). There are also serotonin type 3 (5-HT_3) receptors in the vomiting center. Nausea and the emetic response are produced from these stimuli. Ondansetron and related drugs are 5-HT_3 antagonists. Metoclopramide at high doses also has some 5-HT_3 antagonist activity.
- Vestibular apparatus: Acetylcholine and histamine can stimulate nausea and vomiting (motion sickness). Serotonin and adrenergic receptors may also play a role. Anticholinergic drugs (e.g., scopolamine) and antihistaminic drugs (e.g., diphenhydramine) are less effective antiemetics in dogs than in people with motion sickness.
- CRTZ: When circulating drugs or toxins cause vomiting, it is often via stimulation of the CRTZ, located in the area postrema of the brain—an area that is outside the blood-brain barrier. In the CRTZ, dopamine, serotonin, and acetylcholine all play a role. Histamine is a

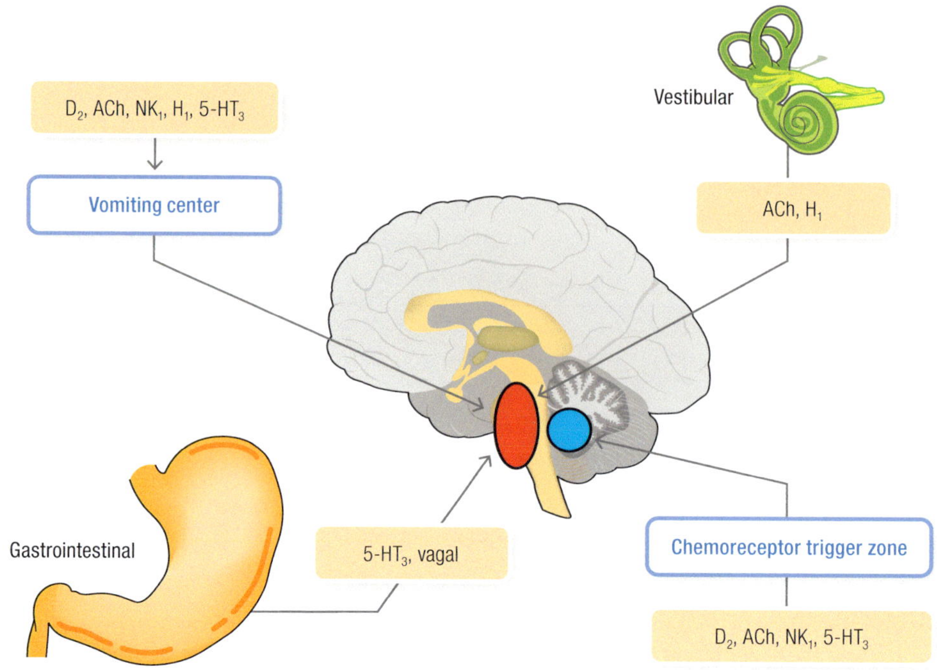

FIG. 32.1 Emetic stimuli, neurotransmitters, and receptors.

more important neurotransmitter in the CRTZ of dogs than in that of cats, but it is a more potent stimulant in people than in dogs.

- Neurokinin-1 (NK_1) receptors: Neurokinin (substance P) is a neurotransmitter from several sources capable of stimulating vomiting. NK_1 receptors are found in the emetic center and the CRTZ. Maropitant is a NK_1 receptor blocker and stops vomiting from several sources.
- Vomiting center: Serotonin (5-HT_3 receptors), histamine (H_1 receptors), acetylcholine (muscarinic M_1 receptors), dopamine (D_2 receptors), and neurokinin (NK_1 receptors) all play some role, although their relative importance varies among species.

Phenothiazine tranquilizers

Phenothiazine tranquilizers, such as chlorpromazine, prochlorperazine, promethazine, and acepromazine, antagonize dopamine (block D_2 receptors) in the central nervous system (CNS) to inhibit vomiting. In addition to their antidopaminergic effects, these drugs can block alpha-adrenergic receptors (α_1) in the emetic center.

Some phenothiazines have overlapping functions and also block histaminic and muscarinic receptors. Because of this broad action, and ability to inhibit vomiting from various stimuli, this group of drugs has been called "broad-spectrum antiemetics". However, clinical use may be limited in some patients by side effects, including sedation, altered involuntary motor activity (extrapyramidal signs), and peripheral α-adrenergic receptor blockade (vasodilation).

Antimuscarinic drugs

Drugs that block muscarinic (M_1) receptors include atropine, scopolamine, aminopentamide, and isopropamide. None of these drugs are commonly used to treat vomiting in dogs, but isopropamide is combined with prochlorperazine in some products. However, they can decrease vomiting from various causes, including vestibular (motion sickness) and CRTZ stimulation. In people, scopolamine is one of the most effective agents for treating motion sickness, but it is less effective in dogs.

Adverse effects of anticholinergic drugs include xerostomia, decreased stomach emptying, ileus, urine retention, constipation, worsening of glaucoma, and excitement in some animals.

Antihistaminic drugs

Histamine H_1 and H_2 receptors are involved in the transmission of vomiting stimuli in the CRTZ and vestibular apparatus, but this mechanism is more prominent in people than in dogs. Antihistamines can also have antimuscarinic effects. Antihistaminic drugs administered to control vomiting include diphenhydramine (the active component of dimenhydrinate), cyclizine, and promethazine (a phenothiazine with antihistamine effects).

Antihistamines are relatively safe drugs. Their most significant side effect is sedation, but this is not necessarily undesirable in most vomiting patients. Sedation occurs because H_1 receptors regulate sleep–wake cycles. Diphenhydramine and dimenhydrinate have the greatest sedative effects.

Metoclopramide

Metoclopramide has antiemetic effects via three mechanisms (see Chapter 32):

- At low doses inhibition of dopaminergic (D_2 receptors) transmission in the CNS, which is similar to the action of phenothiazines.
- Peripheral effects on the GI tract that possibly increase emptying of the stomach and upper duodenum.

- At high doses (1–3 mg/kg) only, inhibition of 5-HT_3 receptors. Metoclopramide can be administered as an intravenous infusion during cancer chemotherapy, although adverse effects are more likely at these high doses.

Metoclopramide is used less commonly in dogs because maropitant has become more popular. However, in head-to-head comparisons, metoclopramide shows equivalent efficacy for treating vomiting in dogs. Indeed, metoclopramide, ondansetron, and maropitant are equally effective in reducing the frequency and severity of vomiting in dogs with parvovirus enteritis.[1]

Metoclopramide has been used in small animal medicine for treating animals that vomit because of drug therapy (e.g., cancer medication) or during the postoperative period. Nevertheless, effectiveness for these indications has not been measured in clinical trials. For control of vomiting caused by cancer drugs the results have been disappointing.[2] See Chapter 31 for information of the prokinetic effects of metoclopramide.

Regarding pharmacokinetics in dogs, the half-life ranges from about 100 to 190 minutes, and the systemic availability of an oral dose is only about 50%.

Being a dopamine antagonist, metoclopramide at high dosages can produce adverse reactions that are similar to those caused by phenothiazines, including excitement and behavior changes. To produce adequate antiemetic effects by blocking 5-HT_3 receptors, high doses are often needed, which increases the risk of extrapyramidal CNS effects attributed to central dopamine antagonism. Because metoclopramide stimulates upper GI motility, it may produce some abdominal discomfort and should not be administered if there is an obstruction. It also produces transient endocrine changes, including an increase in prolactin.

Serotonin antagonists

Selective 5-HT_3 antagonists include ondansetron, granisetron, palonosetron, dolasetron, tropisetron, and azasetron. Of these, ondansetron is the best-known specific serotonin inhibitor in veterinary medicine. It is often used as an antiemetic in dogs during cancer chemotherapy but has become popular for other causes of vomiting. The doses of ondansetron used are 0.5–1.0 mg/kg intravenously or orally 30 minutes prior to the administration of cancer drugs.

The major limitation for ondansetron use in dogs is its poor oral absorption. After oral administration, the concentration in dogs is low or undetectable.[3] Owing to an extensive first-pass metabolism, oral bioavailability is estimated to be less than 10% in dogs,[4] with a short half-life, and high variability.[5] This is lower than in people, in which oral absorption is approximately 60%. However, oral absorption in dogs is better when administered with food, and this could perhaps overcome this limitation to some extent. After intravenous administration, ondansetron was shown to be an effective anti-nausea drug at doses of 0.5 or 1 mg/kg. Both doses were effective, but more dogs responded to the higher dose.[6]

Many clinicians believe that ondansetron is better for decreasing nausea than vomiting and, conversely, that maropitant is better for inhibiting vomiting than as an anti-nausea agent. There is indeed evidence in dogs to suggest that ondansetron is more effective as an anti-nausea drug than as an antiemetic.[7] Oral administration of maropitant 2 hours prior to premedication with hydromorphone reduced both vomiting and nausea in healthy dogs, but, in comparison, oral administration of ondansetron reduced the incidence and severity of nausea but not the incidence of vomiting.[8] However, there are likely overlapping effects, and ondansetron has been reported to be as effective an antiemetic when compared to maropitant or metoclopramide; indeed, the greatest antiemetic and anti-nausea efficacy of these three drugs for cisplatin-induced nausea and vomiting has been described.[9]

Administration of ondansetron (0.5 mg/kg IV) was beneficial for dogs with nausea secondary to acute vestibular syndrome. It substantially and rapidly decreased clinical signs of nausea behavior and stopped emesis.[10]

In dogs with parvovirus enteritis, maropitant (1 mg/kg IV every 24 h) and ondansetron (0.5 mg/kg IV every 8 h) were equally effective in controlling clinical signs.[11] In a similar study, metoclopramide, ondansetron, and maropitant were equally effective in reducing the frequency and severity of vomiting in dogs with parvovirus enteritis.[1]

Therefore, it appears that ondansetron, and likely other 5-HT_3 receptor antagonists, is an effective anti-nausea agent but should be administered intravenously for the best effect. It may also be an effective antiemetic agent, depending on the cause of vomiting. In many cases, clinicians will administer both ondansetron and maropitant for a dual effect of antiemesis and anti-nausea for an optimum effect.

Glucocorticoids

Glucocorticoids, such as dexamethasone, have antiemetic properties, possibly by inhibiting prostaglandin synthesis. These drugs are sometimes used in addition to other drugs for decreasing vomiting, particularly when it is caused by cancer chemotherapy.

NK_1 receptor blockers

NK_1 receptor blockers were approved for use in people for cancer chemotherapy-induced vomiting. Aprepitant was the first substance P (NK_1) receptor antagonist approved for people,[12] and it is used primarily with drugs known to be highly emetic, such as cisplatin. This drug is effective because chemotherapy drugs release substance P, which is highly emetic, and injure the GI tract mucosa, which releases serotonin, inducing nausea and vomiting via afferents to the CRTZ and vomiting center. Maropitant is not used in people because of a concern of cardiac arrhythmias (long QT syndrome), but it has been used successfully in dogs.

The only NK_1 receptor antagonist available for dogs, maropitant, was approved in 2007. It shares the same activity as the human antiemetics aprepitant, fosaprepitant, and rolapitant. Several studies in animals have documented the effects of NK_1 antagonists.[13–20]

Maropitant is an effective antiemetic in both experimental and clinical patients for a variety of stimuli (Box 32.1).

Box 32.1 Causes of vomiting for which maropitant is an effective treatment.[16–23]

- Apomorphine
- Cisplatin
- Copper sulfate
- Enteritis (dietary indiscretion)
- Hydromorphone
- Ipecac
- Morphine
- Pancreatitis
- Parvovirus enteritis

It is available as a 10 mg/mL injection (1 mg/kg once daily subcutaneously or intravenously for up to 5 days) and as a tablet (2 mg/kg per day) in a range of tablet sizes. The tablet can also be used to prevent vomiting caused by motion sickness (8 mg/kg/day for up to 2 days).

The efficacy of maropitant is attributed to its central site of action blocking NK_1 receptors in the nucleus tractus solitarius. Therefore, it blocks input from multiple sources and is broad spectrum in action.

Although maropitant is effective against vomiting, there is some debate about whether it is as effective for reducing nausea. Some animals may not vomit but can still have the discomfort of nausea. This notion is supported by studies in dogs after preoperative administration of hydromorphone, in which maropitant significantly decreased the incidence of vomiting but did not improve signs of nausea unless given 60 minutes prior.[24–27] Yet in a comparison between maropitant (1 mg/kg) and metoclopramide (0.5 mg/kg) in dogs with morphine-induced nausea and vomiting, there was no difference in the incidence of nausea, but vomiting occurred less often in the maropitant-treated group.[28]

There is conclusive evidence that maropitant is an effective antiemetic agent for vomiting caused by a variety of stimuli. As described above, it may not relieve nausea from all sources, so when dogs show persistent signs of nausea despite maropitant administration, ondansetron may be added for a synergistic effect.

Pharmacokinetics

Maropitant is extensively metabolized by the liver and there is little clearance by the kidneys, so no dose adjustments are necessary in patients with compromised renal function. Absorption from subcutaneous administration is rapid and complete (91%), but oral absorption is limited by the first-pass metabolic effects (24% at 2 mg/kg, and 37% at 8 mg/kg).[29] The half-life is 7.75 and 4–5.5 hours after subcutaneous and oral administration, respectively. However, the effects persist for at least 24 hours after a dose, presumably because of binding to the CNS NK_1 receptor that maintains the drug at the site of action. Penetration across the blood-brain barrier has been demonstrated,[16,21] which is necessary for activity in the emetic center.

Adverse effects

There are NK_1, NK_2, and NK_3 receptors throughout the body, but maropitant has little binding affinity to the latter two. This drug does not bind to any other CNS receptors, and although NK_1 receptors are involved in many other physiological and behavioral responses, at doses used for antiemesis there are no adverse effects associated with these other functions.

One of the adverse effects reported is pain or a stinging response when injected subcutaneously. This is caused by the irritant effect of the drug formulation (a molecular inclusion complex with a cyclodextrin) when it dissociates at room temperature. At refrigerated temperatures, however, maropitant remains complexed within a cavity in the cyclodextrin molecule.[30] This provides higher drug solubility and improved injection-site tolerance, as entrapment within the cyclodextrin cavity prevents direct contact of maropitant with biologic membranes by limiting the free drug concentration, thus reducing injection-related local irritation. Consequently, this drug complex will remain intact and is less likely to cause pain from injection if stored in the refrigerator between uses and injected cold.

Maropitant is also approved for intravenous use, which can be used to avoid subcutaneous injection. After intravenous administration, blood pressure may decrease in some dogs, but this has not been widely reported as a problem when used as a preanesthetic agent.[34] Other adverse effects are minimal. Compared to other antiemetic drugs, maropitant has had a very good safety profile in the clinical trials conducted in dogs thus far.

Other uses

Because NK_1 receptors are also involved in transmission of pain, there has been interest in using this substance P antagonist for analgesia and for the treatment of pancreatitis, coughing, and chronic rhinitis, although the evidence of efficacy in these cases is weak.[35]

Cannabinoids

Cannabinoids have been used in people who have not responded to any other antiemetic drugs. They have also been utilized to increase the appetite in patients with terminal diseases. There are two important cannabinoid receptors: CB_1 and CB_2. CB_1 receptors are found in the brain and are responsible for the CNS effects, including appetite stimulation, anti-nausea, and antiemetic properties.

There are approximately 100 cannabinoids in the cannabis plant, but tetrahydrocannabinol (delta-9-THC) is believed to be the most pharmacologically active. In addition to botanical sources, there are two pharmaceutical formulations of cannabinoids: synthetic marijuana (THC) is available as dronabinol and nabilone. There is also a cannabis extract that contains THC and cannabidiol (CBD), which is another major cannabinoid found in cannabis. Pure CBD does not have psychoactive effects compared to the other commercial cannabinoids.

Cannabinoids are relatively well tolerated by people, but side effects include drowsiness, dizziness, ataxia, and disorientation. Withdrawal signs may occur after abrupt discontinuation following repeated doses. Oral absorption of dronabinol is good, but bioavailability is low due to high first-pass effects. It is very lipophilic, producing a high volume of distribution.

In places where medical cannabis is legal, it has also been used in dogs. Please refer to local regulations controlling the use of cannabinoids.[36] Clinical studies have not been published on the use of cannabinoids for nausea and vomiting in dogs, but they have been used by some veterinarians to increase appetite. Recommendations are based on anecdotal observations or small, observational uncontrolled studies.

Suggested doses for dronabinol in animals (but untested in clinical trials) are 5 mg/m^2, increasing as needed up to 15 mg/m^2, for antiemetic administration prior to chemotherapy. For appetite stimulation in animals, suggested dronabinol doses start at 2.5 mg before meals.

KEY POINTS

- A variety of inputs to the vomiting center can trigger the vomiting reflex.
- Neurokinin, dopamine, and serotonin are the most important vomiting-associated neurotransmitters in dogs.
- Metoclopramide blocks dopamine type 2 (D_2) receptors.
- Ondansetron blocks serotonin type 3 (5-HT_3) receptors.
- Maropitant blocks neurokinin-1 (NK_1) receptors.
- Combinations of these antiemetics can be synergistic.

References

1. Yalcin E, Keser GO. Comparative efficacy of metoclopramide, ondansetron and maropitant in preventing parvoviral enteritis-induced emesis in dogs. *J Vet Pharmacol Ther* 40(6):599-603, 2017.
2. Fukui H, Yamamoto M, Sato S. Vagal afferent fibers and peripheral 5-HT_3 receptors mediate cisplatin-induced emesis in dogs. *Jpn J Pharmacol* 59(2):221–226, 1992.
3. Zersen KM, Molli A, Weisbeck BG, et al. Plasma concentrations of oral ondansetron in hospitalized dogs exhibiting clinical signs of nausea. *Vet Sci* 11(3):112, 2024.
4. Saynor DA, Dixon CM. The metabolism of ondansetron. *Eur J Cancer Clin Oncol* 25 Suppl 1:S75–S77, 1989.
5. Baek IH, Lee BY, Kang J, Kwon KI. Pharmacokinetic modeling and Monte Carlo simulation of ondansetron following oral administration in dogs. *J Vet Pharmacol Ther* 38(2):199–202, 2015.
6. Sotelo CK, Shropshire SB, Quimby J, et al. Pharmacokinetics and anti-nausea effects of intravenous ondansetron in hospitalized dogs exhibiting clinical signs of nausea. *J Vet Pharmacol Ther* 45(6):508–515, 2022.
7. Foth S, Meller S, Kenward H, et al. The use of ondansetron for the treatment of nausea in dogs with vestibular syndrome. *BMC Vet Res* 17(1):222, 2021.
8. Burke JE, Hess RS, Silverstein DC. Effectiveness of orally administered maropitant and ondansetron in preventing preoperative emesis and nausea in healthy dogs premedicated with a combination of hydromorphone, acepromazine, and glycopyrrolate. *J Am Vet Med Assoc* 260(S1):S40–S45, 2021.
9. Kenward H, Elliott J, Lee T, Pelligand L. Anti-nausea effects and pharmacokinetics of ondansetron, maropitant and metoclopramide in a low-dose cisplatin model of nausea and vomiting in the dog: a blinded crossover study. *BMC Vet Res* 13(1):244, 2017.
10. Henze L, Foth S, Meller S, et al. Ondansetron in dogs with nausea associated with vestibular disease: A double-blinded, randomized placebo-controlled crossover study. *J Vet Intern Med* 36(5):1726–1732, 2022.
11. Sullivan LA, Lenberg JP, Boscan P, et al. Assessing the efficacy of maropitant versus ondansetron in the treatment of dogs with parvoviral enteritis. *J Am Anim Hosp Assoc* 54(6):338–343, 2018.
12. Dando TM, Perry CM. Aprepitant: a review of its use in the prevention of chemotherapy-induced nausea and vomiting. *Drugs* 64(7):777–794, 2004.
13. Watson JW, Gonsalves SF, Fossa AA, et al. The anti-emetic effects of CP-99,994 in the ferret and the dog: role of the NK_1 receptor. *Br J Pharmacol* 115(1):84–94, 1995.
14. Huskey SE, Dean BJ, Doss GA, et al. The metabolic disposition of aprepitant, a substance P receptor antagonist, in rats and dogs. *Drug Metab Dispos* 32(2):246–258, 2004.
15. Fukuda H, Koga T, Furukawa N, et al. The tachykinin NK_1 receptor antagonist GR205171 abolishes the retching activity of neurons comprising the central pattern generator for vomiting in dogs. *Neurosci Res* 33(1):25–32, 1999.
16. Vail DM, Rodabaugh HS, Conder GA, et al. Efficacy of injectable maropitant (Cerenia) in a randomized clinical trial for prevention and treatment of cisplatin-induced emesis in dogs presented as veterinary patients. *Vet Comp Oncol* 5(1):38–46, 2007.
17. Ramsey DS, Kincaid K, Watkins JA, et al. Safety and efficacy of injectable and oral maropitant, a selective neurokinin$_1$ receptor antagonist, in a randomized clinical trial for treatment of vomiting in dogs. *J Vet Pharmacol Ther* 31(6):538–543, 2008.
18. de la Puente-Redondo V, Tingley FD 3rd, Schneider RP, Hickman MA. The neurokinin-1 antagonist activity of maropitant, an antiemetic drug for dogs, in a gerbil model. *J Vet Pharmacol Ther* 30(4): 281–287, 2007.
19. Sedlacek HS, Ramsey DS, Boucher JF, et al. Comparative efficacy of maropitant and selected drugs in preventing emesis induced by centrally or peripherally acting emetogens in dogs. *J Vet Pharmacol Ther* 31(6):533–537, 2008.
20. Conder GA, Sedlacek HS, Boucher JF, Clemence RG. Efficacy and safety of maropitant, a selective neurokinin 1 receptor antagonist, in two randomized clinical trials for prevention of vomiting due to motion sickness in dogs. *J Vet Pharmacol Ther* 31(6):528–532, 2008.
21. de la Puente-Redondo VA, Siedek EM, Benchaoui HA, et al. The anti-emetic efficacy of maropitant (Cerenia) in the treatment of ongoing emesis caused by a wide range of underlying clinical aetiologies in canine patients in Europe. *J Small Anim Pract* 48(2):93–98, 2007.
22. de la Puente-Redondo VA, Tilt N, Rowan TG, Clemence RG. Efficacy of maropitant for treatment and prevention of emesis caused by intravenous infusion of cisplatin in dogs. *Am J Vet Res* 68(1):48–56, 2007.
23. Benchaoui HA, Siedek EM, De La Puente-Redondo VA, et al. Efficacy of maropitant for preventing vomiting associated with motion sickness in dogs. *Vet Rec* 161(13):444–447, 2007.
24. Claude AK, Dedeaux A, Chiavaccini L, Hinz S. Effects of maropitant citrate or acepromazine on the incidence of adverse events associated with hydromorphone premedication in dogs. *J Vet Intern Med* 28(5):1414–1417, 2014.
25. Hay Kraus BL. Efficacy of maropitant in preventing vomiting in dogs premedicated with hydromorphone. *Vet Anaesth Analg* 40(1):28–34, 2013.
26. Hay Kraus BL. Effect of dosing interval on efficacy of maropitant for prevention of hydromorphone-induced vomiting and signs of nausea in dogs. *J Am Vet Med Assoc* 245(9):1015–1020, 2014.
27. Hay Kraus BL. Efficacy of orally administered maropitant citrate in preventing vomiting associated with hydromorphone administration in dogs. *J Am Vet Med Assoc* 244(10):1164–1169, 2014.
28. Lorenzutti AM, Martín-Flores M, Litterio NJ, et al. A comparison between maropitant and metoclopramide for the prevention of morphine-induced

nausea and vomiting in dogs. *Can Vet J* 58(1): 35–38, 2017.
29. Benchaoui HA, Cox SR, Schneider RP, et al. The pharmacokinetics of maropitant, a novel neurokinin type-1 receptor antagonist, in dogs. *J Vet Pharmacol Ther* 30(4):336–344, 2007.
30. Narishetty ST, Galvan B, Coscarelli E, et al. Effect of refrigeration of the antiemetic Cerenia (maropitant) on pain on injection. *Vet Ther* 10(3):93–102, 2009.
31. Boscan P, Monnet E, Mama K, et al. Effect of maropitant, a neurokinin 1 receptor antagonist, on anesthetic requirements during noxious visceral stimulation of the ovary in dogs. *Am J Vet Res* 72(12):1576–1579, 2011.
32. Kinobe RT, Miyake Y. Evaluating the anti-inflammatory and analgesic properties of maropitant: A systematic review and meta-analysis. *Vet J* 259–260:105471, 2020.
33. Grobman M, Graham A, Outi H, et al. Chronic neurokinin-1 receptor antagonism fails to ameliorate clinical signs, airway hyper-responsiveness or airway eosinophilia in an experimental model of feline asthma. *J Feline Med Surg* 18(4):273–279, 2016.
34. Chi TT, Hay Kraus BL. The effect of intravenous maropitant on blood pressure in healthy awake and anesthetized dogs. *PLoS One* 15(2):e0229736, 2020.
35. Aoki T, Eki K. Comparative study of the effects of antitussive drugs in a canine acute cough model. *Vet Med Sci* 10(5):e1549, 2024.
36. American Veterinary Medical Association. Cannabis use and pets. Available from: https://www.avma.org/resources-tools/animal-health-and-welfare/animal-health/cannabis-use-and-pets. Accessed November 2024.

CHAPTER 33

Antidiarrheal drugs

Mark G. Papich
DVM, MS, DACVCP

Treatment of diarrhea should include fluid therapy, electrolyte replenishment, maintenance of acid–base balance, and control of discomfort (see Chapters 24 and 28). Any intestinal parasites should be treated with antiparasitic agents (see Chapter 30), while dietary modifications, pre- and probiotics, and fecal microbiota transplantation may also be used (see Chapters 25–27). Other specific drugs, and especially antibacterials, are often not indicated (see Chapter 29), although immunosuppressive agents may be used in inflammatory bowel disease if dietary modification is unsuccessful (see Chapter 34). Some nonspecific antidiarrheal agents, such as intestinal protectants and motility modifiers, are sometimes utilized. The pathophysiology of diarrhea is typically multifactorial, but few mechanisms involve hypermotility; therefore, the use of antimotility agents is usually unwarranted.

Mucosal protectants and adsorbents

Kaolin–pectin formulations

Products that are promoted as mucosal protectants, such as mixtures of kaolin and pectin, are commonly available in over-the-counter formulations. Kaolin (clay) is a form of aluminum silicate, with montmorillonite being its most absorbent form. Pectin is a carbohydrate polymer, gelling agent extracted from apples and citrus fruits. Some kaolin–pectin formulations also contain salicylate as one of the active ingredients. Since some animals may be sensitive to salicylates, the salicylate content of the formulation should be considered before administration. Other products may include antibacterials (e.g., neomycin), for which there is little indication.

The manufacturers of kaolin–pectin products claim that they act as demulcents and adsorbents in the treatment of diarrhea. The binding of bacterial toxins (endotoxins and enterotoxins) in the gastrointestinal (GI) tract has also been claimed. However, kaolin–pectin is an ineffective binder of *Escherichia coli* enterotoxin, and clinical studies have failed to show a benefit from administration to patients. These products may have a cosmetic effect, improving the consistency of stool, but they do not decrease fluid or electrolyte loss, nor do they shorten the duration of illness.

Despite the lack of clinical evidence of efficacy, some veterinarians administer kaolin–pectin preparations at a dose of 1–2 mL/kg every 6 hours. Kaolin–pectin is not absorbed, but any salicylate may be.[1] Drug interactions are also possible: kaolin–pectin may adsorb or bind other drugs that are administered orally and decrease their effectiveness.

Bismuth subsalicylate

Although other "mucosal protectants" have questionable efficacy, bismuth subsalicylate is considered by some gastroenterologists to be a useful symptomatic treatment for acute diarrhea. Its efficacy has been proven in controlled clinical trials in humans with acute diarrhea, particularly when caused by enterotoxigenic *E. coli* (also known as traveler's diarrhea).[2] Bismuth may have some ability to adsorb bacterial enterotoxins, may be antibacterial, and may produce a gastric or intestinal protective effect. It does have an anti-*Helicobacter* effect in the stomach, and bismuth-containing products have been included in regimens for treating gastritis.

The salicylate component has an anti-inflammatory action, which is most likely responsible for its observed efficacy. Two tablespoonfuls (~30 mL), the typical human dose, contain almost 300 mg of salicylate. Practically all of this salicylate is absorbed systemically when administered to dogs.[1] Despite the systemic absorption, this amount is unlikely to produce salicylate toxicity.

The dose administered to animals was not derived from clinical studies but extrapolated from human dosages. A total of 1–3 mL/kg/day in divided doses has been administered safely to dogs. Some animals do not like the taste, but otherwise there have not been serious adverse effects reported after administration. Salicylate toxicosis is possible from overdose, and pet owners should be advised to limit the amount administered. Pet owners should also be warned that bismuth may turn the stools black, which should not be confused for melena.

Motility-modifying agents

Anticholinergic drugs

Anticholinergic (antimuscarinic) drugs significantly decrease intestinal motility and secretion. They were included in some older (and outdated) antidiarrheal preparations. These drugs inhibit muscarinic action via their antagonism of either the ganglionic M_1 or peripheral M_3 muscarinic receptors. This parasympatholytic effect decreases segmental and propulsive intestinal smooth muscle contractions. Although they do not alter the course of disease, anticholinergic drugs may decrease the urgency associated with some forms of diarrhea, decrease the fluid secreted into the bowel, and decrease abdominal discomfort associated with intestinal spasms. The actions of these drugs are also associated with important side effects.

The limitation of the use of anticholinergic drugs lies in the questionable efficacy for most forms of diarrhea seen in dogs, as few cases are classified as "hypermotile". In addition, although these agents undeniably decrease intestinal motility, there is no clear evidence that this is necessarily beneficial. Intestinal motility is already impaired in many patients with intestinal disease, and these drugs may worsen the diarrhea by creating a "stove pipe" effect. The use of these drugs should be avoided if the diarrhea is bacterial in origin, as diarrhea is the intestine's way of purging toxins.

Anticholinergics can have profound systemic pharmacological effects. If administered in sufficient doses to affect the bowel, possible adverse effects include ileus, xerostomia, urine retention, cycloplegia, tachycardia, and central nervous system (CNS) excitement. Chronic administration can lead to severe bowel atony. In addition to decreasing bowel motility, anticholinergic drugs decrease stomach emptying, which can lead to stomach distension and discomfort. This is certainly contraindicated in patients with gastritis and vomiting.

Atropine is the best-known anticholinergic drug, but because it has many other systemic effects, it is not ordinarily used for its antidiarrheal properties. To avoid CNS effects, quaternary amines are used because they are charged and their lipophilicity is reduced, so that they do not cross the blood–brain barrier as readily as tertiary amines (Box 33.1).

Anticholinergic drugs such as aminopentamide and diphemanil were included in old and rarely used formulations, and another old combination, marketed in the USA, contained both isopropamide and prochlorperazine. Combination products may also contain hyoscine/scopolamine, atropine, and hyoscyamine, sometimes with phenobarbital. Most of these formulations are outdated and, thankfully, unavailable today.

Opioids

Opioids can have both antisecretory and antimotility actions, as they act on the µ-opiate receptors of the GI tract. They decrease propulsive intestinal contractions and increase segmentation, resulting in an overall constipating effect.[3] They also increase the tone of GI sphincters. In addition to affecting motility, opioids have an antisecretory effect and stimulate absorption of fluid, electrolytes, and glucose. The effects on secretory diarrhea are probably caused by inhibition of calcium influx and decreased calmodulin activity.[4]

The constipating effects of morphine and other opioids are well-known. However, it would be irrational to administer morphine repeatedly to animals simply for its antidiarrheal effect. Instead, opioids with intestinal effects but without systemic action are used. Tincture of opium (paregoric) is an older compound found in some antidiarrheal products (5 mL of paregoric corresponded approximately to 2 mg of morphine); it is now banned in many countries. Eluxadoline is a modern µ-opioid receptor agonist and δ-opioid receptor antagonist. It is used in people to treat irritable bowel syndrome associated with diarrhea but is contraindicated if they have concurrent biliary disease. Its use has not been reported in dogs.

Loperamide and diphenoxylate, two synthetic opioids, are known for their specific action on the GI tract and their effect on secretory diarrhea. Their main effect is the local action on intestinal µ-opioid receptors to produce GI effects without other systemic side effects.

Widely available over-the-counter, loperamide is one of the most common treatments for acute diarrhea in people. The typical dose for small animals is 0.1 mg/kg orally every 12 hours. This dose is extrapolated from human use and is untested in clinical canine studies.

Diphenoxylate is a derivative of meperidine/pethidine and contains 25 µg of atropine per 2.5 mg tablet. This amount of atropine may contribute to some inhibition of intestinal smooth muscle but is present in the formulation primarily to discourage substance abuse by people. This drug is no longer available or used in many countries, but in some it is used as an antitussive for treating collapsing trachea.

Opioids can have potent effects on the GI tract and should be used cautiously. Of note, pet owners may administer over-the-counter loperamide to animals without first consulting a veterinarian. These drugs are generally contraindicated in infectious diarrhea because they may significantly slow GI transit and increase the absorption of bacterial toxins. Loperamide does not normally cause opioid-related CNS effects because the membrane transporter P-glycoprotein helps to remove this drug from the CNS. Dogs that have a mutation in the *ABCB-1* gene (e.g., Collie dogs and other herding breeds) are deficient in P-glycoprotein and may be prone to loperamide neurotoxicity.[5]

Box 33.1 Anticholinergic antidiarrheal drugs.

Tertiary amines:	Quaternary amines:
Atropine	Methscopolamine
Hyoscine butylbromide/scopolamine	Isopropamide
	Propantheline
	Glycopyrrolate

Antimicrobial agents

Routine use of antimicrobials to treat diarrhea is questioned by most gastroenterologists (see Chapter 29). In most cases, a specific bacterial etiology cannot be identified as primary bacterial cases are rare. Even if diarrhea is caused by bacteria, antibiotic therapy may not alter the course of the disease, and there is a lack of well-controlled studies to demonstrate efficacy.[6] Indeed, administration of oral antibiotics can actually cause diarrhea.[7,8] Nevertheless, oral nonabsorbed antibiotics (e.g., neomycin) are sometimes combined with motility modifiers, adsorbents, and intestinal protectants. Some of these are irrational combinations. Antibiotics used in people with traveler's diarrhea and irritable bowel syndrome include rifaximin and rifamycin. Rifamixin has been reported to be as effective as metronidazole in dogs but is not normally indicated.[9]

Antibacterials administered empirically for "antibiotic-responsive diarrhea" in dogs are most often oxytetracycline, tylosin, or metronidazole, although other treatments should be trialed first (see Chapter 29). There is little or no evidence for any benefit of metronidazole, but tylosin has been shown to be effective in a condition known as "tylosin-responsive diarrhea".[10,11]

Tylosin

Tylosin has been effective at improving clinical signs, with or without bacterial pathogens being identified. When administered at 12 mg/kg/day (average dose), dogs respond within 24 hours to 3 days. These benefits appear to be unique to tylosin, because studies by the same investigators showed that tylosin at a dose of 20 mg/kg/day was effective, but other drugs (metronidazole, trimethoprim–sulfonamides, doxycycline, or prednisolone) were not.[10,11]

Off-label use of the powdered form of tylosin for livestock can be mixed with the animal's food at a dosage of 40–80 mg/kg/day (10–40 mg/kg 2–3 times per day), or sometimes lower doses of 20–25 mg/kg per day. After the initial response, it is advised to taper the dose to the lowest possible that will control the disease, often as low as 5 mg/kg per day. One teaspoon contains approximately 3,000 mg, so ¼ teaspoon (750 mg) is enough for many dogs. Some animals may find the bitter taste unpleasant and refuse their food; therefore, drug administration should be tested to identify the method that is best tolerated. Tablets for small animals are available in some countries.

Metronidazole

Metronidazole is active against anaerobic bacteria and *Giardia*. Other agents for *Giardia*, such as fenbendazole, are preferred because they have broader activity against intestinal parasites and do not affect the intestinal microbiome. Metronidazole is potentially neurotoxic at the antiprotozoal dosage of 25 mg/kg every 12 hours. A safe antibacterial dose is 5–10 mg/kg twice daily, and ideally this should not be exceeded. Adverse effects from metronidazole are primarily seen as CNS signs (tremors, seizures, and other CNS disturbances caused by inhibition of γ-aminobutyric acid [GABA]) and are more likely with higher doses.

While lower doses of metronidazole may have activity against other intestinal organisms, its use for treating nonspecific acute or chronic diarrhea has been questioned because of a lack of convincing evidence that it is beneficial. The misuse and lack of efficacy was summarized in a review.[12] In some cases, bowel inflammation may be caused by metronidazole-sensitive bacteria, which act as an attractant for inflammatory cells, and the rationale for administering this drug may be related to this antibacterial activity. The supposed "immunomodulatory" effect of metronidazole in the intestine (decreased cell-mediated response), as cited in some recommendations, comes from only a few isolated studies and has been largely dismissed for lack of evidence.[12]

Metronidazole (with or without combination with ampicillin) was reported to be effective for granulomatous (histiocytic ulcerative) colitis in dogs,[13] but it is no longer effective, as multidrug resistance is now prevalent. While metronidazole was used for acute treatment of nonspecific diarrhea in dogs, it had modest benefit, shortening the duration by an average of only 1.5 days.[14] All dogs in this study improved within 1 week regardless of whether they received metronidazole. In another study, dogs were treated with either metronidazole or a probiotic. Findings failed to provide evidence to support the use of metronidazole in dogs with acute diarrhea.[15] In a randomized controlled study of dogs with colitis, dietary management was superior to treatment with metronidazole, and the latter worsened the dysbiosis index.[16] The authors of this study concluded that their results add to the growing body of evidence that metronidazole is not the optimal management strategy for dogs with noninfectious acute colitis, especially considering the long-lasting effects of metronidazole on the microbiome. Overall, an analysis of all the available studies leads to the conclusion that there is a lack of evidence to support the use of metronidazole for treatment of acute diarrhea, and alterations in the intestinal microbiome from its use may be detrimental.[12]

Crofelemer

Crofelemer is a novel antidiarrheal drug used in people to treat noninfectious diarrhea in adults with HIV/AIDS who take antiretroviral therapy. It is available as a delayed-release tablet and is composed of a botanical compound harvested from the sap of a medicinal tropical plant, the *Croton lechleri* tree. It was conditionally approved by the FDA in 2021 for use in dogs for the treatment of chemotherapy-induced diarrhea at a daily dose of 250 mg for dogs weighing up to 64 kg and 500 mg for dogs weighing more than 64 kg. Before granting full approval, "substantial evidence" of the drug's effectiveness will have to be provided within 5 years. However, the study to establish the conditional approval was a pilot study of 24 shelter-housed dogs with acute diarrhea, with only 12 of them treated.

Secretory diarrhea is caused by excess secretion of chloride into the lumen of the intestine, followed by a flux of sodium, which then produces a flux of fluid into the intestine creating watery diarrhea. The mechanism of action of crofelemer is unique. It acts by inhibiting both cAMP-stimulated CTFR chloride channels (cAMP, cyclic adenosine phosphate; CFTR, cystic fibrosis transmembrane conductance regulator) and calcium-activated chloride channels at the luminal membrane of intestinal epithelial cells, thereby blocking the secretion of chloride ions and the accompanying water loss in secretory diarrhea. Crofelemer acts within the lumen of the GI tract, on the luminal side of the intestinal epithelium, and is not absorbed systemically.

KEY POINTS

- Intestinal protectants and adsorbents are nonspecific antidiarrheal products.
- There is little evidence for efficacy of kaolin–pectin products.
- Bismuth subsalicylate may have an antidiarrheal effect, probably due to its salicylate component.
- Anticholinergic (antimuscarinic) agents are generally not recommended as antidiarrheals.
- Antibacterials are rarely indicated in cases of acute or chronic diarrhea.
- Crofelemer is a novel antidiarrheal drug that inhibits chloride channels in enterocytes.

References

1. Papich MG, Davis CA, Davis LE. Absorption of salicylate from an antidiarrheal preparation in dogs and cats. *J Am Anim Hosp Assoc* 23(2):221–226, 1987.
2. Bierer DW. Bismuth subsalicylate: history, chemistry, and safety. *Rev Infect Dis* 12 Suppl 1:S3–S8, 1990.
3. DeHaven-Hudkins DL, DeHaven RN, Little PJ, Techner LM. The involvement of the mu-opioid receptor in gastrointestinal pathophysiology: therapeutic opportunities for antagonism at this receptor. *Pharmacol Ther* 117(1):162–187, 2008.
4. Hedner T, Cassuto J. Opioids and opioid receptors in peripheral tissues. *Scand J Gastroenterol Suppl* 130:27-46, 1987.
5. Mealey KL, Owens JG, Freeman E. Canine and feline P-glycoprotein deficiency: What we know and where we need to go. *J Vet Pharmacol Ther* 46(1):1–16, 2023.
6. Marks SL, Rankin SC, Byrne BA, Weese JS. Enteropathogenic bacteria in dogs and cats: diagnosis, epidemiology, treatment, and control. *J Vet Intern Med* 25(6):1195–1208, 2011.
7. Bartlett JG. Clinical practice. Antibiotic-associated diarrhea. *N Engl J Med* 346(5):334-339, 2002.
8. Whittemore JC, Moyers TD, Price JM. Randomized, controlled, crossover trial of prevention of antibiotic-induced gastrointestinal signs using a synbiotic mixture in healthy research dogs. *J Vet Intern Med* 33(4):1619–1626, 2019.
9. Menozzi A, Dall'Aglio M, Quintavalla F, et al. Rifaximin is an effective alternative to metronidazole for the treatment of chronic enteropathy in dogs: a randomised trial. *BMC Vet Res* 12(1):217, 2016.
10. Westermarck E, Frias R, Skrzypczak T. Effect of diet and tylosin on chronic diarrhea in beagles. *J Vet Intern Med* 19(6):822–827, 2005.
11. Westermarck E, Skrzypczak T, Harmoinen J, et al. Tylosin-responsive chronic diarrhea in dogs. *J Vet Intern Med* 19(2):177–186, 2005.
12. Ellis C, Odunayo A, Tolbert MK. The use of metronidazole in acute diarrhea in dogs: a narrative review. *Top Companion Anim Med* 56-57:100824, 2023.
13. Mansfield CS, James FE, Craven M, et al. Remission of histiocytic ulcerative colitis in Boxer dogs correlates with eradication of invasive intramucosal *Escherichia coli*. *J Vet Intern Med* 23(5):964–969, 2009.
14. Langlois DK, Koenigshof AM, Mani R. Metronidazole treatment of acute diarrhea in dogs: A randomized double blinded placebo-controlled clinical trial. *J Vet Intern Med* 34(1):98–104, 2020.
15. Shmalberg J, Montalbano C, Morelli G, Buckley GJ. A randomized double blinded placebo-controlled clinical trial of a probiotic or metronidazole for acute canine diarrhea. *Front Vet Sci* 6:163, 2019.
16. Rudinsky AJ, Parker VJ, Winston J, et al. Randomized controlled trial demonstrates nutritional management is superior to metronidazole for treatment of acute colitis in dogs. *J Am Vet Med Assoc* 260(S3):S23–S32, 2022.

CHAPTER 34

Use of immunosuppressants in gastrointestinal disease

Nathaniel Whitley
BVMS, PhD, CertVC, DACVIM (SAIM), DECVIM-CA, FRCVS

Immunosuppressants are used in gastrointestinal (GI) disease when immune dysregulation has caused an inflammatory mucosal infiltrate that is refractory to other treatment modalities, regardless of the region of the GI tract that is affected. These infiltrates are usually dominated by increased numbers of lymphocytes and plasma cells, and affected patients are referred to as having idiopathic inflammatory bowel disease (IBD), a chronic inflammatory enteropathy. Less often, infiltrates are eosinophilic or granulomatous in nature and rarely neutrophilic. Caution is necessary in the use of immunosuppressants in patients with predominantly granulomatous or neutrophilic inflammation unless bacterial pathogens and protozoal disease have been ruled out. IBD classification is often dictated by response to therapeutic trials. Despite textbook definitions, in the real world, this translates into significant fluidity in the classification of IBD types depending on the rigor and willingness of the vet and dog owner to perform therapeutic diet trials and attempts to manipulate the intestinal microbiome. Food-responsive enteropathy is an important category of disease. Historically, other dogs were labeled as having "antibiotic-responsive diarrhea", but such diagnoses merit close scrutiny. Good antibiotic stewardship discourages empirical use of metronidazole and other antibiotics as the primary means of control of any enteropathy, with greater emphasis encouraged on the use of prebiotics, probiotics, and even fecal microbiota transplants. Responsibility lies with the clinician in deciding when these modalities have been exhausted for all practical purposes and immunosuppressants are indicated. Feeding of raw diets is strongly contraindicated in patients receiving immunosuppressants due to the significantly increased risk of intestinal and systemic infectious complications.

General principals of choosing and dosing immunosuppressants

Glucocorticoids ("steroids") are first-line immunosuppressants for GI disease. A second-line immunosuppressant is sometimes added to or substituted for glucocorticoid therapy if the disease is considered steroid-refractory or if steroid side effects are sufficiently severe that accelerated dose reduction or cessation is required. An introductory dose is generally maintained for 2–4 weeks according to the clinical response. This is then tapered over weeks to months, ideally aiming not to reduce the dose by more than one third every 2–4 weeks, with an end goal of complete discontinuation of immunosuppressants provided the condition has not previously relapsed off immunosuppressants. Side effects and availability of different tablet sizes influence timing and magnitude of dose reductions. Specialist advice should be sought before combining more than two immunosuppressants and only one cytotoxic drug should be used at a time.

Glucocorticoids

Glucocorticoids include dexamethasone, prednisolone, methylprednisolone, or budesonide.

- **Mechanism of action:** Numerous cellular receptors give glucocorticoids potent anti-inflammatory and immunosuppressive effects. Key actions of glucocorticoids include inhibition of prostaglandin synthesis by action on phospholipase A2 and alteration of expression of genes involved in innate and adaptive immune responses by action on the transcription factor NF-κB in the cell nucleus.
- **Side effects:** Glucocorticoid side effects are unavoidable due to widespread cellular receptors. They are also dose and duration dependent, with variations between patients and between the preparations used, according to absolute and relative glucocorticoid and mineralocorticoid potency. Box 34.1 lists the potential side effects of immunosuppressant doses of glucocorticoids and includes findings of (iatrogenic) hyperadrenocorticism. The adrenal axis is inhibited by glucocorticoids, which can also be ulcerogenic by inhibiting cytoprotective prostaglandin production. However, GI bleeding is an inherent feature of many enteropathies, with the potential to be resolved with effective glucocorticoid therapy. Hence, preexisting GI bleeding is not an absolute contraindication for glucocorticoid therapy, but new or worsening GI bleeding should prompt dose reduction or cessation, and commencement of any other necessary interventions.

Box 34.1 Potential side effects of immunosuppressant doses of glucocorticoids.

- Polyuria
- Polydipsia
- Polyphagia
- Panting
- Sarcopenia
- Liver enzyme induction
- Hepatomegaly
- Gastrointestinal upset and/or ulceration
- Insulin resistance (diabetogenic)
- Sodium and water retention
- Alopecia
- Predisposition to infection (skin, urinary)
- Impaired wound healing
- Behavior change
- Prothrombotic effect, which can be exacerbated by concurrent ciclosporin use

- **Indications:** GI inflammation refractory to other treatment modalities.
- **Dosage:** Injectable preparations are used only when the patient is unable to tolerate oral dosing.

Prednisolone

Prednisolone is the preferred product. The recommended starting dose is 1–2 mg/kg PO q24h. This can be given once daily or divided twice daily. Once daily dosing may reduce side effects. Noninferiority of (i.e., as good as) once daily dosing has been demonstrated.[1] Heavier dogs experience more adverse effects when dosed based on body weight.[2] For this reason, dosing based on body surface area is recommended in dogs >25 kg, with the dosage not to exceed 50 mg/m^2 q24h.

Budesonide

Budesonide is an oral, high potency glucocorticoid with local activity in the distal small intestine and extensive first-pass metabolism in the liver. Despite this, it is not completely free from systemic side effects and has not shown superiority over prednisolone for canine IBD.[3] An initial dose of 1, 2, or 3 mg PO q24h has been suggested for small, medium, and large dogs respectively.[4]

Second-line immunosuppressants

Second-line immunosuppressants are indicated for steroid-refractory disease or for use in combination with glucocorticoids for a "steroid-sparing effect".

Ciclosporin (cyclosporine)

- **Mechanism of action:** Ciclosporin inhibits calcineurin, reducing interleukin 2 (IL-2)–induced T-lymphocyte activation, hence also reducing B lymphocyte activation. Other cytokines and cells involved in innate immune responses are affected to a much lesser extent. Although ciclosporin concentrates in the intestine through enterohepatic recycling, there is significant variation in response, drug metabolism, and tolerability between individual dogs. Absorption is optimized by administering on an empty stomach. Ciclosporin showed efficacy in one study of steroid-resistant canine IBD.[5]
- **Side effects:** GI upset is common but typically transient. This can be managed by dose reduction, concurrent use of antiemetics, or administering ciclosporin capsules frozen. Other side effects include gingival proliferation, papillomatosis, hirsutism, secondary infection (especially cutaneous fungal infection). Hepatic and renal toxicity are rare. Ciclosporin increases the incidence of some neoplasms and has a mild prothrombotic effect. Drug interactions are common due to cytochrome P450 metabolism.
- **Dosage**: 2.5–5 mg/kg PO q12h.

Cytotoxic second-line immunosuppressants

Azathioprine

- **Mechanism of action:** Purine synthesis inhibitor, impeding nucleic acid synthesis in lymphocytes, which lack salvage pathways. This impairs lymphocyte proliferation and cell-mediated immunity.
- **Side effects**: GI (typically mild), hepatotoxicity (idiosyncratic, reversible), myelosuppression.
- **Dosage:** Not to exceed 2 mg/kg PO q24h, reducing after 2–3 weeks. Hematology and liver enzymes should be monitored at 0, 2, and 4 weeks, then every 1–2 months.

Mycophenolate mofetil

- **Mechanism of action**: Lymphocyte-selective purine synthesis inhibitor, developed to avoid the hepatotoxicity sometimes associated with azathioprine. Use in canine enteropathy has been limited.
- **Side effects:** Diarrhea (dose dependent, can be severe, reversible), myelosuppression (rare).
- **Dosage:** 7.5–10 mg/kg PO q12h. Hematology should be monitored at 0, 2, and 4 weeks, then every 1–2 months.

Leflunomide

- **Mechanism of action:** Pyrimidine synthesis inhibitor, inhibiting T and B lymphocyte proliferation. Use in canine enteropathy has been limited.
- **Side effects:** GI (typically mild), hepatoxicity (rare), myelotoxicity (rare).
- **Dosage:** 2 mg/kg PO q24h. Dosage up to 4 mg/kg has been reported but with an increased incidence of side effects. Hematology and liver enzymes should be monitored at 0, 2, and 4 weeks, then every 1–2 months.

Chlorambucil

- **Mechanism of action:** Cell cycle nonspecific alkylating agent, cross-linking with cellular DNA, inhibiting its replication and function.
- **Side effects**: GI (uncommon), myelosuppression (uncommon), neurotoxicity (rare).
- **Indication:** A prednisolone/chlorambucil combination was suggested to be more effective than prednisolone/azathioprine for management of protein-losing enteropathy.[6]
- **Dosage**: 0.1–0.2 mg/kg or 2–6 mg/m^2 PO q24–48h, or pulse dosed such that the cumulative weekly dose does not exceed 7 times the daily dose. Hematology should be monitored at 0, 2, and 4 weeks, then q1–2 months.

KEY POINTS

- Immunosuppressant therapy is indicated for managing chronic enteropathy when other therapies have been exhausted, typically when lymphoplasmacytic inflammation is present.
- Oral glucocorticoid therapy is the mainstay of treatment, but side effects are common.
- Ciclosporin or cytotoxic immunosuppressants may be added or substituted in glucocorticoid-refractory cases to improve response or assist accelerated weaning of glucocorticoids.
- Cytotoxic immunosuppressants require special handling and hematological monitoring.
- Raw feeding is absolutely contraindicated during immunosuppressant therapy.

References

1. Swann JW, Szladovits B, Threlfall AJ, et al. Randomised controlled trial of fractionated and unfractionated prednisolone regimens for dogs with immune-mediated haemolytic anaemia. *Vet Rec* 184(25):771, 2019.
2. Sri-Jayantha LS, Doornink MT, Urie BK. Increased risk of select glucocorticoid adverse events in dogs of higher body weight. *Can Vet J* 63(1):32–38, 2022.
3. Dye TL, Diehl KJ, Wheeler SL, et al. Randomized, controlled trial of budesonide and prednisone for the treatment of idiopathic inflammatory bowel disease. *J Vet Intern Med* 27:1385–1391, 2013.
4. Hall EJ, Day MJ. Diseases of the Small Intestine. In: Ettinger S, Feldman E, Cote E (eds.). *Textbook of Veterinary Internal Medicine*, 8th ed. Missouri, Elsevier, 2017. p. 1555.
5. Allenspach K, Rufenacht S, Sauter S, et al. Pharmacokinetics and clinical efficacy of cyclosporine treatment of dogs with steroid-refractory inflammatory bowel disease. *J Vet Intern Med* 20:239–244, 2006.
6. Dandrieux JRS, Noble PJM, Scase TJ, et al. Comparison of a chlorambucil-prednisolone combination with an azathioprine-prednisolone combination for treatment of chronic enteropathy with concurrent protein-losing enteropathy in dogs: 27 cases (2007-2010). *J Am Vet Med Assoc* 242:1705–1714, 2013.

Acute hemorrhagic diarrhea syndrome

Stefan Unterer
DVM, Dr Med Vet,
Dr Habil, DECVIM-CA

Mara Holz
Dr. med. vet.

Acute hemorrhagic diarrhea is much more common in dogs than in humans, but the presence of visible blood in feces is a highly specific clinical feature of infectious diarrhea in both species. In addition to various factors potentially causing gastrointestinal (GI) bleeding (see Box 35.1), the two main causes of acute hemorrhagic diarrhea in dogs are canine parvovirosis in puppies and young dogs and acute hemorrhagic diarrhea syndrome (AHDS), previously known as *hemorrhagic gastroenteritis*, in adult dogs. AHDS is characterized by the sudden onset of severe bloody diarrhea and is often accompanied by vomiting.[1] Necrotic enterocolitis in dogs with AHDS is thought to arise from the proliferation of *Clostridium perfringens* type A strains containing the gene that encodes the NetF toxin.[2,3] This overgrowth is then linked to the production and release of the so-called pore-forming toxin NetF, potentially in conjunction with numerous other extracellular enzymes and minor toxins.[4] Their cumulative effect can be profound and leads to destruction of the intestinal mucosa, which is associated with severe fluid loss. With adequate fluid therapy and symptomatic management, most dogs recover within a few days. Thus, the syndrome can be a self-limiting disease.[1,5] Nevertheless, during the acute phase of the disease, characterized by epithelial necrosis and intestinal barrier dysfunction, there is a potential for permanent alterations in mucosal structures and sensitization of the immune system. This possibility is supported by the fact that ~30% of affected dogs develop chronic diarrhea later in life.[6]

Box 35.1 Differential diagnoses for dogs with acute hemorrhagic diarrhea.

- Acute liver or kidney failure
- Acute pancreatitis
- Bacterial enteritis (e.g., *Salmonella* spp., *Campylobacter* spp.); see Chapter 37.
- Coagulopathy
- Conditions resulting in endotoxic or hypovolemic shock (e.g., blood loss or hypotension)
- Drugs/toxins causing mucosal irritation (e.g., nonsteroidal anti-inflammatory drugs, high-dose corticosteroids, or doxycycline)
- Heat stroke
- Hypoadrenocorticism
- Intestinal foreign body or intussusception
- Viral enteritis (e.g., canine parvovirus or circovirus); see Chapter 36.

Etiology

Histologically, AHDS is characterized by acute necrotizing and neutrophilic enterocolitis with the detection of clostridia-like gram-positive bacteria on the necrotic mucosal surface.[3] Notably, because the stomach is not implicated in the pathology of affected dogs with an uncomplicated clinical course, the term *acute hemorrhagic diarrhea syndrome* appears to be more appropriate than the commonly used term *hemorrhagic gastroenteritis*. The mucosal-attached bacteria have been identified by polymerase chain reaction (PCR) as *C. perfringens* type A containing the gene encoding the pore-forming toxin NetF.[3] *In vitro* experiments have revealed a pronounced cytotoxicity of the NetF toxin, and several studies have shown a greater prevalence of *C. perfringens* containing the *NetF* gene in fecal samples from dogs with AHDS than in those from healthy dogs and dogs with other intestinal diseases. In summary, it can be assumed that the proliferation of *C. perfringens* strains in the large intestine, with subsequent growth in the small intestine followed by toxin production with NetF as the likely major virulence factor, explains the extensive lesions in dogs with AHDS.[3,4] It is crucial to emphasize that AHDS is not a contagious infectious disease because clostridial growth only develops in individual dogs and AHDS typically follows a self-limited course. Strains of *C. perfringens* containing the *NetF* gene typically disappear within 1 week of remission without the need for specific antibacterial interventions or intestinal microbiota modulation.[7]

Clinical features

Dogs of various ages and breeds may be susceptible to AHDS, although the syndrome is notably more prevalent in middle-aged dogs (median age, 5.0 years) and those of smaller breeds (median weight, 9.8 kg). The disease typically manifests acutely to peracutely, with vomiting as the initial clinical sign, observed in ~50% of cases, followed

TABLE 35.1 Criteria for the assessment of the canine acute hemorrhagic diarrhea syndrome (AHDS) activity index.

Parameter	0	1	2	3
Activity	Normal	Mildly reduced	Moderately reduced	Severely reduced
Appetite	Normal	Mildly reduced	Moderately reduced	Severely reduced
Vomiting (times/day)	0	1	2–3	>3
Fecal consistency	Normal	Slightly soft	Very soft	Watery diarrhea
Defecation (times/day)	1	2–3	4–5	>5
Dehydration (%)	0	<5	5–10	>10
Total AHDS activity index score	0–3	4–5	6–8	≥9
Clinical significance of disease	Clinically insignificant	Mild AHDS	Moderate AHDS	Severe AHDS

Source: Adapted from Mortier et al. (2015).

by the onset of watery hemorrhagic diarrhea. Physical examination results, such as lethargy, weakness, tachycardia, prolonged capillary refill time, and weak pulse pressure, mirror the signs of hypovolemia. Owing to the peracute onset and a delay in compartmental fluid shifts, skin turgor may appear normal in certain cases. Significant abdominal pain is infrequent, and affected dogs typically exhibit normo- or hypothermia. Clinical assessment can be performed using the AHDS index[1] (Table 35.1).

Clinicopathological findings

In cases of AHDS, there is usually a significant increase in the packed-cell volume (PCV), primarily due to substantial fluid loss from the intestines concentrating the red blood cells in a smaller vascular volume. However, the degree of PCV increase is influenced by the extent of dehydration and blood loss. According to a study encompassing 108 dogs diagnosed with AHDS, the median PCV was 57%, ranging from 33% to 76%.[1] This finding implies that the presence of anemia in a dog presenting with bloody diarrhea is consistently indicative of genuine intestinal bleeding and is not characteristic of AHDS. Changes in the leukogram typically mirror the expected alterations observed in a stress response, characterized by mild neutrophilia, lymphopenia, and eosinopenia. Due to significant mucosal damage, ~50% of dogs with an uncomplicated clinical course and no signs of sepsis may exhibit a mild left shift.[1] Consequently, clinicians should be alert to neutropenia and a significant increase in segmented neutrophil or band numbers because these indicators should prompt an investigation into other potential causes of acute hemorrhagic diarrhea (e.g., canine parvovirosis) or raise suspicions for an enteropathogenic bacterial infection, bacterial translocation, and sepsis. Dogs with hypoadrenocorticism can be presented with acute hemorrhagic diarrhea; thus, this differential diagnosis must be ruled out in dogs exhibiting an absence of a stress leukogram, along with lymphocytosis and eosinophilia, or displaying characteristic electrolyte changes such as hyperkalemia and hyponatremia.[8,9]

Diagnostic imaging

Ultrasound findings are not specific to AHDS and should be interpreted in conjunction with other diagnostic test and clinical findings. Typically, fluid-filled small and large intestinal loops, often displaying decreased motility, are observed. In some dogs, mild thickening of the intestinal wall due to inflammation and edema, as well as a small quantity of abdominal fluid, may be observed because of acute enteritis. Abdominal imaging, including ultrasound, can be especially useful for identifying or excluding other conditions, such as pancreatitis or intestinal obstruction.

Diagnosis (see also Chapter 11)

The diagnosis of AHDS relies on observation of distinctive clinical signs (as mentioned earlier) along with rapid clinical improvement following appropriate supportive care coupled with the exclusion of other established causes of acute hemorrhagic diarrhea. Fecal culture and PCR testing for *C. perfringens* type A strains lack specificity for AHDS. In contrast, a positive fecal PCR test result for *C. perfringens* type A strains that contain the gene encoding the NetF toxin can aid in confirming the diagnosis.[1,3] However, it is important to note that the expression of this NetF toxin diminishes rapidly, potentially resulting in negative test results for dogs presenting later in the disease course.[7] A complete blood count and serum biochemistry profile should be performed as baseline

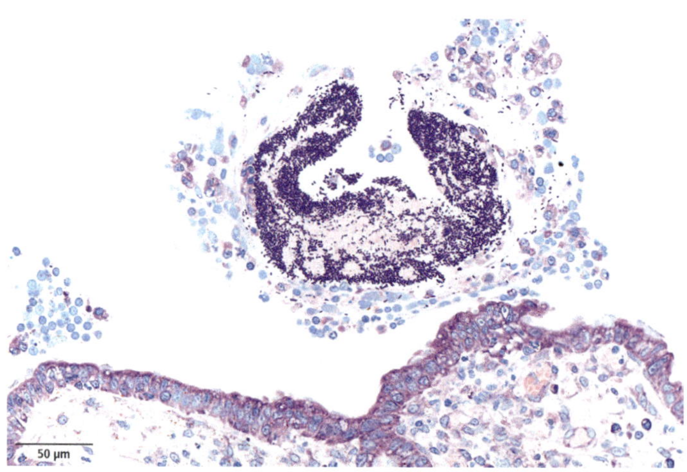

FIG. 35.1 Plump, rod-shaped bacteria (*Clostridium perfringens*) in the necrotic material of the small intestinal mucosa of a dog with acute hemorrhagic diarrhea syndrome. No bacteria adhered to the intact epithelium (Giemsa staining; bar = 50 µm). Image courtesy of Institute of Veterinary Pathology, Ludwig-Maximilians-University, Munich, Germany.

diagnostics in every patient with hemorrhagic diarrhea. Performing a fecal examination to exclude parasites, which could impact the clinical progression of the disease, also may be warranted. In cases where there is a history of suspected stress intolerance (such as prolonged recovery after anesthesia) or vague and nonspecific chronic signs, it is advisable to measure basal cortisol concentrations to exclude Addison's disease; a concentration >55 nmol/L (2 µg/dL) virtually excludes hypoadrenocorticism. To identify potential atypical hypoadrenocorticism or complicating findings, additional tests including an ACTH stimulation test may be necessary (Table 35.2).

Therapy

Severe fluid loss in patients with AHDS frequently leads to significant hypovolemia and disturbances in electrolyte concentrations. Therefore, the administration of fluids plays a crucial role in stabilizing patients (see Chapter 24). To address hypovolemia/hypovolemic shock, an intravenous bolus of 10–20 mL/kg of crystalloids over 10–15 minutes is typically sufficient. Following the bolus, improvements in clinical parameters should be observed within a few minutes. This may manifest as a reduction in tachycardia, improvement in capillary refill time, increased peripheral perfusion, and a clearer mental status. If the initial clinical response is insufficient or diminishes quickly, additional fluid boluses (maximum of three) should be administered until hemodynamic stability is regained.[10] Colloid solutions, such as plasma, albumin, or synthetics such as hydroxyethyl starch, should be limited to select patients with severe hypoalbuminemia or if hypovolemic shock appears refractory to crystalloid resuscitation.[11,12] Fluid therapy that addresses both maintenance requirements (~50 mL/kg q24h) and ongoing losses (up to 10 mL/kg/h in severely affected dogs) must be maintained until the dog can achieve a normal fluid balance through oral intake. Dogs experiencing an uncomplicated course of AHDS typically exhibit rapid and consistent improvement in their condition with fluids, antiemetics (e.g., maropitant, 1 mg/kg intravenously q24h), and analgesics such as buprenorphine (e.g., 0.01 mg/kg intravenously q6–8h) within the initial 2 days. Considering antibiotic stewardship, the use of antibacterial agents should be restricted to dogs that cannot be closely monitored or do not show expected clinical improvement after fluid and symptomatic treatment.[13] Dogs presenting with signs of systemic inflammation/sepsis (e.g., fever, inflammatory leukogram, and hypoglycemia), obvious immunosuppression (e.g., neutropenia), or ineffective clearance of bacteria by the liver (e.g., portosystemic shunt or liver dysfunction) should be administered intravenous bactericidal broad-spectrum antibiotics (e.g., amoxicillin–clavulanate or ampicillin–sulbactam, 20 mg/kg intravenously q6–8h).

TABLE 35.2 Further considerations and diagnostic approaches for complications or atypical findings in dogs with acute hemorrhagic diarrhea syndrome (AHDS).

Possible findings indicating complications or atypical findings requiring additional tests	Additional tests
No improvement after 24–48 hours of treatment	■ Repeat CBC and serum biochemistry profile
Significant abdominal pain, suspicion of foreign body, intussusception, or acute pancreatitis	■ Abdominal ultrasound
Acute abdomen (e.g., mesenteric volvulus), suspicion of foreign body	■ Abdominal radiographs
Significant abdominal pain	■ Pancreatic lipase test (quantitative if SNAP® cPL test is positive)
False-negative tests for CPV may occur if performed too early in the course of infection	■ Repeat fecal lateral-flow or SNAP test or PCR testing if initially negative: ■ In young dogs (< 6 months) ■ In unvaccinated/inadequately vaccinated dogs ■ During an outbreak of acute diarrhea in a dog population ■ In older dogs (>6 months) with neutropenia
False-positive tests for CPV may occur after recent vaccination or with PCR due to environmental contamination	■ Repeat fecal lateral-flow or SNAP test or PCR testing if initially positive: ■ After very recent vaccination ■ In vaccinated dogs without neutropenia ■ With suspected environmental contamination
Suspicion of bacterial translocation/sepsis Significant neutrophilia/left shift, fever	■ Fecal culture ■ Blood culture ■ Culture from enlarged lymph nodes and abdominal fluid sampling (if present) and analysis
Severe hypoalbuminemia	■ Urine protein-to-creatinine ratio
ALT/ALP >3 times upper reference interval	■ Serum bile acids
Anemia at presentation	■ Platelet count ■ Coagulation profile ■ Ultrasonographic imaging of GI tract
Serum basal cortisol <55 nmol/L (<2 mg/dL)	■ ACTH stimulation test

CBC complete blood count; CPV, canine parvovirus; PCR, polymerase chain reaction; ALT, alanine aminotransferase; ALP, alkaline phosphatase; GI, gastrointestinal; ACTH, adrenocorticotropic hormone

Dogs with severe destruction of the intestinal mucosa and thus intestinal barrier dysfunction, as in AHDS, as well as intestinal dysbiosis, have an increased risk of developing a chronic GI disorders later in life.[6] Although the following recommendations are unproven, some clinicians suggest the use of 1) hypoallergenic diets (e.g., hydrolyzed, elemental or parenteral nutrition) to minimize the risk for immune sensitization, 2) early enteral nutrition, 3) specific nutritional constituents (e.g., mucosal nutrients such as glutamine or fiber) or supplements (e.g., high doses of multistrain probiotics, sucralfate, or slippery elm) to improve intestinal barrier function, and 4) fecal microbiota transplantation to restore intestinal microbial homeostasis.[14–16]

KEY POINTS

- Overgrowth of *Clostridium perfringens* strains and the release of their toxins, mainly the pore-forming toxin NetF, are responsible for the pathogenesis of acute hemorrhagic diarrhea syndrome (AHDS).
- AHDS manifests as a sudden onset of severe bloody diarrhea, often accompanied by vomiting as the initial clinical sign.
- Because mucosal necrosis and neutrophilic infiltration are confined to the intestines, the term previously used, *hemorrhagic gastroenteritis*, which implies gastric inflammation, is inappropriate.
- Clinical and laboratory findings indicate hypovolemia due to a significant loss of fluid into the intestinal lumen.
- Diagnosis relies on the characteristic clinical course and the exclusion of other known causes of acute hemorrhagic diarrhea. Additionally, a positive PCR test for the *C. perfringens* gene encoding the pore-forming toxin NetF suggests AHDS.
- Prompt fluid replacement and symptomatic treatment typically result in a short disease duration of 24–72 hours. Antibiotics should be administered only to dogs showing signs of systemic inflammation.

References

1. Mortier F, Strohmeyer K, Hartmann K, Unterer S. Acute haemorrhagic diarrhoea syndrome in dogs: 108 cases. *Vet Rec.* 176(24):627, 2015.
2. Leipig-Rudolph M, Busch K, Prescott JF, et al. Intestinal lesions in dogs with acute hemorrhagic diarrhea syndrome associated with netF-positive *Clostridium perfringens* type A. *J Vet Diagn Invest.* 30(4):495–503, 2018.
3. Sindern N, Suchodolski JS, Leutenegger CM, et al. Prevalence of *Clostridium perfringens* netE and netF toxin genes in the feces of dogs with acute hemorrhagic diarrhea syndrome. *J Vet Intern Med.* 33(1):100–105, 2019.
4. Mehdizadeh Gohari I, Parreira VR, Nowell VJ, et al. A novel pore-forming toxin in type A *Clostridium perfringens* is associated with both fatal canine hemorrhagic gastroenteritis and fatal foal necrotizing enterocolitis. *PLoS One.* 10(4):e0122684, 2015.
5. Unterer S, Busch K, Leipig M, et al. Endoscopically visualized lesions, histologic findings, and bacterial invasion in the gastrointestinal mucosa of dogs with acute hemorrhagic diarrhea syndrome. *J Vet Intern Med.* 28(1):52–58, 2014,
6. Skotnitzki E, Suchodolski JS, Busch K, et al. Frequency of signs of chronic gastrointestinal disease in dogs after an episode of acute hemorrhagic diarrhea. *J Vet Intern Med.* 36(1):59–65, 2022.
7. Ziese AL, Suchodolski JS, Hartmann K, et al. Effect of probiotic treatment on the clinical course, intestinal microbiome, and toxigenic *Clostridium perfringens* in dogs with acute hemorrhagic diarrhea. *PLoS One.* 13(9):e0204691, 2018
8. Busch K, Wehner A, Dorsch R, et al. Acute haemorrhagic diarrhoea as a presenting sign in a dog with primary hypoadrenocorticism. *Tierarztl Prax Ausg K Kleintiere Heimtiere.* 42(5):326–330, 2014.
9. Medinger TL, Williams DA, Bruyette DS. Severe gastrointestinal tract hemorrhage in three dogs with hypoadrenocorticism. *J Am Vet Med Assoc.* 202(11):1869–1872, 1993.
10. Butler AL. Goal-directed therapy in small animal critical illness. *Vet Clin North Am Small Anim Pract.* 41(4):817–838, vii, 2011.
11. Finfer S, Bellomo R, Boyce N, et al. A comparison of albumin and saline for fluid resuscitation in the intensive care unit. *N Engl J Med.* 350(22): 2247–2256, 2004.
12. Martin LG, Luther TY, Alperin DC, et al. Serum antibodies against human albumin in critically ill and healthy dogs. *J Am Vet Med Assoc.* 232(7):1004–1009, 2008.
13. Unterer S, Strohmeyer K, Kruse BD, et al. Treatment of aseptic dogs with hemorrhagic gastroenteritis with amoxicillin/clavulanic acid: a prospective blinded study. *J Vet Intern Med.* 25(5):973–979, 2011.
14. Will K, Nolte I, Zentek J. Early enteral nutrition in young dogs suffering from haemorrhagic gastroenteritis. *J Vet Med A Physiol Pathol Clin Med.* 52(7):371–376, 2005.
15. Gal A, Barko PC, Biggs PJ, et al. One dog's waste is another dog's wealth: a pilot study of fecal microbiota transplantation in dogs with acute hemorrhagic diarrhea syndrome. *PLoS One.* 16(4):e0250344, 2021.
16. Jugan MC, KuKanich K, Freilich L. Clinical response in dogs with acute hemorrhagic diarrhea syndrome following randomized probiotic treatment or fecal microbiota transplant. *Front Vet Sci.* 10:1050538, 2023.

CHAPTER 36

Viral enteritides

Tawny Chandler
MS, PhD

Sarah Caddy
MA, VetMB, PhD, DACVM, FRCVS

Viruses can be detected in approximately 60% of canine diarrhea samples.[1–3] Since 1978, the most widely recognized cause of viral gastroenteritis in dogs has been canine parvovirus, with cases of canine coronavirus, canine rotavirus, and canine distemper virus occasionally reported. However, in recent years several other viruses have been identified in association with canine diarrhea, although it is often not clear if they are the cause of the disease observed.[4] This chapter describes the pathology and epidemiology of each virus associated with gastroenteritis in dogs and discusses ways to diagnose, prevent, and manage viral enteritides.

Common enteric viruses

Canine parvovirus

Canine parvovirus (CPV) was first identified in the late 1970s when outbreaks of severe hemorrhagic gastroenteritis in young dogs were reported around the world.[5] The *Parvoviridae* family is a group of small icosahedral single-stranded DNA viruses, with CPV classified into the genus *Protoparvovirus* within the subfamily *Parvovirinae* (Fig. 36.1).[6] The first strains of CPV were designated CPV-2 to differentiate them from CPV-1, a member of the *Bocaparvovirus* genus in the *Parvovirinae* subfamily. CPV-2 itself was renamed *Carnivore protoparvovirus 1* in 2020, but for the purposes of this text it will continue to be referred to as CPV.

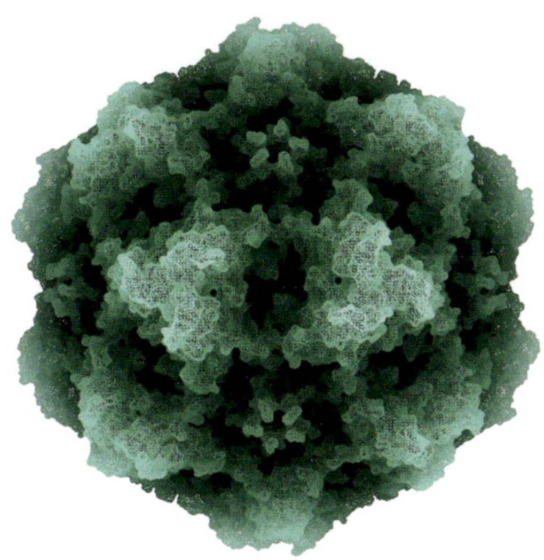

FIG. 36.1 Structural image of canine parvovirus. Image courtesy of Colin Parrish, Baker Institute for Animal Health.

Pathogenesis and clinical signs

Parvoviruses must infect rapidly dividing cells to hijack the host cell DNA replication machinery. This is required to generate double-stranded DNA, which can then be replicated, transcribed, and translated by the cell. Observations of naturally infected dogs and multiple experimental studies performed in the 1970s and 1980s confirmed that parvoviruses target mitotically active cells of the immune system, intestinal epithelia, and, in very young dogs, myocardial cells.[7] After an incubation period of 3–7 days, this results in the clinical signs of severe gastroenteritis in addition to leukopenia or myocarditis in young puppies. Disease severity varies widely, from subclinical to severe and lethal, and is primarily due to viral damage to the small intestine (Fig. 36.2). Mortality rates for puppies that show clinical signs range from 15% to 50% depending on the severity of the infection and treatment given.[8,9]

Emergence of novel strains

CPV is gradually evolving in the face of host-immune pressure. Following the initial appearance of CPV in dogs, a new variant [(CPV type 2a (CPV-2a)] was identified in 1979 which replaced the original virus strain worldwide. Other subsequent antigenic variants have been designated CPV-2b and CPV-2c, which have a single amino acid change of residue 426 in the capsid protein (Asn to Asp, and Asp to Glu, respectively).[10] CPV-2a, 2b, and 2c strains are circulating globally, but country-to-country variation is reported (e.g., CPV-2b appears to predominate in the UK and Australia).[11,12]

It is uncertain whether CPV-2c strains cause greater disease severity than CPV-2a and 2b. Natural CPV-2c infections observed in two litters of dogs had relatively mild clinical disease,[13] whereas there was 50% mortality amongst six dogs experimentally infected with a CPV-2c strain.[14] Similarly, there is some disagreement as to whether vaccines containing non-CPV-2c strains are protective against CPV-2c. Two experimental studies

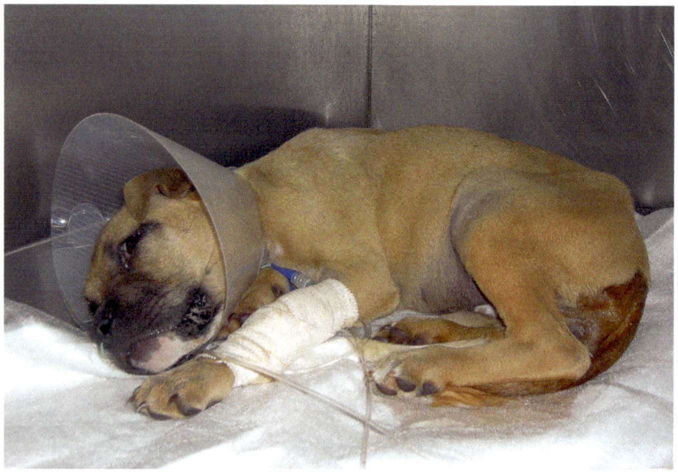

FIG. 36.2 Eight-week-old mixed-breed puppy with canine parvovirus infection confirmed by patient-side testing.

indicate heterologous vaccinations are fully protective,[14,15] whereas in several natural outbreaks of CPV-2c infected dogs were fully vaccinated with the original CPV strain.[16] However, in practice all current commercial vaccines protect effectively against any strains circulating in nature, and the management of clinical CPV cases should be the same regardless of the causative strain.

Canine enteric coronavirus

Canine enteric coronavirus (CECoV) was first isolated from an outbreak of gastroenteritis amongst military dogs in Germany in 1971.[17] CECoV is a member of the *Coronaviridae* family, of the genus *Alphacoronavirus*. Other members of this genus include feline coronavirus (FCoV) and transmissible gastroenteritis virus of swine (TGEV). CECoV is genetically distinct from the causative agent of the COVID-19 pandemic, SARS-CoV-2, which is a coronavirus classified in the genus *Betacoronavirus*.[18] A canine coronavirus responsible for respiratory disease in dogs is also a member of the genus *Betacoronavirus*, alongside the human viruses SARS and Middle Eastern respiratory syndrome (MERS).[19] Coronaviruses are enveloped viruses with a single-stranded positive-sense RNA genome of approximately 30 kb, divided into seven open reading frames.[20]

Pathogenesis of classical strains

Experimental infections with the first strain of CECoV isolated confirmed that this pathogen caused gastroenteritis, with clinical signs developing 4–7 days after inoculation.[21] Disease was mild and self-limiting in these experimental infections, which is comparable to the clinical picture described for most natural infections with the classical strains.[22] However, it has been reported that coinfections with CPV can induce more severe disease.[23] CECoV has often been identified in stool samples from healthy dogs, which indicates that subclinical infections are relatively common.

Emergence of novel strains

Sequence analysis of circulating CECoV strains revealed that two genetic clusters of the virus were circulating in 2002.[24] Unexpectedly, the emerging CECoV strains were found to be more closely related to FCoVs than the reference canine strains. FCoVs had already been differentiated into two subtypes based on serology: type I and type II. As the novel CECoV strains were most similar to type I FCoV by genetic analysis, the emerging strains were designated type I and the reference CECoV strains were classified as type II.[20] Both types of CECoV have now been reported worldwide, although the clinical significance of these two lineages is uncertain.[25] Reports exist of virus outbreaks with increased severity for both type I and type II CECoVs, and coinfections with type I and type II strains can occur.

Following recognition of type I and type II CECoV strains, multiple new strains have recently been identified. It has been proposed that type II CECoVs be further subdivided into type IIa, IIb, and IIc strains, based on the first 300 nucleotides of the spike protein.[26] The clinical implications of these different types is unclear, but each has been reported in multiple countries, and type IIb was identified as the cause of a nationwide outbreak of CECoV in the UK in 2020.[27] It appears that emergence of yet further novel CECoV strains is inevitable, and surveillance for strains with increased pathogenicity is important.

Canine distemper virus

Canine distemper is a highly contagious and lethal viral disease that has been documented in canines for centuries. Recent paleopathological work suggests the disease originated in South America as early as 1735.[28] It is caused by the canine distemper virus (CDV), an enveloped, single-stranded, negative RNA virus of the *Morbillivirus* genus of the *Paramyxoviridae* family. Related morbilliviruses are the causative agents of human measles, mumps, and bronchiolitis. Though CDV is highly contagious, vaccination controls virus spread well, and the disease is usually rare in domestic dog populations. However, CDV continues to emerge in unvaccinated and incompletely vaccinated animals, so it remains a major disease of canines and an important source of morbidity and mortality in animal shelters.

Pathogenesis

CDV has a tropism for epithelial, lymphoid, and neurological tissue. This is largely dependent on the distribution of the viral receptor CD150 (also known as signaling lymphocyte activation molecule, SLAM). As a part of its pathogenesis, CDV can induce fusion of infected cells, leading to syncytia formation (Fig. 36.3).

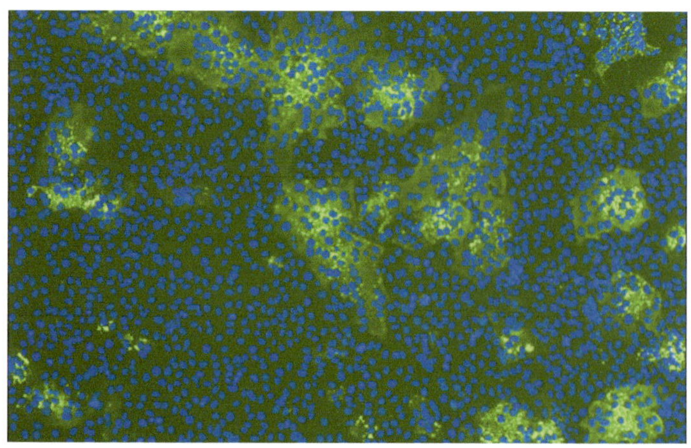

FIG. 36.3 Canine distemper virus (CDV) infection of cells in tissue culture. Vero cells expressing the canine CD150 receptor are susceptible to CDV infection, which results in cell-to-cell fusion and syncytia formation. CDV is stained green, cell nuclei are stained blue. Image courtesy of Lotta Truyen, Baker Institute for Animal Health.

Gastroenteritis is a classical sign of CDV infection, but unlike the other viruses considered in this chapter, additional clinical signs are also highly likely, including both significant respiratory and neurological signs. The leukopenia induced by infection also makes dogs more susceptible to secondary bacterial infections. After a 1–4-week incubation period, CDV is shed in all bodily secretions during active infection. Although this means that diarrhea can transmit CDV, the dominant means of transmission between dogs is via respiratory aerosols.[29] Infectious viruses are usually only shed for a limited period of time, but viral RNA can be detected for months after infection. Mortality rates can be around 50% in unvaccinated dogs.[30]

Epidemiology

CDV has a worldwide distribution. Eleven distinct geographic cocirculating lineages of the virus have been identified by sequencing of the hemagglutinin (H) gene.[31] With large reservoirs (unvaccinated dogs and wildlife), the virus has continued to circulate, and outbreaks in wild animals are becoming increasingly common.[32,33] Reports of infections in new hosts including wild and captive large cats are raising concerns and making the virus a serious threat for wildlife species. The difficulty vaccinating wildlife hosts means the virus is expected to continue to threaten wildlife species.

Canine rotavirus

Rotaviruses are members of the *Reoviridae*, a family of viruses with segmented double-stranded RNA genomes approximately 18.5 kb in length. Rotaviruses can cause gastroenteritis in young animals of a wide range of domestic species, including horses, cattle, and pigs. The first reports of rotaviruses in dogs appeared in the late 1970s, when viral particles with rotavirus morphology were identified in canine stool samples.[34] With the development of sequencing techniques, it was later possible to classify rotaviruses into different subgroups based on their two outer capsid proteins. Classification into G and P genotypes is dependent on the nucleotide sequences of the capsid proteins VP7 and VP4, respectively; there are over 40 described G genotypes and more than 55 P genotypes. The majority of rotavirus strains isolated from dogs have been classified as G3P[3]. Canine rotavirus strains are distinct from the major genotypes prevalent in human populations, but isolated reports of G3P[3] strain infections in humans exist, suggestive of zoonotic transmission of disease.[35]

Pathology

The ability of rotaviruses to induce gastroenteritis in dogs has been confirmed by experimental infections. Gnotobiotic puppies inoculated with canine rotavirus isolated from a young dog with fatal diarrhea all developed clinical signs of gastroenteritis after 24 hours.[36] The genotype of the inoculating strain in this first experimental setting was not known, but later experimental infections with a canine rotavirus strain classified as G3P[3] showed that gastroenteritis was also induced.[37] In contrast, experimental infections of dogs with bovine strains of rotaviruses showed evidence of viral replication but no induction of clinical disease.[38]

Epidemiology

A number of epidemiological surveys have sought to determine the prevalence of rotavirus shedding in dog populations. A survey of canine gastroenteritis in Japan and Florida, USA, both found canine rotavirus in 2% of diarrheic samples.[39,40] A serological survey of UK dogs presenting at a veterinary hospital demonstrated a seroprevalence of 86%.[41] Overall, this suggests that canine rotavirus infections are rarely detected, as many dogs have developed immune responses to the virus. Continued surveillance for this enteric virus is deemed valuable, as the segmented RNA genome enhances continued evolution of this viral genera.

Emerging viruses

Many new viruses have been identified in association with gastroenteritis in dogs over the past two decades. Development of next-generation sequencing approaches has enabled identification and characterization of previously unknown viruses from diarrheic stool samples. However, whether these newly discovered viruses are the primary cause of clinical disease in each case is difficult to determine. It is important to note that detection of a viral genome does not always mean that infectious viral particles are present. Table 36.1 presents key questions to be considered when aiming to ascertain whether a new virus can cause gastroenteritis. The majority of newly identified viruses are related to human gastroenteric viruses, which is often the reason why interest in a new virus first arises. Epidemiological surveys are valuable for examining whether detection of the virus is positively associated with disease, but different surveys often generate conflicting results depending on geographic areas. Finally, whilst experimental infections are the gold standard approach to confirming whether a virus can cause disease, none have yet been reported for any of the emerging viruses in this section.

Canine astrovirus

Astroviruses are star-shaped viruses that were first identified in human diarrheic fecal samples in 1975.[42] Canine astrovirus (CaAstV) was first reported in dogs in 1980 in Ohio, USA.[43] There was then a lull in reports until 2009, when CaAstV was identified in Italy. CaAstV has since been identified at low levels in dogs across multiple continents.[4]
At present it is unclear whether CaAstV is clinically important in dogs. It is known that related human astroviruses cause ~10% of diarrhea cases in children worldwide, indicating that astroviruses can cause gastrointestinal pathology. Epidemiological studies have largely found a positive association between the presence of this virus and diarrhea in dogs; for example a British study found CaAstV in 4/63 dogs with severe gastroenteritis, and 0% in healthy controls.[44] A similar association with disease was reported in several subsequent studies, although surveys from France and Hungary did not find a difference between diarrheic

TABLE 36.1 Key questions to ascertain if a new virus identified in association with diarrhea in dogs is pathogenic.

Question	Example
Does a related virus cause diarrhea in another species?	Human norovirus causes gastroenteritis in people, so it is possible that canine norovirus causes gastroenteritis in dogs
Is the virus found more commonly in dogs with diarrhea than in healthy dogs?	Epidemiological studies show a higher prevalence of virus in dogs with clinical signs than in healthy animals
Do dogs experimentally infected with the purified virus show clinical signs of gastroenteritis?	Canine parvovirus has been shown to cause disease when administered to healthy dogs in experimental conditions

administered to adult dogs is now advised to be no more than once every 3 years. There is evidence that geriatric dogs will have a weaker immune response to vaccines if primary vaccination is administered in old age, but most older dogs have good immunological memory to core vaccines. Serological testing of dogs to identify and measure the presence of virus-specific antibodies is now becoming routine in some practices. Antibody or "titer" testing can be performed on a serum sample to determine if a vaccine has been effective more than 4 weeks after it was administered. Alternatively, testing can be performed to determine if a booster vaccine is required. The most accurate results are obtained from antibody tests performed in a diagnostic laboratory, but rapid patient-side tests are now more widely available. It is important that clinicians are aware that patient-side tests have variable accuracy.[76]

Aside from vaccines specific for CPV and CDV, the only other pathogen that can induce gastroenteritis in dogs for which a vaccine is available is CECoV. However, the WSAVA does not recommend the use of this vaccine, as there is insufficient evidence that CECoV can cause significant disease in domestic dog populations. There is also no evidence at present that the existing CECoV vaccines would protect against any new strains that emerge with a higher pathogenicity.

No vaccines are currently being developed for any of the other viruses discussed in this chapter that are associated with gastroenteritis. The low pathogenicity of rotavirus does not warrant vaccination, and there is currently not enough evidence that any of the emerging viruses cause disease.

Case management

Due to the high transmissibility of most fecal–oral pathogens, an essential aspect of managing suspect or confirmed cases of viral gastroenteritis is strict isolation from uninfected dogs (Box 36.1 and Fig. 36.5). With the absence of readily available tests for many viruses associated with gastroenteritis, it is prudent to assume that a case with suspicious signs is infectious.

Box 36.1 Isolation protocols for dogs with viral gastroenteritis.

- Ensure a fully equipped isolation ward is available at all times to house suspect infectious disease cases. If a separate self-contained facility is not available, then there must be a detailed standard operating procedure (SOP) in place to explain how infectious cases are to be dealt with, or cases should be referred elsewhere.
- Full personal protective equipment (PPE) must be worn whenever entering the isolation ward, including disposable gloves, disposable shoe covers, and ideally a disposable suit.
- Clear protocols for items leaving the isolation unit must exist, including disposal of clinical waste, washing of soiled linen, and sterilization of any necessary equipment. Protocols for thorough disinfection of kennels in between patients must also be established.

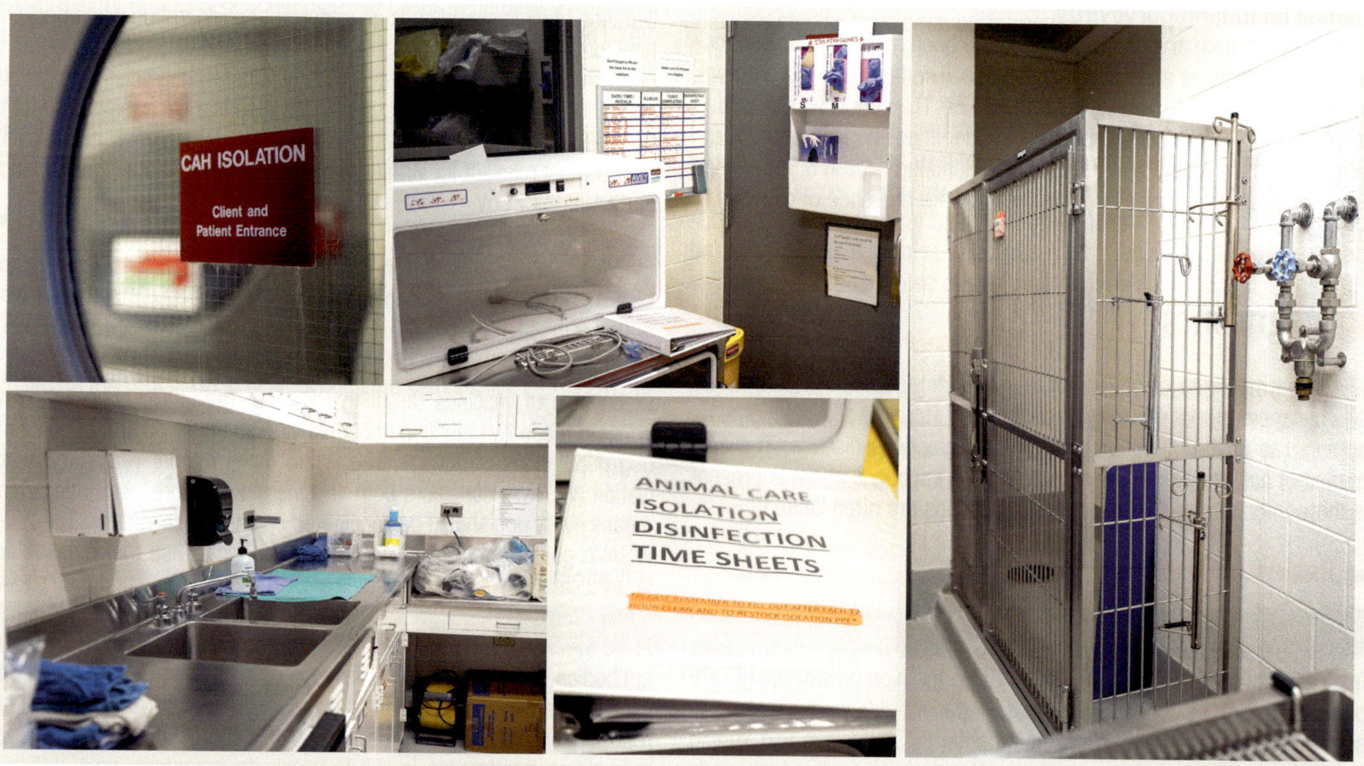

FIG. 36.5 Isolation facilities at Cornell University Hospital for Animals, Ithaca, New York. Images courtesy of Carol Jennings and the Cornell College of Veterinary Medicine.

Treatment of all canine viral gastroenteritis cases requires extensive supportive therapy of clinical signs. Detailed recommendations for the different supportive therapies are provided in Chapters 24-26, 32 and 33. One additional management strategy that has been stringently tested in dogs with CPV is fecal microbiota transplantation (see Chapter 27). Rectal administration of 10 g of stool from a healthy dog diluted into 10 mL saline was shown to reduce hospitalization times and result in faster resolution of diarrhea in CPV cases.[79]

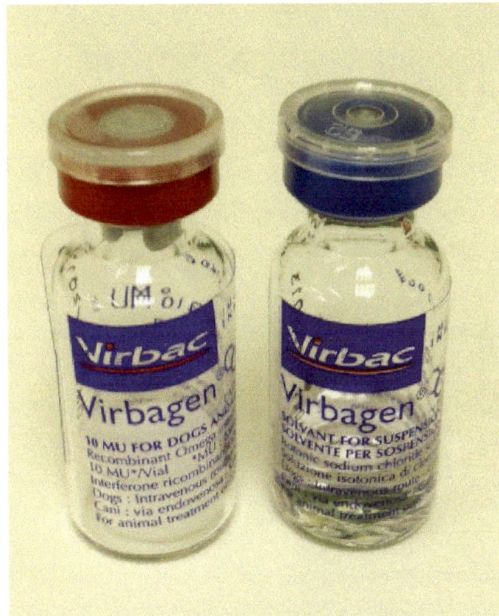

FIG. 36.6 Recombinant interferon feline omega (rfIFNω).

Antiviral therapies

Specific treatments available to effectively treat canine enteric viral infections are extremely limited. One immunomodulatory agent that has been shown to be useful in viral gastroenteritis is recombinant feline interferon omega (rfIFNω). Published studies showed a 4.4-fold reduction in mortality with CPV in a trial involving 94 dogs given 2.5 million IU/kg once daily for three consecutive days.[80] In Europe, rfIFNω is licensed for use against CPV in dogs over 1 month old (**Fig. 36.6**), although in practice this drug is not often used due to financial restrictions.

A potential breakthrough in the field of antiviral therapy for dogs was the approval of a canine parvovirus monoclonal antibody (CPMA) in 2023. Monoclonal antibodies are purified antibodies that are highly specific for a single target. CPMA binds to CPV and blocks ongoing infection. CPMA was conditionally approved in the USA following a successful clinical trial where 28 beagles were infected with CPV-2b, and CPMA was administered intravenously to 21 dogs 4 days after infection. All dogs receiving CPMA made a full recovery, whereas 4 of 7 dogs receiving the saline control were euthanized due to disease severity.[9] The efficacy of CPMA in practice is still being established, but this is an exciting development in the field of canine infectious diseases.

KEY POINTS

- Canine parvovirus continues to be the major viral cause of gastroenteritis in dogs.
- New viruses are being detected in stool samples of dogs with diarrhea at increasing frequency, but these are often also found in asymptomatic animals.
- The clinical relevance and zoonotic potential of many emerging canine viruses is unclear, and ongoing research is needed to determine if veterinarians and pet owners should be concerned.
- Strict hygiene and isolation procedures should be observed for any dogs with gastroenteritis and an index of suspicion for an infectious cause.

References

1. Dema A, Tallapally MR, Ganji VK, et al. A comprehensive molecular survey of viral pathogens associated with canine gastroenteritis. *Arch Virol* 168(2):36, 2023.
2. Godsall SA, Clegg SR, Stavisky JH, et al. Epidemiology of canine parvovirus and coronavirus in dogs presented with severe diarrhoea to PDSA PetAid hospitals. *Vet Rec* 167(6):196–201, 2010.
3. Gizzi AB, Oliveira ST, Leutenegger CM, et al. Presence of infectious agents and co-infections in diarrheic dogs determined with a real-time polymerase chain reaction-based panel. *BMC Vet Res* 10:23, 2014.
4. Caddy SL. New viruses associated with canine gastroenteritis. *Vet J* 232:57-64, 2018.
5. Hoelzer K, Parrish CR. The emergence of parvoviruses of carnivores. *Vet Res* 41(6):39, 2010.
6. Pénzes JJ, Söderlund-Venermo M, Canuti M, et al. Reorganizing the family *Parvoviridae*: a revised taxonomy independent of the canonical approach based on host association. *Arch Virol* 165(9):2133–2146, 2020.
7. Parrish CR. Pathogenesis of feline panleukopenia virus and canine parvovirus. *Baillieres Clin Haematol* 8(1):57–71, 1995.
8. Horecka K, Porter S, Amirian ES, Jefferson E. A decade of treatment of canine parvovirus in an animal shelter: a retrospective study. *Animals (Basel)* 10(6):939, 2020.

9. Larson L, Miller L, Margiasso M, et al. Early administration of canine parvovirus monoclonal antibody prevented mortality after experimental challenge. *J Am Vet Med Assoc* 262(4):506–512, 2024.
10. Buonavoglia C, Martella V, Pratelli A, et al. Evidence for evolution of canine parvovirus type 2 in Italy. *J Gen Virol* 82(Pt 12):3021–3025, 2001.
11. Kwan E, Carrai M, Lanave G, et al. Analysis of canine parvoviruses circulating in Australia reveals predominance of variant 2b and identifies feline parvovirus-like mutations in the capsid proteins. *Transbound Emerg Dis* 68(2):656–666, 2021.
12. Smith SL, Afonso MM, Roberts L, et al. A virtual biobank for companion animals: A parvovirus pilot study. *Vet Rec* 189(6):e556, 2021.
13. Decaro N, Desario C, Campolo M, et al. Clinical and virological findings in pups naturally infected by canine parvovirus type 2 Glu-426 mutant. *J Vet Diagn Invest* 17(2):133–138, 2005.
14. Spibey N, Greenwood NM, Sutton D, et al. Canine parvovirus type 2 vaccine protects against virulent challenge with type 2c virus. *Vet Microbiol* 128 (1-2):48–55, 2008.
15. Siedek EM, Schmidt H, Sture GH, Raue R. Vaccination with canine parvovirus type 2 (CPV-2) protects against challenge with virulent CPV-2b and CPV-2c. *Berl Munch Tierarztl Wochenschr* 124(1-2):58–64, 2011.
16. Decaro N, Buonavoglia C. Canine parvovirus—a review of epidemiological and diagnostic aspects, with emphasis on type 2c. *Vet Microbiol* 155(1): 1–12, 2012.
17. Binn LN, Lazar EC, Keenan KP, et al. Recovery and characterization of a coronavirus from military dogs with diarrhea. *Proc Annu Meet U S Anim Health Assoc* (78):359–366, 1974.
18. Wu F, Zhao S, Yu B, et al. A new coronavirus associated with human respiratory disease in China. *Nature* 579(7798):265–269, 2020.
19. Erles K, Toomey C, Brooks HW, Brownlie J. Detection of a group 2 coronavirus in dogs with canine infectious respiratory disease. *Virology* 310(2):216–223, 2003.
20. Pratelli A. The evolutionary processes of canine coronaviruses. *Adv Virol* 2011:562831, 2011.
21. Keenan KP, Jervis HR, Marchwicki RH, Binn LN. Intestinal infection of neonatal dogs with canine coronavirus 1-71: studies by virologic, histologic, histochemical, and immunofluorescent techniques. *Am J Vet Res* 37(3):247–256, 1976.
22. Greene CE (ed.). *Infectious Diseases of the Dog and Cat*, 4th ed. St. Louis, Missouri: Elsevier; 2012.
23. Pratelli A, Tempesta M, Roperto FP, et al. Fatal coronavirus infection in puppies following canine parvovirus 2b infection. *J Vet Diagn Invest* 11(6):550–553, 1999.
24. Pratelli A, Martella V, Decaro N, et al. Genetic diversity of a canine coronavirus detected in pups with diarrhoea in Italy. *J Virol Methods* 110(1): 9–17, 2003.
25. Decaro N, Buonavoglia C. An update on canine coronaviruses: viral evolution and pathobiology. *Vet Microbiol* 132(3-4):221–234, 2008.
26. Licitra BN, Duhamel GE, Whittaker GR. Canine enteric coronaviruses: emerging viral pathogens with distinct recombinant spike proteins. *Viruses* 6(8):3363–3376, 2014.
27. Radford AD, Singleton DA, Jewell C, et al. Outbreak of severe vomiting in dogs associated with a canine enteric coronavirus, United Kingdom. *Emerg Infect Dis* 27(2):517–528, 2021.
28. Uhl EW, Kelderhouse C, Buikstra J, et al. New world origin of canine distemper: Interdisciplinary insights. *Int J Paleopathol* 24:266–278, 2019.
29. Appel MJ, Summers BA. Pathogenicity of morbilliviruses for terrestrial carnivores. *Vet Microbiol* 44(2-4):187–191, 1995.
30. Bruyette DS. Canine distemper. In: Bruyette DS, Bexfield N, Chretin JD, et al. (eds.). *Clinical Small Animal Internal Medicine*, 1st ed. Wiley; 2020.
31. Wang H, Guo H, Hein VG, et al. The evolutionary dynamics history of canine distemper virus through analysis of the hemagglutinin gene during 1930–2020. *Eur J Wildl Res* 69(3):56, 2023.
32. Garigliany M, Sarlet M, Franssen M, et al. Re-emergence of canine distemper in wildlife in Belgium. *Vet Rec* 182(15):439, 2018.
33. Monne I, Fusaro A, Valastro V, et al. A distinct CDV genotype causing a major epidemic in Alpine wildlife. *Vet Microbiol* 150(1-2):63–69, 2011.
34. Eugster AK, Sidwa T. Rotaviruses in diarrheic feces of a dog. *Vet Med Small Anim Clin* 74(6): 817–819, 1979.
35. Martella V, Bányai K, Matthijnssens J, et al. Zoonotic aspects of rotaviruses. *Vet Microbiol* 140(3-4):246–255, 2010.
36. Johnson CA, Fulton RW, Henk WG, Snider TG 3rd. Inoculation of neonatal gnotobiotic dogs with a canine rotavirus. *Am J Vet Res* 44(9):1682–1686, 1983.
37. Kang BK, Song DS, Jung KI, et al. Genetic characterization of canine rotavirus isolated from a puppy in Korea and experimental reproduction of disease. *J Vet Diagn Invest* 19(1):78–83, 2007.
38. Dagenais L, Schwers A, Pastoret PP, Chappuis G. Propagation of bovine rotavirus by dogs. *Vet Rec* 109(9):187, 1981.
39. Tupler T, Levy JK, Sabshin SJ, et al. Enteropathogens identified in dogs entering a Florida animal shelter with normal feces or diarrhea. *J Am Vet Med Assoc* 241(3):338–343, 2012.
40. Mochizuki M, Hashimoto M, Ishida T. Recent epidemiological status of canine viral enteric infections and *Giardia* infection in Japan. *J Vet Med Sci* 63(5):573–575, 2001.
41. Tennant BJ, Gaskell RM, Jones RC, Gaskell CJ. Prevalence of antibodies to four major canine viral diseases in dogs in a Liverpool hospital population. *J Small Anim Pract* 32(4):175–179, 1991.
42. Madeley CR, Cosgrove BP. Letter: 28 nm particles in faeces in infantile gastroenteritis. *Lancet* 2(7932):451–452, 1975.
43. Williams FP Jr. Astrovirus-like, coronavirus-like, and parvovirus-like particles detected in the diarrheal stools of beagle pups. *Arch Virol* 66(3): 215–226, 1980.
44. Caddy SL, Goodfellow I. Complete genome sequence of canine astrovirus with molecular and epidemiological characterisation of UK strains. *Vet Microbiol* 177(1-2):206–213, 2015.
45. Grellet A, De Battisti C, Feugier A, et al. Prevalence and risk factors of astrovirus infection in puppies from French breeding kennels. *Vet Microbiol* 157(1-2):214–219, 2012.
46. Mihalov-Kovács E, Martella V, Lanave G, et al. Genome analysis of canine astroviruses reveals genetic heterogeneity and suggests possible inter-species transmission. *Virus Res* 232:162–170, 2017.
47. Kapoor A, Simmonds P, Dubovi EJ, et al. Characterization of a canine homolog of human Aichivirus. *J Virol* 85(21):11520–11525, 2011.
48. Li L, Pesavento PA, Shan T, et al. Viruses in diarrhoeic dogs include novel kobuviruses and sapoviruses. *J Gen Virol* 92(Pt 11):2534–2541, 2011.
49. Carmona-Vicente N, Buesa J, Brown PA, et al. Phylogeny and prevalence of kobuviruses in dogs and cats in the UK. *Vet Microbiol* 164(3-4): 246–252, 2013.
50. Martella V, Lorusso E, Decaro N, et al. Detection and molecular characterization of a canine norovirus. *Emerg Infect Dis* 14(8):1306–1308, 2008.
51. Azevedo M, Mullis L, Vegas E, et al. Detection of norovirus in dogs in Arkansas. In: American Society of Virology Conference; 2012. pp. 23–30.
52. Caddy S, Emmott E, El-Attar L, et al. Serological evidence for multiple strains of canine norovirus in the UK dog population. *PLoS One* 8(12):e81596, 2013.
53. Bodnar L, Lorusso E, Di Martino B, et al. Identification of a novel canine norovirus. *Infect Genet Evol* 52:75-81, 2017.
54. Mesquita JR, Barclay L, Nascimento MS, Vinjé J. Novel norovirus in dogs with diarrhea. *Emerg Infect Dis* 16(6):980-982, 2010.
55. Summa M, von Bonsdorff CH, Maunula L. Pet dogs—a transmission route for human noroviruses? *J Clin Virol* 53(3):244–247, 2012.
56. Caddy SL, de Rougemont A, Emmott E, et al. Evidence for human norovirus infection of dogs in the United Kingdom. *J Clin Microbiol* 53(6): 1873–1883, 2015.
57. Charoenkul K, Nasamran C, Janetanakit T, et al. Human norovirus infection in dogs, Thailand. *Emerg Infect Dis* 26(2):350–353, 2020.
58. Kapoor A, Dubovi EJ, Henriquez-Rivera JA, Lipkin WI. Complete genome sequence of the first canine circovirus. *J Virol* 86(12):7018, 2012.
59. Li L, McGraw S, Zhu K, et al. Circovirus in tissues of dogs with vasculitis and hemorrhage. *Emerg Infect Dis* 19(4):534–541, 2013.
60. Decaro N, Martella V, Desario C, et al. Genomic characterization of a circovirus associated with fatal hemorrhagic enteritis in dog, Italy. *PLoS One* 9(8):e105909, 2014.

61. Kotsias F, Bucafusco D, Nuñez DA, et al. Genomic characterization of canine circovirus associated with fatal disease in dogs in South America. *PLoS One* 14(6):e0218735, 2019.
62. Anderson A, Hartmann K, Leutenegger CM, et al. Role of canine circovirus in dogs with acute haemorrhagic diarrhoea. *Vet Rec* 180(22):542, 2017.
63. Lempp C, Jungwirth N, Grilo ML, et al. Pathological findings in the red fox (*Vulpes vulpes*), stone marten (*Martes foina*) and raccoon dog (*Nyctereutes procyonoides*), with special emphasis on infectious and zoonotic agents in Northern Germany. *PLoS One* 12(4):e0175469, 2017.
64. Hsu HS, Lin TH, Wu HY, et al. High detection rate of dog circovirus in diarrheal dogs. *BMC Vet Res* 12(1):116, 2016.
65. Stamelou E, Giantsis IA, Papageorgiou KV, et al. First report of canine Astrovirus and Sapovirus in Greece, hosting both asymptomatic and gastroenteritis symptomatic dogs. *Virol J* 19(1):58, 2022.
66. Soma T, Nakagomi O, Nakagomi T, Mochizuki M. Detection of *Norovirus* and *Sapovirus* from diarrheic dogs and cats in Japan. *Microbiol Immunol* 59(3):123–128, 2015.
67. Melegari I, Marsilio F, Di Profio F, et al. Seroprevalence of sapovirus in dogs using baculovirus-expressed virus-like particles. *Virus Res* 251:1–5, 2018.
68. Bodewes R, Lapp S, Hahn K, et al. Novel canine bocavirus strain associated with severe enteritis in a dog litter. *Vet Microbiol* 174(1-2):1–8, 2014.
69. Sobhy NM, Armién AG, Pilot J, et al. Detection and molecular characterization of astro and bocaviruses in dogs in Minnesota. *Comp Immunol Microbiol Infect Dis* 81:101740, 2022.
70. Martella V, Lanave G, Mihalov-Kovács E, et al. Novel parvovirus related to primate bufaviruses in dogs. *Emerg Infect Dis* 24(6):1061–1068, 2018.
71. Charoenkul K, Thaw YN, Phyu EM, et al. First detection and genetic characterization of canine bufavirus in domestic dogs, Thailand. *Sci Rep* 14(1):4773, 2024.
72. Fahsbender E, Altan E, Seguin MA, et al. Chapparvovirus DNA found in 4% of dogs with diarrhea. *Viruses* 11(5):398, 2019.
73. Piewbang C, Lohavicharn P, Nguyen TV, et al. Carnivore chaphamaparvovirus-1 (CaChPV-1) infection in diarrheic dogs reveals viral endotheliotropism in intestine and lung. *Vet Q* 43(1):1–10, 2023.
74. Desario C, et al. Canine parvovirus infection: which diagnostic test for virus? *J Virol Methods* 126 (1–2):179–85, 2005.
75. Allen C, Ellis A, Liang R, et al. Prolonged persistence of canine distemper virus RNA, and virus isolation in naturally infected shelter dogs. *PLoS One* 18(1):e0280186, 2023.
76. Squires RA, Crawford C, Marcondes M, Whitley N. 2024 guidelines for the vaccination of dogs and cats—compiled by the Vaccination Guidelines Group (VGG) of the World Small Animal Veterinary Association (WSAVA). *J Small Anim Pract* 65(5):277–316, 2024.
77. Gillespie JH, Baker JA, Burgher J, et al. The immune response of dogs to distemper virus. *Cornell Vet* 48(2):103–126, 1958.
78. Pollock RV, Carmichael LE. Maternally derived immunity to canine parvovirus infection: transfer, decline, and interference with vaccination. *J Am Vet Med Assoc* 180(1):37–42, 1982.
79. Pereira GQ, Gomes LA, Santos IS, et al. Fecal microbiota transplantation in puppies with canine parvovirus infection. *J Vet Intern Med* 32(2): 707–711, 2018.
80. de Mari K, Maynard L, Eun HM, Lebreux B. Treatment of canine parvoviral enteritis with interferon-omega in a placebo-controlled field trial. *Vet Rec* 152(4):105–108, 2003.

CHAPTER 37

Bacterial enteritides

Cameron Prior
BVSc, MSc, PgCert CertAVP, DECVIM-CA, MRCVS

Fergus Allerton
BSc, BVSc, CertSAM, DECVIM-CA, FRCVS

The number of shark attacks at American beaches increases as the sales of ice cream increase. Although this statement may be true and repeatable, it obviously should not prompt bans on selling ice cream or vilification of ice cream sellers. The tenet that correlation does not mean causation is just as relevant when evaluating the clinical significance of bacterial enteropathogens in gastrointestinal (GI) disease. Many putative disease-causing bacteria are isolated at similar frequencies in animals with and without diarrhea.[1] Cautious interpretation of fecal culture and other organism-identifying diagnostic modalities is required to determine whether any detected enteric bacteria are pathogenic, a consequence of the associated disease process, or merely an incidental finding.

Because any antibiotic use may promote the development of antimicrobial resistance, clinicians are regularly encouraged to establish a bacterial etiology before reaching for antibiotic therapy. This step is particularly challenging in the context of GI disease because of the question of causality. This chapter focuses on several common bacterial enteritides, attempts to define the clinical relevance of enteric bacteria, and supports evidence-based decision making. The zoonotic potential of certain bacteria (e.g., *Campylobacter jejuni* and *Salmonella* spp.), especially toward children and immunocompromised individuals, may influence the diagnostic and therapeutic approach and also will be discussed.

Diagnostic and treatment approach

The clinical manifestations of bacterial enteritis are nonspecific and include acute and chronic presentations with combinations of vomiting, diarrhea of small and/or large intestinal origin (with or without the presence of blood), and a variety of other systemic signs. Similarly, physical examination findings, clinical pathology results, and imaging changes overlap considerably with noninfectious pathologies. Nonetheless, appropriate investigations are useful to stage the severity of presentation and to guide treatment decisions. Dogs and cats that exhibit markers of sepsis, such as neutropenia, hypoglycemia, and hypotension unresponsive to fluid resuscitation, require aggressive supportive measures and are candidates for early instigation of broad-spectrum antibiosis. Consequently, the clinical status of the pet typically exerts a greater influence over treatment decisions than identification of specific organisms. The diagnosis of bacterial enteritis relies on methodologies to detect and identify salient enteropathogens, including fecal cytology, fecal culture, polymerase chain reaction (PCR), fluorescent *in situ* hybridization, and immunodetection of elaborated toxin. Although individual treatment decisions may be best made based on clinical parameters, demonstration of the presence of particular bacteria can affect infection-control measures (e.g., need for barrier hygiene precautions, housing within isolation facilities, and implementation of disinfection protocols).

Escherichia coli

Etiology and pathogenesis

Escherichia coli are gram-negative facultative rod-shaped anaerobes that are part of the normal fecal flora. Classifications of strains of *E. coli* have been described based on virulence properties that reflect their mechanism of pathogenicity (e.g., toxin production, adhesion and effacement, or mucosal invasion).

A contributory role to chronic diarrhea may be inferred from the inclusion of *E. coli* among the 7 bacterial taxa included in the dysbiosis index (see Chapters 19 and 20). An increased abundance of *E. coli* will increase the dysbiosis index and has been found in dogs with chronic enteropathy and in dysbiosis secondary to antibiotic administration. However, causality is again uncertain, and the proportional change in *E. coli* numbers may be consequent to dysbiosis rather than a driving force. Mucosally invasive *E. coli* have been causally linked to granulomatous (histiocytic ulcerative) colitis. This serious condition primarily affects young Boxers and French bulldogs (see Chapter 48).

Although considered to be commensal bacteria, *E. coli* can cause opportunistic systemic infections in animals and humans. *E. coli* also may serve as a reservoir for genes conferring antimicrobial resistance that can be shared horizontally with pathogenic bacteria. Consequently, hygiene measures are important to prevent the transmission of *E. coli* between companion animals and humans. Careful attention to regular hand washing and proper cleaning and disinfection should be applied when handling all pets with GI signs.

Clinical signs

Pets with different *E. coli* pathovars may present with a variety of overlapping clinical syndromes (many of which may not be directly attributable to the presence of *E. coli*). Clinical signs are inherently variable and feature a range of diarrheic manifestations. Dogs with granulomatous colitis due to *E. coli* have predominantly large intestinal diarrhea with tenesmus, hematochezia and/or mucoid stools, and increased defecation frequency alongside inappetence and weight loss.

Diagnosis

The demonstration of *E. coli* in a fecal culture has little diagnostic value (Table 37.1). Differentiation between *E. coli* pathovars is not typically performed because it requires specialized molecular testing and still would not warrant specific management changes for the individual animal. Among the *E. coli* pathovars, *E. coli* O157 poses the greatest zoonotic threat (low infective dose and risk of severe disease in people). An outbreak affecting 4 people in the United Kingdom (including 1 fatality) was traced back to raw-fed dogs,[2] highlighting a potential role for epidemiological surveillance in public health.

Immunohistochemistry or fluorescent *in situ* hybridization (FISH) can detect. the presence of intramucosal enteroinvasive *E. coli* within the lamina propria, colonic submucosa, and colonic mucosa of endoscopic biopsies and is a key diagnostic criterion for granulomatous colitis (Fig. 37.1).

TABLE 37.1 Comparative aspect of data showing the prevalence rates of different pathogens in dogs (D) and cats (C) with and without diarrhea.

Pathogen	Animals with diarrhea (%)	Healthy animals (%)	References
Escherichia. coli	34 (C)	47 (C)	22*
Campylobacter spp.	0–87	0–87	6, 23, 23–25
Salmonella spp.	0–3.6 (D)	0–3.6 (D) and 0–8.6 (C)	11, 12
Clostridioides difficile	10–21	0–58 (D and C)	17
Clostridium perfringens	80–100 (D)	80–100 (D) and 63 (C)	17
Clostridium perfringens enterotoxin	34 (D)	5–14 (D)	17
Clostridium perfringens enterotoxin gene (*cpe*)	36.3 (D)	33.8 (D)	17

* No studies in dogs.

Treatment

For most animals presenting with acute or chronic diarrhea, no antibiotic treatment is warranted, and supportive measures to maintain hydration status are sufficient (see Chapter 29). Antibiotics should be reserved for animals with severe disease and suspected or confirmed sepsis, independent of the presence or absence of *E. coli*. The single exception to this recommendation is the need for antibiotic therapy to manage granulomatous colitis. In these cases, enrofloxacin (10 mg/kg PO q24h) for a duration of 6 to 8 weeks has been proposed to ensure sufficient intracellular antibiotic concentration to eliminate bacteria within macrophages.[3] Inadequate treatment duration can foster fluoroquinolone resistance and has been observed in ~50% of cases, justifying routine susceptibility testing on biopsy samples and adapted antibiotic selection.

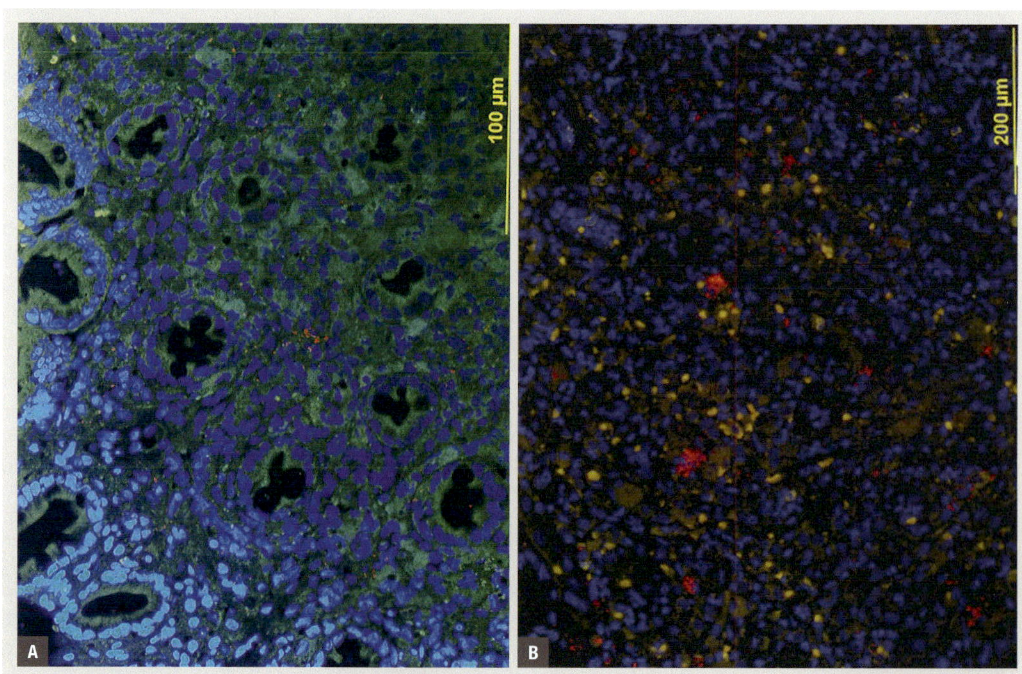

FIG. 37.1 Fluorescent *in situ* hybridization of colonic biopsies showing multifocal clusters of *Escherichia coli* in a dog with granulomatous colitis (red clusters) in the lamina propria: (**A**) colonocyte nuclei are labeled in blue, and mucosal autofluorescence in green; (**B**) a higher-magnification microscopic view shows multiple clusters of red-staining bacteria (*Escherichia coli*). Images courtesy of Kenneth Simpson.

Campylobacter spp.

Etiology and pathogenesis

The *Campylobacter* genus includes multiple species of small microaerophilic gram-negative rod-shaped bacteria including *C. upsaliensis*, *C. helveticus*, *C. coli*, and *C. jejuni*. *Campylobacter* spp. are the most common cause of bacterial enteritis in people. Although most infections in people are from food-borne transmission, pet ownership is an important risk factor, especially if the pet is young. Because transmission occurs via the fecal–oral route, prevalence is higher in closely housed animals (e.g., in kennels or shelters), where environmental hygiene is suboptimal, or among pets that are raw fed.[4] Young animals (<6 months old) have higher carriage and infection rates, attributed to a lack of immunity from prior exposure.

Campylobacter-induced diarrhea hinges on its adhesion to and invasion of the intestinal epithelium, followed by the release of toxins that disrupt normal enterocyte function. This disruption triggers an inflammatory response, characterized by the influx of inflammatory cells and the secretion of proinflammatory cytokines, further exacerbating tissue damage and GI dysfunction.

Isolation rates of *Campylobacter* spp. from canine fecal samples have ranged from 0–76% and depend on seasonality (i.e., shedding is greater during the summer and autumn), geographical location, and sample methodology, but they are *not* dependent on the presence or absence of diarrhea. *C. upsaliensis* accounted for 98% of *Campylobacter* spp. isolates in a UK cross-sectional study, with the remainder being *C. jejuni*. Younger dogs were more likely to carry *C. upsaliensis* and may be an important source of infection in people.[5] A mean prevalence of 24.7% in household cats and dogs was found after a meta-analysis of 34 studies.[6]

Clinical signs

Infections are usually subclinical in dogs. Young animals or those with comorbidities are more prone to infection and may present more severe clinical signs.[1] Affected dogs commonly exhibit mild to moderate diarrhea (watery ± blood or mucus), tenesmus, lethargy, dehydration, and inappetence. Pyrexia, vomiting, and abdominal discomfort are occasionally present. Clinical signs typically develop within 3 days of oral challenge, reflecting the short incubation time. Non-GI conditions also have been reported, including cholangiohepatitis, cholecystitis, reproductive issues, and neurological disorders such as polyradiculoneuritis.[7]

Diagnosis

Direct examination of a Gram-stained fecal smear can demonstrate bacteria with morphological characteristic of *Campylobacter* spp., although this offers no information as to species and other *Campylobacter*-like organisms (e.g., enteric *Helicobacter* spp. may appear similar; Fig. 37.2). Furthermore, detection of suspect organisms does not imply causality. Optimal plating conditions (i.e., microaerophilic environment and incubation at 37–42°C) using modified charcoal–cefoperazone–deoxycholate agar facilitate the growth of this fastidious organism (Fig. 37.3). Organisms take on a seagull morphology within the colonic glandular crypt on histopathology (Fig. 37.4). The inclusion of antimicrobial agents in selective media (e.g., cefoperazone, amphotericin, or teicoplanin) improves recovery rates, especially of *C. upsaliensis*, without preferentially selecting for resistant strains. Biochemical assays can permit differentiation of isolated *Campylobacter* spp. which may have important implications in an outbreak situation or to assess zoonotic potential. PCR assays and matrix-assisted laser desorption/ionization time-of-flight mass spectrometry (MALDI-TOF MS) also can be performed for speciation and have largely replaced phenotypic testing in commercial diagnostic laboratories.

Treatment

Most *Campylobacter* spp. infections are either asymptomatic or self-limited, and they resolve with supportive therapy alone. Antibiotic therapy is rarely warranted and should only be considered in animals that are exhibiting severe (suspicion of sepsis) or persistent clinical signs. Owners should be offered advice around hygiene (*Campylobacter* spp. are susceptible to many disinfectants) and quarantine measures to protect at-risk individuals (e.g., young children, pregnant women, or immunocompromised individuals in the household), and they should be cautioned that shedding of bacteria can persist for several months.

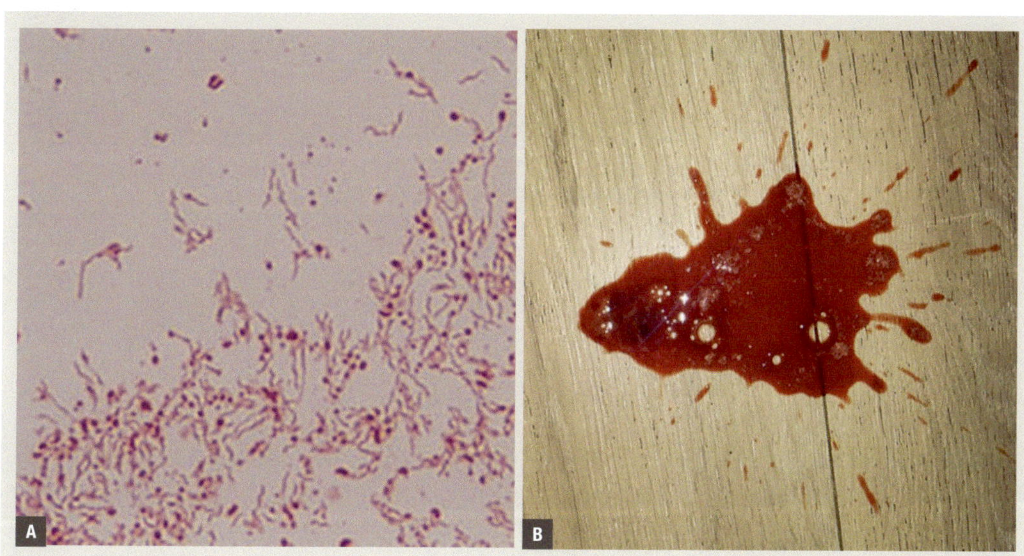

FIG. 37.2 (A) Direct cytological examination of a Gram-stained fecal smear demonstrating bacteria with morphology characteristic of *Campylobacter* spp; (B) hemorrhagic diarrhea from a dog in which *Campylobacter* spp. were isolated. Images courtesy of Joe Rubin.

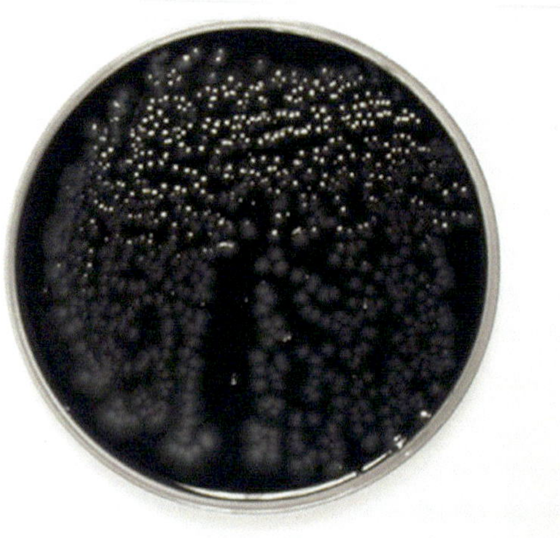

FIG. 37.3 Petri dish with typical *Campylobacter jejuni* colonies on a modified charcoal–cefoperazone–deoxycholate agar. Image courtesy of Els Acke.

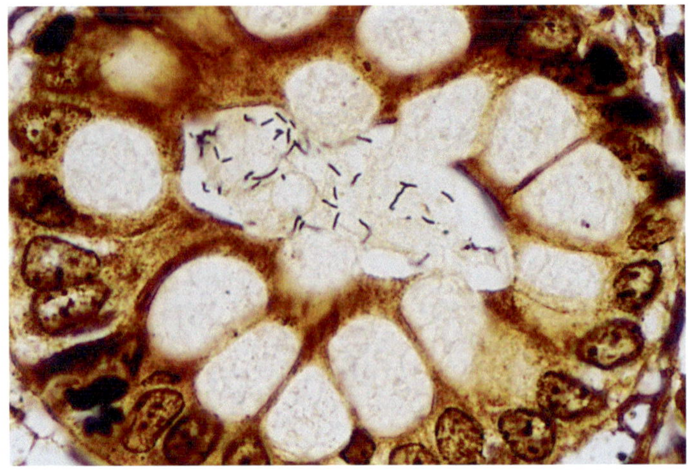

FIG. 37.4 Intestinal biopsy from a case of *Campylobacter* enterocolitis in a puppy with large intestinal diarrhea. Organisms with a seagull appearance are noted within the colonic glandular crypt (Wartin–Starry argyrophilic stain; ×100). Image courtesy of Dr. Marco Colaceci in 2000 via Fabio Del Piero.

Where antibiotic therapy is deemed necessary, macrolides (e.g., erythromycin or azithromycin) are typically preferred. Erythromycin (10–20 mg/kg PO q8h) is suggested as a first-line option, but GI upset (especially vomiting) is not uncommon, and resistance rates of up to 11.8% have been described.[8] Treatment should not extend beyond clinical resolution (typically <7 days). The use of fluoroquinolones is inappropriate given increasing rates of resistance fueled by high *de novo* mutation and the categorization of fluoroquinolones among the European Medicines Agency's Antimicrobial Advice Ad Hoc Expert Group Category B ("Restrict") class of antibiotics.

Salmonella spp.

Salmonella enterica and *Salmonella bongori* (previously known as subspecies V), the 2 species from the *Salmonella* genus (Enterobacteriaceae family), are gram-negative rod-shaped facultative anaerobes. The genus is further divided into 6 subspecies and >2600 serotypes with varying impact on human and animal health. Ingestion of *Salmonella* spp. in contaminated food (especially raw food), water, or other fomites represents the main route of transmission. *Salmonella* spp. have been isolated from 17–80% of raw-meat diets, underscoring the importance of good food hygiene practices. Dogs fed a raw-meat diet are almost 30 times more likely to be positive for *Salmonella* spp. than dogs on a conventional diet.[9] Multidrug resistance has been identified in 43% of *Salmonella* spp. isolates obtained from household dogs and cats.[10]

Pathogenesis

After ingestion, *Salmonella* serovars attach to the mucosal membrane of intestinal villi, invading microfold cells in Peyer's patches and enterocytes. Various virulence factors enable the bacteria to evade host defenses (e.g., Vi antigen), adhere to intestinal epithelial cells (fimbriae and pili), move around (flagellae), and finally invade, survive, and spread beyond the small intestine (essential genes encoded in *Salmonella* pathogenicity islands), leading to colonization. The host's inflammatory response causes epithelial injury and sloughing, provoking a secretory and/or hemorrhagic diarrhea. *Salmonella* spp. can persist in enterocytes and phagocytic cells within the liver, spleen, and intestinal lymph nodes, enabling disease recrudescence should the animal subsequently become immunocompromised or stressed. Fecal shedding may persist for 3–6 weeks after resolution of diarrhea.

Clinical signs

In most cases, pets infected with *Salmonella* spp. are subclinical or experience mild, self-limited illness; carriage rates of between 1 and 36% have been reported in clinically healthy animals.[11] More seriously affected animals may present with diarrhea (watery, mucoid, and/or hemorrhagic) with or without vomiting alongside systemic signs (e.g., pyrexia, lethargy, anorexia, and weight loss) or extra-GI disease (e.g., endocarditis, abortion, or prostatitis). *Salmonella*-associated sepsis has been reported in dogs.[12]

Diagnosis

Salmonella spp. can be cultured from fecal samples on specific agar types after selective enrichment. Genus and species–level identification typically involves biochemical testing or MALDI-TOF MS, although PCR and agglutination tests with specific antisera can be used for serotyping.

Treatment

Most *Salmonella* spp. infections are self-limited and will resolve with supportive therapy alone but adapted to the severity of presentation. Antibiotic therapy should be avoided unless the animal is showing clinical signs consistent with sepsis because treatment aggravates GI dysbiosis, can prolong fecal shedding of this zoonotic pathogen leading to the development of a carrier state, and increases the risk of acquiring plasmid-mediated resistance. Where possible, antibiotic treatment should be guided by antimicrobial susceptibility testing. Empiric choices (pending culture results) should be broad spectrum and effectively penetrate phagocytic cells. Trimethoprim-sulfonamide, amoxicillin-clavulanate, and fluoroquinolones are suitable choices.

Clostridial enteritides

Clostridium perfringens and *Clostridioides difficile* are gram-positive anaerobic spore-forming rod-shaped bacteria. Five biotypes (A–E) of *C. perfringens* are described based on the presence of 4 major toxins (alpha, beta, epsilon, and iota). Although *C. difficile* is the most common cause of healthcare-associated diarrhea in people and causes significant morbidity and even mortality, the pathogenic role of both *C. perfringens* and *C. difficile* in dogs and cats is uncertain.

Pathogenesis

Sporulation of all biotypes of *C. perfringens* (particularly Type A strains) is coregulated with the expression of *C. perfringens* enterotoxin gene (*cpe*). Both events can be triggered by an abrupt diet change, antibiotic administration, or intestinal inflammation. However, *cpe* gene carriage is not ubiquitous among *C. perfringens*, and other virulence factors (e.g., β_2 toxin or pore-forming Type A toxins netE, netF, and netG) may play a more significant role in disease pathogenesis, particularly in acute hemorrhagic diarrhea syndrome (AHDS) (see Chapter 35).[13–16]

In *C. difficile*, enterotoxin A and cytotoxin B have been implicated in disease pathogenesis in a dose-dependent and synergistic manner. Toxin A creates unregulated pores within the intestinal cell membrane and disrupts normal cellular function. Toxin B also causes cellular dysfunction and has cytotoxic effects. A further binary toxin (CDT) is also produced by certain strains of *C. difficile*, although its role is unclear.

Diagnosis

Fecal culture has no diagnostic value for *C. perfringens* because the organism is often detected in fecal samples from healthy animals, and *C. perfringens* was found in all sampled dogs (healthy and diarrheic) via quantitative PCR, suggesting a commensal role for this microorganism.[17] The enterotoxin CPE can be detected in feces via enzyme-linked immunosorbent assay (ELISA) but has been detected in healthy animals. For dogs with AHDS, CPE levels did not correlate with the severity of clinical signs, the duration of hospitalization, or outcome. Testing for netF is also not recommended because a positive result would not change treatment.[15] The enterotoxin gene (*cpe*) can be detected in feces via PCR but was detected at similar levels in dogs that were healthy and dogs with GI disease, questioning the significance of a positive result.[17] Current suggested protocols for *C. perfringens* detection are to perform both a CPE ELISA and PCR for the presence of the *cpe* gene.

C. difficile can be detected in 0–58% of healthy dogs and cats without GI signs, rendering a positive fecal culture of no clinical value.[1] Detection of toxins A and B via ELISA or PCR tests for the associated toxigenic genes (*tcdA* and *tcdB*) are the preferred diagnostic approaches, although test sensitivity and specificity are variable. Human immunoassays for these toxins should be avoided.

Treatment

Treatment recommendations should follow the algorithm for management of acute diarrhea; that is, antibiotic therapy should be used only if the animal is showing clinical signs consistent with sepsis. This recommendation applies equally to dogs with AHDS. Research evaluating the potential benefit of fecal microbiota transplantation is ongoing and, if adopted as a therapeutic measure, would mirror current guidelines for *C. difficile* management in people.

Providencia alcalifaciens

Providencia alcalifaciens, another rod-shaped gram-negative member of the Enterobacteriaceae family, has been linked to diarrhea in both humans and animals. *P. alcalifaciens* was detected in the feces of 41% of dogs with AHDS in an outbreak from Norway in 2019.[18] Non-culture-based methods (16S rRNA gene amplicon sequencing) indicated greater abundance of *Providencia* spp. in fecal samples from dogs with AHDS compared with healthy control dogs.[19] Further evidence supporting a potential etiological role has come from *in vitro* studies showing the potential of *P. alcalifaciens* to invade mammalian epithelial cells.[20] However, more work is required to establish *P. alcalifaciens* as a genuine canine enteropathogen.

Conclusion

Instances of both acute and chronic GI disease in cats and dogs can be attributed to the nefarious effects of enteric bacteria. However, their precise role in individual animals can be difficult to ascertain. Testing for bacterial enteropathogens is not routinely recommended in animals with GI disease because it is unlikely that the findings would prompt any change to the treatment plan. Fecal testing may be considered if the pet is presenting severe disease (e.g., potentially septic animal); in animals fed a raw diet, where carriage rates of zoonotic bacteria are higher; or when individuals in a household (either the pet or the owner) are immunocompromised. An awareness of common enteric pathogens also can offer epidemiological information in shelter or kennel situations that may guide infection-control measures. Targeted microbiological testing in such scenarios could include *C. difficile* (PCR for toxigenic genes and ELISA for toxins A and B), *C. jejuni* (PCR or MALDI-TOF MS), and *Salmonella* spp. (PCR or culture). *C. perfringens* is part of the microbiota in healthy dogs, and although netF toxin has been linked to AHDS, routine testing is not recommended because a positive result would not alter treatment recommendations. Similarly, testing for *E. coli* in feces has no value given its common presence in healthy dogs.

Most enteric bacterial infections are self-limited and will resolve within 3–5 days with appropriate supportive therapy. Antibiotic treatment is not recommended for the management of acute diarrhea unless there are signs of sepsis.[21] The high incidence of enteropathogenic and multidrug-resistant bacteria isolated from dogs consuming raw food, as well as directly from the food itself, is a significant concern. Owners should be discouraged from adopting raw-food diets due to the risk from zoonotic pathogens and should be educated about proper hygiene practices.

KEY POINTS

- Bacterial enteropathogens are found at similar frequencies in animals with and without GI disease, questioning their role in disease pathogenesis and the need for antibiotic therapy.
- Routine fecal testing for enteropathogens in fecal culture is not recommended because it does not offer actionable information to guide treatment.
- *Campylobacter* spp. and *Salmonella* spp. are significant zoonotic pathogens that may be acquired from exposure to pets, highlighting the importance of good hygiene practices.
- Raw feeding is associated with an increased risk of carriage of enteric bacteria.

References

1. Marks SL, Rankin SC, Byrne BA, Weese JS. Enteropathogenic bacteria in dogs and cats: diagnosis, epidemiology, treatment, and control. *J Vet Intern Med.* 25:1195–1208, 2011.
2. Kaindama L, Jenkins C, Aird H, et al. A cluster of Shiga toxin-producing *Escherichia coli* O157:H7 highlights raw pet food as an emerging potential source of infection in humans. *Epidemiol Infect.* 149:e124, 2021.
3. Craven M, Mansfield CS, Simpson KW. Granulomatous colitis of boxer dogs. *Vet Clin North Am Small Anim Pract.* 41:433–445, 2011.
4. Acke E. Campylobacteriosis in dogs and cats: a review. *N Z Vet J.* 66:221–228, 2018.
5. Parsons BN, Porter CJ, Ryvar R, et al. Prevalence of *Campylobacter* spp. in a cross-sectional study of dogs attending veterinary practices in the UK and risk indicators associated with shedding. *Vet J.* 184:66–70, 2010.
6. Pintar KDM, Christidis T, Thomas MK, et al. A systematic review and meta-analysis of the *Campylobacter* spp. prevalence and concentration in household pets and petting zoo animals for use in exposure assessments. *PLoS One.* 10:e0144976, 2015.
7. Martinez-Anton L, Marenda M, Firestone SM., et al. Investigation of the role of *Campylobacter* infection in suspected acute polyradiculoneuritis in dogs. *J Vet Intern Med.* 32:352–360, 2018.
8. Acke E, McGill K, Quinn T, et al. Antimicrobial resistance profiles and mechanisms of resistance in *Campylobacter jejuni* isolates from pets. *Foodborne Pathog Dis.* 6:705–710, 2009.
9. Viegas FM, Ramos CP, Xavier RGC, et al. Fecal shedding of *Salmonella* spp., *Clostridium perfringens*, and *Clostridioides difficile* in dogs fed raw meat-based diets in Brazil and their owners' motivation. *PLoS One.* 15:e0231275, 2020.
10. Srisanga S, Angkititrakul S, Sringam P, et al. Phenotypic and genotypic antimicrobial resistance and virulence genes of *Salmonella enterica* isolated from pet dogs and cats. *J Vet Sci.* 18:273–281, 2017.
11. Usmael B, Abraha B, Alemu S, et al. Isolation, antimicrobial susceptibility patterns, and risk factors assessment of non-typhoidal *Salmonella* from apparently healthy and diarrheic dogs. *BMC Vet Res.* 18:37, 2022.
12. Dow SW, Curtis CR, Jones RL, Wingfield WE. Bacterial culture of blood from critically ill dogs and cats: 100 cases (1985–1987). *J Am Vet Med Assoc.* 195:113–117, 1989.
13. Mehdizadeh Gohari I, Unterer S, Whitehead AE, Prescott JF. NetF-producing *Clostridium perfringens* and its associated diseases in dogs and foals. *J Vet Diagn Invest.* 32:230–238, 2020.
14. Leipig-Rudolph M, Busch K, Prescott JF, et al. Intestinal lesions in dogs with acute hemorrhagic diarrhea syndrome associated with netF-positive *Clostridium perfringens* type A. *J Vet Diagn Invest.* 30:495–503, 2018.
15. Sindern N, Suchodolski JS, Leutenegger CM, et al. Prevalence of *Clostridium perfringens* netE and netF toxin genes in the feces of dogs with acute hemorrhagic diarrhea syndrome. *J Vet Intern Med.* 33:100–105, 2019.
16. Ziese AL, Suchodolski JS, Hartmann K, et al. Effect of probiotic treatment on the clinical course, intestinal microbiome, and toxigenic *Clostridium perfringens* in dogs with acute hemorrhagic diarrhea. *PLoS One.* 13:e0204691, 2018.
17. Minamoto Y, Dhanani N, Markel ME, et al. Prevalence of *Clostridium perfringens*, *Clostridium perfringens* enterotoxin and dysbiosis in fecal samples of dogs with diarrhea. *Vet Microbiol.* 174:463–473, 2014.
18. Jørgensen HJ, Valheim M, Sekse C, et al. An official outbreak investigation of acute haemorrhagic diarrhoea in dogs in Norway points to *Providencia alcalifaciens* as a likely cause. *Animals (Basel).* 11:3201, 2021.
19. Herstad KMV, Trosvik P, Haaland AH, et al. Changes in the fecal microbiota in dogs with acute hemorrhagic diarrhea during an outbreak in Norway. *J Vet Intern Med.* 35:2177–2186, 2021.
20. Janda JM, Abbott SL, Woodward D, Khashe S. Invasion of HEp-2 and other eukaryotic cell lines by Providenciae: further evidence supporting the role of *Providencia alcalifaciens* in bacterial gastroenteritis. *Curr Microbiol.* 37:159–165, 1998.
21. Scahill K, Jessen LR, Prior C, et al. Efficacy of antimicrobial and nutraceutical treatment for canine acute diarrhoea: a systematic review and meta-analysis for European Network for Optimization of Antimicrobial Therapy (ENOVAT) guidelines. *Vet J.* 303:106054, 2024.
22. Watson VE, Jacob ME, Flowers JR, et al. Association of atypical enteropathogenic *Escherichia coli* with diarrhea and related mortality in kittens. *J Clin Microbiol.* 55:2719–2735, 2017.
23. Hald B, Pedersen K, Wainø M, et al. Longitudinal study of the excretion patterns of thermophilic *Campylobacter* spp. in young pet dogs in Denmark. *J Clin Microbiol.* 42:2003–2012 2004.
24. Parsons BN, Cody AJ, Porter CJ, et al. Typing of *Campylobacter jejuni* isolates from dogs by use of multilocus sequence typing and pulsed-field gel electrophoresis. *J Clin Microbiol.* 47:3466–3471, 2009.
25. Hascall KL, Kass PH, Saksen J, et al. Prevalence of enteropathogens in dogs attending 3 regional dog parks in Northern California. *J Vet Intern Med.* 30:1838–1845, 2016.

CHAPTER 38

Fungal, pseudofungal, and algal enteritides

Alyssa M. Sullivant
DVM, MS, DACVIM (SAIM)

Among the several types of infectious enteropathies are those caused by fungal, pseudofungal, and algal organisms. These infections may affect other organ systems apart from the gastrointestinal (GI) tract. The incidence varies by region, depending on the geographical distribution of the causative organisms. The most common fungal enteritis is caused by *Histoplasma capsulatum*. GI involvement is rare in cryptococcosis, coccidiomycosis, and blastomycosis. There are sporadic case reports of GI disease caused by saprophytic opportunistic fungal infections, such as basidiobolomycosis and mucormycosis. *Aspergillus fumigatus* primarily causes opportunistic sinonasal fungal infections, but GI aspergillosis has been reported rarely in immunocompromised dogs. Protothecosis is an uncommon algal infection that may affect the GI tract, particularly the large intestine. The fungal-like organism *Pythium insidiosum* may cause extensive GI disease.

Considering these infectious causes of enteritis as differentials is important when approaching cases of canine GI disease. The clinical features of deep mycotic and algal infections are similar and may mimic those of numerous other GI diseases. These infections can be challenging to treat, with some having a grave prognosis. Nevertheless, an early diagnosis may improve the clinical outcome. See Table 38.1 for a summary of the clinical highlights of fungal, pseudofungal, and algal enteritides.

Histoplasmosis

Etiology

H. capsulatum is a dimorphic fungus found worldwide, especially in subtropical and temperate regions. It is most commonly found along the Mississippi, Ohio, Missouri, and Tennessee river valleys in the USA but has also been reported in other US states, including Colorado and California.[1,2] Infection also occurs in Australia, Mexico, and Central and South America and has been reported in countries worldwide.[1,3] The fungus is found in the soil, especially in humid environments. Bats are the primary reservoir, but the organism can be found in decaying feces of birds as well.[1] Dogs (and cats) may become infected after exposure to bat guano or intestines or to decaying material contaminated with the mycelial form.[1] Infection occurs via inhalation of microconidia, which become yeasts over the next few weeks. The yeasts are phagocytosed by alveolar macrophages, which may contain the infection, or the organisms may spread via lymphatics and the bloodstream to cause disseminated disease. In addition to this classic route of infection, ingestion of microconidia may lead to GI infection.[4]

Clinical presentation

Young to middle-aged dogs are more likely to be affected. Hunting, sporting, and working dogs may be more predisposed, simply due to increased exposure to infected soil or bat feces, but English Pointers, Brittany Spaniels, and Weimaraners may be at increased risk.[5] Toy breeds may be more likely to develop GI histoplasmosis than the pulmonary form.[4]

H. capsulatum initially replicates in the lungs, where the infection may be eliminated by the immune system or remain subclinical.[6] In case of clinical infection, pulmonary signs such as coughing and tracheobronchial lymphadenopathy may ensue. Infection may be limited to the lungs, or it may disseminate via lymphatics or the bloodstream to the liver, spleen, eyes, bone marrow, skin, lymph nodes, bone, small and large intestine, and/or the central nervous system (CNS), where the organism incites pyogranulomatous inflammation. Clinical signs vary based on the organ system affected but include fever, lethargy, lymphadenopathy, hepatosplenomegaly, ascites, ocular pathology (e.g., uveitis, chorioretinitis), cutaneous lesions, icterus, and GI signs.[5,7,8] Seizures or tetraparesis may occur if the CNS is infected.[7,8] Patients may have GI disease with or without involvement of other organ systems. Both the small and large intestine may be affected, causing a variety of GI signs such as malabsorption, vomiting, diarrhea, hyporexia/anorexia, weight loss, diarrhea, and melena. Patients with large bowel involvement may have tenesmus, dyschezia, frequent defecation, hematochezia, and increased mucus in the stool. Histoplasmosis affecting the GI tract presents remarkably similar to inflammatory bowel disease. Physical examination findings in patients with the GI form may include thin body condition, lymphadenopathy, icterus, ascites, or abdominal pain. Clinical signs may

TABLE 38.1 Clinical highlights of fungal, pseudofungal, and algal enteritis.

Disease	Causative organism	Common gastrointestinal features	Diagnosis	Treatment
Histoplasmosis	Dimorphic fungus *Histoplasma capsulatum*, found in soil and bat droppings	Chronic small or large bowel signs, wall thickening or loss of wall layering	Cytology, serology, histopathology	Itraconazole or fluconazole Amphotericin B for disseminated disease Complete remission possible
Pythiosis	Oomycete *Pythium insidiosum*, found in aquatic and marginal plant environments	Chronic small or large bowel signs, regurgitation, GI obstruction, weight loss, transmural masses, wall thickening or loss of wall layering	Cytology, serology, histopathology, tissue PCR	Aggressive surgical resection followed by itraconazole and terbinafine Without surgery or with incomplete resection: itraconazole, terbinafine, prednisone, and mefenoxam Variable treatment success
Zygomycosis	Saprophytic fungi, including *Conidiobolus* spp., *Rhizopus* spp., and *Basidiobolus* spp.	Acute or chronic small or large bowel signs, mass lesions, wall thickening or loss of wall layering	Cytology, histopathology, culture, tissue PCR	Itraconazole or amphotericin B Limited treatment success
Protothecosis	Achlorophyllous algae *Prototheca* spp., found in various water sources, sewage, tree slime, and decaying organic matter	Hematochezia, tenesmus, dyschezia, mucus in stool, colonic wall thickening or loss of wall layering	Cytology, histopathology, culture	Itraconazole or amphotericin B Limited treatment success

be acute or chronic, and many patients have signs for months before a diagnosis is made.

Clinicopathological findings

Anemia is found in >50% of dogs with histoplasmosis due to GI hemorrhage, chronic inflammation, or bone marrow involvement.[7–9] Thrombocytopenia or neutropenia may occur due to bone marrow infection, sequestration, or consumption. Other complete blood count findings may include neutrophilia and eosinophilia.[7–9] Clotting times (prothrombin and/or partial thromboplastin times) may be prolonged in more advanced cases with disseminated intravascular coagulation or hepatic dysfunction.

Hypoalbuminemia is a common finding, seen in >75% of patients, and may be due to GI losses, hepatic dysfunction, malabsorption, and/or proteinuria.[4] Hyperglobulinemia may also occur. Hepatic enzyme (alanine aminotransferase, alkaline phosphatase, gamma-glutamyltransferase) activity increases and hyperbilirubinemia may occur in case of hepatic involvement. Hypoglycemia, low blood urea, and hypocholesterolemia may be present in patients with liver dysfunction. Pleural or peritoneal effusion is possible and is usually a transudate or modified transudate. Urinalysis may reveal proteinuria due to glomerular involvement.

Diagnosis

A definitive diagnosis of histoplasmosis may be achieved via cytology, serology, or histopathology on surgical or endoscopic biopsies, depending on the location of the lesions. The yeasts are 2–4 µm in diameter, have an oval shape and a basophilic center, and can be extracellular or intracellular within macrophages.[1] They have a characteristic clear halo surrounding them.[1] Cytology of lymph nodes, liver, spleen, GI lesions, rectal scrapes (Fig. 38.1), and effusions inconsistently yields the organism but often reveals the associated pyogranulomatous, suppurative, or granulomatous inflammation.

If a cytological diagnosis cannot be made, or if there is any doubt about the type of fungus seen, serology is indicated. Specifically, an enzyme immunoassay for *Histoplasma* antigen in the urine of dogs has a sensitivity of 89.5% and a specificity for fungal vs. nonfungal disease as high as 100%.[10] The assay detects galactomannan in the fungal cell wall, but the specificity depends on the geographical region. Cross-reactivity with *Blastomyces* spp., *Paracoccidioides* spp., *Coccidiodes* spp., *Aspergillus* spp., and *Penicillium mameffei* occurs, but given that GI histoplasmosis is significantly more common than GI infection by any of these other organisms, a positive result in a patient with GI signs is most consistent with histoplasmosis.[10] This is the preferred serological test in dogs (and cats) for detection of *Histoplasma* and for serial monitoring during therapy. Detection of anti-*Histoplasma* serum antibodies via enzyme immunoassay is helpful in 5–10% of patients without detectable *Histoplasma* antigen in the urine, with a diagnostic sensitivity of 77% and specificity of 93% in dogs.[11] Culturing tissue or fluid for *Histoplasma* may take several weeks for results and is not routinely recommended or performed.

Endoscopic findings are nonspecific and may include mucosal granularity and ulcerations of the small or large intestine. Histopathology of surgical or endoscopic tissue samples of the GI tract reveals pyogranulomatous or granulomatous inflammation surrounding *Histoplasma* yeasts. Periodic acid–Schiff or Gomori's methenamine silver stain improves detection of *Histoplasma* organism in tissues.

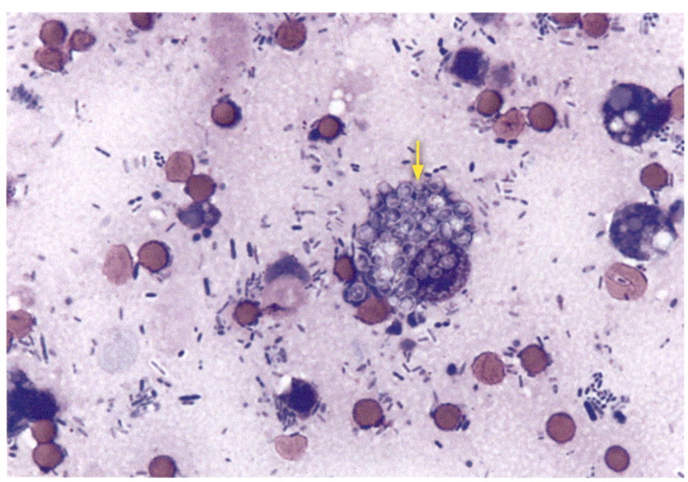

FIG. 38.1 Rectal scrape cytology showing *Histoplasma* organisms (arrow).

Diagnostic imaging findings

Pulmonary histoplasmosis manifests radiographically as an interstitial, alveolar, or bronchial pattern. Sternal and tracheobronchial lymphadenopathy and pleural effusion may be evident. Abdominal radiographs may show peritoneal effusion and hepatosplenomegaly. Bony lesions may also be seen on radiographs.

Ultrasound findings vary from diffuse or regional wall thickening (mucosal, submucosal, and/or muscularis layers) to abnormal wall layering (Fig. 38.2).[9] Abnormalities associated with infiltrative GI disease may be diffuse, multifocal, or focal. In a report of 19 dogs with GI histoplasmosis, 18 had abnormal findings in the GI tract on ultrasonography.[9] Colonic thickening and abnormal wall layering were the most frequent (16/19) findings. Colonic wall thickness ranged from 0.36 to 1.2 cm. Peritoneal effusion was noted in 8 dogs, and abdominal lymphadenopathy was also common, with some lymph nodes measuring ≥2 cm.

Treatment

Systemic antifungals are the treatment of choice and are necessary for at least 6 months; although some chronic cases may require treatment for more than 12 months. Itraconazole (5 mg/kg PO q12h or 10 mg/kg PO q24h) or fluconazole (5–10 mg/kg PO q12h) are preferred.[4] Prognosis is similar with either drug, and the rate of relapse does not differ.[4] In case of ocular or CNS involvement, fluconazole should be chosen because of better drug penetration. Short-term administration of an anti-inflammatory dose of glucocorticoids to mitigate the overwhelming inflammation associated with organism die-off early in therapy has been a common practice; however, no benefit has been shown to support steroid use. Hepatotoxicity may occur with either azole; therefore, liver values should be monitored. Amphotericin B should be administered to patients with severe pulmonary, disseminated, or CNS disease, followed by itraconazole or fluconazole. Newer azoles, posaconazole and voriconazole, are effective in cases of feline histoplasmosis, and future studies may prove them effective in dogs.

Therapeutic drug monitoring is available for itraconazole and should be considered if treatment response is slow or minimal. The author monitors antigenuria via enzyme immunoassay 1 month into therapy, and every 3 months thereafter. Treatment should be continued for 1 month beyond resolution of clinical signs and radiographic/ultrasonographic lesions and until resolution of antigenuria. In a group of dogs with pulmonary, disseminated, or GI histoplasmosis, the remission rate was 67%.[4] Relapses occurred in 21% of cases. Negative prognostic factors reported by this study included the Great Pyrenees breed, icterus, dyspnea, need for oxygen supplementation, anemia, hypercalcemia, and palpable abdominal organomegaly.

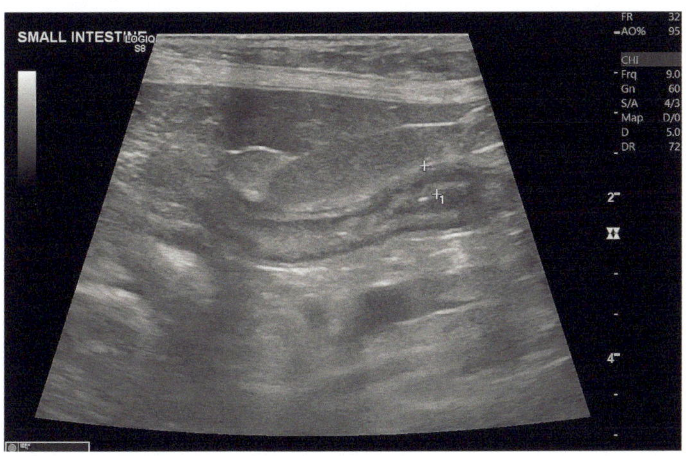

FIG. 38.2 Ultrasonographic image of small intestinal wall thickening of the serosal, mucosal, and muscularis layers caused by histoplasmosis.

Protothecosis

Etiology

Prototheca species are achlorophyllous, saprophytic algae ubiquitous in nature, especially in warm, humid climates in water sources where decaying organic matter is found. They are predominantly distributed in southern and southeastern USA, northeastern Australia, and parts of Europe and Japan.[12] Sources of infection include fish tanks, soil, sewage, tree slime, fresh or saltwater, and animal waste.[13] There are several known species that affect the skin or cause systemic disease. Protothecosis in dogs is rare, but it may affect the skin or, more commonly, the GI tract, eyes, and CNS. The disseminated and GI forms in dogs are caused by *Prototheca zopfii*. Ingestion or cutaneous inoculation and subsequent hematogenous or lymphatic dissemination are the most likely routes of infection.

Clinical presentation

Most dogs with protothecosis are not immunosuppressed.[12] Collies and Boxers may be predisposed.[14,15] GI protothecosis predominantly affects the large intestine, causing acute or chronic hematochezia, diarrhea with mucus, tenesmus, and dyschezia. Affected dogs eventually become thin and hyporexic or anorexic. Severe ocular and neurological signs may also be present, and dissemination to other organ systems occurs.[14,15] Small bowel diarrhea, melena, or vomiting may be seen if the small intestine, pancreas, or liver are affected.

Clinicopathological findings

Patients with GI protothecosis often have a normal complete blood count. Anemia may be present due to hematochezia or chronic disease. Neutrophilia or eosinophilia may be present. Serum biochemistry panels may reveal hypoalbuminemia and hyperglobulinemia.

Diagnosis

Prototheca organisms are readily seen on cytology of affected lymph nodes or rectal scrapes (Fig. 38.3), or even in urine sediment.[12] They may appear similar to *Blastomyces*, *Coccidioides*, or *Cryptococcus*. The organisms are bean-shaped, ovoid, or elliptical, with a thick cell wall that does not stain. *Prototheca* species range in size from 1.5 to 30 μm.[16] Multiple daughter cells may be seen inside the cell. *Prototheca* grows readily within days on routine culture media. Culturing affected tissue or aspirates is recommended to confirm the diagnosis. Colonoscopy findings are nonspecific and may include friable, inflamed, irregular, or ulcerated mucosa. Histopathology of colonic mucosal biopsies reveals numerous sporulating or nonsporulating organisms, surrounded by mild to severe mixed or granulomatous inflammation.[12,14] Gomori's methenamine silver or periodic acid–Schiff stain improves visualization of the organisms (Fig. 38.3).

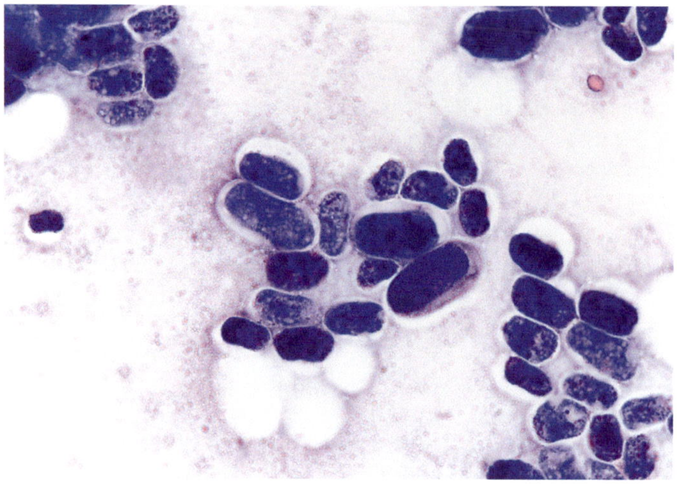

FIG. 38.3 Rectal scrape cytology showing *Prototheca* organisms in a patient with hematochezia. Wright's stain.

Diagnostic imaging findings

Thickened colonic walls and loss of colonic wall layering are typical ultrasonographic findings, along with abdominal lymphadenopathy. However, ultrasound may reveal no significant abnormalities.

Treatment

Treatment of disseminated or GI protothecosis is very challenging. Success with oral azoles alone is rare, but itraconazole with or without amphotericin B has proven effective in a limited number of cases.[14] Amphotericin B is the treatment of choice in dogs with disseminated disease. While remission is possible, relapse is almost inevitable, and the disease is nearly always fatal, with patients succumbing to disease within weeks to several months of diagnosis.[14,15] Supportive therapy for *Prototheca* colitis may include sulfasalazine, fiber, and pain control.

Pythiosis and zygomycosis

Etiology

P. insidiosum and *Lagenidium* spp. are water molds of the class Oomycetes. Clinically, they cause deep mycotic infections, affecting the skin and/or GI tract of dogs (and cats), although lagenidiosis has not been reported in the canine GI tract. Because these organisms lack ergosterol in their cell walls, they are not true fungi; therefore, the disease is referred to as a pseudofungal infection.

P. insidiosum is found globally in tropical and subtropical climates, including Southeast Asia, South America, and eastern Australia.[17] In the USA, the disease occurs most often in the Gulf Coast and the Southeast; however, it has been reported in the East Coast, the Midwest, and the western states.[18] The infective zoospores are found in aquatic environments near plant material and enter via skin wounds or via the GI tract by ingestion of contaminated water or plants/grass.[17] Infection occurs when zoospores encyst and cause progressive, severe cutaneous or GI disease.

Zygomycetes are true saprophytic fungi which are often grouped with *P. insidiosum* and *Lagenidium* spp. due to the similarities in their clinical presentation and histological findings. However, it is very important to distinguish pythiosis and lagenidiosis from zygomycosis, because the therapeutic approaches and prognoses differ significantly. Organisms that cause zygomycosis, such as *Basidiobolus* spp., *Conidiobolus* spp., and *Mucor* spp., have recently been reclassified, and the infections they cause are now called entomophthoromycosis and mucormycosis (although the term *zygomycosis* is still commonly used to refer to infection with these emerging pathogens).[17] Infections are rare, but case reports of basidiobolomycosis and conidiobolomycosis (two types of entomophthoromycoses) and mucormycosis affecting the GI tract have been published.[19–21]

These fungi live in soil, stagnant water, and the GI tract of some fish, amphibians, reptiles, and bats[17,20,21] and may cause infection of the skin, GI tract, or other organ systems if the spores are inoculated into the skin, ingested, or inhaled, respectively. GI lesions caused by *Basidiobolus* spp., *Rhizopus* spp., and *Conidiobolus* spp. have been reported in dogs.[19–21] Immunosuppression may predispose dogs to these infections but is not a consistent risk factor among affected patients.[19–21]

Clinical presentation

Young, large-breed outdoor dogs are predisposed to pythiosis. Most affected patients have either cutaneous manifestations (ulcerations, draining tracts, and/or nodular lesions) or the GI form. Esophageal, pharyngeal, and pulmonary pythiosis have also been reported in dogs.[22–24] GI pythiosis is characterized by severe, segmental transmural thickening of the wall of the stomach, intestines, colon, or rectum.[23,25,26] Lesions progress to large granulomatous masses that are often palpable and cause partial or complete GI obstruction, with some lesions measuring several centimeters in diameter.[25] The pyloric region, proximal duodenum, ileocolic junction, and descending colon are the most frequently affected sites.[26,27] Mesenteric lymph node involvement is common and may cause severely enlarged, palpable lesions. Patients are frequently thin or cachexic, with a chronic history of weight loss (Fig. 38.4), anorexia/hyporexia, vomiting, small or large bowel diarrhea, hematochezia, melena, fever, and/or regurgitation.

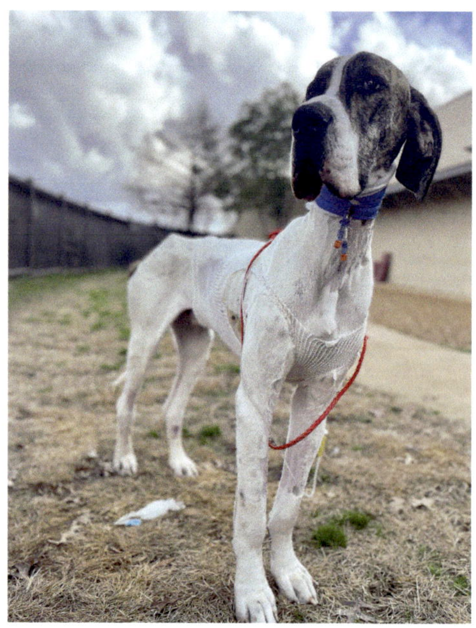

FIG. 38.4 Cachexic 1-year-old male Great Dane with gastroduodenal and colonic pythiosis.

Clinicopathological findings

Complete blood count and serum biochemistry panels in patients with pythiosis frequently reveal eosinophilia, anemia, hyperglobulinemia, and hypoalbuminemia.[17,25] In 10 dogs with GI pythiosis from California, 7/9 had a mild nonregenerative anemia and eosinophilia.[25] In the same cohort of dogs, 9/9 had hypoalbuminemia ranging from 16 to 29 g/L (reference range 30–44 g/L) and 8/9 had mild to moderate hyperglobulinemia. Hypercalcemia appears to be uncommon in patients with GI pythiosis. Laboratory abnormalities in cases with GI zygomycosis are not well-defined, but case reports indicate that eosinophilia and hyperglobulinemia are common findings.[19–21]

Diagnosis

Aspiration cytology, fluid cytology, or impression smear analysis of lymph nodes or lesions associated with pythiosis, entomophthoromycosis, and mucormycosis show pyogranulomatous and eosinophilic inflammation, with large, broad, nonseptate hyphae that are negatively staining to slightly basophilic and have nonparallel walls and acute to right-angle branching (Fig. 38.5).[17,28] *P. insidiosum* hyphae measure 3–8 µm in diameter and have rounded, tapered ends.[28] The hyphal diameter of *Basidiobolus* spp. and *Conidiobolus* spp. is larger, at 5–30 µm and 5–15 µm, respectively.[20,21,28] Some cytological features may help distinguish these organisms, but additional testing is recommended due to their similar cytological appearance but significant differences in treatment and outcome.

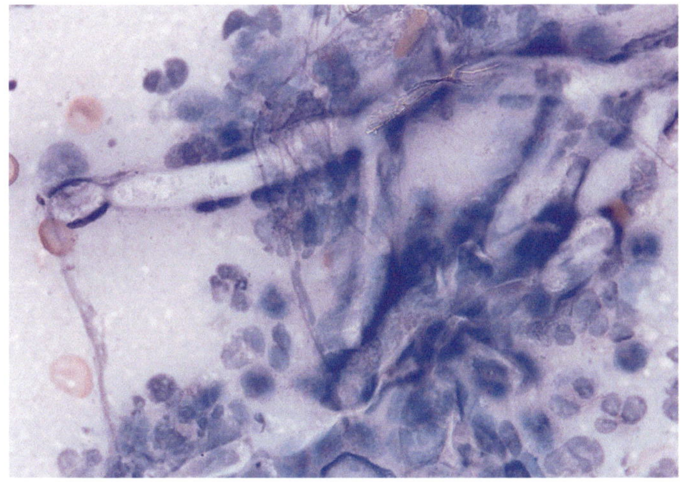

FIG. 38.5 Aspiration cytology of a gastric mass showing pyogranulomatous inflammation and negatively stained *Pythium insidiosum* hyphae.

Serological testing is widely used in the diagnosis of pythiosis. ELISA for the detection of antibodies against *P. insidiosum* is highly sensitive. Antibody titers decrease with successful therapy.[29] This assay is not very specific due to cross-reactivity with *Lagenidium* spp., zygomycetes, and other fungi.[17,20,21,29] Therefore, a combination of ELISA, histopathology, and PCR methodologies that identify genus and species is recommended to maximize the chance of an accurate diagnosis. Culture of fresh diseased GI or lymph node tissue for detection of *P. insidiosum* is possible, but special handling and culture techniques by laboratories with experience in culturing oomycetes are required. Fungal culture with subsequent sequencing for species identification is helpful in the diagnosis of zygomycosis and should be performed at laboratories with expertise and experience with these organisms. A species-specific panfungal PCR assay with variable sensitivity may be performed on fresh, frozen, or paraffin-embedded tissues or cultured isolates.[30]

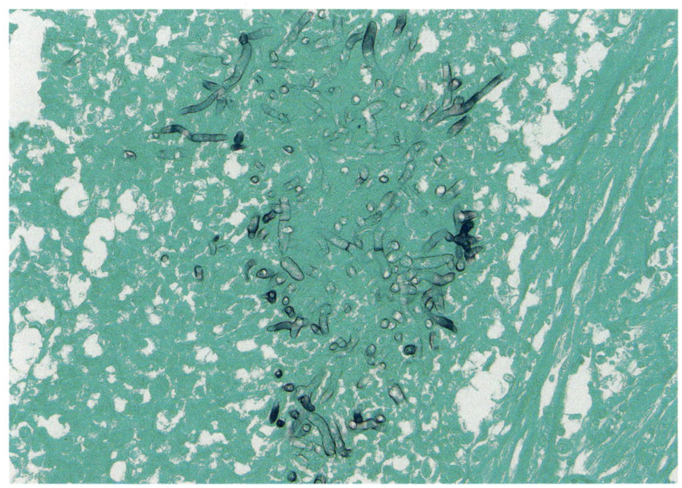

FIG. 38.6 *Pythium insidiosum* hyphae demonstrated with Gomori's methenamine silver stain in a biopsy of a colonic mass.

Histopathological features of *P. insidiosum* include granulomas in the wall of the GI tract and intense eosinophilic and granulomatous inflammation within the mucosal, submucosal, and muscularis layers. These deeper structures may be missed with endoscopic mucosal biopsies. Hyphae do not stain well, or at all, with routine hematoxylin and eosin, but they are readily visible with Gomori's methenamine silver stain (Fig. 38.6). Cytological and histological features of zygomycosis are almost indistinguishable from those of pythiosis, except for a few hyphal characteristics. Zygomycetes have a much wider eosinophilic sleeve surrounding the hyphae than *P. insidiosum*.[17]

Diagnostic imaging findings

Abdominal imaging is vital for localizing lesions caused by these organisms, especially those caused by *P. insidiosum*. Radiography may show mass lesions and possibly GI obstructions. Ultrasound findings include severe segmental, transmural thickening with loss of wall layering and lymphadenopathy (Fig. 38.7).[26] Computed tomography findings in

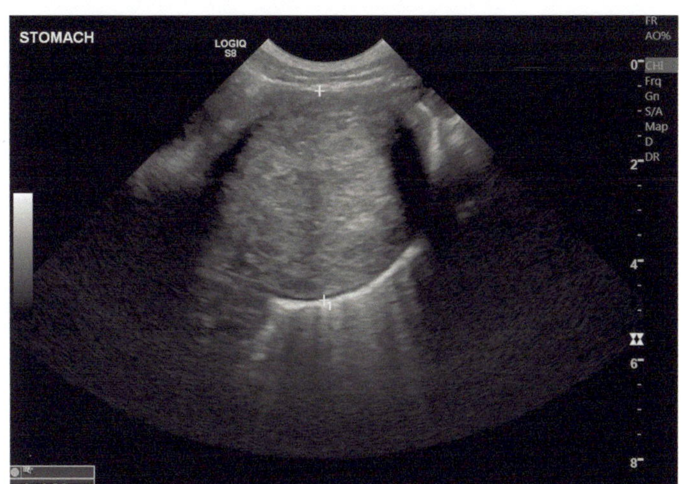

FIG. 38.7 Ultrasonographic image of a gastric mass caused by *Pythium insidiosum*, showing transmural thickening and loss of wall layering.

noncutaneous pythiosis have recently been well described. Lesions were intramural in 23/23 dogs and were usually focal (14/23), well-defined, smoothly marginated, and heterogeneously contrast enhancing.[27] In 12/19 dogs, two or more regions of the GI tract were affected.[27] For zygomycosis, reported abdominal imaging findings are similar to those of pythiosis or histoplasmosis, including wall thickening, loss of wall layering, and mass lesions centered around the submucosa.

Treatment

Treatment for pythiosis has evolved over the last years. The mainstay of therapy has been aggressive surgical resection with 4–5 cm margins plus medical management with antifungals for several months to treat microscopic disease and prevent recurrence.[31] The combination of itraconazole (10 mg/kg PO q24h) and terbinafine (5–10 mg/kg PO q24h) is recommended for 2–6 months after surgery. ELISA serology is used to monitor for recurrence and treatment success. Therapy should not be discontinued until antibody titers decrease at least 50%.[17]

Medical therapy should be considered in patients that do not undergo surgery or if aggressive surgical resection is not possible or would require a procedure associated with increased morbidity and mortality (e.g., Billroth II). Success with antifungals alone is limited because the cell wall of *P. insidiosum* lacks ergosterol, the primary target of azole antifungals and amphotericin B. Over the last years, the addition of steroids and mefenoxam to the treatment regimen of itraconazole and terbinafine has improved survival times. Three cases of nonresectable colonic pythiosis treated with prednisone, terbinafine, and itraconazole achieved remission as determined by decreasing serological titers and ultrasonographic resolution of lesions.[32] These patients were still alive years after diagnosis. Prednisone alone has also achieved resolution of GI pythiosis in a few anecdotal cases.[17] Because of this apparent benefit, treatment recommendations for nonresectable GI pythiosis include itraconazole, terbinafine, and prednisone. Ultrasound should be repeated after approximately 1 month, and if improvement is noted, prednisone is continued at the same dose, and eventually tapered slowly.[17] Antifungals are given for at least 6 months, and serial monitoring using ELISA serology is recommended to gauge treatment success or relapse.

Mefenoxam is an agricultural antifungal and antioomycete compound that impairs RNA synthesis in fungal zoospores.[33] Successful outcomes have been reported with the addition of 8 mg/kg/day oral mefenoxam to the itraconazole and terbinafine regimen, with or without surgical resection.[34] In a case series of five dogs with GI pythiosis, patients that underwent surgical resection followed by therapy with mefenoxam, itraconazole, and terbinafine (three dogs) were alive at the end of the follow-up period (287–443 days).[34] Two of the dogs had Billroth procedures performed, but with incomplete margins. Of the two dogs treated with mefenoxam, itraconazole, and terbinafine alone, one was alive 210 days after initiation of therapy. Successful treatment with mefenoxam alone has not yet been reported. A retrospective study summarized the use of mefenoxam in GI pythiosis from 2013 to 2020 and found that, when given with other therapeutic interventions, a 31% cure rate was achieved.[34] Most of the dogs received a combination therapy with minocycline, terbinafine, and steroids. No adverse effects were noted, but pharmacokinetic and safety studies with mefenoxam are needed. Based on the current literature, mefenoxam may be beneficial for the treatment of nonresectable or partially resected GI pythiosis when combined with antifungals and steroids.

Another therapy for pythiosis is minocycline, which has in vitro efficacy against *P. insidiosum*. However, efficacy as a sole therapy has not been proven, and further investigation is needed. Immunotherapy improves the outcome of equine cutaneous cases but has shown no benefit in dogs and is therefore not recommended at this time.

Treatment with antifungals, such as itraconazole, terbinafine, and amphotericin B, has been attempted in patients with GI, cutaneous, and disseminated zygomycosis, with success reported rarely. Prognosis is typically grave for the GI and disseminated forms. Further research and treatment trials are needed in this area of emerging diseases in dogs.

KEY POINTS

- Histoplasmosis is the most common cause of fungal enteritis in dogs. The stomach and/or intestine may be affected, and clinical signs may be present for weeks or months prior to diagnosis. Diagnosis is obtained by cytology or histopathology as well as urine antigen testing. Treatment with azole antifungals may achieve complete remission. Serial monitoring of urine antigen is helpful during treatment.
- Pythiosis may cause severe gastrointestinal lesions in dogs. The esophagus, stomach, intestine, and/or rectum may be affected. Patients have chronic vomiting, diarrhea, and weight loss. Diagnosis is made through a combination of cytology, histopathology with special stains, serology, and PCR. Wide surgical resection followed by itraconazole and terbinafine is the mainstay of therapy. If surgery is not possible or resection is incomplete, medical therapy with itraconazole, terbinafine, and prednisone should be considered. Mefenoxam is an agricultural fungicide that may be added to the treatment protocol. Remission is possible, but treatment success varies.
- *Zygomycosis* is a term historically used to describe infections with certain saprophytic fungi. Cytological and histopathological features are almost indistinguishable from those caused by *Pythium insidiosum*; therefore, culture and PCR are recommended for diagnosis. Case reports of gastrointestinal zygomycosis are sporadic, and most cases are fatal.
- Protothecosis primarily affects the large intestine and is diagnosed via rectal scrape cytology, histopathology, and tissue culture. Treatment success using itraconazole or amphotericin B is limited. Most cases are fatal.

References

1. Reagan KL, Sykes JE. Histoplasmosis. In: Sykes JE (ed.). *Greene's Infectious Diseases of the Dog and Cat*, 5th ed. London: Elsevier. pp. 1003–1013; 2022.
2. Johnson LR, Fry MM, Anez KL, et al. Histoplasmosis infection in two cats from California. *J Am Anim Hosp Assoc* 40(2):165–169, 2004.
3. Mackie JT, Kaufman L, Ellis D. Confirmed histoplasmosis in an Australian dog. *Aust Vet J* 75(5):362–363, 1997.
4. Wilson AG, KuKanich KS, Hanzlicek AS, Payton ME. Clinical signs, treatment, and prognostic factors for dogs with histoplasmosis. *J Am Vet Med Assoc* 252(2):201–209, 2018.
5. Selby LA, Becker SV, Hayes HW Jr. Epidemiologic risk factors associated with canine systemic mycoses. *Am J Epidemiol* 113(2):133–139, 1981.
6. Emmons CW, Rowley DA, Olson BJ, et al. Histoplasmosis; proved occurrence of inapparent infection in dogs, cats and other animals. *Am J Hyg* 61(1):40–44, 1955.
7. Mitchell M, Stark DR. Disseminated canine histoplasmosis: a clinical survey of 24 cases in Texas. *Can Vet J* 21(3):95–100, 1980.
8. Clinkenbeard KD, Cowell RL, Tyler RD. Disseminated histoplasmosis in dogs: 12 cases (1981-1986). *J Am Vet Med Assoc* 193(11):1443–1447, 1988.
9. Chávez-Peón Berle E, KuKanich K, Biller D. Ultrasonographic findings of gastrointestinal histoplasmosis in dogs. *Vet Radiol Ultrasound* 62(1):108–115, 2021.
10. Cunningham L, Cook A, Hanzlicek A, et al. Sensitivity and specificity of *Histoplasma* antigen detection by enzyme immunoassay. *J Am Anim Hosp Assoc* 51(5):306–310, 2015.
11. Tims R, Hanzlicek AS, Nafe L, et al. Evaluation of an enzyme immunoassay and immunodiffusion for detection of anti-*Histoplasma* antibodies in serum from cats and dogs. *J Vet Intern Med* 37(3):1007–1014, 2023.
12. Sykes JE. Protothecosis and chlorellosis. In: Sykes JE (ed.). *Greene's Infectious Diseases of the Dog and Cat*, 5th ed. London: Elsevier. pp. 1126–1134; 2022.
13. Pore RS, Barnett EA, Barnes WC Jr, Walker JD. Prototheca ecology. *Mycopathologia* 81(1):49-62, 1983.
14. Stenner VJ, Mackay B, King T, et al. Protothecosis in 17 Australian dogs and a review of the canine literature. *Med Mycol* 45(3):249–266, 2007.
15. Vince AR, Pinard C, Ogilvie AT, et al. Protothecosis in a dog. *Can Vet J* 55(10):950–954, 2014.
16. Whipple KM, Wellehan JF, Jeon AB, et al. Cytologic, histologic, microbiologic, and electron microscopic characterization of a canine *Prototheca wickerhamii* infection. *Vet Clin Pathol* 49(2):326–332, 2020.
17. Grooters AM. Pythiosis, lagenidiosis, paralagenidiosis, entomophthoromycosis, and mucormycosis. In: Sykes JE (ed.). *Greene's Infectious Diseases of the Dog and Cat*, 5th ed. London: Elsevier. pp. 1105–1117; 2022.
18. Nguyen D, Vilela R, Miraglia BM, et al. Geographic distribution of *Pythium insidiosum* infections in the United States. *J Am Vet Med Assoc* 260(5):530–534, 2021.
19. Alves RC, Ferreira JS, Alves AS, et al. Systemic and gastrohepatic mucormycosis in dogs. *J Comp Pathol* 175:90–94, 2020.
20. Black A, Wiertek M, Ferguson S, et al. Case report: Localized coloproctitis caused by novel *Basidiobolus arizonensis* in a dog. *Front Vet Sci* 11:1427496, 2024.
21. Mackey PE, Cappe KG, Mani R, et al. Disseminated *Conidiobolus incongruus* in a dog: A case report and literature review. *Med Mycol Case Rep* 8:24–28, 2015.
22. Patton CS, Hake R, Newton J, Toal RL. Esophagitis due to *Pythium insidiosum* infection in two dogs. *J Vet Intern Med* 10(3):139–142, 1996.
23. Helman RG, Oliver J 3rd. Pythiosis of the digestive tract in dogs from Oklahoma. *J Am Anim Hosp Assoc* 35(2):111–114, 1999.
24. Kepler D, Cole R, Lee-Fowler T, et al. Pulmonary pythiosis in a canine patient. *Vet Radiol Ultrasound* 60(2):E20–E23, 2019.
25. Berryessa NA, Marks SL, Pesavento PA, et al. Gastrointestinal pythiosis in 10 dogs from California. *J Vet Intern Med* 22(4):1065–1069, 2008.
26. Graham JP, Newell SM, Roberts GD, Lester NV. Ultrasonographic features of canine gastrointestinal pythiosis. *Vet Radiol Ultrasound* 41(3):273–277, 2000.
27. Hamlin AN, Locker S, Huguet E, et al. Computed tomographic characteristics of confirmed and presumed noncutaneous pythiosis in 25 dogs. *Vet Radiol Ultrasound* 65(2):87–98, 2024.
28. Dehghanpir SD. Cytomorphology of deep mycoses in dogs and cats. *Vet Clin North Am Small Anim Pract* 53(1):155–173, 2023.
29. Grooters AM, Leise BS, Lopez MK, et al. Development and evaluation of an enzyme-linked immunosorbent assay for the serodiagnosis of pythiosis in dogs. *J Vet Intern Med* 16(2):142–146, 2002.
30. Meason-Smith C, Edwards EE, Older CE, et al. Panfungal polymerase chain reaction for identification of fungal pathogens in formalin-fixed animal tissues. *Vet Pathol* 54(4):640–648, 2017.
31. Schmiedt CW, Stratton-Phelps M, Torres BT, et al. Treatment of intestinal pythiosis in a dog with a combination of marginal excision, chemotherapy, and immunotherapy. *J Am Vet Med Assoc* 241(3):358–363, 2012.
32. Reagan KL, Marks SL, Pesavento PA, et al. Successful management of 3 dogs with colonic pythiosis using itraconzaole, terbinafine, and prednisone. *J Vet Intern Med* 33(3):1434–1439, 2019.
33. Billings P, Walton S, Shmalberg J, Santoro D. The use of mefenoxam to treat cutaneous and gastrointestinal pythiosis in dogs: a retrospective study. *Microorganisms* 11(7):1726, 2023.
34. Cridge H, Hughes SM, Langston VC, Mackin AJ. Mefenoxam, itraconazole, and terbinafine combination therapy for management of pythiosis in dogs (six cases). *J Am Anim Hosp Assoc* 56(6):307, 2020.

CHAPTER 39

Protozoal infections

Ian Wright
BVMS, BSc, MSc, MRCVS

A wide range of intestinal protozoa with an ample global geographic distribution commonly infect dogs. The most common with clinical significance are *Giardia* spp., flagellant protozoa inhabiting the small intestine, and members of the Apicomplexan group, including *Cystoisospora* and *Cryptosporidium* species. Although flagellates and apicomplexan protozoa are very different parasites, they share the potential to cause primary intestinal disease through the presence of developing life stages or to contribute to multifactorial gastrointestinal (GI) disease. The zoonotic potential should also be considered in the case of *Giardia* and *Cryptosporidium* infections.

Giardia duodenalis

Giardia duodenalis (also known as *G. intestinalis*) is a flagellate protozoan that inhabits the intestines of a wide variety of both domestic and wild animals. Many infections are subclinical in nature, and the prevalence in host populations is high.[1] This can make it difficult to establish the significance of infection when it is found in animals with GI signs. With possible *Giardia* resistance developing to chemotherapeutic agents,[2] considering whether treatment is required, and how to make it as effective as possible, is vital before embarking on a treatment program for this parasite.

Life cycle and zoonotic risk

Giardia spp. live in the small intestine as flagellate trophozoites dividing by binary fission. These trophozoites will intermittently form infective cysts, which are passed in the feces. Transmission then occurs via the fecal–oral route. Cysts may enter environments contaminated by feces, contaminate food, or adhere to the coat of pets soiled with feces. Cysts have the potential to be long-lived in the environment, especially in cool, damp conditions. Many species of *Giardia* are species-specific, but *G. duodenalis* infects a wide variety of mammals, including humans, cats, and dogs. It is currently classified into ten subgroups or assemblages, with each assemblage infecting one or more host species, although cross infections can occur in immunocompromised hosts. Dog and cat assemblages are relatively species-specific. In contrast, human infection most commonly occurs with assemblages A and B, which can also infect cats and dogs if they are exposed to environmental contamination from human infection. This enables human infection to be cycled through pets, allowing zoonotic exposure. Anyone infected with *Giardia* should maintain strict hygiene with their pets and avoid contact with cats and dogs if possible until their infection has been resolved.

Canine giardiasis

Many infections in otherwise healthy dogs are subclinical, but *Giardia* has the potential to cause GI disturbances or contribute to multifactorial intestinal disease. There are no pathognomonic clinical signs for giardiasis, but the most common sign is chronic, small intestinal diarrhea that may be intermittent in nature. This diarrhea is often foul smelling and accompanied by flatulence. Occasional involvement of the large bowel and tenesmus may be seen. Clinical disease is most likely to occur in young or immunosuppressed animals. The clinical picture can be complicated by concurrent GI disease. Mixed infections of *Giardia*, *Campylobacter*, and *Cystoisospora* are common in puppies. The prognosis for clinical cases is generally very favorable, although young, debilitated, geriatric, or immunocompromised dogs are more likely to be severely affected. *Giardia* should be considered as a differential diagnosis in the investigation of all diarrhea cases in dogs, but it should not be assumed to be the sole cause of disease if identified.

Diagnosis

The following methods can be used in the diagnosis of infection with *Giardia*:

- Direct smear examination of fresh feces: Direct smears can be used for the detection of *Giardia* trophozoites and cysts in the feces. A small quantity (about the size of a match head) of fresh (warm) feces is mixed with warm saline. Active trophozoites may then be identified. These have a "falling leaf" motion, have a concave sucker, and are binucleate. Fresh feces need to be kept warm and examined immediately or cysts are more likely to be observed. Cysts are small (approximately 15 µm), with a flagellum sometimes visible crossing the ova in an S shape. The sensitivity of direct smear examination in detecting *Giardia* cysts is low, and fecal flotation techniques are required to improve sensitivity.

- Fecal flotation: Fecal samples should be collected for three consecutive days to increase sensitivity, as shedding of cysts is often intermittent. Concentration methods such as SAFC (sodium acetate–acetic acid–formalin-concentration) or MIFC (merthiolate–iodine–formalin concentration) result in a higher sensitivity, but when performed with centrifugation, simple flotation techniques can be performed in-house with reasonable sensitivity. Commercial zinc sulphate preparations with slightly lower specific gravity than those used for worm ova flotations will improve *Giardia* detection rates, as there will be less distortion of the cysts (see Fig. 19.1F).
- Antigen detection in feces: Fecal antigen ELISA tests have a high sensitivity, are relatively cheap, and are rapid to perform. They will, however, detect recently treated as well as current infections. They may also detect extremely low parasite burdens, which are of no clinical relevance.
- PCR: PCR tests for *Giardia* infection also have a high sensitivity and specificity and may also give false positives for a short period of time after infection has cleared. Some PCR tests have the advantage of being able to assess the zoonotic potential of infections by identifying the specific assemblage, which may be useful when deciding whether to treat in subclinical cases.

The tendency for flotation techniques to underestimate clinical infection and for both antigen and PCR testing to overestimate them means that there are benefits of using flotation in combination with one of these two tests. This allows potential infection to be detected with a high sensitivity while seeing if cyst shedding is taking place. Repeat testing in dogs after treatment assesses whether shedding is still taking place and, if clinical signs have not improved, to establish if infection may still be contributing. This should be done within 3 days after the completion of treatment to rule out infection having recurred from contaminated environments or from the coat of the animal. The Companion Animal Parasite Council (CAPC) recommends fecal flotation with centrifugation rather than fecal antigen tests alone, as the latter may still be positive immediately after infection, even if infection has been eliminated. This is because fecal antigen tests may remain positive even after treatment for variable periods of time even if signs have resolved.

Treatment

Fenbendazole (directly or after metabolism of its prodrug febantel) remains the first-line treatment of giardiasis in cats and dogs. Products in some countries are licensed for a 3-day course of treatment. This, however, is often insufficient, and treatment at 50 mg/kg daily for five consecutive days is required. Cases of suspected resistance to fenbendazole have been reported in North America; therefore, to limit the risk of further resistance developing, treatment of individual pets to attempt elimination of infection is not advised. Rather, the aim of treatment should be to resolve clinical signs. Treatment for 5 days should be sufficient to achieve this, and if signs persist, then other causes of diarrhea should be investigated.

Metronidazole can also be used to treat dogs with *Giardia* infection but is generally less effective than fenbendazole, with often high-end therapeutic doses (25 mg/kg twice daily) having to be used. These doses increase the risk of adverse side effects such as vomiting and central nervous system toxicity leading to nystagmus, ataxia, proprioceptive deficits, head tilt, and seizures. Its use should be reserved for the treatment of canine giardiasis when fenbendazole has failed to control clinical infection or when the volumes of fenbendazole required to treat large dogs are impractical. Resistance to metronidazole has been reported in human cases but has yet to be a significant issue in companion animals.[3] Metronidazole is particularly useful when utilized in combination with fenbendazole to improve outcomes in refractory cases. Fenbendazole at 50 mg/kg every 24 hours should be used with metronidazole at 25 mg/kg every 12 hours for 5 days. A low-residue, highly digestible diet may also be beneficial to help to reduce diarrhea during treatment. Diets should be low in carbohydrates and high in protein to inhibit excessive growth of *Giardia* in the intestine.

Clinical signs may recur due to reinfection from environmental contamination. In these situations, further courses of treatment with management of environmental contamination by cysts is required. Pets should be regularly cleaned to remove fecal contamination from the coat and clipped to reduce the risk of contamination building up. Feces should be picked up daily and disposed of responsibly, and pet bedding should be hot washed to at least 60°C.

Cystoisospora spp.

Cystoisospora spp. (previously *Isospora* spp.) are host-specific protozoans, with *C. canis*, *C. ohioensis*, and *C. burrowsi* infecting the small and large intestine of dogs. Although many infected dogs are subclinical carriers, *Cystoisospora* is a common cause of diarrhea in puppies.

Life cycle and zoonotic risk

Multiplication of the intestinal stages takes place intracellularly, and oocysts are shed in the feces 6–10 days after infection. Oocysts are not immediately infective but need to mature in the environment. This takes several days and is influenced by temperature and humidity. Once mature, infection can take place by the fecal–oral route or through the consumption of rodents and small ruminants acting as paratenic hosts. The period during which oocysts are passed in the feces is highly variable but is typically 5–10 days. Infection most commonly occurs during the suckling period between 3 and 8 weeks of age via ingestion of oocysts from contaminated environments, with oocysts building up in kennels, catteries, and breeding establishments with a high density of dogs. Oocysts can remain viable in the environment for several months, so very high densities can be reached. As a result of these factors, clinical cases are most commonly seen in puppies with no acquired immunity exposed to high levels of infection. The highly host-specific nature of the parasite means there is no zoonotic risk.

Clinical signs

Clinical cystoisosporiasis most commonly presents as diarrhea in puppies. The most severe infections lead to significant morbidity and can even be fatal, although this is uncommon with prompt treatment and environmental management. Intestinal signs can be exacerbated by coinfections such as giardiasis and campylobacteriosis, and also by sudden dietary changes. Often, clinical presentation is associated with viral, helminth, or bacterial coinfections and if there have been changes in the diet (e.g., puppies receiving solid food). Reinfection can rapidly occur through contaminated environments, but clinical signs rarely reoccur and oocyst shedding is minimal.

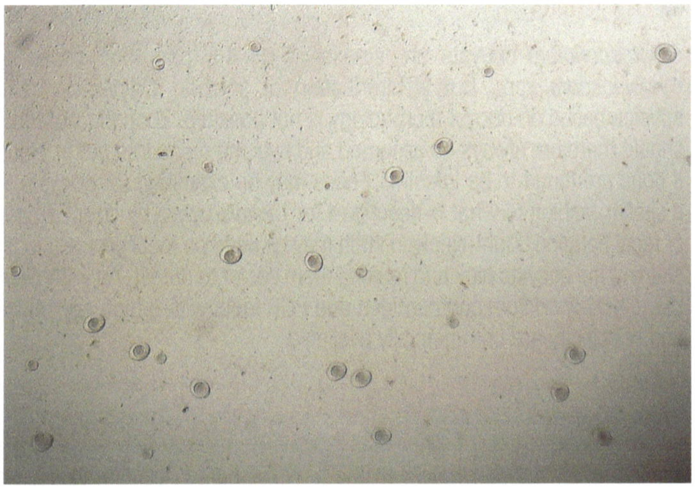

FIG. 39.1 Photomicrograph of unsporulated oocysts (sporoblasts) of *Cystoisospora* spp. in a fecal flotation of a fresh sample.

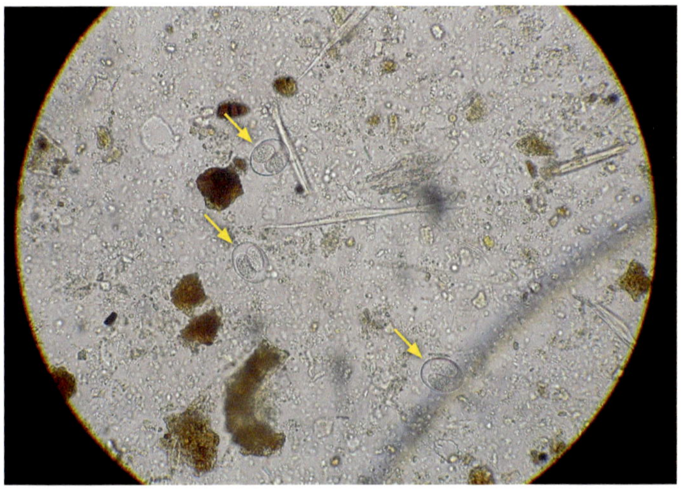

FIG. 39.2 Photomicrograph of mature oocysts of *Cystoisospora* spp. (arrows) in a fecal sample, each containing two round sporocysts.

Diagnosis

Clinical signs commence shortly after oocysts begin to be shed in the feces. These can be detected by direct smear or fecal flotation concentration methods, with the latter being more sensitive. Shedding of oocysts can be intermittent, so pooled fecal samples collected over 3 days will increase sensitivity. The oocysts of *Cystoisospora* spp. in fresh feces contain a large sporoblast (Fig. 39.1). In older fecal samples, the oocyst matures and two round sporocysts may be seen (Fig. 39.2). Oocyst size varies depending on species, with *C. burrowsi* typically being 21 × 18 µm, *C. canis* 39 × 32 µm, and *C. ohioensis* 24 × 20 µm. As with *Giardia*, *Cystoisospora* coproantigen and PCR tests with a high sensitivity and specificity are commercially available.

Treatment

Where puppies and young dogs are living in groups with close proximity, treatment at an early stage after the onset of clinical signs is essential to limit oocyst shedding into the environment. Several chemotherapeutic options have been demonstrated to be effective in reducing oocyst shedding and resolving clinical signs (Table 39.1). It is also important to reduce oocyst buildup in the environment by the daily removal of feces from housing and kennel runs and thorough cleaning and disinfection of living areas and breeding units. Steam cleaning and chemical disinfection using oocidal compounds, such as cresols, are required to inactivate oocysts in the environment. Sleeping and exercise areas should be kept as dry as possible to limit oocyst development.

Cryptosporidium spp.

Cryptosporidium species are apicomplexan protozoa-like organisms that infect a wide variety of vertebrate hosts. They live in the small intestine, and while infections can be subclinical they can also lead to GI disturbances.

Life cycle and zoonotic risk

Most species are host-specific, but some cross infection can occur in immunocompromised hosts. *C. parvum*, however, is capable of infecting a wide range of mammalian immunocompetent hosts, including humans. Humans are most commonly infected by the host-specific *C. hominis* or by *C. parvum*. The zoonotic risk is therefore generally low, unless individuals are immunocompromised or *C. parvum* is involved. Dogs are most commonly infected by their own host-specific species, *C. canis*, but can also be infected by *C. parvum*, allowing cross infection between dogs and humans in outbreaks.[4]

The life cycle is similar to that of *Cystoisospora*, with intracellular division of the parasite taking place in the small intestinal enterocytes.

TABLE 39.1 Chemotherapeutic agents with efficacy against *Cystoisospora* in dogs.

Therapeutic agent	Dose	Treatment frequency	Treatment duration
Sulfadimethoxine	50–60 mg/kg	Every 24 h	7–21 days
Sulfaguanidine	100–200 mg/kg	Every 8 h	5 days
Sulfadimethoxine + ormetoprim	55 mg/kg of sulfadimethoxine and 11 mg/kg of ormetaprim	Every 24 h	7–21 days
Toltrazuril	10–30 mg/kg	Every 24 h	1–3 days
Ponazuril	20 mg/kg	Every 24 h	1–3 days

Clinicopathological findings

Changes on routine blood work are often nonspecific. Anemia and neutrophilia are the most commonly reported hematological abnormalities. Cases may present as a protein-losing enteropathy (see Chapter 13), with hypoalbuminemia being the most common biochemical abnormality seen.[1,4,7,9] Less commonly, mild increases in liver enzymes are reported. A low cobalamin concentration is reported in up to 70% dogs with low-grade small-cell AL[4,7] but is rarely reported in high-grade AL. Despite the high prevalence of T-cell phenotypes AL, the incidence of hypercalcemia appears to be very low.[4,9]

Diagnostic imaging

Radiography is often nonspecific in AL, but abdominal radiography may demonstrate abdominal masses and loss of serosal detail due to abdominal effusion. Thoracic radiography may show sternal lymphadenomegaly. Abdominal ultrasound is the more useful imaging modality to assess the GI tract, associated lymph nodes, and adjacent organs for AL. Ultrasound can be useful to exclude other common differential diagnoses for GI signs (e.g., partial obstruction/foreign body and intussusception).

Common findings in AL include GI wall thickening, loss of wall layering, mass lesions, and enlarged mesenteric lymph nodes, all of which are suggestive of neoplasia (Fig. 42.1). Lesions are variable in appearance and may be focal, multifocal, or diffuse. Loss of intestinal wall layering in particular is very suggestive of alimentary cancer rather than IBD,[5,10] although this differentiation may be less clear in low-grade small-cell lymphoma patients, who typically have more diffuse disease. In studies, up to 38% of patients with low-grade AL had no changes identified on abdominal ultrasound.[5,7] Less commonly, ascites and/or hepatosplenomegaly may be seen.

Staging of AL is unlikely to alter treatment options or prognosis, and most would be classified as Stage V (extranodal site) and Substage b (unwell at diagnosis). In dogs that were fully staged, no bone marrow involvement was noted with high-grade AL.[9]

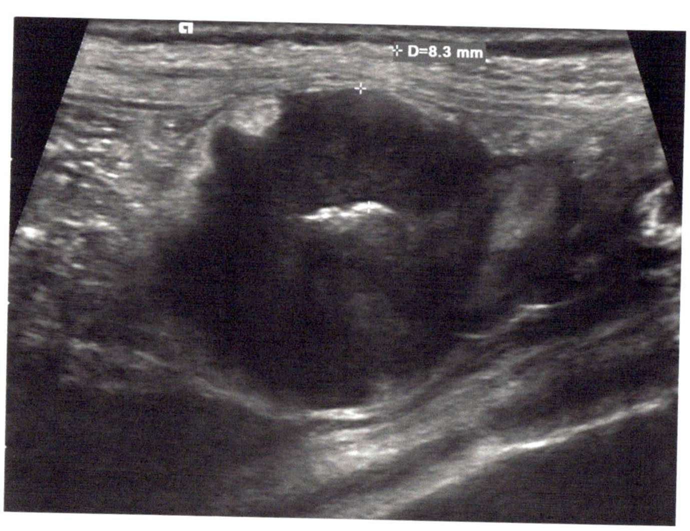

FIG. 42.1 Ultrasonographic cross-sectional image of the jejunum with wall thickening and loss of layering in a dog with high-grade intestinal lymphoma.

Diagnostic tests

Diagnosis of AL requires cytological and/or histological evaluation of lesions with or without lymph nodes. Additional testing such as polymerase chain reaction for antigen receptor rearrangement (PARR), immunocytochemistry, immunohistochemistry, flow cytometry, and other biomarkers may assist in particular to differentiate between low-grade AL and LPE.[4,7,11] A diagnostic algorithm for high- and low-grade AL is provided in Figure 42.2.

Cytology

In many cases, the diagnosis of high-grade AL is achievable cytologically by the identification of a monomorphic population of intermediate to large lymphocytes in mass lesions, enlarged lymph nodes, or enlarged liver and/or spleen. Care must be taken when obtaining needle samples because neoplastic lymphocytes are fragile and can easily be disrupted with the use of suction and/or poor smearing technique. Ninety-four percent of enlarged lymph nodes sampled cytologically were diagnostic of high-grade AL.[6] Cytology from endoscopic biopsies is reported to have good sensitivity. In a study of 167 dogs, cytology of squash–smear preparations taken from endoscopic biopsies were in complete agreement with histopathological findings in 81% cases, in which 93 dogs were diagnosed with LPE, 45 dogs with small-cell lymphoma, 24 dogs with large-cell lymphoma, and 5 dogs with eosinophilic enteritis.[12] A rapid cytological diagnosis benefits patients by enabling prompt initiation of treatment without the need for surgery.

Endoscopic biopsy

Most dogs selected for endoscopy following appropriate clinicopathological investigations are likely to have IBD, with studies suggesting that <5% of dogs are diagnosed with AL.[13] The most common endoscopic features of AL reported are a cobblestone appearance to the mucosa and visualization of a mass, although the gross appearance of intestinal lesions at endoscopy does not correspond with the severity of histopathological lesions or help in differentiating between IBD and intestinal lymphoma. Upper and lower endoscopies are essential because many dogs with AL have ileal lesions. Improvements in histopathological and immunophenotypic techniques are assisting the diagnosis of AL from endoscopic biopsies.

In a small number of patients, neoplastic infiltrates present below the mucosa and submucosa may be missed by endoscopic biopsy. However, most high-grade T-cell ALs involve the mucosa, and up to 60% show epitheliotropism.[4]

Full-thickness biopsy

Histopathology via full-thickness biopsies is considered the "gold standard" for the diagnosis of intestinal lymphoma. Biopsies can be taken via exploratory laparotomy or laparoscopically (Fig. 42.3).

Surgical biopsies may be most appropriate in patients with obstructive lesions requiring resection and anastomosis, in patients with peritonitis, and in patients whose lesions are predominantly located in the ileum or a solitary mass lesion is present (Fig. 42.4). Full-thickness biopsies of the large bowel should be avoided if possible due to the high risk of complications. Studies suggest a mortality rate of up to 10% following exploratory laparotomy in dogs with AL, but some of these patients presented with peritonitis due to spontaneous perforation.[6]

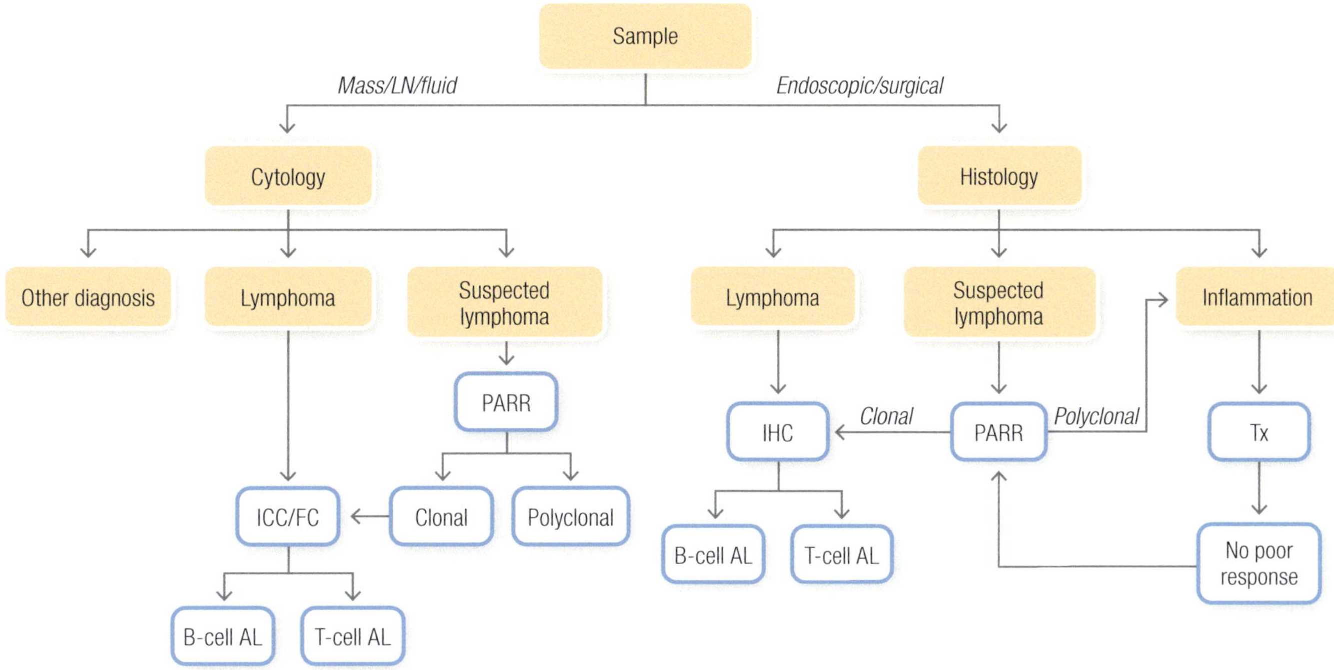

LN, lymph node; PARR, polymerase chain reaction for antigen receptor rearrangement; ICC/FC, immunocytochemistry/flow cytometry; IHC, immunohistochemistry; Tx, treatment; AL, alimentary lymphoma .

FIG. 42.2 Diagnostic algorithm for alimentary lymphoma.

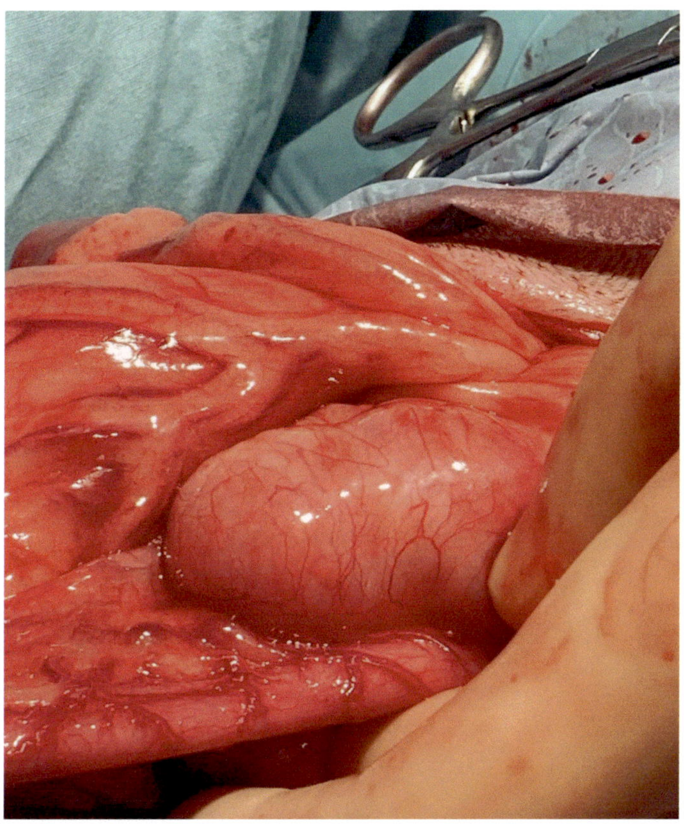

FIG. 42.3 Significantly enlarged mesenteric lymph node in a dog diagnosed with high-grade alimentary lymphoma.

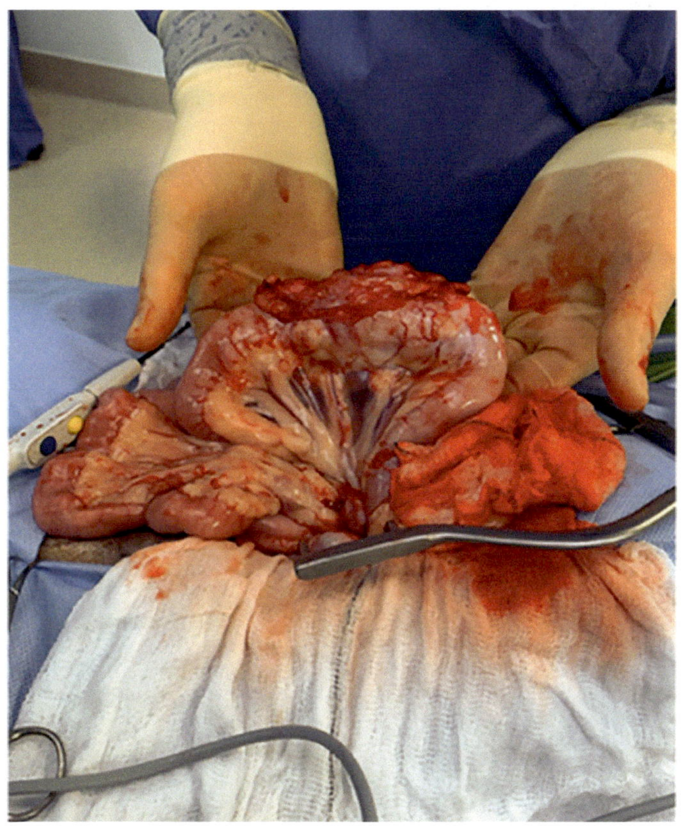

FIG. 42.4 High grade intestinal lymphoma at exploratory laparotomy.

Additional testing

The PARR test amplifies the highly variable T- or B-cell antigen receptor genes and is used to detect clonal expansion of lymphocytes. PARR testing in canine multicentric lymphoma is well established. Its usefulness in differentiating between lymphoplasmacytic enteritis and small-cell lymphoma in intestinal biopsies is less clear. Studies suggest that the sensitivity and specificity of PARR are significantly lower in intestinal biopsies compared with lymph node biopsies.[11]

Therefore, given the low incidence of AL compared with IBD, additional testing for clonality should only be undertaken in cases where there is significant clinical, cytological, or histological concern for neoplastic disease or a poor response to treatment in patients with severe IBD.

Immunophenotyping identifies antigens present on a population of cells. The differing antigens seen on T and B cells can be identified using fluorescent antibodies. Common antigens seen on T cells include CD3, CD4, and CD8. Common B-cell antigens include CD20, CD79a, and CD21. Immunophenotyping can be performed to differentiate between B and T-cell lymphomas. Occasional neoplastic cells show aberrant expression; for example, they have neither T- nor B-cell antigens or both T- and B-cell antigens.

Demonstrating that cells express the same immunophenotype does not prove that they are genetically clonal, and therefore, the results of immunophenotyping should not be considered in isolation. Abnormal patterns of antibody staining are suggestive of neoplasia.

Immunophenotyping can be undertaken on cytological samples by immunocytochemistry or flow cytometry or on fixed histological preparations using immunohistochemistry. Immunophenotyping lymphoma can provide prognostic information and guide therapeutic decision making regarding chemotherapy drug choices, with particular reference to high-grade AL.

Flow cytometry is commonly used to phenotype high-grade multicentric lymphomas in dogs but has been little used in intestinal lymphoma. Histology-guided mass spectrometry has been used in cats to differentiate between LPE and small-cell lymphoma (EATL-2), but there is little evidence of its clinical utility in dogs.[14] Cell-free DNA is becoming used as a cancer biomarker in dogs, but its ability to differentiate between small-cell lymphoma and LPE has not been documented.

Antigen Kiel 67 (Ki-67) is an indicator of the growth fraction of a population of cells. It is widely used as a prognostic marker in many cancers. Ki-67 may have some relevance in differentiating between LPE and AL because patients with lymphomas tend to have higher KI-67 values than dogs with LPE,[11] although most cases of AL in this series were high grade (EATL-1). MicroRNAs may offer a test to discriminate between AL and intestinal inflammation (see Chapter 20).

All results should be interpreted in the clinical context, and overreliance on the results of a single test should be avoided. In some cases, despite extensive testing, it still may be difficult to differentiate between low-grade lymphoma and LPE

Treatment and prognosis

High-grade AL

Multidrug chemotherapy is the treatment of choice in high-grade T-cell alimentary lymphomas. Initial studies suggested that the prognosis invariably was poor despite chemotherapy, with average survival times of 62–77 days.[6,9,15] This may be due in part to patients presenting with advanced disease or the use of drug combinations that are less efficacious for T-cell lymphoma. Most retrospective studies report poor survival using cyclophosphamide, doxorubicin hydrochloride (hydroxydaunorubicin), vincristine sulfate, and prednisone (CHOP)–based protocols or vincristine, L-asparaginase, cyclophosphamide, and doxorubicin.

Multidrug resistance mutation (MDR1) expression is higher in GI lymphoma than in other anatomical forms of lymphoma, suggesting that drugs exported by MDR1 (e.g., doxorubicin and vincristine) would be of less benefit than drugs not affected by MDR1 (i.e., alkylating agents).[16]

The optimal chemotherapy protocols for EATL-1 are not well established, Colorectal high-grade B-cell lymphoma carries a far better prognosis than other anatomical forms of alimentary lymphoma and is treated with CHOP/cyclophosphamide, vincristine (Oncovin), and prednisolone (COP)–based protocols, with progression-free survival time of 1318 days reported.[2] Miniature dachshunds with high-grade B-cell AL have a median survival time of 1503 days.[3]

Low-grade AL

Dogs with low-grade small-cell AL can achieve prolonged survival with treatments including steroids and alkylating agents, with median survival times of between 424 and 628 days reported and response rates of around 70%.[4,7] The most common drugs used are prednisolone with chlorambucil. This drug combination also may be effective in treating LPE.[17] Prospective studies are lacking with regard to the most effective treatments for low-grade AL, with other alkylating agents (e.g., cyclophosphamide and lomustine) also being used. Low-grade B-cell AL is invariably treated the same as low-grade T-cell AL.

Prognostic factors

Patients that are unwell at the time of diagnosis (Substage b) are expected to have a poorer prognosis than patients judged clinically well, although dogs with colorectal lymphoma Substage b can do well. Anemia and peritonitis and progressive disease despite drug therapy are poor prognostic features. Patients achieving rapid remission are likely to exceed average survival times. Several studies suggest that younger dogs may have a better prognosis with some forms.[2,3] The advantage of prognostication using biomarkers over clinical response has not been elucidated for AL.

KEY POINTS

- Alimentary lymphoma (AL) is rare in dogs.
- Various anatomical, morphological, and phenotypic forms are described.
- High-grade intestinal T-cell AL is the most common form in dogs.
- Cytological or histological diagnosis is straightforward in most high-grade cases.
- Diagnosis of low-grade AL often requires additional clonality testing and immunohistochemistry.
- Prognosis is generally poor for high-grade T-cell AL despite multidrug chemotherapy, although a few patients can do well on protocols tailored for T-cell lymphomas.
- High-grade B-cell colorectal lymphoma and Mott-cell (B-cell) lymphoma in young dogs can have prolonged survival with multidrug chemotherapy.
- Low-grade AL has good prognosis with combined prednisolone–alkylating agents.

References

1. Couto CG, Rutgers HC, Sherding RG, Rojko J. Gastrointestinal lymphoma in 20 dogs, a retrospective study. *J Vet Intern Med.* 3(2):73–78, 1989.
2. Desmas I, Burton JH, Post G, et al. Clinical presentation, treatment and outcome in 31 dogs with presumed primary colorectal lymphoma (2001–2013*). Vet Comp Oncol.* 15(2):504–517, 2017.
3. Rimpo K, Hirabayashi M, Tanaka A. Lymphoma in miniature dachshunds: a retrospective multicenter study of 108 cases (2006–2018) in Japan. *J Vet Intern Med.* 36(4);1390–1397, 2002.
4. Lane J, Price J, Moore A, et al. Low-grade gastrointestinal lymphoma in dogs: 20 cases (2010–2016). *J Small Anim Pract.* 2018;59(3):147–153.
5. Frances M, Lane AE, Lenard ZM. Sonographic features of gastrointestinal lymphoma in 15 dogs. *J Small Anim Pract.* 54(9);468–474, 2013.
6. Sogame N, Risbon R, Burgess K. Intestinal lymphoma in dogs: 84 cases (1997–2012). *J Am Vet Med Assoc.* 252(4);440–447, 2018.
7. Couto KM, Moore PF, Zwingenberger AL, et al. Clinical characteristics and outcome in dogs with small cell intestinal lymphoma. *J Vet Comp Oncol.* 16(3):337–343, 2018.
8. Stranahan L, Whitley D, Thaiwong T, et al. Anaplastic large T-cell lymphoma in the intestine of dogs. *J Vet Pathol.* 56(6):878–884, 2019.
9. Rassnick KM, Moore AS, Collister KE, et al. Efficacy of combination chemotherapy for treatment of gastrointestinal lymphoma in dogs. *J Vet Intern Med.* 23(2):317–322, 2009.
10. Penninck D, Smyers B, Webster CRL, et al. Diagnostic value of ultrasonography in differentiating enteritis from intestinal neoplasia in dogs. *Vet Radiol Ultrasound.* 44(5):570–575, 2003.
11. Carrasco V, Rodríguez-Bertos A, Rodríguez-Franco F, et al. Distinguishing intestinal lymphoma from inflammatory bowel disease in canine duodenal endoscopic biopsy samples. *Vet Pathol.* 52(4):668–675, 2015.
12. Maeda S, Tsuboi M, Sakai K, et al. Endoscopic cytology for the diagnosis of chronic enteritis and intestinal lymphoma in dogs. *Vet Pathol.* 54(4):595–604, 2017.
13. Ivasovic F, Ruetten, Kook PH. Prevalence of inflammatory versus neoplastic lesions in dogs with chronic gastrointestinal sings undergoing gastroduodenoscopy: 195 cases (2007–2015). *Res Vet Sci.* 146(2022): 28–33, 2022.
14. Marsilio S, Newman SJ, Estep JS, et al. Differentiation of lymphocytic-plasmacytic enteropathy and small cell lymphoma in cats using histology-guided mass spectrometry. *J Vet Intern Med.* 34(2):669–677, 2020.
15. Frank JD, Reimer SB, Kass PH, Kiupel M. Clinical outcomes of 30 cases (1997–2004) of canine gastrointestinal lymphoma. *J Am Anim Hosp Assoc.* 44(6):313–321, 2007.
16. Moore AS. Treatment of T cell lymphomas in dogs. *Vet Record.* 179(11):264–288, 2016.
17. Dandrieux J, Noble PJM, Scase TJ, et al. Comparison of a chlorambucil-prednisolone combination with an azathioprine-prednisolone combination for treatment of chronic enteropathy with concurrent protein-losing enteropathy in dogs: 27 cases (2007–2010). *J Am Vet Med Assoc.* 242(12):1705–1714, 2013.

of patients with functional ileus; therefore, additional agents should be added. Both erythromycin and cisapride may be effective as second-line drugs. Use of erythromycin in this context may present problems from an antibiotic stewardship perspective, while availability of cisapride may be impacted by the need for compounding and manufacturing variables and may lead to concerns about the legal implications of off-label use of pharmaceuticals. Clinically, there is no strong data to suggest superiority of either of these two compounds.

Nonpharmacological interventions are also valuable in the management of patients with GI motility disorders. In humans, an intervention as simple as chewing gum has been shown to decrease the duration of postoperative ileus.[9] In veterinary patients there is growing evidence to support early enteral nutrition in many disease processes, and planning for early feeding is recommended in all hospitalized animals. When a patient has already developed GI dysmotility, it may be necessary to provide nutritional support via tube feeding and slow constant rate infusion to reduce the risk of vomiting/regurgitation from bolus feeding. Trickle feeding is generally well tolerated, and entry of food into the GI tract, even in small quantities, may stimulate the return of normal GI motility.

Other patient management actions, such as encouraging early ambulation (if possible), maintenance of adequate fluid and electrolyte balance, multimodal pain control, and anxiolysis, may all contribute to improved GI function in hospitalized animals, but there is no specific data regarding the efficacy of these interventions in veterinary patients.

Dysautonomia

Given the crucial role that the autonomic nervous system plays in the overall regulation of GI function (Table 43.1), it is not surprising that autonomic nervous system dysfunction is associated with compromised GI motility. Dysautonomia in dogs is recognized sporadically worldwide,[10] with occasional case clusters reported in the literature.[11] Histologically, dysautonomia is characterized by neuronal degeneration in autonomic ganglia; this is usually a postmortem diagnosis. In some cases, an antemortem diagnosis may be made by detecting characteristic lesions within the ganglia of the enteric nervous system on full-thickness biopsy samples.

Several underlying causes have been suggested for dysautonomia in dogs, with the sporadic cluster diagnoses suggesting that environmental factors may be important. However, there is no clear overall pattern suggesting any specific causative agent.

With the critical importance of the autonomic nervous system in general homeostasis, patients with dysautonomia present with a constellation of clinical signs impacting not only the GI tract. In dogs, GI signs were the most common presenting clinical sign in one study, with vomiting or regurgitation reported in 94% of animals, while hyporexia was present in all dogs.[10] In most cases, ocular signs, such as reduced tear production, altered pupillary light responses, mydriasis, and third eyelid protrusion, were noted. Lower urinary tract signs were common in dogs (cats commonly show constipation and nasal discharge as well).

In dogs, a combination of GI signs and ocular abnormalities (e.g., reduced tear production, poor pupillary light responses, third eyelid protrusion) warrants the consideration of dysautonomia as an underlying diagnosis. Unfortunately, this condition generally carries a poor to grave prognosis, with many patients euthanized within days of the diagnosis due to poor response to therapy. Some cases, however, show symptomatic improvement with medical therapy to address GI dysmotility, urinary retention, and ocular tear film. Recovery times can be prolonged, and complete recovery may not occur even in patients initially responding to symptomatic therapy.

Visceral neuropathy and myopathy

Visceral neuropathy (myenteric plexus ganglionitis)[12] and visceral myopathy (intestinal leiomyositis)[13] are rare, typically devastating inflammatory disorders affecting the enteric nervous system and intestinal smooth muscle, respectively. One case of combined visceral neuropathy and myopathy in a dog has been documented in the literature.[14] In all cases reported to date, clinical signs of GI dysmotility, predominantly intermittent to persistent vomiting, diarrhea, intermittent regurgitation, and weight loss, were the most prominent findings, with clinical durations ranging from days to approximately 5 months. Diagnostic imaging (abdominal ultrasound), when reported, commonly reveals gastric dilation with decreased gastric motility and small intestinal dilation. Abdominal radiography often shows massive, diffuse dilation of intestinal loops, which may be mistaken for mechanical obstruction (see Fig. 47.11). Thus, an alternative name for these conditions is chronic intestinal pseudo-obstruction (CIPO). Histological assessment of full-thickness GI biopsies shows mixed mononuclear inflammation and loss of intestinal myocytes in visceral myopathy, and loss of autonomic neurons in visceral neuropathy. It should be noted that detecting lesions at this level within the GI wall requires full-thickness biopsies, as endoscopic biopsy specimens do not reliably sample deeply enough to include the myenteric plexus and tunica muscularis.

The great majority of cases with visceral ganglionitis and leiomyositis in the veterinary literature were euthanized shortly after diagnosis due to poor response to therapy. However, successful management of dogs with these diseases via immunosuppressive therapy has been reported rarely.[14,15] It is possible that the poor outcomes for most reported cases are skewed due to poor response to therapy, late-stage diagnosis, and the need for full-thickness intestinal biopsy samples leading to the diagnosis. Given that full-thickness biopsy is necessary to document these lesions, and immunosuppressive therapy is commonly used in animals with working diagnoses of immune-mediated chronic enteropathies based solely on endoscopic biopsy samples and response to therapy, the true prevalence of these conditions may be underestimated in veterinary patients.

KEY POINTS

- Gastrointestinal motility disorders can be difficult to recognize and manage and are likely underdiagnosed in companion animal patients.
- In patients with gastrointestinal dysmotility or ileus, efforts should be made to identify, and manage, the primary disease process.
- Patients in critical care, trauma patients, and patients undergoing anesthesia for significant surgical procedures are at a higher risk for ileus. In these cases, patient management should be planned to preemptively reduce this risk, including minimal handling of the gastrointestinal tract and multimodal analgesia.
- Pharmacological and nonpharmacological strategies can be used to manage animals with gastrointestinal motility disorders, but there is limited data on their efficacy in veterinary patients.
- Dysautonomia and visceral neuropathy/myopathy carry a poor prognosis, but symptomatic or immunosuppressive therapy may be beneficial in some dogs.

References

1. Whitehead K, Cortes Y, Eirmann L. Gastrointestinal dysmotility disorders in critically ill dogs and cats. *J Vet Emerg Crit Care (San Antonio)* 26(2): 234–253, 2016.
2. Sharma A, Thompson MS, Scrivani PV, et al. Comparison of radiography and ultrasonography for diagnosing small-intestinal mechanical obstruction in vomiting dogs. *Vet Radiol Ultrasound* 52(3):248–255, 2011.
3. Wyse CA, McLellan J, Dickie AM, et al. A review of methods for assessment of the rate of gastric emptying in the dog and cat: 1898–2002. *J Vet Intern Med* 17(5):609–621, 2003.
4. Chalmers AF, Kirton R, Wyse CA, et al. Ultrasonographic assessment of the rate of solid-phase gastric emptying in dogs. *Vet Rec* 157(21):649–652, 2005.
5. Tittel A, Schippers E, Anurov M, et al. Shorter postoperative atony after laparoscopic-assisted colonic resection? An animal study. *Surg Endosc* 15(5):508–512, 2001.
6. Schippers E, Ottinger AP, Anurov M, et al. Laparoscopic cholecystectomy: a minor abdominal trauma? *World J Surg* 17(4):539–543, 1993.
7. Camilleri M, Lembo A, Katzka DA. Opioids in gastroenterology: treating adverse effects and creating therapeutic benefits. *Clin Gastroenterol Hepatol* 15(9):1338–1349, 2017.
8. Hill TL. Gastrointestinal tract dysfunction with critical illness: clinical assessment and management. *Top Companion Anim Med* 35:47–52, 2019.
9. Li S, Liu Y, Peng Q, et al. Chewing gum reduces postoperative ileus following abdominal surgery: a meta-analysis of 17 randomized controlled trials. *J Gastroenterol Hepatol* 28(7):1122–1132, 2013.
10. Clarke KE, Sorrell S, Breheny C, et al. Dysautonomia in 53 cats and dogs: retrospective review of clinical data and outcome. *Vet Rec* 187(12):e118, 2020.
11. Harkin KR, Andrews GA, Nietfeld JC. Dysautonomia in dogs: 65 cases (1993–2000). *J Am Vet Med Assoc* 220(5):633–639, 2002.
12. Willard MD, Mullaney T, Karasek S, Yamini B. Diarrhea associated with myenteric ganglionitis in a dog. *J Am Vet Med Assoc* 193(3):346–348, 1988.
13. Zacuto AC, Pesavento PA, Hill S, et al. Intestinal leiomyositis: a cause of chronic intestinal pseudo-obstruction in 6 dogs. *J Vet Intern Med* 30(1):132–140, 2016.
14. Kopke MA, Ruaux CG, Gal A. Myenteric ganglionitis and intestinal leiomyositis in a Jack Russell terrier. *J Small Anim Pract* 61(12):772–775, 2020.
15. Olivarez MP, Williams J, Udomteerasuwat N, et al. Case report: successful treatment of intestinal leiomyositis in a dog using adjunctive intravenous immunoglobulin. *Front Vet Sci* 11:1373882, 2024.
16. Husnik R, Gaschen F. Gastric motility disorders in dogs and cats. *Vet Clin North Am Small Anim Pract* 51(1):43–59, 2021.
17. Washabau RJ. Gastrointestinal motility disorders and gastrointestinal prokinetic therapy. *Vet Clin North Am Small Anim Pract* 33(5):1007–1028, 2003.

TABLE 44.2 Conditions affecting the oropharynx and salivary glands in dogs.

Vascular	None
Infectious	■ Dental disease (refer to dentistry textbooks) ■ Stomatitis ■ Tonsillitis ■ Sialadenitis
Trauma	■ Trauma/foreign body
Anatomical	■ Cricopharyngeal achalasia ■ Craniomandibular osteopathy ■ Calvarial hyperostosis ■ Temporomandibular joint dysplasia ■ Cleft palate ■ Sialadenosis (phenobarbitone-responsive)
Metabolic	■ Fibrous osteodystrophy (renal secondary hyperparathyroidism) ■ Uremia ■ Gingival hyperplasia ■ Sialolithiasis
Inflammatory Immune mediated	■ Dental disease (refer to dentistry textbooks) ■ Stomatitis ■ Tonsillitis ■ Sialadenitis ■ Masticatory myositis
Neoplasia Nutritional	■ Epulis, fibrosarcoma, squamous cell carcinoma, melanoma, osteosarcoma ■ Fibrous osteodystrophy (nutritional hyperparathyroidism)
Degenerative	■ Temporomandibular joint osteoarthritis

Electric/thermal burns

Electrical burns usually occur due to chewing of electrical cords and are most common in puppies. Dogs can develop severe systemic signs (e.g., seizures, non-cardiogenic pulmonary edema), but local signs such as oral burns, halitosis, and ptyalism also may develop over the subsequent 24 hours. Dogs also may suffer from thermal burns if they steal very hot food or when a carer tries to encourage the dog to eat by warming up the food. Because of this risk, care must be taken when warming up meals for pets not to overheat them.

Caustic substances

Caustics can be acidic or alkaline. The latter may be more dangerous because they do not cause immediate discomfort, and this may result in a more prolonged exposure, so even if oral damage is not present, esophageal damage may be. Damage from acidic substances becomes apparent shortly after exposure, whereas it may take several hours after exposure to alkaline substances. On top of oral signs, systemic signs also can occur, such as pneumonitis or gastrointestinal (GI) ulceration.

Pine and oak processionary moth caterpillars

The caterpillars of pine and oak processionary moths[2] (*Thaumetopoea pityocampa* and *T. processionea*, respectively) can cause severe problems in dogs if they are contacted or ingested. In the past, they were more common in the Mediterranean area and south Atlantic coast, but due to global warming, their distribution has expanded, and the oak processionary moth now has been found in southeast England.

Contact with these caterpillars can cause anaphylactic reactions. However, the most commons signs are glossitis (e.g., tongue lesions including ulcers, superficial necrosis, and sloughing) and ptyalism. The toxicity of these caterpillars is due to their poisonous hairs (setae), which cause mechanical irritation and release multiple allergens. In the most recent retrospective study of 109 affected dogs in France, most of the cases of *T. pityocampa* envenomation occurred between March and May.[2] Tongue lesions and vomiting were the most common clinical signs, but ocular and dermatological signs can also occur.

History and physical exam

A good history is fundamental for raising a suspicion of traumatic damage. Oral examination is key in these cases. However, in most cases, evaluation of the mouth in a conscious patient is not possible (due to pain or demeanor). Sedation/anesthesia is often required to be able to properly examine the oral cavity fully.

Clinicopathological findings

Hematological and biochemical findings are nonspecific and may not even be present in most cases. Neutrophilia and monocytosis compatible with ongoing inflammation can be present. C-reactive protein also can be increased. Hypokalemia due to decreased food intake and hyperglobulinemia and mild hypoalbuminemia due to a negative acute-phase protein response (secondary to inflammation) may be present.

Diagnostic imaging

Advanced imaging (the author's preference is computed tomography) can help in finding a foreign body and assessing the extent of the damage and identifying the need and planning for surgery, that is, the most convenient surgical approach. Depending on the presentation or suspected cause, esophagoscopy to assess the esophagus is also recommended to determine the extent of any damage and the need for placing a gastrostomy feeding tube (e.g., percutaneous endoscopic gastrostomy tube). In the case of exposure to corrosive substances, endoscopy should be performed after 12–24 hours because that is when the lesions become more apparent.

Diagnosis

A strong suspicion is usually present after collecting the clinical history. Oral examination is fundamental for confirmation (Fig. 44.2), but sedation/anesthesia is usually required.

Treatment

Depending on the extent of the damage, surgical management may be required. Supportive treatment with analgesia and assisted nutrition (e.g., esophageal or gastrostomy tubes) is fundamental.

- Antibiotics may be used in cases of foreign bodies/penetrating injuries while waiting for bacterial culture results.
- When a dog has been exposed to a corrosive substance, emesis or gastric lavage should not be attempted due to the risk of re-exposure and perforation. Activated charcoal shouldn't be used either because it might interfere with the healing process. Dilution with water or milk should be performed when the exposure is recent.
- For caterpillar exposure, flushing of the affected areas is the most important treatment and needs to be done as early as possible after exposure, and the prognosis is usually good. Changes in the color of the tongue are predictive of tongue necrosis at a later stage.

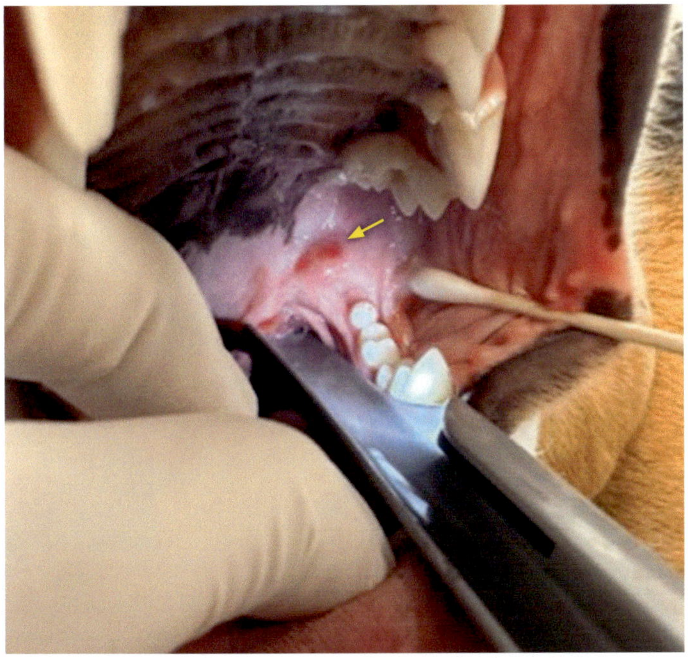

FIG. 44.2 Middle-aged beagle that presented because of anorexia and an inability to open its mouth. The yellow arrow shows a hyperemic area, which was lanced, releasing hemorrhagic/purulent content. A penetrating injury was suspected.

Anatomical

Cricopharyngeus muscle dysfunction

Etiology

The cricopharyngeus muscle is fundamental for a correct function of the upper esophageal sphincter and consequent swallowing. The muscle can suffer from a failure to relax (achalasia) or an incoordination between pharyngeal contraction and the upper esophageal sphincter (asynchrony). These problems can be congenital or acquired, but in the author's opinion, it is more common for the congenital form to be responsible for an exclusively dysphagic presentation. The definitive underlying mechanism has not been confirmed but is suspected to be some sort of neuropathy. Cranial neuropathy, myasthenia gravis, and polymyositis are possible acquired conditions that also may cause cricopharyngeus muscle dysfunction.

Clinicopathological findings

Any hematological and biochemical abnormalities are nonspecific and are not present in most cases. Neutrophilia and monocytosis and increased C-reactive protein can be present if there is concomitant aspiration pneumonia. Hypokalemia due to decreased food intake and mild hypoalbuminemia due to a negative acute-phase protein response (secondary to inflammation) may be present.

Neurological exam and investigations

Depending on the history and neurological exam—which always should be performed—different tests may be considered to screen for neuropathies and myopathies. Some examples include an evaluation for antibodies against acetylcholine receptors to diagnose myasthenia gravis and creatine kinase evaluation to raise a suspicion for myopathy/muscular dystrophy if increased. Other tests that are more invasive but may be necessary in some cases (e.g., if there is no response to treatment or to confirm a diagnosis) are electromyography and muscle biopsies. In this case, consultation with a neurology specialist is recommended prior to performing such tests.

Diagnostic imaging

A fluoroscopic swallowing study (Video 44.1) is the test of choice to confirm this pathology. Different food consistencies (e.g., dry and wet) and water can be tested during the study because individual dogs may struggle with different consistencies. One of the main challenges when performing this test is to get the dog to eat. Extended periods of withholding food and the use of appetite stimulants may be considered. It is recommended to create a comfortable and stress-free environment for the dog after a habituation period with the place, position, machinery, and operators. Syringe feeding should be avoided if possible.

Thoracic radiography (at least two orthogonal views) is recommended to screen for evidence of aspiration pneumonia, which is a common complication in these cases due to the impaired swallowing.

Treatment

Surgical treatment is the definitive treatment for cricopharyngeus muscle dysfunction—myotomy or myectomy of the cricopharyngeus muscle (as described in surgical textbooks). Other therapies that have been described are endoscopic carbon dioxide laser myotomy of the muscle or injection of botulinum toxin into the muscle. The latter provides only temporary control of the disease (~3–4 months) but does assess whether the patient would benefit from surgery. It's important to know whether there is concomitant pharyngeal weakness because such patients may not improve as expected or may even worsen after surgery.

Craniomandibular osteopathy

Etiology

Craniomandibular osteopathy (CMO) is a rare, nonneoplastic osteoproliferative disease that affects the ventral and caudal aspects of the mandible, temporomandibular joint, and tympanic bullae bilaterally. It's a condition that usually affects young (3–8 months old) small breeds, in particular West Highland White Terriers In this breed, an autosomal recessive mode of inheritance has been suggested.

Clinical signs

Clinical signs include a reluctance to open the mouth, prehension difficulties, anorexia, and fever.

Imaging

Imaging reveals irregular new bone formation in the affected areas (Fig. 44.3). Usually, there is bilaterally asymmetrical involvement. The disease can affect the temporomandibular joint(s).

Video 44.1

Video of a dog with cricopharyngeal achalasia where there is a clear impairment of the bolus moving from the oropharynx to the esophagus. Video courtesy of Virgine de Busscher.

Diagnosis
Diagnosis is usually by a combination of signalment, physical examination, and imaging. Biopsy is only recommended in nonterrier breeds or dogs with unilateral involvement.

Treatment
CMO is usually a self-limiting disease once individuals reach maturity. Nonsteroidal anti-inflammatory drugs (NSAIDs) or corticosteroids, analgesia, and nutritional support should be implemented while signs are present. The prognosis is usually good, but if the temporomandibular joint is affected, difficulties in opening the mouth may remain lifelong.

Calvarial hyperostosis

Etiology
This is a very rare non-neoplastic, self-limiting condition characterized by proliferation of the flat bones of the skull. Its pathogenesis is not understood, and it most commonly affects young bull mastiffs. However, it has been reported in other breeds, such as the Dalmatians,[3] Weimaraners, and American Pit Bulls, among others, and in general, it tends to be a condition of large breed dogs.

Clinical signs
Signs include painful swelling of the skull, pain, exophthalmos, fever, and local lymphadenomegaly.

Imaging
Advanced imaging can be used, but radiography is generally successful in helping to reach or confirm a diagnosis. The bone growth is usually unilateral with asymmetrical thickening of several skull bones, and there is no temporomandibular joint or mandibular involvement. This last feature, along with the specific breed, helps to differentiate it from CMO.

Histology
Histology can be useful to confirm the diagnosis and differentiate it from CMO and neoplasia. However, the differences at histological level between calvarial hyperostosis and CMO are subtle.

Diagnosis
Diagnosis is usually based on signalment, physical exam, and imaging. In some cases, biopsy is performed to give supporting evidence to a clinical suspicion.

Treatment
This condition is usually self-limiting once the dog reaches skeletal maturity, but while in the active phase, it can be painful and symptomatic. NSAIDs or steroids can be used along with analgesia. The medications are tapered/discontinued once the dog is close to reaching skeletal maturity.[3] Sometimes it's difficult to distinguish the clinical findings from a focal osteomyelitis, and some authors advocate for a trial of antibiotics along with the anti-inflammatory drugs as a precaution.

Sialadenosis

Etiology
Sialadenosis is a non-inflammatory, non-painful enlargement of the salivary glands that may be related to an alteration in the innervation of the salivary glands.[4] Phenobarbitone-responsive (idiopathic) sialadenosis is the best-known form in dogs, and it is suspected to be some sort of limbic epilepsy based on the electroencephalogram and the response to antiepileptic medication.

Clinical signs
This condition usually affects young-adult to middle-aged small breed dogs. Common clinical signs are lip smacking, ptyalism, inappetence, gagging, retching, and vomiting. On physical exam, bilateral nonpainful enlargement of the submandibular salivary glands is the most common finding.

Clinicopathological abnormalities
Mild hypokalemia may be reported due to decreased intake and chronic vomiting.

Advanced imaging
Computed tomography (CT) of the head to visualize the salivary glands is useful to assess any changes that could suggest an alternative differential diagnosis such as neoplasia.

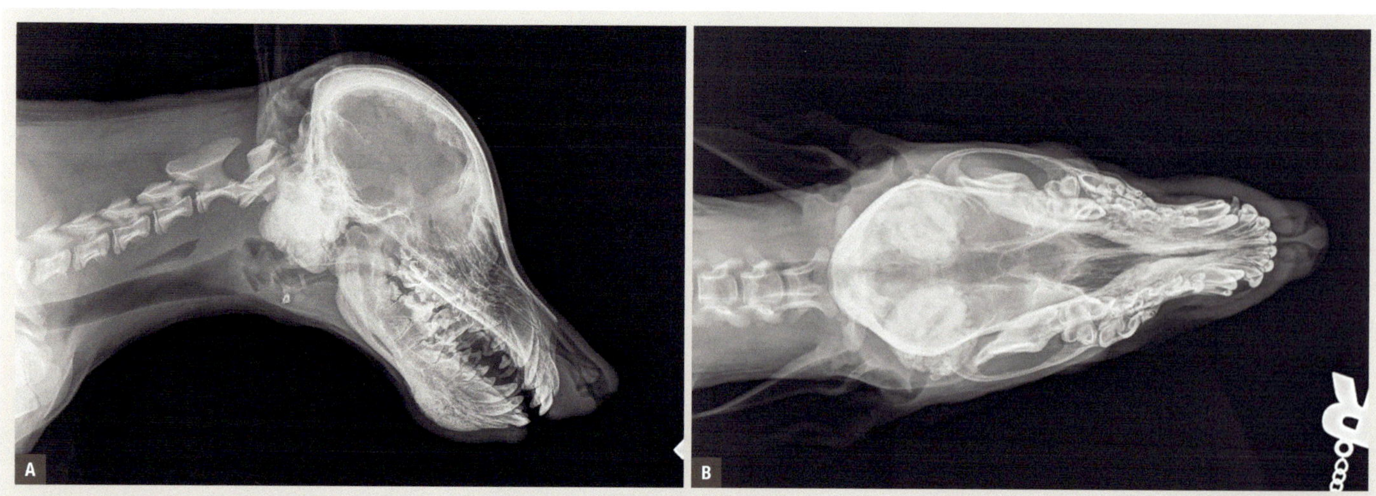

FIG. 44.3 Radiographs of a dog with craniomandibular osteopathy. Note the proliferative bone on the mandible and around the bullae. Images courtesy of Claudia Mallol.

Cytology/histology

Sampling of the salivary glands may be unremarkable but is indicated in some cases to exclude other differential diagnoses such as sialadenitis and neoplasia.

Diagnosis

A presumptive diagnosis of phenobarbitone-responsive sialadenosis is reached by exclusion and confirmed once an improvement on phenobarbitone is seen. Other diseases that can cause vomiting, regurgitation, or nausea should be ruled out. Necrotizing sialometaplasia is an inflammatory variant and one of the main differential diagnoses for sialadenosis along with spirocercosis and granulomatous giant cell sialadenosis.

Treatment

A good response to phenobarbitone is usually seen. In other cases, potassium bromide and levetiracetam have been used. Necrotizing sialometaplasia also shows a response to phenobarbitone.

Sialocele

A sialocele (also known as a *salivary mucocele*) is an extravasation of saliva from the salivary ducts or glands. The sublingual and cervical regions are affected more commonly. This extravasation may be painless but can cause inflammation in the tissues and consequently pain in some dogs. Swallowing and breathing difficulties can occur. The formation of a sialocele has been associated with foreign bodies, trauma, and sialoliths, but on many occasions a definitive trigger cannot be identified. Diagnosis is based on physical examination and fine-needle aspiration of the swelling and advanced imaging if necessary. Surgical management is the treatment of choice.

Metabolic

Gingival hyperplasia

Gingival hyperplasia (Fig. 44.4) can be a side effect of medications such as ciclosporin and amlodipine. It is important to be aware of these possible side effects because, for example, ciclosporin is commonly used for the management of GI, hematological, and dermatological conditions. Usually, this condition is asymptomatic. However, it's noticeable to the carer, who may then seek veterinary advice. Resolution occurs when the drugs are discontinued.

Fibrous osteodystrophy

Etiology

This is a consequence of hyperparathyroidism, most commonly due to renal secondary hyperparathyroidism in chronic kidney disease (CKD). Usually, in dogs with CKD, it appears in International Renal Interest Society (IRIS) stage 3 or stage 4 disease. It also can be caused by nutritional secondary hyperparathyroidism in young dogs fed calcium-deficient foods such as unbalanced homemade or all-meat diets. These dogs have generalized osteopenia, which more commonly affects jaw bones (maxilla and mandible), leading to tooth mobility, facial swelling, and malleable jaw bones ("rubber jaw").

Clinicopathological abnormalities

Most of the time, these patients already have a diagnosis of CKD, and there will be some degree of azotemia and alteration of electrolytes such as hyper- or hypocalcemia, hyperphosphatemia, and hypokalemia. Proteinuria or evidence of infection may be present in the urine on urinalysis.

Diagnostic imaging

Skull radiographs reveal osteopenia, and because there is usually a strong suspicion based on the history and physical exam, advanced imaging is not normally necessary.

Diagnosis

Diagnosis is usually based on the clinical history (e.g., history of CKD or nutritional deficiencies) and confirmed by radiography.

Treatment

If the disease is due to nutritional deficiency, the key is to start the dog on a well-balanced diet (commercial or homemade) because the prognosis may be good. In cases of CKD, guidance for treatment should be based on the IRIS guidelines, but the prognosis is very poor.

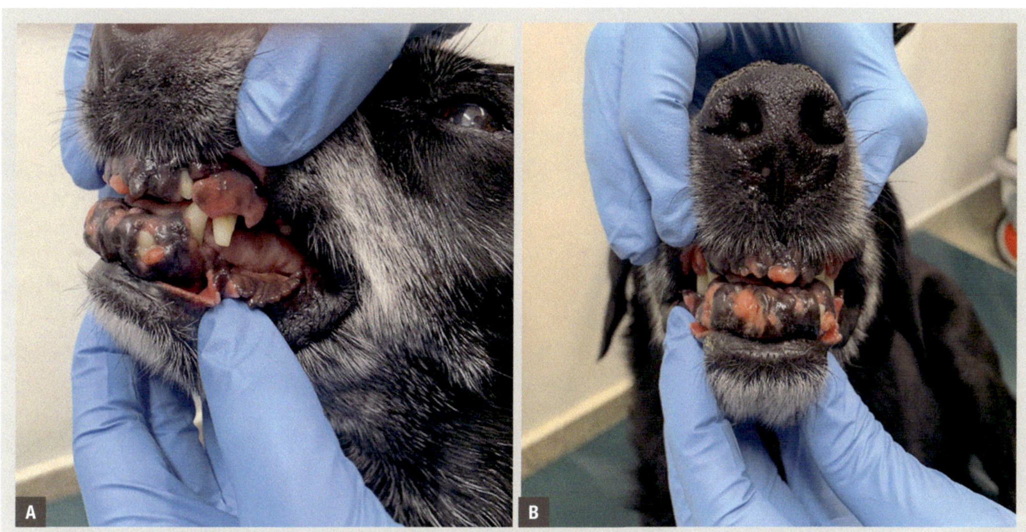

FIG. 44.4 Gingival hyperplasia in a dog treated with amlodipine. The carer noticed the changes and sought veterinary advice.

Ulceration secondary to uremia

Oral ulcerations and halitosis (i.e., odor of ammonia) can occur when dogs suffer from advanced kidney disease. These ulcers are more commonly located in the labial and buccal mucosa, lateral margins of the tongue, and lateral lip frenula. They may cause oral-preparatory dysphagia due to odynophagia (i.e., oral pain). Supportive treatment (e.g., change of food consistencies and feeding tubes) and treatment of the underlying cause are necessary. Topical mouthwashes with sucralfate and lidocaine may be useful to alleviate the pain, and diluted chlorhexidine rinse may help to avoid secondary infections in necrotic areas.

Sialolithiasis

Etiology
Sialolithiasis is the formation of salivary stones, or sialoliths. It's a rare condition in dogs. The underlying mechanism for stone formation is unknown. Sialoliths have been considered triggering factors for the formation of sialoceles.

Imaging
A mineral opacity on radiographs and a mineral-attenuating structure on CT scan can identify sialoliths. Sialography also can be performed to define the morphology of the salivary ducts.

Treatment
Surgical removal is the treatment of choice.

Miscellaneous systemic diseases associated with oral signs

Hypothyroidism also can cause vasculitis and petechiation of the tongue and gingiva.
Hypervitaminosis A can cause gingival enlargement and delayed development and early exfoliation of the incisor teeth. Deficiencies of nutrients such as protein, niacin, and biotin from feeding unbalanced home-cooked diets can cause oral ulcerations (mainly of the tongue), lip scaling, and salivation.

Inflammatory/infectious/immune mediated

Inflammation/infection: oral cavity/tonsils/salivary glands

Etiology
Periodontal disease is common in dogs, whereas localized or generalized stomatitis (inflammation of the oral cavity) and tonsillitis are less common in dogs than in cats. Periodontal disease may include gingivitis and periodontitis, that is, inflammation of the gingiva, periodontal ligament, alveolar bone, and cementum. Inflammation can occur due to trauma (including foreign bodies), toxins, infection, periodontal disease, or neoplasia.
Sialodenitis, inflammation of the salivary glands, is more common in middle-age and older dogs. The zygomatic salivary gland is most commonly affected. Causes for sialodenitis may include sialoliths, bacterial infections, and immune-mediated processes.

Clinical signs
Physical exam may reveal painful swelling in the orbital/retrobulbar area causing exophthalmos. Mandibular lymphadenomegaly may be present, and reluctance to open the mouth may be described. Fever may be present in more severe cases.

Clinicopathological findings
Hematological and biochemical findings are nonspecific and may not even be present in most cases. Neutrophilia and monocytosis and increased C-reactive protein can be present due to the inflammatory process. Hypokalemia (due to decreased food intake), hyperglobulinemia, and mild hypoalbuminemia due to a negative acute-phase protein response (secondary to inflammation) may be present.

Diagnosis
Presumptive diagnosis is made based on physical examination, but cytology/histology may be useful to confirm a clinical suspicion (i.e., to confirm tonsillitis as the cause of anorexia) and exclude other differential diagnoses such as neoplasia. The samples should be sent for bacterial culture to tailor the antibiotic therapy, if used. However, the interpretation of any culture results may be challenging because a healthy mouth is not a sterile area.

Diagnostic imaging
Advanced imaging such as CT or magnetic resonance imaging may be useful to exclude/raise suspicion for other differential diagnoses such as foreign bodies and neoplasia. Ultrasonographic assessment of the area may be more effective on detecting foreign bodies and allowing drainage of abscesses and ultrasound-guided aspirates.

Treatment
Treatment is based on analgesia, anti-inflammatory of drugs such as NSAIDs or corticosteroids, antibiotics (ideally chosen based on bacterial culture), and assisted feeding, if required. Drainage of mucopurulent content may be needed in some cases. Broad-spectrum antibiotics may be used in some cases, ideally after taking samples for bacterial culture. Dental cleaning, polishing, and tooth extraction are indicated in cases of periodontal disease.

Eosinophilic granuloma complex

Etiology
Eosinophilic granuloma complex is a dermatological syndrome that is suspected to be due to an underlying hypersensitivity reaction characterized by an eosinophilic infiltrate on histopathology. In dogs, it usually affects mucosae (i.e., lips, tongue, and palate). It can affect breeds such as Alaskan Malamutes and Siberian Huskies. There is a reported form in Cavalier King Charles Spaniels called *eosinophilic ulcerative palatitis*. Clinically, signs depend on the affected area but can include anorexia and ptyalism.

Clinicopathological abnormalities
Hematological and biochemical findings are nonspecific and may not even be present in most cases. Eosinophilia is present in some cases, but its absence does not exclude the condition. Neutrophilia and monocytosis and increased C-reactive protein can be present due to the inflammatory process. Hypokalemia due to decreased food intake and hyperglobulinemia and mild hypoalbuminemia due to a negative acute-phase protein response (secondary to inflammation) may be present.

Cytology/histology

Cytology can reveal eosinophilic inflammation, but histopathology is the test of choice to confirm the condition and exclude other differential diagnoses such as neoplasia.

Treatment

Some cases may respond to an exclusion diet, but treatment is usually based on immunosuppression. The first-line treatment is corticosteroids such as prednisolone. Some authors advocate for the use of antibiotics if a secondary bacterial infection is reported on cytological examination and/or bacterial culture. In some cases, if a foreign body is suspected, surgical exploration may be considered.

Masticatory myositis

Etiology

Masticatory myositis is an autoimmune disorder where antibodies target the masticatory muscles, that is, the temporalis, masseter, and pterygoid muscles.[5] These muscles have a different type of myosin isoform and myofiber type (type 2M) and are antigenically different from other striated muscles. This difference may explain why they are targeted specifically. The disease tends to affect large breeds more, in particular German shepherds. A juvenile form has been described in Cavalier King Charles Spaniels.

Clinical signs

Signs include swelling of the masticatory muscles, which may shift from one side to another; trismus and the inability to open the mouth (i.e., locked jaw); or pain leading to the inability to eat or oral dysphagia. Fever and exophthalmos also can occur.

Clinicopathological abnormalities

Hematological and biochemical findings are nonspecific and may not even be present in most cases. Neutrophilia and monocytosis and increased C-reactive protein can be present due to the inflammatory process. Hypokalemia due to decreased food intake and hyperglobulinemia and mild hypoalbuminemia due to a negative acute-phase protein response (secondary to inflammation) may be present. Creatine kinase activity also can be increased.

Diagnosis

Diagnosis is based on the presence of antibodies against type 2M myofibers, but in many cases a diagnosis can be made clinically. The sensitivity of the 2M antibody test is high, but false-negative results may occur, for example, due to the use of corticosteroids before taking the sample and in chronic cases.

Diagnostic imaging

CT and magnetic resonance imaging may reveal changes in the masticatory muscles: contrast enhancement, changes in size, and focal changes in attenuation of the affected muscles (Fig. 44.5). Advanced imaging is also useful to rule out other differential diagnoses such as temporomandibular joint disorders.

Electromyography

Electromyography may reveal changes such as fibrillation potentials and sharp waves.

Muscle biopsies

Muscle biopsies may be considered if the result of the 2M antibody titer is negative, but there is still a clinical suspicion. However, if the patient is having biopsies taken, it is important to emphasize the need to be prepared for a challenging tracheal intubation because in some cases, even under anesthesia, it may be really difficult to open the mouth of the patient, and small endotracheal tubes and equipment for an emergency tracheostomy should be prepared. Biopsies reveal mixed inflammatory infiltrates (usually lymphocytes, macrophages, and histiocytes and, less frequently, eosinophils). A report of muscle necrosis and phagocytosis is usually predictive of a worse outcome.

Diagnosis

A strong suspicion can be based on the clinical history and physical exam. Evaluation of the antibodies against type 2M myofibers, muscle biopsies, and/or advanced imaging can strengthen the diagnosis.

Treatment

Therapy is based on immunosuppressants, with prednisolone usually being the first line. Some board-certified neurologists recommend the initial use of second-line immunosuppressants such as ciclosporin or azathioprine in

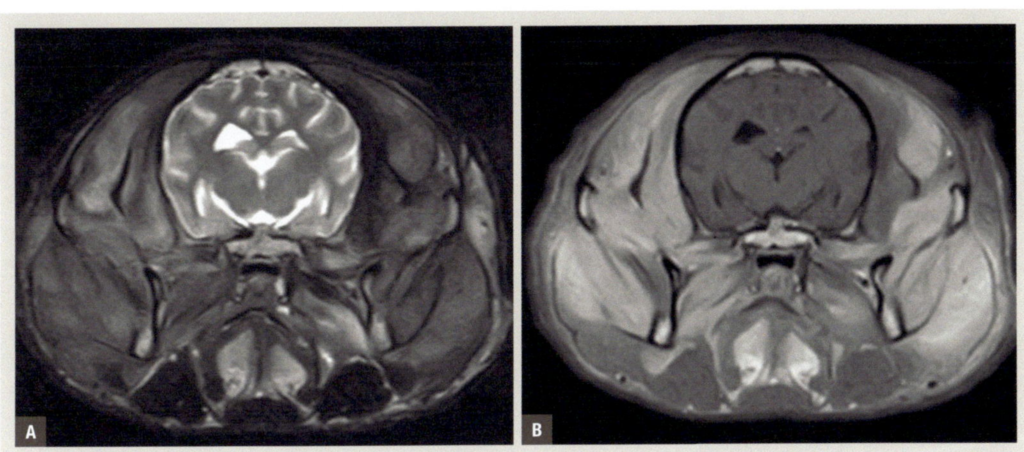

FIG. 44.5 Magnetic resonance imaging of a dog with severe masticatory myositis. Transverse T2-weighted (T2W) (**A**) and T1-weighted postcontrast (**B**) magnetic resonance imaging of a dog's head at the level of the caudal diencephalon. There are bilateral, ill-defined, patchy, T2W hyperintense, contrast-enhancing areas within the masticatory muscles. The bellies of these muscles show an increased volume.

very severe cases based on the history and imaging. Prognosis is usually good, but decreased function may remain.

Temporomandibular disorders

Etiology

The most common type of temporomandibular disorder is osteoarthritis,[6] but other conditions can occur, such as congenital dysplasia, trauma, and neoplasia.

Diagnosis

The diagnostic approach consists of a compatible clinical history (e.g., witnessed trauma or road traffic accident) and diagnostic imaging. The treatment and prognosis depend on the underlying cause.

Neoplasia of the oral cavity and salivary glands

Oral tumors are common in dogs, accounting for 6% of all tumors (in particular in male dogs), and are much more common than in cats.[7] Some breeds that are overrepresented are German Shepherds, Cocker Spaniels, Weimaraners, and Miniature Poodles. The most common malignant oral tumors in a descending order of frequency are malignant melanoma, squamous cell carcinoma, and fibrosarcoma.

Salivary gland tumors are rare in dogs but were the most common reported diagnosis in a study of salivary gland biopsies.[1] They are usually malignant epithelial neoplasms, with simple adenocarcinoma the most common. These tumors can cause clinical signs such the presence of a mass, anorexia, ptyalism, dysphagia, exophthalmos, Horner's syndrome, and dysphonia. Please refer to oncology textbooks for further discussion about the biology and management of oral and salivary gland neoplasias.[7]

KEY POINTS

- In cases of suspected dysphagia, observing the dog eating may help identify the type of dysphagia and facilitate appropriate differential diagnoses.
- Oral-preparatory dysphagia, ptyalism, halitosis, and pain when manipulating/opening the mouth and anorexia are common clinical signs of oropharyngeal and salivary gland disorders.
- History, physical examination (with an emphasis on the oral examination), and imaging usually lead to a diagnosis. In some cases, cytology/histology are required for diagnosis and better management.
- Treatment aimed at the underlying cause is needed, but supportive treatment regarding analgesia and nutrition is frequently necessary.

References

1. Aldelaimi AA, Enezei HH, Aldelaimi TN, et al. Salivary gland diseases: a retrospective clinicopathological study of 159 cases. *Cureus*, 14(9):e29589, 2022.
2. Pouzot-Nevoret C, Cambournac M, Violé A, Goy-Thollot I, Bourdoiseau G, Barthélemy A. Pine processionary caterpillar Thaumetopoea pityocampa envenomation in 109 dogs: a retrospective study. *Toxicon*. 132:1–5, 2017.
3. Planas C, Novellas R, Espada Y, et al. Calvarial hyperostosis syndrome in a dalmatian dog. *Clin Case Rep*. 11(6):e7596, 2023.
4. Alcoverro E, Tabar M, Lloret A, et al. Phenobarbital-responsive sialadenosis in dogs: case series. *Top Companion Anim Med*. 29(4):109–112, 2014.
5. Dewey CW, Da Costa RC. *Practical Guide to Canine and Feline Neurology*. Wiley Blackwell; 2016.
6. Arzi B, Cissell DD, Verstraete FJM, et al. Computed tomographic findings in dogs and cats with temporomandibular joint disorders: 58 cases (2006–2011). *J Am Vet Med Assoc*. 132:1–5, 2017.
7. Vail DM, Thamm DH, Liptak JM. *Withrow & MacEwen's Small Animal Clinical Oncology*. 6th ed. Missouri: Elsevier; 2020.

CHAPTER 45

Esophageal diseases

Megan Grobman
DVM, MS, PhD,
DACVIM (SAIM)

The esophagus is a dynamic muscular tube that conducts swallowed food and oral secretions to the stomach for digestion. Conversely, during vomiting and regurgitation, the esophagus allows retrograde passage of gastric and intestinal contents. The esophagus, as a part of the aerodigestive tract, also provides significant protection against aspiration. This dual role of digestion and defense places a large burden on the esophagus, with dysfunction resulting in substantial patient morbidity and mortality.

Anatomy of the esophagus

The body of the esophagus is composed, from inside to outside, of the mucosa, submucosa, muscularis, and adventitial layers. The muscular body of the esophagus is bracketed on either end by the high-pressure zones of the upper esophageal sphincter (UES) and lower esophageal sphincter (LES). The muscular composition of the esophageal body is variable across species, with the functional canine esophagus being entirely striated muscle. Smooth muscle within the lamina muscularis mucosa, although present, does not contribute to esophageal peristalsis. It may, however, contribute to LES tone by providing muscular support to the esophageal gastric junction (EGJ). The muscularis is comprised of outer longitudinal and inner circumferential layers. During normal swallowing these layers exhibit coordinated contractions. Contraction of the longitudinal layer reduces wall stress and compliance of the contracted segment, while relaxation ahead of the contracted segment helps accommodate the bolus. The circumferential layer provides sequential peristaltic contractions which conduct the bolus into the stomach.

The esophagus receives innervation from the vagus and spinal nerves. Vagal afferents have cell bodies in the nodose ganglia and terminate in the *nucleus tractus solitarius*. Spinal afferents have cell bodies in the dorsal root ganglia and terminate in the spinal column and brain stem. Vagal afferents respond to chemical, thermal, and mechanical stimuli, while spinal afferents are involved in nociception. Motor activity relies on vagal efferent innervation which arises from the *nucleus ambiguus*. The esophagus also possesses some intrinsic innervation: the myenteric plexus lying between the circumferential and longitudinal muscle layers.[1] Even though more research is needed, functional studies in animal models support an inhibitory effect on vagally induced muscle contraction. In people, discordant longitudinal and circumferential muscular contraction and loss of neurons from the myenteric plexus are thought to contribute to several esophageal motility disorders, including esophageal achalasia, a condition recently described in dogs.[2]

The composition of the UES and LES differs from that of the esophageal body. The UES is comprised of the cricopharyngeus and thyropharyngeus muscles and cranial cervical esophagus. The cricopharyngeus muscle demonstrates significant variations in tone during swallowing and breathing. It possesses distinct anatomical features, such as muscle fibers not strictly arranged in parallel (as with most other striated muscles) and larger amounts of elastic connective tissues (e.g., elastin, sarcolemma). These features allow this muscle to maintain a basal tone without active contraction. In addition, distension of the cricopharyngeus muscle increases muscular tension, generating tone behind the bolus consistent with Starling forces. All of this is important to prevent aerophagia as well as reflux from the esophagus into the pharynx. Innervation of the UES is as for the esophageal body.

The LES is part of a high-pressure zone at the EGJ which also includes the crura of the diaphragm, an oblique entrance of the esophagus into the stomach, and rugal folds. The LES itself is comprised of smooth muscle rather than striated.[3] Motor innervation of the LES arises from the dorsal motor nucleus of the vagus nerve. The LES and other components of the EGJ high-pressure zone maintain a pressure of $\approx$30 mmHg as a protective mechanism against reflux. Modulation of LES tone is coordinated by myogenic, neurohormonal, and neuronal factors. For example, gastric distention is associated with increased LES tone via the gastroesophageal reflex. This reflex is protective against reflux during periods of increased intragastric pressure (e.g., coughing, sneezing, defecation, micturition, postprandial gastric distention). The oblique angle of entry of the esophagus into the stomach also prevents reflux by forming a gastroesophageal "flap valve" which prevents gastric contents from flowing back into the esophagus with gastric distention.

Physiology of swallowing

Swallowing is divided into three sequential phases: the oral/preparatory phase, the pharyngeal phase, and the esophageal phase. The former is voluntary and is responsible for prehension, lubrication, mastication, and conduction of the food bolus to the valleculae, which are ventral depressions bounded rostrally by the base of the tongue, caudally by the elevated epiglottis, and dorsally by the soft palate. The bolus in the oropharynx, as well as the levator veli palatini muscle, causes the soft palate to elevate and close the nasopharynx off from the oropharynx to prevent nasopharyngeal reflux.

The pharyngeal and esophageal phases are involuntary once triggered. Pharyngeal swallowing may follow an oral/preparatory phase or occur spontaneously (i.e., reflexive swallow). Reflexive swallows are triggered by stimulation of the larynx and pharynx or by esophageal stimulation or distention (e.g., reflux). Stimulation of the larynx and pharynx is transmitted via the cranial laryngeal nerve and, to a lesser extent, the recurrent laryngeal and glossopharyngeal (cranial nerve IX) nerves. The cranial laryngeal and recurrent laryngeal nerves are branches of the vagus nerve (cranial nerve X). These signals are transmitted to the *nucleus tractus solitarius* and *nucleus ambiguus* to initiate the downstream contraction of the pharyngeal musculature, which propels the bolus through the UES.

The passage of the bolus through the UES triggers the start of the esophageal swallowing phase. Pharyngeal swallow stimulates primary peristalsis and relaxation of the LES to accommodate the bolus. The strength of the peristaltic contraction and rate of transit varies with bolus size and consistency and body position. At baseline (i.e., between swallows), the muscles are generally relaxed, except the UES and LES, which remain tonically contracted. In normal dogs, esophageal peristalsis may be modified while drinking liquids. For example, in deglutitive inhibition (Video 45.1), pharyngeal swallow proceeds as normal, but primary peristalsis is inhibited, and the LES remains relaxed until after the last pharyngeal swallow before returning to baseline. During deglutitive inhibition, secondary peristalsis may still occur. Secondary peristalsis is triggered by esophageal distention, which may occur secondary to food left behind after primary peristalsis or by refluxed content from the stomach into the esophagus. In addition to dilating in response to primary or secondary peristalsis, the LES may also open transiently independent of peristalsis (e.g., transient LES relaxations). While transient LES relaxations are important as a part of the eructation reflex, they are also considered significant contributors to gastroesophageal reflux in both dogs and people.

Video 45.1

Cine loop from a videofluoroscopic swallow study in a 6-year-old spayed female mixed-breed dog freely consuming a liquid test meal containing a non-ionic, low-osmolar contrast agents (iohexol 350 mg/ml), showing normal swallowing with deglutitive inhibition. Oral/preparatory and pharyngeal swallows are unremarkable. Contrast material accumulates in the esophagus before being cleared by secondary peristalsis without incident.

Esophageal disease as aerodigestive disease

Aerodigestive disease occurs when the coordinated interactions between the respiratory and alimentary tracts are disrupted. The aerodigestive tract includes the pharynx, larynx, trachea, bronchi, bronchioles as well as the esophagus and EGJ. For many components of the alimentary tract, airway protection remains a key, but underrecognized, function. The esophagus plays an important role in airway protection, such that most forms of esophageal disease are considered "aerodigestive diseases."[4]

Airway protection is a complex process involving breath–swallow coordination (i.e., "gatekeeping") as well as basal and response elements (Table 45.1). Swallowing and breathing are under the control of central pattern generators in the brainstem: the swallow and respiratory central pattern generators. Cross communication between both of them coordinates swallowing such that it occurs preferentially during specific phases of the respiratory cycle. Timing of swallowing in the respiratory cycle varies with species. In awake or anesthetized dogs, nearly 90% of swallows are initiated during the inspiratory phase. In people, swallowing typically occurs during the expiratory phase, and increases in inspiratory phase swallowing is associated with aspiration. Regardless of the phase of respiration, pharyngeal swallowing is associated with transient apnea caused by powerful laryngeal adduction and contraction of the diaphragm, resulting in airflow dropping nearly to zero during this period.[5]

Basal elements are barriers to aspiration that are present independent of stimulation. The specific mechanisms encountered depend on the source of aspiration (gastroesophageal vs. oropharyngeal). In case of gastroesophageal reflux, gastric contents must span two high-pressure zones (i.e., UES and LES) and overcome the residual volume of the esophagus (i.e., the volume that can be contained by the esophagus before overflowing into the pharynx or airways). Response elements, unlike basal elements, become active in response to stimulation. They fall into one of five categories: reflexes that clear volume, reflexes that increase the pressure of the LES, reflexes that increase the pressure of the UES, reflexes that cause laryngeal closure, and reflexes that remove material from the airways. The esophagus features prominently in both the basal and response elements of airway protection. The increased risk of aspiration in patients with esophageal disease reflects, in part, failures of these protective mechanisms.[4]

Clinical assessment

The clinical approach to esophageal disease begins with careful consideration of the dog's signalment and history. Some forms of esophageal dysfunction have documented breed or familial predispositions (Table 45.2). Dogs with an established lineage may have information regarding affected parents or littermates. The age of onset of clinical signs is variable. For dogs with congenital disease, signs are usually present from birth or weaning. Acquired esophageal dysfunction may develop variably throughout life depending on the underlying cause.

The acuity, frequency, and progression of the clinical signs provide important information. Persistent regurgitation may be associated with chronic conditions such as megaesophagus (ME), vascular ring anomalies, diverticula, mature strictures, and masses. Acute signs may result from esophageal foreign bodies (FBs), esophagitis, or gastroesophageal intussusception (GEI). Intermittent or progressive regurgitation may be associated with sliding hiatal hernia (SHH), reflux, or a developing esophageal stricture. The timing, frequency, and severity of regurgitation depends on the location and severity of the abnormality as well as the residual volume of the dilated esophagus. A massively dilated esophagus may contain significant residual volume from ingesta and swallowed oral secretions such that regurgitation can occur hours after eating. Even though dogs with regurgitation may have a good appetite, anorexia may be seen in patients with esophagitis and odynophagia (i.e., swallowing discomfort or pain).

TABLE 45.1 Summary of basal and response mechanisms of airway protection.

Basal mechanisms		LES	■ Smooth muscle band that in combination with the crura of the diaphragm, rugal folds, and angle of entry of the esophagus into the stomach results in a high-pressure zone at the esophageal gastric junction ■ Basal LES pressure varies with body position and degree of consciousness (e.g., tone lowered with sedation or anesthesia)
		UES	■ Barrier between the pharynx and esophagus ■ Tonic closure prevents aerophagia and reflux of material from the esophagus into the pharynx
		Residual volumes (esophagus and pharynx)	■ Volume that the pharynx and esophagus can contain without spilling over into the pharynx and/or airways
		Mucociliary apparatus	■ Ciliated epithelium and associated mucus layer that traps and clears aspirated material
		Innate immunity	■ Defense mechanism involving leukocytes and airway epithelium
Response mechanisms	Volume clearing	Reflexive pharyngeal swallow	■ Removes debris and residue from the entrance of the respiratory tract, without being preceded by an oral/preparatory phase ■ Thought to play a significant role in airway protection during sleep
		Primary esophageal peristalsis	■ Esophageal peristalsis triggered by pharyngeal swallowing
		Secondary esophageal peristalsis	■ Esophageal peristalsis triggered by luminal distention of the esophagus
	LES pressure	Gastroesophageal reflex	■ Increased LES tone in response to increased intragastric pressure
	UES pressure	Esophago-UES contractile reflex	■ Increased UES tone in response to slow, distal esophageal distention ■ Typically followed by peristalsis to clear esophageal volume
		Esophago-UES relaxation reflex	■ Decreased UES tone in response to rapid esophageal distention consistent with eructation
		Pharyngo-UES contractile reflex	■ Increased UES tone in response to pharyngeal stimulation ■ Ablated by topical anesthetics in experimental models
		Laryngo-UES contractile reflex	■ Increased UES tone in response to laryngeal stimulation
	Laryngeal closure	Esophagolaryngeal closure reflex	■ Laryngeal closure in response to esophageal distention ■ Reduction in this response due to esophagitis has been documented in animal models
		Pharyngeal–laryngeal adduction reflex	■ Laryngeal adduction in response to pharyngeal stimulation
		Laryngeal adductor reflex	■ Laryngeal adduction in response to laryngeal stimulation
	Particulate clearing	Cough and throat clear	■ Clearance of inhaled particulate, irritants, debris, and fluid from the respiratory tract

LES, lower esophageal sphincter; UES, upper esophageal sphincter.

TABLE 45.2 Breed predispositions for selected esophageal disorders.

Esophageal disorder	Predisposed breeds
Idiopathic esophageal dysmotility	Chinese Shar Pei, Bouvier des Flandres, terriers
Vascular ring anomalies	German Shepherd Dog, Irish Setter, Boxer, Labrador Retriever
Gastroesophageal intussusception	German Shepherd Dog, Chinese Shar Pei
Hiatal hernia	Brachycephalic breeds (e.g., French Bulldog), Chinese Shar Pei
Congenital segmental dysmotility	Chinese Shar Pei, Newfoundland
Congenital megaesophagus	Labrador Retriever, Newfoundland, Chinese Shar Pei, Great Dane, German Shepherd Dog, Irish Setter, goldendoodles, Miniature Dachshund, Miniature Schnauzer
Familial megaesophagus	Great Dane, German Shepherd Dog, Labrador Retriever, Irish Setter, Chinese Shar Pei, Newfoundland, Fox Terrier, Miniature Schnauzer

Additional relevant information includes difficulty eating a particular consistency of ingesta (kibble vs. liquid), recent dietary changes, association with activity, travel history (e.g., *Spirocerca lupi*, dysautonomia), recent anesthesia, drug exposure (e.g., vincristine), environmental exposure (e.g., lead), and any associated clinical signs, including those specific to the respiratory tract (e.g., cough, worsening of signs related to brachycephalic obstructive airway syndrome [BOAS], dysphonia).

Clinical signs

Regurgitation is the hallmark of esophageal dysfunction. It is critically important that regurgitation be distinguished from vomiting, oropharyngeal dysphagia, and expectoration (see Chapters 8–10). The timing, frequency, and appearance of regurgitated material is highly variable, and these features should be used cautiously when discriminating between regurgitation and vomiting. The appearance of the regurgitated material is rarely helpful in distinguishing regurgitation from vomiting, unless bile is present (although bile may also be seen in dogs with gastroduodenal–esophageal reflux). Careful observation of feeding behavior and of the act of regurgitation/vomiting itself may be needed to distinguish between these processes. Video recordings may be helpful, especially if a patient refuses to eat during examination. Vomiting and regurgitation may occur in the same patient (e.g., vomiting with secondary reflux esophagitis); in this case, the dominant and/or initial signs should be determined. Other signs of esophageal disease include ptyalism, halitosis, extension of the head and neck, repetitive "dry" swallowing (i.e., not associated with eating or drinking), odynophagia, intermittent epigastric pain, nighttime restlessness, weakness, and weight loss (e.g., decreased body condition score, sarcopenia).

It is important to recognize that dogs with esophageal dysfunction may present without signs of alimentary disease. Several studies have documented esophageal diseases (e.g., ME, SHH, esophageal hypomotility) in dogs with exclusively respiratory signs.[6,7] Dogs with esophageal dysfunction are also at increased risk of developing aspiration-associated respiratory syndromes (e.g., aspiration pneumonia, pneumonitis, diffuse aspiration bronchiolitis).[4] Aspiration pneumonia/pneumonitis is the leading cause of death in dogs with ME. In human medicine, *aspiration pneumonia* specifies bacterial infection, whereas sterile inflammation secondary to aspiration is referred to as *aspiration pneumonitis*. In veterinary medicine, *aspiration pneumonia* is often used to refer to both syndromes collectively, even though they are discrete processes. For the purposes of this chapter, aspiration pneumonia (AP) will refer to both syndromes, unless specified otherwise. Any dog with a history of AP, especially recurrent AP, should be evaluated for esophageal dysfunction.

Physical and neurological examination

Physical examination findings are variable. Complete physical and neurological examinations should be performed in all dogs with suspected esophageal disease. Dogs may have evidence of polyneuropathy (e.g., conscious proprioceptive deficits), myopathy (e.g., muscle atrophy), laryngeal dysfunction (e.g., dysphonia, stridor), cranial nerve deficits, and/or upper airway obstruction (e.g., laryngeal paralysis, BOAS). Harsh lung sounds (e.g., AP) and fever (e.g., AP, inflammatory myopathy) may be present in some patients. In dogs with ME, a fluid-filled esophagus may present as a bulge along the left side of the neck.

Diagnostic approach

The diagnostic approach to dogs with esophageal disease focuses on identifying the underlying cause and the consequences (e.g., AP) of esophageal disease.

Laboratory testing

A complete evaluation of systemic health is recommended for all patients. Initial testing should include a complete blood count with smear evaluation, serum biochemical profile including electrolytes and creatine kinase, and urinalysis. Specific testing is recommended based on the results of preliminary diagnostic tests (e.g., diagnostic imaging). Adrenocorticotropic stimulation testing and thyroid testing (thyroxine, thyroid-stimulating hormone, ± free thyroxine) may be appropriate if Addison's disease and hypothyroidism are suspected, respectively. The

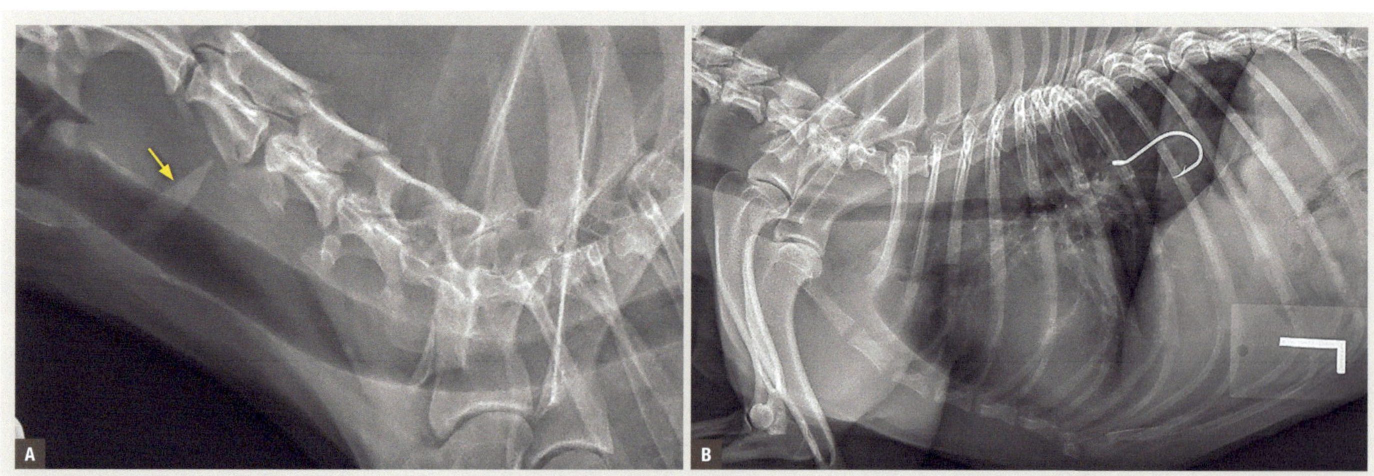

FIG. 45.1 (A) Right lateral cervical radiograph of a 3-year-old castrated male Chihuahua mix with an osseus foreign body (arrow) in the proximal esophagus. There is no evidence of perforation or subcutaneous emphysema. (B) Left lateral thoracic radiograph of a 2.5-year-old spayed female French Bulldog with a metallic foreign body (fishhook) in the distal esophagus. A small volume of fluid is present in the distal esophagus consistent with reflux. No evidence of either perforation or aspiration is identified. In both patients, the foreign body was successfully removed via endoscopy.

association between esophageal dysfunction and hypothyroidism, although frequently commented upon in the literature, is unclear. Euthyroid sick syndrome may complicate the interpretation of test results in some animals, particularly in those with concurrent severe illness.

Measuring acetylcholine receptor antibodies by radioimmunoassay is the criterion standard to diagnose acquired myasthenia gravis (MG) in dogs. Testing for MG is recommended for animals with generalized ME that lack another obvious underlying cause. In addition to esophageal dysfunction, dogs with MG may also demonstrate concurrent laryngeal paresis/paralysis and/or pharyngeal dysphagia. False negatives may occur with focal MG, in dogs receiving immunosuppressive medication, and in acute disease. Repeat titers 1–2 months after a negative test may be recommended. Seronegative generalized MG is reported in 2% of dogs. Acetylcholine receptor antibody testing is not recommended in dogs with suspected congenital MG (<6 months of age). An edrophonium response test may not be fruitful in dogs with focal MG.

Testing for infectious organisms, including *Neospora caninum*, *Spirocerca lupi*, *Pythium insidiosum*, and canine distemper virus, may be considered if appropriate. Persistently and markedly increased creatine kinase may be suggestive of an inflammatory, necrotizing, or dystrophic myopathy. Focal, chronic, or noninflammatory muscular diseases may result in mildly increased creatine kinase or values within the reference range.

Radiographs

Thoracic radiography is an important first-line diagnostic imaging modality for dogs with esophageal disease. Radiographs should include at least three projections of the thorax and one projection of the lateral neck (from at least T1 to the caudal aspect of the skull). Three thoracic projections are recommended because atelectasis of the dependent lung lobes may mask disease or be incorrectly interpreted as pneumonia. If sedation or anesthesia is required to take the radiographs, the former may be preferred, as it is less associated with atelectasis. In a single study in dogs, the mean percentage of atelectasis on thoracic radiographs was reported to be 6.67% for general anesthesia, compared to 0.01% for sedation. Concurrent pathology should be addressed (e.g., thoracocentesis for pleural effusion) prior to radiography to improve the quality of the images as well as patient stability. Imaging of the neck is important because collimation of the thorax does not extend substantially beyond the thoracic inlet, and pathology of the cervical esophagus may greatly contribute to clinical signs (Fig. 45.1). Careful attention should be paid to positioning and technique, as rotation and improper head position can significantly hamper interpretation.

AP is a leading cause of morbidity and mortality in dogs with esophageal disease. Interstitial–alveolar infiltrates in the dependent lung fields (e.g., right middle, right cranial, left caudal) are the conventional diagnostic criteria for AP in dogs. However, the position of the patient during aspiration dictates radiographic findings. For example, dogs aspirating while in dorsal recumbency demonstrated radiographic changes predominantly in the caudal lung lobes. Other aspiration-associated respiratory syndromes, such as bronchiectasis (i.e., irreversible dilation of the airway walls due to chronic inflammation), may also be identified.[4] Bronchiectasis seen in ventrally dependent lobar bronchi should prompt suspicion of aspiration.

Radiographs are not without limitations, however. Lesions in the pharynx or retropharyngeal space and radiolucent and tissue-dense foreign material (e.g., plastic, sticks) can be difficult to visualize. Additionally, radiographs may underestimate the severity of pulmonary lesions. Computed tomography (CT) provides improved resolution and lesion localization compared to thoracic radiographs in many cases, including bronchiectasis and diffuse aspiration bronchiolitis. Radiographs are also limited in their ability to detect and characterize dynamic/functional diseases (e.g., reflux, SHH, esophageal hypomotility). In fact, several recent studies have documented dogs with esophageal dysfunction despite normal thoracic and cervical radiographs.[7,8]

Contrast radiographs

Contrast radiography may be useful if additional imaging is needed to fully characterize a lesion observed on survey radiographs (Fig. 45.2). The type of contrast medium to be utilized depends on the circumstances. Non-ionic, low-osmolar contrast agents (e.g., iohexol 350 mg/ml) are often favored for intraluminal esophageal lesions or if perforation is suspected. Since the rheological properties of non-ionic contrast agents are comparable to those of water, these agents are preferred by some practitioners for videofluoroscopic swallow studies (VFSSs). Liquid barium (60% weight/volume) may also be used in place of non-ionic contrast agents for swallow studies; however, the difference in viscosity may impact objective metrics of swallowing.[9] Barium suspensions may be preferred for dogs with a suspected esophageal fistula due to their viscosity and ability to highlight defects and irregularities in the esophageal mucosa. However, barium is not recommended for patients with suspected esophageal perforation because of the potential to cause a granulomatous reaction. Perforation may be suspected if survey radiographs show gas in the cervical soft tissues or mediastinum, which may be accompanied by a pleural effusion. As such, survey radiographs should always precede contrast radiographs; this will also prevent FBs and pulmonary pathology from being masked by the contrast medium. Sedation should be avoided for contrast radiographs due to the risk of aspiration and the effect of sedation on swallowing function.

Videofluoroscopic swallow studies and respiratory fluoroscopy

The criterion standard in dogs for diagnosis of many types of esophageal disease is VFSSs. This technique allows real-time imaging of all phases of swallowing. Multiple methods for performing a VFSS are reported. Techniques in which patients are positioned in lateral recumbency and force-fed were the historical standard in some parts of the world. However, free-feeding techniques have gained prominence due to the ability to mimic normal feeding practices, including physiologically relevant bolus sizes and body position. Free-feeding protocols also limit the risk of aspiration to what a dog would experience at home, which is important in patients already at high risk. Free-feeding techniques are limited by patient compliance, but one study reported an approximately 80% acceptance rate using published techniques and recipes.[9] Overnight food restriction, preparation of test food immediately before use, and an acclimation period after the dog enters the testing area may improve compliance.

Different consistencies are fed during a VFSS to highlight specific conditions (e.g., liquid for aspiration and aerophagia, kibble for pharyngeal weakness). Images are collected at 30 frames per second. Three to five swallows per food consistency, including multiple swallows in series, is considered ideal. Objective metrics for normal swallowing are published but depend on the collection technique.[9] For example, increased stimulation of primary peristalsis and faster rate of bolus transit through the cervical esophagus was identified in dogs swallowing in sternal recumbency, compared to those in lateral recumbency.[10] Sedation and

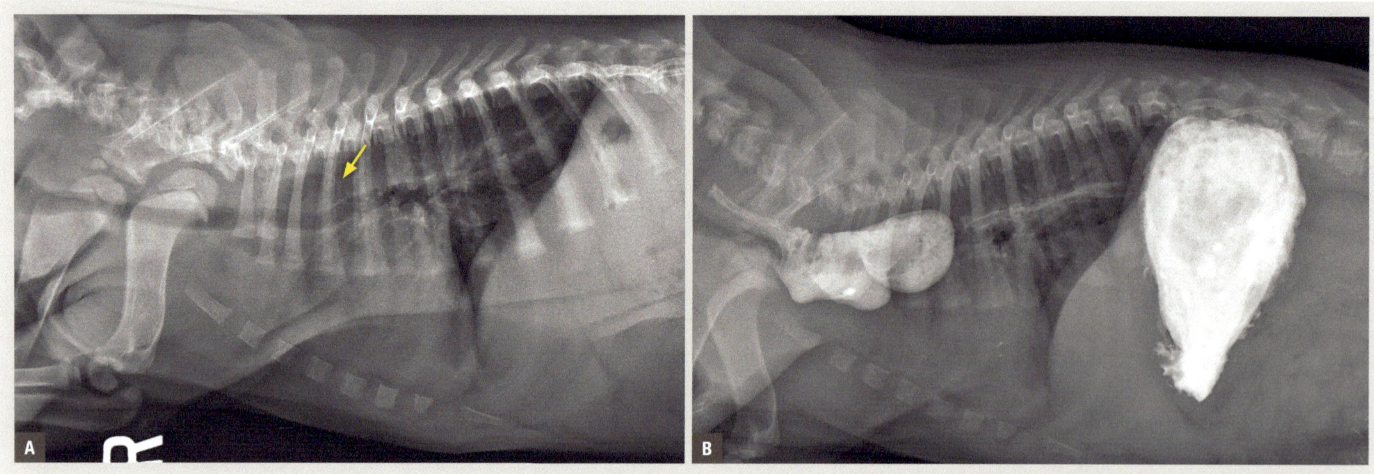

FIG. 45.2 Right lateral thoracic radiographs of a 7-week-old intact female Staffordshire Terrier diagnosed with a persistent right aortic arch. (A) Survey radiograph showing mild ventral deviation of the cranial intrathoracic trachea and proximal esophageal gas dilation at the level of the heart base (arrow). (B) Barium contrast radiograph highlighting the dilated proximal esophagus (i.e., focal megaesophagus). A small portion of the barium-containing bolus can pass through the narrowed esophageal lumen.

restraint can also impact results (e.g., decreased LES tone with sedation), but deglutitive inhibition is a normal finding in dogs consuming liquids. A distinction should also be made between pathological and physiological reflux (see below).

Respiratory fluoroscopy can be performed to look for dynamic changes in the respiratory tract. Movement of airway structures should be evaluated in the context of the phase of respiration to avoid missing subtle forms of upper airway obstruction (e.g., pharyngeal collapse, epiglottic retroversion). Upper airway obstruction has been linked to several esophageal and aerodigestive conditions, including reflux, aerophagia, and SHH. Respiratory fluoroscopy should precede VFSSs to avoid structures being masked by the contrast medium. Images are collected at 30 frames per second both during quiet breathing and with coughing.

Endoscopy

Endoscopy is a useful diagnostic and therapeutic modality in dogs with esophageal strictures, ulcers, or FBs or to identify mucosal lesions that may be missed on radiography or VFSSs. Biopsy collection, FB retrieval, and balloon dilation of an esophageal stricture can be performed at the time of evaluation. Endoscopy is not recommended in areas with residual contrast material (e.g., barium) due to the risk of damaging the endoscope. Conventional endoscopy is performed under general anesthesia, which carries increased risk of aspiration and reflux. Capsule endoscopy has been validated in people with esophageal disease, but the utility of this technique for esophageal disease in dogs is unknown. Further, treatment of lesions identified on capsule endoscopy would require a separate procedure under anesthesia. Consequently, conventional endoscopy is preferred for dogs with esophageal disease.

Computed tomography

CT is an important adjunct to conventional radiography for detection of lesions in both the lungs and esophagus and is superior to radiography for detecting pulmonary pathology. CT evaluation of the lungs is best performed under anesthesia, with inspiratory and expiratory breath holding. This reduces atelectasis, highlights air trapping, and diminishes movement artifact.[11] CT is also useful for evaluating diseases of the esophagus and EGJ. For example, CT angiography may be recommended when assessing vascular ring anomalies. Additionally, CT is used to characterize and determine the extent of esophageal perforations, diverticula, abscesses, tracheo- and bronchoesophageal fistulas, *Spirocerca lupi* granulomas, traumatic esophageal injury, and esophageal masses. Limitations of CT include the need for anesthesia or sedation. Further, imaging the lumen of the esophagus can be challenging. A study in healthy dogs found that esophageal insufflation CT may help visualize the esophageal lumen at an insufflation pressure of 5 mmHg. Even though no dogs in this study exhibited adverse effects, similar studies in dogs with esophageal disease are lacking.

Ultrasonography

Conventional ultrasonography can be used to visualize the cervical and intrabdominal esophagus as well as the gastric cardia. The abdominal esophagus and the cardia can be seen through the acoustic window of the left hepatic lobe, with esophageal layering being adequately visualized in 89% of dogs. Ultrasound of the intrathoracic esophagus is uncommon, although it is reported in dogs with the aid of endoscopy. Esophageal ultrasonography is limited by availability and the need for specialist equipment and training; however, indications include fistula, diverticula, mural infiltration, and esophageal/periesophageal masses.

Scintigraphy

Nuclear scintigraphy has been used to measure mucociliary clearance and diagnose esophageal perforations and fistulas. However, it can also be utilized to measure reflux and small volume aspiration. Detecting reflux and aspiration using scintigraphy is noninvasive, can be performed without anesthesia, and is not reliant on gastric pH. A study has validated this technique in dogs using a meal containing colloidal technetium-99m phytate. Reflux was defined as counts $\geq$200% of background activity with a corresponding decrease in gastric counts. Scintigraphy may be more sensitive than VFSSs for detecting small-volume reflux events but is currently limited to tertiary referral facilities.

High-resolution manometry

High-resolution manometry is the preferred diagnostic test for esophageal motility disease in human medicine. It assesses motility patterns in the esophagus by measuring contractile and relaxation events over time. A catheter incorporating up to 36 pressure sensors along its length is placed transnasally as far as the stomach (1–3 cm distal to the diaphragm). Pressure changes at baseline and during swallowing are recorded to show the pressure topography of the esophagus. Although this technique is not widely available in veterinary medicine, its use in specialty referral and research centers has provided important information on esophageal motility patterns in dogs, including changes in response to therapy (e.g., metoclopramide, cisapride). From a One Health perspective, high-resolution manometry has also been used to characterize diseases common between dogs and people, including LES achalasia (Fig. 45.3).

Endoluminal functional lumen imaging probe

Endoluminal functional lumen imaging probe (EndoFLIP) assesses the cross-sectional area and pressure of the LES during contraction (i.e., impedance planimetry). Collectively this allows measurement of LES distensibility and compliance. Although this technique is frequently used in people to evaluate diseases of the EGJ, it is not widely available in veterinary medicine, but it has been used to measure LES tone in dogs with SHH and in dogs with pneumoperitoneum. Broader applications may be identified as this technique becomes more widespread.

Esophageal pH and impedance

This technique measures changes in esophageal pH over time. Ambulatory pH monitoring is minimally invasive and has been used to identify reflux in dogs following anesthesia and in dogs with SHH and to optimize the treatment of gastroesophageal reflux disease (GERD) by evaluating changes in gastric pH in response to antacid therapy. In addition to being more comfortable, ambulatory pH monitoring is superior to transnasal pH catheters because it collects data over a longer period (up to 96 hours) and allows the dog to adopt multiple body positions and activity levels. This may be superior for detecting episodic reflux events.

The monitoring of esophageal pH has several limitations, including not being useful for detecting reflux in patients receiving acid suppressive medications or in those with nonacidic reflux. Monitoring of pH is also unable to detect cumulative or superimposed reflux (i.e., reflux event that occurs before a preceding event is cleared) or to distinguish between pathological and physiological reflux. Further, ambulatory pH probe placement requires anesthesia. The addition of impedance monitoring may address some of these limitations by increasing detection of nonacidic or only weakly acidic reflux events. This measures electrical impedance differences between different materials (high impedance: air; low impedance: liquid) and so can track bolus movement. In people, impedance is combined with high-resolution manometry to assess both esophageal pressure and bolus movement. This technique is not yet available in veterinary medicine. Photocolorimetric monitoring of esophageal bile (e.g., duodenogastroesophageal reflux) has been reported in people but has not been investigated in dogs.

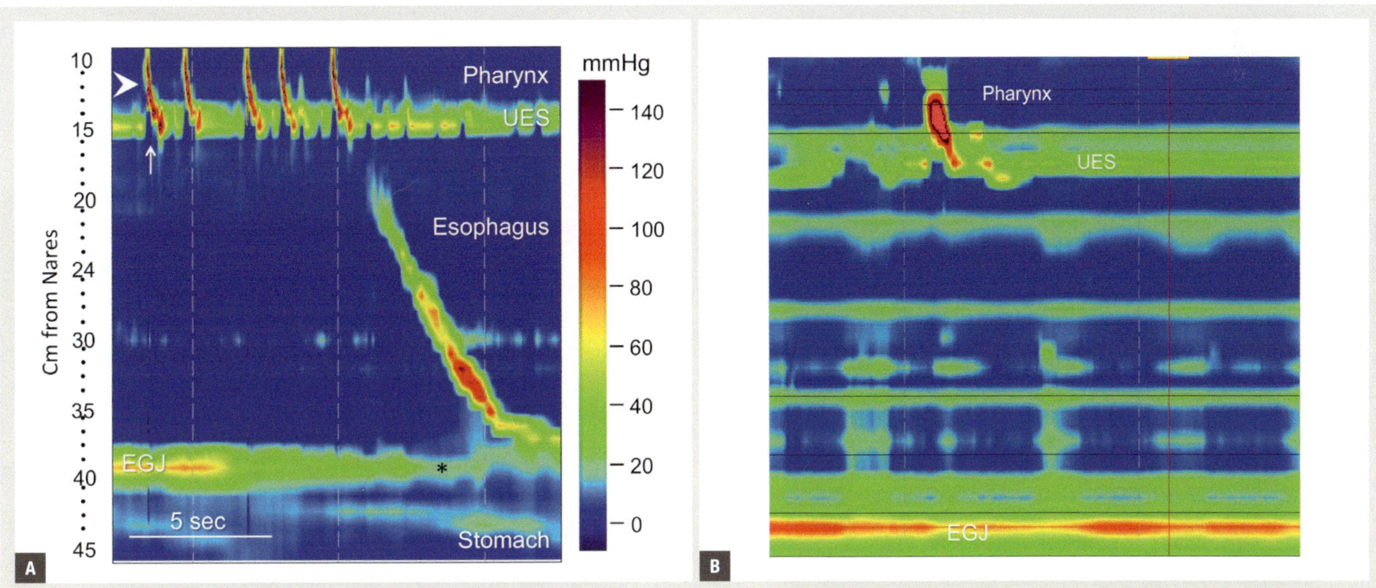

FIG. 45.3 Representative high-resolution esophageal topography profiles of esophageal motor activity generated by the administration of a single liquid bolus (5 mL of water) in a healthy 7.2 kg mixed-breed Terrier (A) and in a 9.4 kg Cairn Terrier with megaesophagus and esophageal achalasia (B). Pressure is represented by color-coding (interpreted based on the color bar on the right). Time is on the x-axis, and sensor location (distance from the nares) is on the y-axis. (A) In the healthy animal, resting upper esophageal sphincter (UES) and esophageal gastric junction (EGJ), or lower esophageal sphincter, pressures are seen as horizontal bands of color that are several centimeters in width. Their hues indicate pressures that are greater than those in the adjacent portion of the pharynx, esophagus, or stomach. Opening of the UES (arrow) and EGJ (asterisk) are depicted as color changes to hues that represent lower pressures. The diagonal bars of color in the pharynx (arrowhead) represent pharyngeal peristaltic contractions produced by swallows of liquid. A diagonal band of color running from just below the UES to the EGJ represents the esophageal peristaltic pressure wave generated by the swallows of liquid. (B) In the diseased animal, the profile is notable for the 100% failure of primary and secondary peristalsis following pharyngeal contraction and relaxation of the UES. In addition, the integrated relaxation pressure, an indication of residual EGJ pressure during swallow-induced relaxation, is persistently above 15 mmHg, which is consistent with a diagnosis of type 1 esophageal achalasia. Images courtesy of Prof. Dr. Stanly Marks, UC Davis College of Veterinary Medicine.

Electrodiagnostic testing and muscle and nerve biopsies

Electromyography and nerve conduction velocity testing are performed to detect myopathies and neuropathies in dogs. They are usually used in combination and in the context of the neurological examination to discriminate between different disease states. Although direct esophageal electrodiagnostic testing has been performed in experimental settings, in routine practice it is used when esophageal dysmotility is thought to be part of a generalized process. Electrodiagnostic tests may inform the best place for biopsy collection. Ideally, samples should be collected contralateral to the site of electrodiagnostic testing to avoid artifact from needle insertion.

Muscle and nerve biopsies may provide a histopathologic diagnosis as well as prognostic information for a variety of myopathies and neuromuscular diseases. End-stage disease, extensive damage, fibrosis, and fiber loss make achieving a diagnosis challenging and are associated with a less favorable overall prognosis. As such, muscle and nerve biopsies are ideally collected from an affected but functional muscle/nerve in the acute phase of disease and prior to starting corticosteroid therapy. Samples should be evaluated by a pathologist experienced in cases of muscular/neuromuscular disease.

Functional upper airway examination

There is a strong link between upper airway obstruction and pharyngeal and esophageal disease.[12] This includes neuromuscular conditions, such as geriatric onset laryngeal paralysis polyneuropathy and MG, as well as reflux and SHH, among others. Reflux is associated with laryngeal paresis, laryngeal collapse, inflammatory laryngeal polyps, and BOAS. Importantly, studies in brachycephalic dogs have documented improvement in GI signs with correction of BOAS and reduction in BOAS signs with treatment for reflux.[13] Given this interrelatedness, evaluating patency and function of the upper airway is an important part of assessing dogs with esophageal disease. This is particularly true if signs of upper airway obstruction are identified.

A comprehensive functional upper airway examination involves evaluating the external structures of the head and neck and assessing nasal airflow. When examining the inside of the oral cavity, particular attention should be paid to the hard and soft palate, tongue, teeth, and pharynx in addition to the larynx. A laryngeal function examination should be performed under a very light plane of anesthesia. Administration of doxopram has been recommended to reduce the risk of a false-positive diagnosis. Laryngeal adduction corresponds to inspiration, so movement should be interpreted considering the respiratory phase. Minimizing traction placed on the tongue will improve detection of epiglottic retroversion. Even though performing a functional upper airway examination is relatively simple, the risk of airway obstruction, reflux, and aspiration warrants appropriate planning and staffing during the procedure.[14]

Bronchoscopy and bronchoalveolar lavage

Bronchoscopy can be helpful when evaluating dogs with respiratory disease secondary to aspiration. A tracheal stripe sign (i.e., proximal tracheal erythema dissipating toward the carina) may be seen in dogs with aspiration. Bronchiectasis and inhaled foreign material (e.g., dog food) can be identified via bronchoscopy. Thoracic radiographs and/or CT are recommended prior to bronchoscopy to target the most affected areas. Bronchoalveolar lavage fluid collection for culture (aerobic ± anaerobic) ± PCR for mycoplasma, and cytology is important to diagnose inflammatory airway disease and to distinguish between AP and pneumonitis. Recent studies have documented inflammatory airway disease without AP in dogs with dysphagia and aspiration on VFSSs.[6]

Functional/motility disorders of the esophagus

Esophageal dysmotility

Etiology

Esophageal dysmotility is defined as ineffective peristalsis with esophageal bolus retention or prolonged esophageal transit time leading to regurgitation. This may occur in the absence of ME. Causes are suspected to be very similar to those of ME and may precede esophageal dilation in these cases (see below). Familial esophageal dysmotility has been reported in several dog breeds (see Table 45.2). Delayed esophageal maturation resulting in esophageal dysmotility without ME has been identified in multiple breeds, although Terrier breeds may be overrepresented. In these cases, motility may continue to improve for up to 1 year due to continued maturation of the neuromuscular system. Esophageal dysmotility may also be seen transiently following anesthesia, which impairs clearance of reflux events and likely contributes to postanesthetic esophagitis.

Clinical features

Clinical features and clinicopathological findings are like those for ME, and similar efforts should be made to identify an underlying cause. Some dogs may be asymptomatic depending on the degree of impairment.

Clinicopathological findings

Clinicopathological findings vary with the underlying cause.

Diagnosis

Generalized or segmental esophageal dilation may be identified on thoracic radiography. However, unremarkable thoracic radiographs do not rule out esophageal dysmotility. Evidence of AP, bronchiectasis, and/or other aspiration-associated respiratory syndromes may be observed. VFSSs are the most accurate means to diagnose esophageal dysmotility in dogs, which is defined as abnormal primary peristaltic waves that fail to propel a bolus aborally more than 5 cm or secondary peristaltic waves that fail to clear residual esophageal volume.

Treatment

Therapy for esophageal dysmotility is as for ME (see below). Radiographs or VFSSs may be considered every 2–3 months to monitor progression.

Megaesophagus

Etiology

ME is diagnosed by the presence of esophageal dilation with concurrent esophageal dysmotility. It may be described as generalized (i.e., the entire esophagus) or focal (i.e., a discrete region of the esophagus) and as congenital or acquired. Breed and familial predispositions are well-known (Table 45.2). ME should be distinguished from transient esophageal dilation secondary to aerophagia, sedation, or anesthesia, which may not be accompanied by persistent esophageal dysfunction.[15] Representative causes, diagnostics, and treatments for ME are presented in Table 45.3. It is important to recognize that "idiopathic" ME is a diagnosis of exclusion. Congenital idiopathic ME in German Shepherd Dogs has been recently identified as a sex-differentiated trait due to mutations in the melanin-concentrating hormone receptor 2 gene. Overall, identifying the underlying cause of ME may allow for targeted interventions and an improved outcome.

Clinical features

Clinical features of ME are similar to those of other forms of esophageal disease. Specific clinical and clinicopathological features are often related to the underlying etiology (e.g., clinical signs consistent with lower motor neuron disease).

Clinicopathological findings

Relevant clinicopathological findings are specific to the underlying cause. Specific diagnostic tests should be selected based on the patient's age, signalment, and diagnostic imaging findings.

Diagnosis

Thoracic radiographs are the first-line diagnostic test for ME. Radiographic findings include generalized or focal dilation of the esophagus containing gas, fluid, or ingesta (see Fig. 21.3). Survey radiographs will help identify AP; however, as previously mentioned, radiographs may underestimate the distribution and severity of AP and lack the sensitivity to diagnose other aspiration-associated respiratory syndromes compared to CT. Radiographs may help provide evidence of thymic enlargement,

TABLE 45.3 Representative causes, diagnostics, and treatment for generalized and focal megaesophagus in dogs.

Causes		Diagnosis	Treatment
Generalized megaesophagus			
Idiopathic	Congenital	Diagnosis of exclusion	Supportive care ± sildenafil
	Acquired	Diagnosis of exclusion	Supportive care ± sildenafil
LES achalasia		VFSS, manometry	Balloon dilation and LES botulinum toxin A injections, modified Heller myotomy with Dor fundoplication, ± sildenafil
Endocrine	Hypothyroidism (possible association, not causation)	T_4 + TSH, ± free T_4, supportive physical examination and biochemical findings (e.g., hypercholesterolemia)	Levothyroxine
	Hypoadrenocorticism	ACTH stimulation test	Glucocorticoid ± mineralocorticoid supplementation
Neuromuscular	Myasthenia gravis	AChR antibody titers ± EMG ± clinical response to edrophonium	Pyridostigmine ± prednisone
	Polyradiculoneuritis	Ruling out other causes of LMND	Rehabilitation therapy, ventilator support as needed
	Tick paralysis	Finding a tick or tick pit (recent bite) on dog with supportive clinical signs (e.g., LMND)	Removal of all ticks, treatment with topical acaricide, supportive care
	Glycogen storage disease II	Muscle biopsy, liver biopsy, urine metabolic screening	Supportive care
	Dysautonomia	Clinical signs, supportive travel history, ± dilute pilocarpine response test, atropine response test, or intradermal histamine	Supportive care
	Immune-mediated polymyositis	CK, muscle biopsy, ± EMG	Immune suppression (e.g., prednisone 1–2 mg/kg every 24 h)
	Generalized inflammatory myopathy	CK, muscle biopsy, ± EMG	Immune suppression (e.g., prednisone 1–2 mg/kg every 24 h)
	Preneoplastic syndrome (e.g., lymphoma, myeloid leukemia)	Identification and sampling of potential preneoplastic lesions	Treating underlying cause
	LP-PNC and GOLPP	Functional upper airway examination, EMG, NCV test	Supportive care ± laryngeal tie-back
	Dermatomyositis	Skin and muscle biopsy	Pentoxifylline, immune suppression, vitamin E
	Demyelinating polyneuropathy	Muscle and nerve biopsy, EMG, NCV test	Supportive care
	Cervical vertebral instability with leukomalacia	MRI	Addressing underlying cause, supportive care
	Brainstem lesions	MRI	Addressing underlying cause, supportive care
	Systemic lupus erythematosus	Antinuclear antibody titers, skin biopsy	Immune suppression (e.g., prednisone 1–2 mg/kg every 24 h)

(continues)

TABLE 45.3 Representative causes, diagnostics, and treatment for generalized and focal megaesophagus in dogs.

Causes		Diagnosis	Treatment
Generalized megaesophagus			
Toxicity	Lead	Hematology (e.g., basophilic stippling), blood lead concentration, known exposure	Decontamination, chelation (e.g., EDTA ± thiamine), supportive care
	Thallium	Thallium concentration in blood and hair	Decontamination, supportive care
	Organophosphates	Whole blood cholinesterase activity	Decontamination (e.g., gastric lavage, careful bathing), atropine sulfate, pralidoxime chloride, or 2-pyridine aldoxime methochloride
	Botulism	History of exposure to carrion, toxin assay (serum, feces, gastrointestinal contents, or food), ± EMG and NCV test	Supportive care, ventilator support as needed
	Envenomation (e.g., elapid snakes)	Supportive exposure, bite wound	Antivenom
	Acrylamide	History of exposure, muscle and nerve biopsies, acrylamide measurement in food	Supportive care
	Vincristine	History of administration	Supportive care
Infectious agents	*Spirocerca lupi*	Endoscopy with biopsy, CT, fecal flotation/sedimentation	Doramectin, milbemycin oxime, and moxidectin; surgery in dogs with malignant transformation
	Neospora caninum	Serology, muscle biopsy	Clindamycin, trimethoprim–sulfonamide, pyrimethamine, ponazuril (combinations of drugs frequently prescribed)
	Canine distemper virus	CSF tap, antibody titers, conjunctival scraping	Supportive care
Esophageal obstruction	Distal esophageal stricture	VFSS, endoscopy	Balloon dilation, bougienage, ± triamcinolone or mitomycin C
	Distal esophageal mass	Radiography (survey or contrast), VFSS, ultrasound, CT	Surgical excision
	Hiatal hernia (types 1 and 2)	Radiography (survey or contrast), VFSS, endoscopy	Surgical correction, medical management (see "Reflux" section below)
	Gastric dilatation and volvulus	Abdominal radiography	Surgical correction
	Gastroesophageal intussusception	Radiography (survey or contrast), VFSS, endoscopy	Surgical correction
Esophagitis		Endoscopy	Antacid therapy, mucosal protection, prokinetic therapy (see "Reflux" section below)
Paraneoplastic syndromes (e.g., thymoma)		Radiography, CT, fine needle aspiration/biopsy	Surgical resection
Pituitary dwarfism		Growth hormone stimulation test, genetic testing	Supportive care, hormone supplementation
Focal megaesophagus			
Vascular ring anomaly		Radiography (survey or contrast), VFSS, CT angiogram	Surgical correction
Esophageal stricture		Radiography (contrast), VFSS, endoscopy	Balloon dilation, bougienage, ± triamcinolone or mitomycin C
Esophageal mass		Radiography (survey or contrast), VFSS, CT, endoscopy, biopsy	Surgical resection, chemotherapy
Esophageal foreign body		Radiography (survey or contrast), endoscopy	Endoscopic or surgical removal

AChR, acetylcholine receptor; ACTH, adrenocorticotropic hormone; CK, creatine kinase; CSF, cerebrospinal fluid; CT, computed tomography; EDTA, ethylenediaminetetraacetic acid; EMG, electromyography; GOLPP, geriatric onset laryngeal paralysis polyneuropathy; LES, lower esophageal sphincter; LMND, lower motor neuron disease; LP-PNC, laryngeal paralysis–polyneuropathy complex; MRI, magnetic resonance imaging; NCV, nerve conduction velocity; T_4, thyroxine; TSH, thyroid-stimulating hormone; VFSS, videofluoroscopic swallow study.

masses, or other discrete lesions specific to the underlying disease process. A VFSS may show hypo- or aperistalsis, help define LES function (normal vs. achalasia), and is recommended for most cases of generalized ME. Endoscopy may be a useful adjunctive diagnostic and therapeutic tool, particularly if causes of mechanical obstruction (e.g., strictures, masses, FBs) are suspected.

Treatment

In addition to treating the underlying cause, supportive care is a critical part of managing dogs with ME. Upright feeding (e.g., Bailey chair) and small frequent meals can help promote bolus transit into the stomach. Dogs should be kept upright for 10–20 minutes after feeding. Feeding trials with different consistencies are recommended, as no single consistency is superior in all cases. If feeding by mouth is not possible due to refractory signs, gastrostomy/percutaneous endoscopic gastrostomy (PEG) tubes may be considered to ensure adequate consumption of calories. Studies evaluating sildenafil showed clinical improvement, including weight gain and reduced frequency of regurgitation, in dogs receiving 1 mg/kg PO every 12 hours. However, many practitioners recommend administering sildenafil every 8 hours due to the drug's short half-life. The response to metoclopramide and cisapride is variable, with many animals having worse signs with increases in LES tone. Prokinetics are most likely to be helpful in dogs with ME secondary to reflux esophagitis.

Repeated aspiration of oral secretions and retained esophageal volume may be a significant problem despite supportive management. In these cases, a fenestrated esophagostomy tube may be considered. Antibiotics should be judiciously used in dogs with ME. Although, hypothetically, ME may be associated with increased risk of bacterial AP, the use of antibiotics should be considered on a case-by-case basis to avoid developing antibiotic resistance.[16] Educating pet owners about managing dogs with ME is critical given the significant risks of aspiration, dehydration, and malnutrition in the long run.

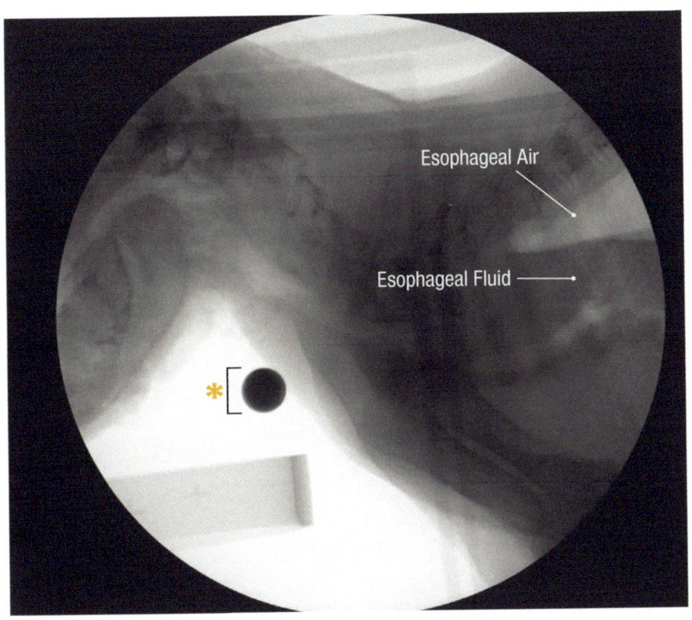

FIG. 45.4 Still image from a videofluoroscopic swallow study in a 7-year-old castrated male mixed-breed dog with lower esophageal sphincter achalasia and megaesophagus. Severe esophageal dilation with marked esophageal fluid retention can be seen despite a 12-hour fast. The asterisk denotes a 1 cm size marker.

Monitoring is recommended every 1–2 months to evaluate the progression of esophageal dilation. Spontaneous remission of congenital ME is possible before 1 year of age. The overall prognosis for dogs with ME is guarded but varies with the underlying disease process, available targeted interventions, and development of secondary complications.

Lower esophageal sphincter achalasia

Etiology

LES achalasia, with or without ME, is a recently identified cause of esophageal dysmotility in dogs. It occurs due to a failure of the LES to relax in response to a pharyngeal swallow. The hypertonic LES acts as a barrier to esophageal clearance, causing clinical signs consistent with esophageal dysfunction. The underlying cause of LES achalasia in dogs is unknown, although individual cases secondary to MG and LES denervation have been identified.

Clinical features

Clinical signs are similar to those shown by most dogs with esophageal disease.

Clinicopathological findings

There are no discriminating clinicopathological features for LES achalasia.

Diagnosis

LES achalasia is a functional disorder that cannot be diagnosed by radiography alone. A diagnosis is achieved by VFSSs or manometry (Fig. 45.3). On a VFSS, the LES must be evaluated for appropriate relaxation during pharyngeal swallowing. An elongated contrast column in the esophagus terminating in an elongated taper, referred to as a "bird beak", is characteristic of achalasia in both people and dogs. The hypertonic LES is also associated with substantial accumulation of fluid in the esophagus even after a prolonged fast (Fig. 45.4).

Treatment

Importantly, dogs with LES achalasia may respond favorably to treatment targeting the LES, including balloon dilation and local botulinum toxin A injections or a modified Heller myotomy with Dor fundoplication.[2,17]

Hiatal hernia

Etiology

A hiatal hernia is the protrusion of any abdominal viscera through an enlarged diaphragmatic esophageal hiatus and/or due to stretching of the phrenoesophageal ligaments. Four types of hiatal hernias are recognized:

- Type 1 (i.e., sliding hernia) is the most common hiatal hernia in dogs and occurs when the esophageal hiatus widens and allows forward movement of the LES and gastric cardia into the thoracic cavity.
- Type 2 (i.e., paraesophageal hernia) is associated with herniation of a portion of the stomach (usually the fundus) alongside the thoracic esophagus, while the LES and cardia remain in place.
- Type 3 is a combination of types 1 and 2.
- Type 4 is a combination of type 3 with the herniation of organs other than the stomach.

Herniation is frequently associated with significant reflux, esophagitis, and changes in esophageal motility. In SHH, reflux is likely due to the decreased tone of the EGJ with displacement of the LES.

Congenital hiatal hernia has been described in the Chinese Shar Pei, English Bulldog, and Chow Chow. This form arises from incomplete fusion of the diaphragm during embryonic development and is anecdotally associated with more severe clinical signs. Acquired hiatal hernia may occur in any breed, although the French Bulldog is overrepresented. This form may be seen secondary to increases in intra-abdominal pressure (e.g., trauma), neuromuscular dysfunction of the diaphragm (e.g., tetanus), esophageal dysmotility, and upper airway obstruction (e.g., BOAS, laryngeal paralysis). Brachycephalic dogs are considered predisposed, as upper airway obstruction secondary to BOAS increases negative intrathoracic pressure. In one study, brachycephalic dogs with a SHH were younger and more likely to present in respiratory distress than nonbrachycephalic dogs with a SHH.[8]

Clinical features

Clinical signs associated with a hiatal hernia may be intermittent and include regurgitation, ptyalism, vomiting, nighttime restlessness, abdominal pain, and nasal discharge. Severe herniation may be associated with coughing, AP, and respiratory distress. A hiatal hernia may also be identified in asymptomatic dogs. A lack of classical signs does not necessarily indicate that the process is benign. The reflux and esophageal dysmotility that accompany a hernia may put these dogs at increased risk for future esophagitis or other forms of aerodigestive disease.

Clinicopathological findings

There are no discriminating clinicopathological findings between types or causes of hiatal hernia.

Diagnosis

Survey thoracic radiographs should be taken in all dogs with a suspected hiatal hernia. A soft tissue or mixed opacity (i.e., soft tissue and gas) may be identified in the caudodorsal lung fields (Fig. 45.5). Unfortunately, survey radiography is poorly sensitive for diagnosing SHHs due to the intermittent nature of herniation events. Contrast radiography may highlight the relative positions of the EGJ and diaphragmatic hiatus, but abdominal compression may be needed to induce a hernia in some dogs. Radiographs will also help identify AP if present. A VFSS is more sensitive than radiography for detecting a SHH, any accompanying reflux (i.e., physiological vs. pathological), and esophageal dysmotility.[8] In dogs with a SHH, esophageal dilation may be observed without concurrent herniation, resulting in a misdiagnosis of idiopathic ME.

Endoscopy can also be used to identify a SHH. Increasing transdiaphragmatic pressure gradients under anesthesia has been shown to improve detection of SHHs compared to conventional radiography.[18] Manipulations under anesthesia include manual pressure to the abdomen, temporary complete endotracheal tube obstruction, and Trendelenburg position (30° head down in left lateral recumbency). Endoscopy of the esophagus may also diagnose esophagitis. Manometry and EndoFlip have also been used successfully to identify SHHs in dogs.

Treatment

Medical management is recommended for asymptomatic dogs with pathological reflux on VFSSs, dogs with mild to moderate clinical signs, or dogs with severe signs awaiting surgery. Surgery should be considered in dogs with congenital disease, those that do not respond to medical management, or those with severe regurgitation, reflux disease, and/or recurrent AP. Medical management is as for reflux disease (see below).

For dogs requiring surgery, esophagopexy, left fundic tube gastropexy, and diaphragmatic crural apposition are often sufficient. Laparoscopic techniques, although not widely available, may be associated with less patient morbidity. Surgical correction of upper airway obstruction (e.g., laryngeal paralysis, BOAS) should be considered if this disorder is suspected to have contributed to the hernia, as dogs with severe upper airway obstruction may be at higher risk for failure of the hernia repair. Despite surgical correction, GERD may persist, requiring lifelong medical management.

Gastroesophageal intussusception

Etiology

GEI refers to the invagination of the stomach, with or without other abdominal organs, into the lumen of the caudal esophagus. It is typically identified in dogs <3 months of age. Male dogs, German Shepherd Dogs, and Shar Peis are overrepresented. GEI may occur intermittently because of laxity at the esophageal hiatus, esophageal dysmotility, and ME. It has also been identified with *Spirocerca lupi* infection and in one dog following balloon dilation and esophageal botulinum toxin A

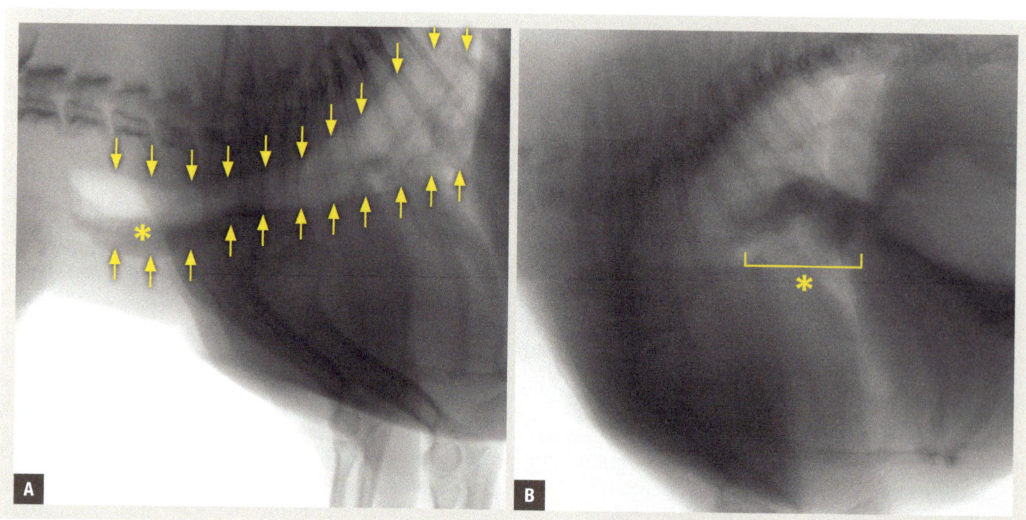

FIG. 45.5 Still images from a videofluoroscopic swallow study in a 4-year-old castrated male French Bulldog that presented for regurgitation, cranial abdominal pain, and exacerbations in clinical signs associated with brachycephalic obstructive airway syndrome. (A) Megaesophagus (arrows) with severe aerophagia and contrast material (asterisk) within the proximal esophagus, reflecting pathological reflux. (B) The stomach (asterisk) can be seen extending through the diaphragm into the thorax, consistent with a sliding hiatal hernia.

injections for esophageal achalasia. In one study, 50% of dogs with GEI had preexisting esophageal abnormalities.

Clinical features

Affected dogs may have a history of regurgitation or other clinical signs of esophageal disease, including vomiting, respiratory distress, hematemesis, and abdominal pain. Without rapid intervention, this may progress to shock, respiratory/cardiac arrest, and death.

Diagnosis

A GEI is identified radiographically if the stomach is displaced at the time of the radiograph. Survey radiographs may show severe esophageal dilation with a distal esophageal mass effect within the lumen and no evidence of the stomach in the abdomen (Fig. 45.6). Rugal folds may be highlighted by contrast radiography. GEI may be diagnosed endoscopically if rugal folds are identified in the caudal esophagus. This may be seen concurrently with esophagitis, esophageal obstruction, and ME.

Treatment

A GEI is a true surgical emergency, and stabilization should be followed by endoscopic or surgical reduction. Left-sided or bilateral gastropexy may be performed to prevent recurrence. When identified during endoscopy, a small GEI may be reduced through maximal esophageal insufflation and pressure on the rugal folds by the endoscope. Placement of a PEG tube may achieve a "gastropexy" in these dogs. Regurgitation may persist after surgical correction due to underlying esophageal dysmotility.

Reflux

Etiology

The term *reflux* is used broadly to describe GERD (i.e., the pathological movement of gastric contents from the stomach into the esophagus). Reflux in dogs is thought to occur secondary to increased negative intrathoracic pressure (e.g., BOAS) and decreased LES tone (e.g., transient LES relaxations). However, this is a limited view of reflux and ignores important distinctions between physiological and pathological reflux, GERD and extraesophageal reflux disease (EERD), and acidic and nonacidic reflux.

Physiological reflux occurs in 41% of healthy dogs on VFSSs and 100% of dogs on nuclear scintigraphy. This type of reflux is similarly reported in people, occurs without apparent clinical consequence, and complicates the diagnosis of pathological reflux. Ultimately, the presence or absence of reflux is likely to be less important than the content, volume, frequency, retention, and margination of the refluxate. Pathological reflux is typically larger in volume, occurs spontaneously (i.e., not during feeding), is retained for longer in the esophagus, and extends beyond the distal third of the esophagus in patients with supportive clinical signs (Videos 45.2 and 45.3).

Pathological reflux also includes EERD, which is the extension of the refluxate beyond the esophagus into the pharynx and upper respiratory tract (Fig. 45.7). It is important to note that pathological reflux (either GERD or EERD) may present without evidence of GI disease (i.e., occult or atypical reflux disease).

Pathology and clinical signs attributable to low pH refluxate are referred to as acidic reflux. However, disease can also be caused by digestive enzymes (e.g., pepsin, bile acids, trypsin) at a neutral or weakly acidic pH (non-acidic reflux). Acidic and non-acidic components of reflux are believed to work synergistically to cause tissue injury.

Anesthesia is the most well-established risk factor for reflux in dogs. Reflux during anesthesia is associated with up to 65% of benign esophageal strictures and is the most common cause of high-grade esophagitis. Changes in LES tone can be seen with both injectable preanesthetic and inhalant anesthetic agents. Even short-duration anesthetic events should be considered to increase risk.

Clinical features

Clinical signs can be broken into typical and atypical manifestations of reflux disease. Typical signs include ptyalism, halitosis, abdominal discomfort/pain, repetitive "dry" swallowing (i.e., not during feeding), lip licking, neck extension, anorexia, regurgitation, and vomiting. Signs may be more prominent after lying down due to increased intra-abdominal pressure and may appear more frequently at night or early in the morning based on the results of one study. Nighttime restlessness and panting are also reported.

Atypical clinical signs reflect the link between reflux, swallow, and respiratory dysfunction. They are usually linked to EERD or aspiration,

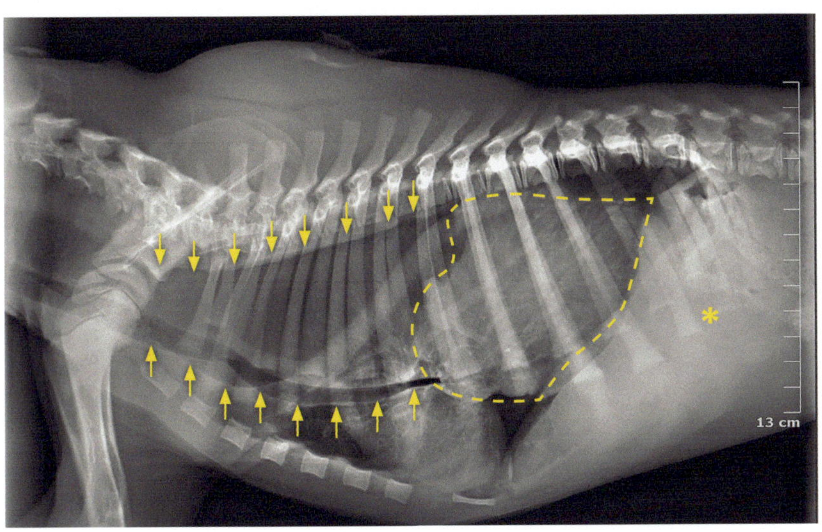

FIG. 45.6 Right lateral thoracic radiograph of a 7-month-old German Shepherd Dog presenting for regurgitation, lethargy, and abdominal pain. Marked generalized megaesophagus (arrows) is present with a large soft tissue opacity within the distal esophagus (dashed line). The asterisk marks the normal location of the stomach, which cannot be visualized in this image. These cumulative findings are consistent with a gastroesophageal intussusception.

Video 45.2

Cine loop from a videofluoroscopic swallow study in a 7-year-old spayed female Labrador Retriever with pathological reflux after consuming a test meal (liquid, puree, and kibble). Puree and liquid contained non-ionic contrast material (iohexol), and the kibble was impregnated with barium.[9] A spontaneous high-volume reflux event extending past the distal third of the esophagus is seen.

Video 45.3

Cine loop from a videofluoroscopic swallow study in a 3-year-old castrated male mixed-breed dog freely consuming a puree test meal containing non-ionic contrast material (iohexol), showing physiological reflux. A small volume of food is seen moving orad through the lower esophageal sphincter during feeding. This bolus is cleared by a subsequent food bolus and does not extend beyond the distal third of the esophagus.

including reverse sneezing, cough, nasal discharge, dysphonia, and upper respiratory noise (i.e., stridor or stertor). Reflux and other upper digestive tract abnormalities have been linked to lymphoplasmacytic rhinitis in dogs.[19] In severe cases of reflux and aspiration, patients may present in respiratory distress secondary to AP or upper airway obstruction. Anecdotally, otitis media, sleep apnea, and vasovagal syncope (secondary to nasopharyngeal reflux) have also been reported.

Diagnosis

Diagnostic modalities for detecting GERD and EERD in veterinary medicine incorporate a combination of pet owner surveys, treatment trials, esophagoscopy, VFSSs, and, less commonly, esophageal manometry and ambulatory pH probes. Survey radiographs are not typically helpful in diagnosing reflux. Fluid in the distal esophagus is difficult to interpret on radiographs, particularly in a sedated animal. A VFSS is preferred to diagnose reflux in dogs.

Treatment

Medical and dietary management make up the mainstay of treatment in dogs with pathological reflux. Surgical interventions (e.g., Dor or Nissen fundoplication) are more common in severely affected people but have been used sporadically in dogs. "Preventative" medical management (i.e., pre- and intraoperative treatment for reflux) may be recommended for at-risk dogs undergoing anesthesia. Treatment trials for GERD are multimodal and may take up to 6–8 weeks, particularly in dogs with atypical reflux.

Histamine type 2 receptor antagonists and proton pump inhibitors (PPIs) are the most used antacids in dogs, but the former are generally considered inferior for increasing gastric pH (see Chapter 46). Coadministration of both types of drugs is not recommended, as this significantly decreases the efficacy of the PPI. PPIs are also considered acid labile, so crushing tablets or opening capsules is not recommended. There is currently no conclusive evidence that one PPI is superior to another. Although studies in dogs are lacking, long-term administration of PPIs may result in rebound hyperacidemia secondary to a lack of negative feedback inhibition on gastrin. As such, it is recommended to taper rather than abruptly discontinue omeprazole if administered for ≥4 weeks.

As acid blockers only address a single component of reflux and do not reduce the frequency of reflux events, treatment with antacids should be coupled with prokinetics and dietary modification. Metoclopramide and cisapride are used to promote gastric emptying and increase LES tone. Metoclopramide is used successfully in clinical practice; however, its actions are largely considered to be less effective than those of cisapride. A study demonstrated that orally administered cisapride increased LES tone in dogs compared to placebo, while oral metoclopramide did not. Small, frequent meals consisting of a low-fat diet may encourage gastric emptying, and feeding right before bed is discouraged.

Sucralfate is recommended for esophagitis. Its action is considered multifactorial and includes coating of the damaged esophageal mucosa and interfering with pepsin. However, retention of sucralfate in the esophagus is limited, and in nonacidic conditions sucralfate is rapidly cleared. As such, sucralfate is not considered protective against future esophagitis. Sucralfate administration should be separated from other drugs by 1–2 hours to avoid impacting on their bioavailability.

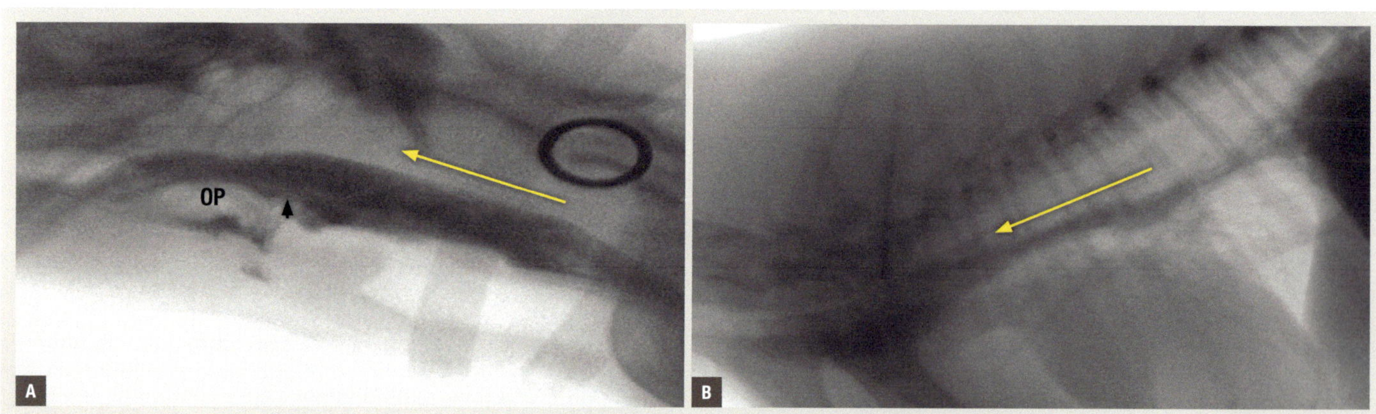

FIG. 45.7 Still images from two patients with pathological reflux undergoing videofluoroscopic swallow studies. (A) A 6-year-old female Labrador Retriever presenting for recurrent aspiration pneumonia with reflux (arrow) extending beyond the upper esophageal sphincter (arrowhead) into the oropharynx (OP). (B) A 7-year-old mixed-breed dog presenting for repetitive swallowing and gagging with pathological reflux (i.e., refluxate [arrow] extending past the distal third of the esophagus).

Esophagitis

Etiology

Esophagitis is a common consequence of esophageal disease. It is frequently associated with reflux either alone or in combination with other motility disorders. Decreased esophageal motility (e.g., during anesthesia) increases mucosal contact time with refluxate (acidic and non-acidic) and increases the risk of esophagitis. Esophagitis is also associated with esophageal FBs, trauma, ingestion of caustic substances (acidic, alkaline, or oxidant), chronic vomiting, irritation caused by feeding tubes, and neoplasia.

Granulomatous necrotizing esophagitis caused by *Pythium insidiosum* has been reported in dogs in the southeastern United States. Other infectious causes of esophagitis include *Candida albicans* and *Spirocerca lupi*. Regardless of the underlying cause, a consequence of esophagitis is decreased esophageal motility and decreased LES tone, which establishes a vicious circle of injury and may predispose dogs to more severe disease, aspiration, and esophageal strictures.

Barrett's esophagus (i.e., transformation of the normal squamous epithelial mucosa into columnar epithelium in response to chronic inflammation) is considered a precursor to adenocarcinoma. This is well established in people, but there is only a single case report in dogs (see Video 22.4).

Clinical features

Clinical features of esophagitis vary with severity. With mild inflammation, dogs may be asymptomatic. In case of moderate to severe disease, however, clinical signs are similar to those seen in dogs with typical reflux. Respiratory signs may be seen in patients with concurrent atypical reflux or AP.

Clinicopathological findings

There are no discriminating clinicopathological features specific to esophagitis.

Diagnosis

Thoracic radiographs may be unremarkable or show diffuse or segmental esophageal dilation in case of severe disease. Radiographic changes consistent with AP may also be observed. As for reflux, fluid in the distal esophagus is difficult to interpret on radiographs and may be seen in normal dogs. A definitive diagnosis of esophagitis is made by visualization of an erythematous or eroded/ulcerated esophageal mucosa on endoscopy (Fig. 45.8). Biopsy or brush cytology may be considered, particularly if there is significant mucosal atypia (e.g., nodular/granular changes, mass) or when infectious esophagitis (e.g., pythiosis, candidiasis, spirocercosis) is suspected. For infectious esophagitis, adjunctive diagnostics (e.g., *Pythium* serology, fecal evaluation) may also be recommended. A VFSS is helpful to diagnose underlying motility disorders. However, mild primary esophageal dysmotility may be difficult to distinguish from dysmotility caused by esophagitis. A diagnosis of Barrett's esophagus requires biopsy with histopathology.

Treatment

Unless an infectious agent is identified, therapy for esophagitis is as for reflux. Sucralfate and other mucosal protectants should be considered. Treatment for 1–2 weeks is recommended after a known event (e.g., esophageal FB retrieval). Temporarily withholding oral feeding in dogs with esophagitis is controversial, and the current recommendation is to feed a soft, ideally low-fat, diet as soon as it is tolerated. For dogs with severe disease or prolonged anorexia, a gastrostomy or PEG tube should be considered.

Mechanical disorders of the esophagus

Esophageal stricture

Etiology

An esophageal stricture is a discrete intraluminal narrowing of the esophagus. It most commonly results from circumferential injury and fibrosis during healing; however, congenital strictures are also reported. Anesthesia is the most well recognized risk factor for esophageal strictures in dogs. Other risk factors include esophageal FBs, accidental ingestion of caustic substances, and GERD.

Clinical features

Clinical signs are consistent with other causes of esophageal disease. The severity of signs varies with the degree of esophageal obstruction and esophageal dysmotility. Dogs may have a history of progressive

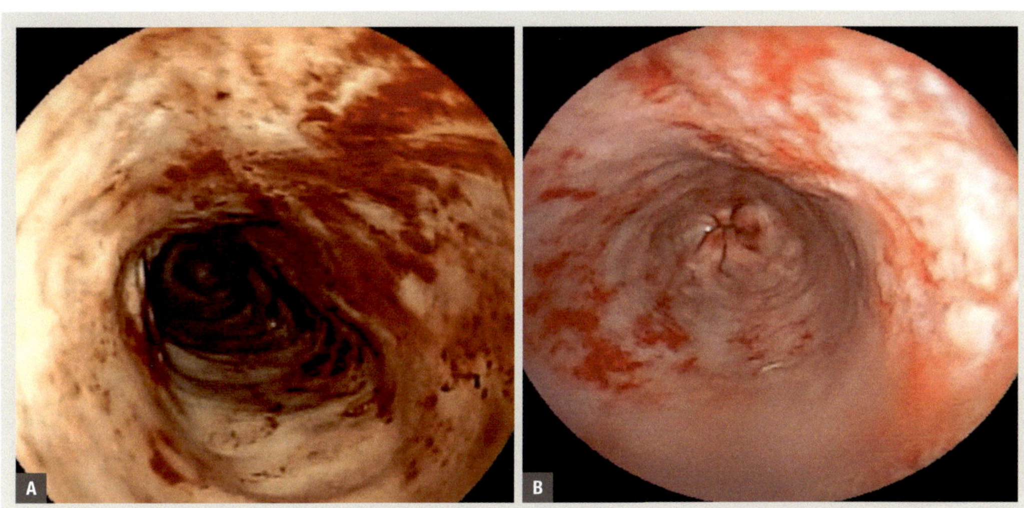

FIG. 45.8 Endoscopic images of the distal esophagus demonstrating severe (A) and moderate–severe (B) esophagitis with esophageal erosions and hemorrhage secondary to gastroesophageal reflux.

regurgitation with different consistencies. Generally, soft food and liquids are better tolerated than kibble because they pass more easily through the narrowed esophageal lumen.

Clinicopathological findings

There are no discriminating clinicopathological features specific to an esophageal stricture.

Diagnosis

Survey radiographs may be normal or show focal ME and/or a diverticulum orad to the site of the stricture. Contrast radiography or VFSSs may highlight the site of luminal narrowing and identify accompanying esophageal dysmotility or reflux. The length of the stricture cannot be confirmed on radiographs, as the esophagus distal to the stricture is not maximally distended. Additionally, esophageal spasm and edema may make the stricture appear longer. A very distal esophageal stricture may cause generalized esophageal dilation and be mistaken for generalized ME. A possible stricture must be differentiated from other causes of esophageal obstruction (e.g., vascular ring anomaly, neoplasia).

Endoscopy is needed to diagnose an esophageal stricture, determine its length, and identify concurrent esophagitis (reported in 40% of cases). Overall, 80% of strictures in dogs are in the intrathoracic esophagus, with the heart base and EGJ being overrepresented sites. A stricture is generally described as a thin band of fibrotic tissue; however, chronic strictures may be associated with thick fibrotic tissue and variable amounts of orad esophageal dilation or architectural distortion. The length of a stricture is variable but may reach up to 15 cm. Strictures may be single (≈80%) or multifocal (≈20%) (Fig. 45.9).

Treatment

Mechanical dilation by balloon dilation or bougienage is the treatment of choice. This may be performed under endoscopic guidance, with videofluoroscopy, or a combination of these. Endoscopy is generally preferred because it allows direct observation of the esophagus during dilation. Multiple redilations may be required every 1–2 weeks until the stricture is sufficiently resolved to allow normal eating and drinking. Transendoscopic injections of triamcinolone or topical mitomycin C may be recommended in dogs with severe or recurrent strictures. Treatment for esophagitis (see "Reflux" section above) following dilation is recommended.

Pet owners should be counseled that most strictures require between two and four dilations and that "successful" treatment may still require changes in feeding practices. This might include softening kibble, converting to a soft food diet, and upright feeding depending on the degree of esophageal dysmotility. Risks of mechanical dilation include esophageal tearing and perforation. An increased risk of tearing may be associated with bougienage compared to balloon dilation. Surgical resection is reported but is not generally recommended (except in cases of malignant strictures) due to poor wound healing and tension at the anastomosis. Esophageal stenting is reported in dogs with refractory esophageal strictures but is not considered a first-line therapy. A gastrostomy or PEG tube may be required in animals unable to intake food or water. Esophageal balloon dilation feeding tubes (B-tubes) have been reported with moderate success but may require careful patient selection and pet owner education before prescribing.

Esophageal foreign bodies

Etiology

Esophageal FBs are identified relatively frequently in dogs, with bones, needles, fishhooks, and sticks being the most common. FBs tend to lodge at the least distensible regions of the esophagus: the thoracic inlet, base of the heart, and EGJ, although 16.7% are identified rostral to the thoracic inlet. The damage to the esophagus depends on the size and shape of the object and on the duration of the esophageal obstruction. Esophageal FBs can lead to impaction, pressure necrosis, mucosal laceration, and perforation.

Clinical features

An acute onset of clinical signs of regurgitation, repetitive swallowing, and ptyalism is suggestive of a potential esophageal FB. Large FBs causing complete obstruction tend to be associated with more acute, and more severe clinical signs. Halitosis may be associated with tissue necrosis or rotting material. Dogs with perforation may present with fever, pleural effusion, and respiratory distress. A large FB in the cervical esophagus may be able to be palpated, but diagnostic imaging is still required for confirmation.

Clinicopathological findings

There are no discriminating clinicopathological features specific to esophageal FBs.

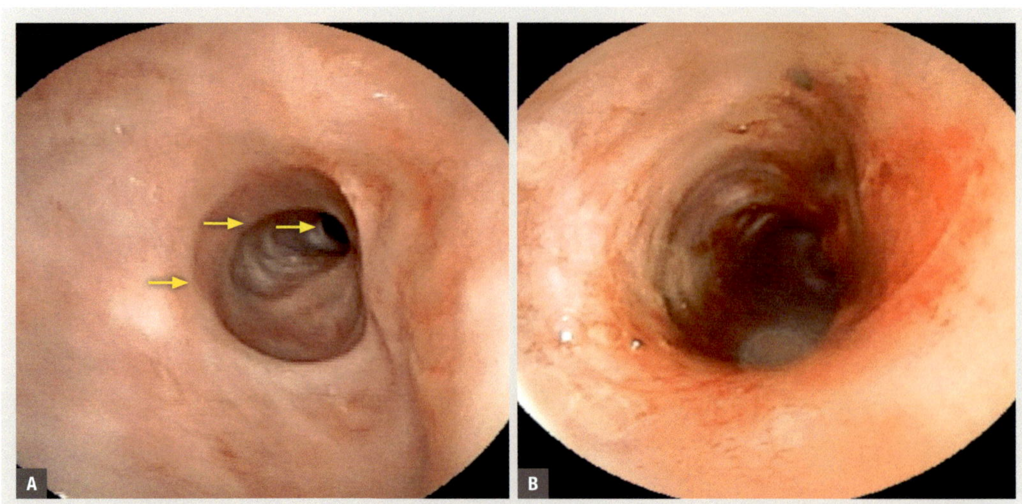

FIG. 45.9 Endoscopic images of a 1.5-year-old intact male Doberman Pinscher mix presented for severe regurgitation and weight loss of 1-month's duration following surgical removal of a gastric foreign body. (**A**) Multifocal esophageal stricture (arrows). (**B**) Esophagus following successful balloon dilation.

Diagnosis
Most FBs can be detected by survey thoracic and cervical radiographs. Contrast radiographs or VFSSs may help identify rarer radiolucent FBs. Evaluation for esophageal perforation is important and may be suggested by identifying an esophageal FB with concurrent pleural effusion, pneumomediastinum, or emphysema. Pleural fluid should be collected via thoracocentesis and submitted for cytology and culture and sensitivity testing. Endoscopy is indicated to evaluate the degree of esophageal damage and to remove foreign material (Fig. 45.10).

Treatment
Esophageal FBs are considered emergencies, as prolonged retention is associated with increased likelihood of perforation. Rigid or flexible endoscopy can be used for FB retrieval. Despite being operator choice, a rigid sigmoidoscope may be preferred for removal of large proximal esophageal FBs, while flexible endoscopy is preferred for smaller distal esophageal FBs. Large FBs that cannot be extracted via the mouth may be pushed into the stomach and removed via gastrotomy. Moving a FB into the stomach may also allow the endoscopist to find a better angle to grasp and remove the FB than can be achieved in the esophagus. After the FB is removed, the mucosa should be evaluated for esophagitis, perforation, and fistulas. Fasting is recommended for 24–48 hours following FB removal in dogs with severe esophagitis or esophageal necrosis. A gastrostomy/PEG tube may be considered in some patients. Treatment for esophagitis is recommended for 1–4 weeks following FB retrieval, as dogs with ulceration involving more than 180° are at increased risk of developing an esophageal stricture. Longer treatment duration is recommended with more severe disease. Surgery is indicated if the FB cannot be removed endoscopically or if there is evidence of perforation. Small perforations may respond to medical management with antimicrobial therapy, PPIs, and supportive care based on a small case series.

Esophageal neoplasia

Etiology
Primary esophageal neoplasia is rare in dogs, accounting for less than 0.5% of canine tumors. The most common primary malignant tumors include squamous cell carcinoma, leiomyosarcoma, and fibrosarcoma. Primary esophageal tumors tend to be locally invasive, with metastasis to local lymph nodes. *Spirocerca lupi* is associated with malignant transformation (to fibrosarcoma and osteosarcoma). Leiomyoma is the most common benign esophageal tumor and often arises near the EGJ in dogs. Gastric tumors at the cardia (e.g., extramedullary plasmacytoma) may result in signs of esophageal disease by obstructing bolus flow from the esophagus into the stomach. Metastatic neoplasia and lymphoma are more common (≈3×) than primary esophageal neoplasia and are also capable of causing esophageal outflow obstruction.

Clinical features
Most animals with esophageal cancer are older, and no breed or sex predisposition is reported. Clinical signs may be progressive and often occur late in disease, when the mass causes obstruction or disruption of esophageal motility. Paraneoplastic syndromes are reported, including hypoglycemia (leiomyomas and leiomyosarcomas) and hypertrophic osteopathy (*Spirocerca lupi* sarcomas). Bleeding tumors may be associated with hematemesis or melena.

Clinicopathological findings
Clinicopathological abnormalities are specific to the tumor, such as hypercalcemia (e.g., lymphoma), hypoglycemia (e.g., leiomyoma, leiomyosarcoma), and monoclonal gammopathy (e.g., extramedullary plasmacytoma). Dogs with bleeding tumors may develop anemia with or without thrombocytosis.

Diagnosis
A soft tissue mass with or without mineralization may be visible on survey radiographs in addition to concurrent metastasis or AP. Contrast radiographs, VFSSs, or CT may be used to highlight suspicious esophageal lesions and distinguish them from other causes of an esophageal mass effect (e.g., GEI, SHH, FB) (Fig. 45.11). Endoscopy with biopsy may help achieve a definitive diagnosis when the mass extends into the esophageal lumen. Thoracic CT or magnetic resonance imaging may be useful in characterizing intramural lesions, including leiomyomas. Additional imaging, such as abdominal ultrasonography and fine needle aspiration, may be useful for complete tumor staging.

Treatment
Treatment is specific to the tumor type. Surgical treatment for esophageal neoplasia is challenging due to limited access, tension at any anastomosis, and risk of strictures at the surgical site. The most favorable prognosis is

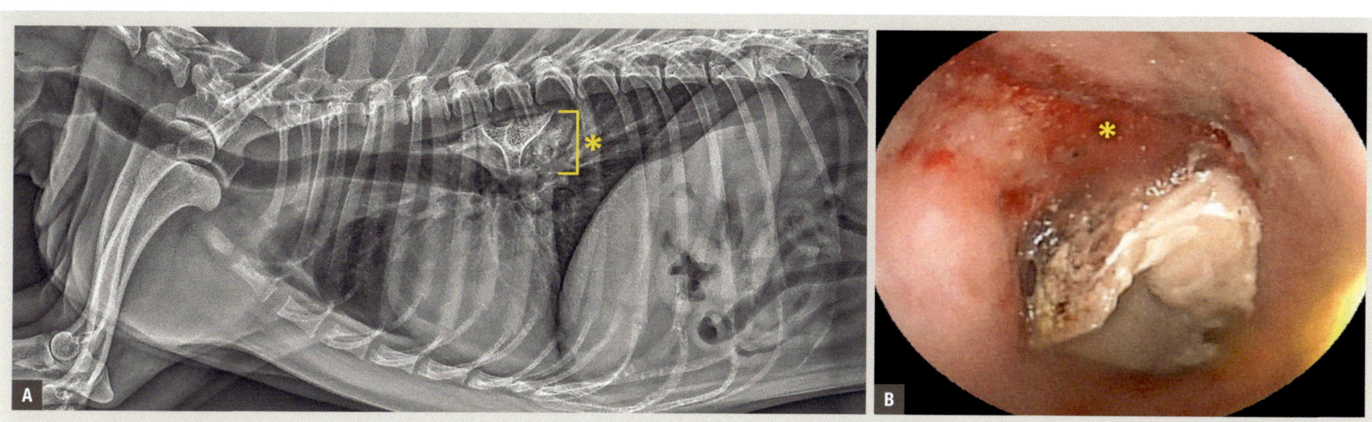

FIG. 45.10 (A) Right lateral thoracic radiograph of a 5-year-old castrated male Shih Tzu with an osseus esophageal foreign body (asterisk) in the thoracic esophagus. Pulmonary parenchyma is normal, with no evidence of aspiration pneumonia. (B) Endoscopic image of the same dog showing the bone foreign body and associated esophageal ulceration (asterisk). The foreign body was successfully removed via endoscopy.

associated with en bloc resection; however, submucosal resection to debulk the mass may be considered in some instances. Esophageal stenting is not routinely performed in dogs with esophageal neoplasia but has been reported. Gastrostomy or PEG tubes may be considered following surgery or as a palliative measure.

Esophageal diverticula

Etiology

Esophageal diverticula are uncommon and may be congenital or acquired. A breed predisposition has been proposed in Cairn Terriers. The congenital form is very rare and occurs as a result of a defect in the muscularis which allows herniation of the mucosa. Acquired esophageal diverticula are subclassified as traction or pulsion. Traction diverticula are caused by inflammatory periesophageal adhesions to adjacent tissues that distort the esophagus. They are usually caused by abscesses or migrating FBs (e.g., grass awns) and may be seen in combination with esophagobronchial fistulas. Pulsion diverticula are caused by intraluminal distention/pressure caused by esophageal injury, dysmotility, or obstruction. Pulsion diverticula in the distal esophagus are referred to as epiphrenic diverticula and are mostly associated with previous FB impaction.

Clinical features

Clinical signs are similar to those of other forms of esophageal disease. Rarely, weakening and perforation of the diverticula is reported and may be associated with signs of sepsis and respiratory distress.

Clinicopathological findings

There are no discriminating clinicopathological features specific to esophageal diverticula.

Diagnosis

A diverticulum can be identified on survey radiographs as an air- or fluid-filled outpouching. This should be distinguished from a redundant deviation of the esophagus, which can be seen in normal brachycephalic and Shar Pei dogs. A redundant esophagus should disappear with neck extension. Contrast radiography or VFSSs can highlight lesions or identify an underlying cause (e.g., esophageal dysmotility). On endoscopy, a diverticulum may appear as a sac-like outpouching often containing food and fluid (Fig. 45.12). Careful suctioning of food and fluid may be needed for visualization; however, the wall of the diverticula is thin and at high risk of perforation. Evaluation for perforation is as for esophageal FBs.

Treatment

Small diverticula may be managed by upright feeding a liquid or semiliquid diet to minimize food impaction. Diverticulectomy is the treatment of choice for large diverticula or those associated with repeated esophageal impaction. For pulsion diverticula, treatment of the underlying cause (e.g., stricture) is necessary.

Esophageal fistula

Etiology

Esophageal fistulas are the abnormal communication between the esophagus and surrounding structures. They may be congenital or acquired. The former are caused by incomplete separation of the digestive tract from the respiratory tract during embryonic development. Acquired forms include esophagoaortic, tracheoesophageal, bronchoesophageal, and esophagopulmonary fistulas. Bronchoesophageal fistulas are the most common in dogs. Most acquired fistulas arise from esophageal perforation (e.g., bone FB) or inflammation of surrounding tissue. Healing of the esophageal lesions leads to a communicating tract and contamination of the airways with esophageal contents. There is an association between esophageal fistulas and traction diverticula in dogs. As for esophageal diverticula, a breed predisposition has been proposed in Cairn Terriers.

Clinical features

Most clinical signs of an esophageal fistula are respiratory, including coughing, nasal discharge, and respiratory distress, and may be exacerbated by eating or drinking. Dogs with an esophageal fistula may also have a history of recurrent pneumonia.

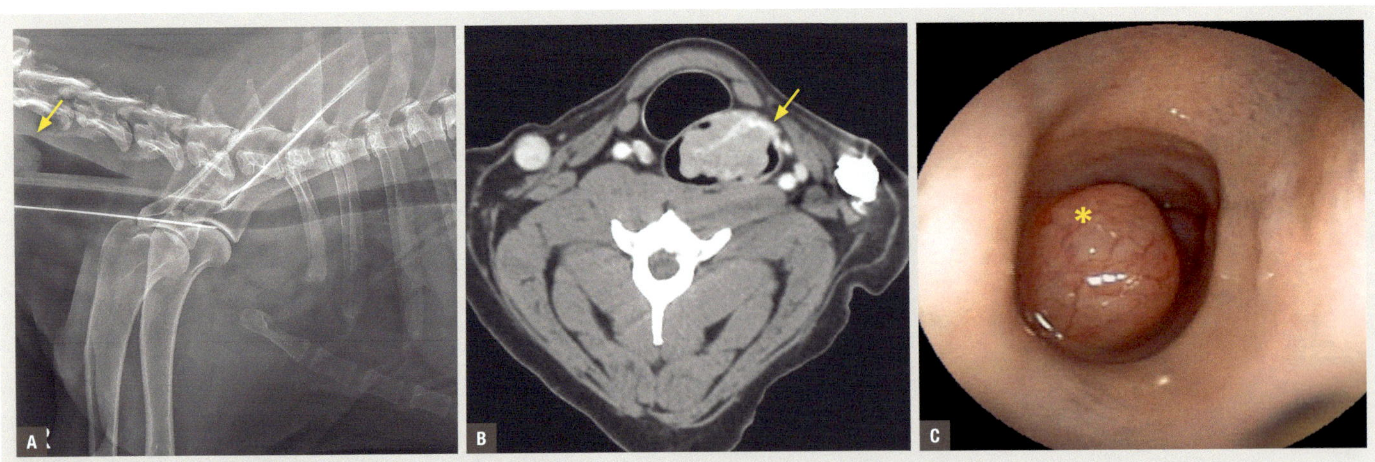

FIG. 45.11 (A) Right lateral thoracic radiograph of a 12-year-old castrated male Border Collie diagnosed with an extramedullary plasmacytoma in the proximal esophagus. The caudal border of a mass effect is just visible in the cervical esophagus (arrow). (B) Axial computed tomography image of the same dog showing a heterogeneously contrast-enhancing mass (arrow) obstructing the lumen of the proximal esophagus. (C) Endoscopic image of a 12-year-old spayed female Chihuahua with a distal esophageal mass suspected to be a leiomyoma (asterisk).

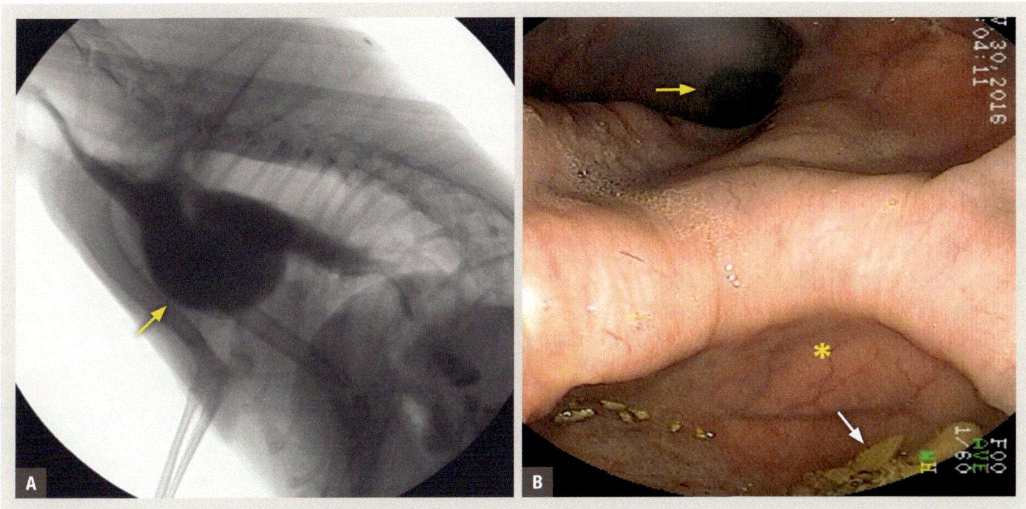

FIG. 45.12 (**A**) Still image from a videofluoroscopic swallow study in a 3-year-old castrated male mixed-breed dog with lower esophageal achalasia and an esophageal diverticulum (arrow yellow). (**B**) Endoscopic image from the same dog showing the interior of the diverticulum (asterisk) with ingested boney material (arrow white). The yellow arrow is pointing towards the lower esophageal sphincter.

Clinicopathological findings

There are no discriminating clinicopathological features specific to esophageal fistulas.

Diagnosis

Survey radiographs may reveal an interstitial–alveolar or bronchial pattern. The distribution of respiratory lesions depends on the connection between the esophagus and the respiratory tract. Most bronchoesophageal fistulas are associated with the right caudal and right middle lobar bronchi. On endoscopy, a fistula appears as a small opening in the wall of the esophagus or airway (trachea or bronchi). This may be accompanied by purulent or hemorrhagic fluid. Scintigraphy, contrast radiography, VFSSs, and histopathology may also be used to confirm a fistula. For contrast studies, thin barium is preferred because it may be less irritating to the airways compared to non-ionic contrast agents.

Treatment

Surgery is the treatment of choice for dogs, including excision of the fistula and repair of the defect in the esophageal wall. Lung lobectomy may be needed depending on the degree of pathology and location of the fistula. Broad-spectrum antibiotics are recommended following surgery.

Vascular ring anomalies

Etiology

Vascular ring anomalies are congenital malformations of the embryonic great vessels leading to entrapment of the esophagus and other intrathoracic structures. A persistent right aortic arch makes up 95% of vascular ring anomalies diagnosed in dogs and occurs when the esophagus is entrapped between the ligamentum arteriosum (dorsal), pulmonary artery (left), heart (ventral), and aorta (right). Other reported vascular ring anomalies include persistent right or left subclavian arteries, persistent right dorsal aorta, double aortic arch, left aortic arch, aberrant intercostal arteries, and right ligamentum arteriosum. Esophageal compression from an aberrant left subclavian artery occurs because of compression from the subclavian and brachiocephalic arteries. Predisposition has been reported for several breeds (see Table 45.2).

Clinical features

Puppies usually present just after birth or weaning with regurgitation or failure to thrive. Dogs are typically thin and may have respiratory signs related to regurgitation and aspiration.

Clinicopathological findings

There are no discriminating clinicopathological features specific to vascular ring anomalies. Clinicopathological abnormalities consistent with malnutrition may be observed.

Diagnosis

Focal ME proximal to the heart base associated with moderate to marked leftward tracheal deviation on dorsoventral or ventrodorsal radiographs are consistent with a vascular ring anomaly. A diverticulum orad to the stricture may be present, especially with chronic disease. CT angiography may be needed to diagnose atypical vascular ring anomalies. Endoscopy may be useful if survey and contrast radiographs are inconclusive and to rule out causes of intraluminal compression. As extraluminal compression is caused by great vessels, pulsations against the esophageal wall may be noticed endoscopically at the site of luminal narrowing.

Treatment

Surgical correction is recommended for vascular ring anomalies. For a persistent right aortic arch, this is performed by transection of the ligamentum arteriosum. Dogs with severe malnutrition may require nutritional support before and after surgery. Early correction should be carried out, as chronic obstruction may lead to permanent esophageal dysmotility. Upright feeding as for ME may be recommended in dogs with permanent esophageal dysmotility.

Esophageal varices

Etiology

Esophageal varices (i.e., abnormal esophageal venous dilation in response to increased resistance to portal or caval blood flow) are uncommon in dogs. Reported etiologies in dogs include thrombi (portal, pulmonary), portal hypertension, space-occupying masses, bronchoesophageal arterial hypertrophy, and arteriovenous fistulas, among others.

Clinical features

Despite being a frequent consequence of esophageal varices in people, affected dogs rarely exhibit hemorrhage (i.e., hemoptysis, hematemesis, melena). Signs of hepatic encephalopathy (e.g., head pressing), GI disease (e.g., vomiting), and respiratory disease (e.g., cough and syncope) were more common in dogs with esophageal varices based on a single retrospective study.

Clinicopathological findings

There are no discriminating clinicopathological features specific to esophageal varices. Clinicopathological abnormalities are usually associated with the underlying cause (e.g., portal hypertension in cirrhotic liver disease).

Diagnosis

Direct visualization of prominent esophageal vessels may be possible during endoscopy (see Video 22.10). However, the definitive diagnosis and characterization of esophageal varices require CT with contrast and possibly an angiogram. Subclassifications are based on the direction of blood flow, whether the flow is arterial or venous, and the location of collateral vessels. Additional imaging may be needed depending on the suspected etiology (e.g., echocardiogram, abdominal ultrasound/CT).

Treatment

Direct treatment of esophageal varices is rarely indicated. Treatment is generally focused on the underlying etiology. The use of angiotensin-converting enzyme inhibitors may be beneficial in patients with esophageal varices due to arteriovenous communications based on a single case report.

KEY POINTS

- Dogs with esophageal disease may present exclusively with gastrointestinal or respiratory signs, or a combination of both.
- Regurgitation must be distinguished from vomiting, oral preparatory and pharyngeal dysphagia, and expectoration.
- Videofluoroscopic swallow studies may be required to diagnose functional esophageal diseases, including reflux, sliding hiatal hernia, and lower esophageal sphincter achalasia.
- Idiopathic megaesophagus is a diagnosis of exclusion, and prognosis may improve with targeted interventions.

References

1. Neuhuber WL, Wörl J. Enteric co-innervation of striated muscle in the esophagus: still enigmatic? *Histochem Cell Biol* 146(6):721–735, 2016.
2. Grobman ME, Schachtel J, Gyawali CP, et al. Videofluoroscopic swallow study features of lower esophageal sphincter achalasia-like syndrome in dogs. *J Vet Intern Med* 33(5):1954–1963, 2019.
3. Rinaldo JA Jr, Levey JF, Smathers HM, et al. An integrated anatomic, physiologic and cineradiologic study of the canine gastroesophageal sphincter. *Am J Dig Dis* 16(6):556–565, 1971.
4. Grobman M, Reinero C. A One Health review of aerodigestive disease in dogs. *J Vet Intern Med* 37(3):817–834, 2023.
5. Bautista TG, Sun QJ, Pilowsky PM. The generation of pharyngeal phase of swallow and its coordination with breathing: interaction between the swallow and respiratory central pattern generators. *Prog Brain Res* 212:253–275, 2014.
6. Howard J, Grobman M, Lever T, Reinero CR. Videofluoroscopic swallow study abnormalities identify aerodigestive disorders in dogs with respiratory disease versus healthy controls. *J Vet Intern Med* 37(3):1166–1178, 2023.
7. Grobman ME, Masseau I, Reinero CR. Aerodigestive disorders in dogs evaluated for cough using respiratory fluoroscopy and videofluoroscopic swallow studies. *Vet J* 251:105344, 2019.
8. Luciani E, Reinero C, Grobman M. Evaluation of aerodigestive disease and diagnosis of sliding hiatal hernia in brachycephalic and nonbrachycephalic dogs. *J Vet Intern Med* 36(4):1229–1236, 2022.
9. Harris RA, Grobman ME, Allen MJ, et al. Standardization of a videofluoroscopic swallow study protocol to investigate dysphagia in dogs. *J Vet Intern Med* 31(2):383–393, 2017.
10. Bonadio CM, Pollard RE, Dayton PA, et al. Effects of body positioning on swallowing and esophageal transit in healthy dogs. *J Vet Intern Med* 23(4):801–805, 2009.
11. Masseau I, Reinero CR. Thoracic computed tomographic interpretation for clinicians to aid in the diagnosis of dogs and cats with respiratory disease. *Vet J* 253:105388, 2019.
12. Petchell WHR, Noble PM, Broome HAO, Burrow R. Incidence of alimentary and respiratory disease in brachycephalic dogs presenting to primary care veterinary practices participating in the SAVSNET project. *Vet Rec* 191(7):e1685, 2022.
13. Poncet CM, Dupre GP, Freiche VG, Bouvy BM. Long-term results of upper respiratory syndrome surgery and gastrointestinal tract medical treatment in 51 brachycephalic dogs. *J Small Anim Pract* 47(3):137–142, 2006.
14. Loewen JM, Bach JF. Performing an upper airway examination in dogs. *J Vet Emerg Crit Care (San Antonio)* 32(S1):16–21, 2022.
15. Grobman M, Reinero C, Lee-Fowler T, Lever TE. Incidence and characterization of aerophagia in dogs using videofluoroscopic swallow studies. *J Vet Intern Med* 38(3):1449–1457, 2024.
16. Lappin MR, Blondeau J, Boothe D, et al. Antimicrobial use guidelines for treatment of respiratory tract disease in dogs and cats: Antimicrobial Guidelines Working Group of the International Society for Companion Animal Infectious Diseases. *J Vet Intern Med* 31(2):279–294, 2017.
17. Winston JM 3rd, Mann FAT, Dean L. Management and outcomes of 13 dogs treated with a modified Heller myotomy and Dor fundoplication for lower esophageal sphincter achalasia-like syndrome. *Vet Surg* 52(2):315–329, 2023.
18. Broux O, Clercx C, Etienne AL, et al. Effects of manipulations to detect sliding hiatal hernia in dogs with brachycephalic airway obstructive syndrome. *Vet Surg* 47(2):243–251, 2018.
19. Gianella P, Roncone S, Ala U, et al. Upper digestive tract abnormalities in dogs with chronic idiopathic lymphoplasmacytic rhinitis. *J Vet Intern Med* 34(5):1845–1852, 2020.

CHAPTER 46

Gastric diseases

Katherine Tolbert
DVM, PhD, DACVIM
(SAIM & Nutrition)

Vomiting is a common sign of gastric disease although it's not unique to gastric disease. Moreover, pet owners often struggle to accurately distinguish true vomiting from other acts such as regurgitation or immediate food ejection. Therefore, when evaluating a dog reported by the owner to be vomiting, the veterinarian should first verify that the owner actually observed true vomiting. Once vomiting is confirmed, the clinician must determine if it is gastrointestinal (GI) in origin or if it is caused by an extra-GI stimulus (Table 46.1). A detailed algorithm on how to evaluate and approach dogs presented for acute or chronic vomiting can be found in Chapter 10.

Other clinical signs that can be attributed to gastric disease include abdominal pain, lip licking, hypersalivation, change in appetite or food-seeking behavior (dysorexia), weight loss, behavioral changes (including hiding or aggression), melena, bloating, early satiety, or, rarely, regurgitation due to pyloric outflow obstruction and other causes of delayed gastric emptying. Major causes of gastric disease, including inflammatory diseases, neoplasms, and motility disorders, are discussed in this chapter.

Gastritis

The inflammation causing gastritis typically does not confine itself to the stomach but is also frequently identified in the upper small intestine and beyond. When dogs develop gastroenteritis, they typically suffer from additional signs such as excessive gas, decreased energy, or diarrhea. Guidelines for the histopathologic evaluation of GI inflammation are available from the World Small Animal Veterinary Association (WSAVA) International Gastrointestinal Standardization Group.[1] However, histopathologic evaluation is not always performed, especially in the acute setting, and, therefore, gastritis is commonly categorized by the duration of the clinical signs as acute or chronic.

Acute gastropathy

Acute gastropathies are defined by their signs lasting less than 2 weeks. They commonly affect dogs of any age or breed and often resolve on their own with just basic supportive treatment. There are many causes of acute gastropathies including ingestion of foreign objects or inappropriate foods, food intolerances, various drugs including antibiotics or NSAIDs, among others (Table 46.1). Additionally, certain metabolic conditions (such as hypoadrenocorticism) or conditions that restrict blood flow (such as abdominal organ torsions) can cause acute gastritis or gastric erosions and ulceration. However, these conditions typically present with additional serious signs beyond vomiting.

Even though infectious agents are more often causes of chronic gastritis, some infections can present acutely, such as those caused by the helminths *Physaloptera* spp. and, very infrequently, *Ollulanus* spp. and *Gnathostoma* spp.; the oomycete. *Pythium* spp.; the fungus *Histoplasma* spp.; the bacteria *Salmonella* spp., *Campylobacter jejuni*, and *Helicobacter* spp.; and, very infrequently without concurrent diarrhea, parvovirus and canine distemper virus. Bacteria rarely trigger gastric inflammation although dogs may be at a higher risk of bacterial gastritis if they consume raw foods. Dogs with enteropathogenic infections generally present with severe signs of illness (e.g., fever, hypovolemia). Anaphylactic reactions and/or envenomations are also infrequent causes of vomiting, which can appear immediately (within seconds to minutes) or be delayed (hours to days); therefore, pet owners should be questioned about the possible exposure of the dog to insects or snakes.

A thorough medical history, including full diet history and history of recent travels, combined with a complete physical examination, are essential for determining the most appropriate diagnostic tests and treatment plan. The extent of testing and treatment needed depends on how severe the signs are and what the physical examination reveals. For example, the clinical signs of dogs with vomiting from dietary indiscretion can rapidly resolve with supportive care. However, cases involving prolonged vomiting, behavioral changes like sudden aggression, vomiting blood, or physical signs such as changed mental status, severe abdominal pain, or low blood pressure require immediate stabilization and a more detailed evaluation.

Veterinarians should ask owners about possible exposure to foreign objects such as baby or pet toys or bathroom trash. The veterinarian should also obtain a complete list of medications to which the dog could be exposed. The timing of the signs (e.g., they appear after feeding or

TABLE 46.1 Potential causes of vomiting in the dog.

Category	Causes
Primary gastric structural or inflammatory	■ Dietary indiscretion ■ Foreign body ■ Food-responsive gastroenteropathy ■ Steroid-responsive gastroenteropathy ■ Gastric neoplasia (e.g., adenocarcinoma, leiomyoma, leiomyosarcoma, mast cell tumor) ■ Eosinophilic gastroenteritis ■ Benign gastric hypertrophy ■ Bilious vomiting syndrome
Systemic	■ Anaphylactoid reaction ■ Hepatic failure ■ Acute kidney injury ■ Chronic kidney disease ■ Hypoadrenocorticism ■ Pancreatitis
Infectious	■ Viral (e.g., parvovirus) ■ Bacterial (e.g., *Helicobacter* spp.) ■ Fungal (e.g., *Histoplasma capsulatum*) ■ Helminthic (*Gnathostoma* spp., *Ollulanus* spp., *Physaloptera* spp., *Toxocara canis*) ■ Oomycetal (*Pythium* spp.)
Environmental	■ Nonsteroidal anti-inflammatory drugs ■ Antibiotics ■ Chemotherapeutics ■ Other drugs ■ Household chemicals ■ Plants
Hyperacidity	■ Pancreatic gastrinoma ■ Mastocytosis
Stress, exercise induced	■ Surgery ■ High-intensity exercise

outdoor exercise) should also be considered. While viruses rarely cause vomiting as the only clinical sign, they should be considered when multiple dogs in the same environment are affected or when young animals display additional signs compatible with a virus such as bloody diarrhea (see Chapter 36).

The physical examination findings in dogs with an acute gastropathy can range from normal to severe. Some dogs may appear to be healthy while others might display severe abdominal pain, excessive drooling, prolonged capillary refill time, or hypotension. The examination should include a rectal examination and evaluation of the feces for mucus, frank or digested blood, or parasites. Examination of the vomited material for blood, bile, and parasites (which are sometimes easier to spot in vomit than in stool) is also important. In cases of acute gastropathy with the absence of comorbidities, the patient's body and muscle condition should be normal.

The reader is referred to Chapter 10 for a more detailed review of the diagnostic and therapeutic approach to the acutely vomiting dog. For mild cases without dehydration, a brief fasting period (under 12 hours) with supportive care and gradual introduction of water is advised. Once the dog can keep water down, small, frequent meals using a easily digestible, low-fat, moisture-rich diet should be introduced. The dog's previous diet can then be reintroduced over a period of 3-5 days, assuming no chronic condition is suspected. Fasting for more than 72 hours is not advised unless vomiting or other complications of gastric disease cannot be controlled. In these cases, consultation with a veterinary nutritionist and administration of parenteral nutrition until enteral nutrition can be instituted are warranted. Correction of fluid and electrolyte deficits is required in dogs with more severe signs. In some patients, symptomatic treatment with antiemetic drugs may be needed while evaluating the cause of the vomiting. Antiemetics (see Chapter 32) should be administered once mechanical obstruction or toxicity have been ruled out, as these conditions might require different management strategies (e.g., emesis, endoscopy, surgery). Deworming is advised, especially for younger animals or those without regular parasite prevention. Since stomach worms (like *Physaloptera*) can be hard to diagnose, it is reasonable to administer a broad-spectrum dewormer such as pyrantel pamoate before pursuing additional diagnostic tests. Gastric acid suppressants or cytoprotective drugs (e.g., histamine type 2 receptor antagonists, proton pump inhibitors [PPIs], sucralfate) should not be used in every dog with vomiting. Rather, these drugs should be reserved for patients in which gastric erosion or ulceration is suspected due to the presence of hematemesis or melena, as discussed below.

Chronic gastritis

The underlying cause of a chronic gastropathy often remains unknown. While some cases can be traced to specific triggers – such as parasites or neoplasms – many cases have no identifiable cause. If these causes are determined to be unlikely, the condition is labeled as idiopathic, and a food-responsive gastroenteropathy is prioritized as the cause. Certain dog breeds appear to be more susceptible to developing chronic gastritis, including the Norwegian Lundehund, German Shepherd dog, and Rottweiler. Chronic gastritis is characterized by persistent or intermittent clinical signs, such as vomiting, for >2 weeks duration. Because inflammation can impair gastric motility and delay gastric emptying, animals with chronic gastritis can display clinical signs of vomiting and early satiety. Following collection and routine histopathologic evaluation of mucosal biopsies, the gastritis can be classified based on the inflammatory cellular infiltrate (i.e., lymphocytic, lymphoplasmacytic, eosinophilic), the presence of morphological changes (i.e., hypertrophy, atrophy, mineralization, ulceration, edema, glandular nesting, fibrosis), and lesion severity (i.e., normal, mild, moderate, marked, severe).

The most common inflammatory infiltrate in dogs with chronic gastritis is lymphoplasmacytic.[2] However, mild to moderate degrees of such lymphoplasmacytic inflammation can appear in dogs without clinical signs. Therefore, veterinarians must consider both clinical signs and other diagnostic findings in conjunction with biopsy results when deciding whether treatment is necessary. Lymphocytic and lymphoplasmacytic gastritis do not warrant immediate steroid therapy, as they can be observed with food-responsive gastroenteropathies, *Helicobacter* spp. colonization, or in working dogs. *Helicobacter* spp. are frequently identified in the stomach of dogs with or without gastric inflammation and regardless whether clinical signs of disease are present; therefore, the role of these bacteria as a potential pathogen in dogs remains unclear. Treatment of *Helicobacter* spp., as described later, is often recommended when these bacteria are associated with inflammation in animals that are refractory to other therapies, such as dietary modification.

Eosinophilic gastritis is often accompanied by abnormal eosinophil accumulation in other organs, including the esophagus, small intestine, or colon, and can also be found as part of a mixed inflammatory disease with other inflammatory cells.[3] When allergies or parasites have been ruled out, this condition falls under the broader category of chronic inflammatory gastroenteropathies. This form typically affects younger dogs, with Rottweilers being particularly susceptible. While the inflammation usually affects only the mucosa, it can sometimes penetrate into the muscle layers or serosa. The condition can cause the rugal folds to enlarge, and the damaged tissue may develop ulcers, leading to hemorrhage and protein loss. High blood eosinophil counts are common but vary widely. Some dogs may also show signs of allergic reactions, such as hives. Before concluding that the condition is immune-mediated, veterinarians should rule out parasites, infections, and tumors (particularly mast cell tumors). Treatment for eosinophilic gastritis typically starts with deworming medications and dietary modification. Commercial dietary options that are reasonable to consider for dogs with eosinophilic gastritis include partially or extensively hydrolyzed, limited-ingredient, or amino acid–based diets. Home-prepared diets are also excellent options but require the supervision of a board-certified veterinary nutritionist to ensure the diet is complete and balanced if it is then to be continued as the maintenance diet. Several dietary trials, in which the pet owner feeds the diet exclusively, are often needed before clinical signs resolve. If GI signs are going to improve with the selected diet, they will generally do so within 1–2 weeks of feeding with an elimination diet trial. For dogs that do not respond to deworming and dietary changes, medications that modulate the immune system such as corticosteroids or ciclosporin may prove effective.

Helicobacter-associated gastritis

Helicobacter spp. are gram-negative, curved- to spiral-shaped bacteria that predominantly colonize the stomach; however, they can also be found in the oral cavity, intestine, and hepatobiliary system. The Helicobacter-like organisms found in dogs' stomachs are typically large spiral shapes that, while indistinguishable under standard microscopy, are different from the smaller *Helicobacter pylori* found in humans.[4] There is a high prevalence of gastric Helicobacter-like organisms (GHLO) in asymptomatic dogs, particularly in shelter or colony environments, suggesting living conditions influence infection rates. While the exact transmission method remains unclear, these GHLOs likely spread through oral-to-fecal or oral-to-oral contact.

Unlike in humans, where treating *H. pylori* infections with antibiotics can eliminate the inflammation, the relationship between *Helicobacter* and illness in dogs is less clear. Most dogs with naturally acquired *Helicobacter* colonization, however, are healthy, and an obvious relationship between *Helicobacter* infection and the presence of clinical signs is difficult to prove. Moreover, gastric inflammation can persist even after eradication of the organism. Noninvasive tests, such as serology by ELISA or Western blotting, have little utility in dogs because non-*H. pylori* species predominate.

To definitively diagnose Helicobacter colonization, veterinarians must examine gastric tissue samples or confirm findings through culture or DNA testing (PCR). A quick screening test called the rapid urease test can help identify potential infections by detecting the bacteria's ability to break down urea, causing a visible color change within 1–24 hours, though this method is less reliable than cytologic examination.[4] Using special staining techniques (such as Warthin-Starry silver, toluidine blue, or Giemsa) help make the bacteria more detectable on microscopic examination. Because these organisms are not evenly distributed throughout the stomach, multiple tissue samples from different areas of the stomach should be examined. While growing Helicobacter in laboratory cultures is specific, it is also the most challenging and least sensitive test.

Treatment

Triple therapy with two antibiotics and an acid blocker (e.g., amoxicillin 20 mg/kg PO q8–12 h, metronidazole 20 mg/kg PO q8–12 h, omeprazole 1 mg/kg PO q12–24 h) can be attempted for dogs that do not respond to other therapies and have evidence of moderate to severe gastric inflammation associated with *Helicobacter*-like organisms. Unfortunately, most dogs will experience treatment failure or reinfection, and the inflammation often persists despite organism eradication.[5]

Parasitic and infectious gastritis

Vomiting is the most common clinical sign of stomach worm infection, although regurgitation is also infrequently reported.[6] Although *Physaloptera* spp. have a worldwide distribution, only in regions where infections are commonly reported (i.e., tropical, subtropical, USA) should infection be ruled out prior to more invasive and expensive diagnostic tests. Diagnosis of stomach worms using routine centrifugal fecal flotation can be falsely negative due to a low worm burden. Identification of *Physaloptera* spp. in the vomitus or endoscopic visualization of stomach worms (1–6 cm in length, stout, cream-colored to white, straight or coiled) can help confirm disease. Empirical treatment with an appropriate anthelminthic agent is recommended for any dog with chronic idiopathic vomiting; however, treatment failure or reinfection is possible. Evaluation for the presence of other parasites and infectious agents (e.g. *Gnathostoma*, *Spirocerca*, *Histoplasma capsulatum*, *Heterobilharzia americana*) should be considered based on the dog's environment and travel history. Pythium can also cause GI signs in dogs and is discussed elsewhere (see Chapter 38).[7]

Diagnostic approach to chronic gastritis

Extra-GI causes of chronic vomiting should be ruled out through evaluation of history, physical examination, and blood work, including a complete blood count, serum chemistry panel, urinalysis, and urine sediment examination, and also hypoadrenocorticism testing when appropriate. In older dogs, especially those of susceptible breeds which are underweight and have high concentrations of C-reactive protein, or those with low blood folate, veterinarians should strongly consider gastric cancer as a possibility and pursue more thorough diagnostic testing.[8] Additionally, conditions affecting the pancreas (pancreatitis or exocrine pancreatic insufficiency) or liver and biliary system can mimic the signs of chronic gastritis. Therefore, when bloodwork suggests these conditions may be present, additional tests such as pancreatic lipase assay and abdominal imaging should be considered.

For dogs with mild signs, starting with a fecal evaluation, such as centrifugal fecal flotation or fecal antigen assays, and deworming treatment is a reasonable first step (see Chapter 19). However, dogs showing more severe signs, concerning blood test results, or those not responding to initial treatment should undergo abdominal imaging. Using contrast material during radiography can help better reveal gastric abnormalities. When ultrasound shows thickening of the gastric wall, this may indicate neoplasia, but often reflects gastric edema, which can be seen in cases of pancreatic inflammation or low blood protein. Conversely, dogs with either gastritis or gastric neoplasia can have an ultrasonographically normal stomach and small intestine.

When blood work and abdominal imaging reveal no abnormalities, further testing is recommended based on patient signalment, history, clinical signs, and initial diagnostic tests. These may include standard radiography, testing for hypoadrenocorticism, or testing for appropriate infectious diseases. For chronic vomiting in dogs, enteropathogen panel testing is only warranted when the animal shows systemic illness signs often accompanied by diarrhea, or consumes raw food, or comes from a high-density housing environment such as an animal shelter. If anthelmintic or dietary interventions fail, GI biopsies can be obtained via endoscopy (Fig. 46.1) or surgery for histopathologic examination. Endoscopy allows for direct visualization and sampling of luminal and mucosal abnormalities (see Chapter 22) and is particularly beneficial for evaluating gastric mucosa because imaging and exploratory surgery might miss ulcerative lesions. Surgery, however, provides full-thickness samples, the ability to resect lesions, and access to areas that are difficult to reach by endoscopy such as the mid-jejunum.

Therapeutic approach to chronic gastritis

When no cause can be identified despite a thorough diagnostic evaluation, anthelmintic and dietary management should be the first treatments employed. Food-responsive gastroenteropathies encompass more than adverse food reactions to dietary protein. For suspected food-responsive conditions, dietary interventions may include feeding a highly digestible, high-moisture, and/or lower fat diet to accelerate gastric emptying; limited-ingredient diets with a single protein and carbohydrate source (preferably novel); or hydrolyzed-protein diets to minimize GI and cutaneous adverse food reactions (see Chapter 41). Most food-responsive cases show improvement after a strict two-week dietary trial. In young animals especially, multiple diet trials targeting different nutritional strategies should be attempted before determining the dog to be non-food responsive. Absence of response to one hydrolyzed diet, even to one that is extensively hydrolyzed (i.e., oligopeptides, amino acids), does not rule out food-responsive GI disease.

Immunomodulatory therapies are pursued when dietary interventions fail, when imaging and infectious disease tests are negative or inconclusive, or when owners decline endoscopy or surgery. Initial treatment typically involves prednisone or prednisolone at 1 mg/kg/day, with large to giant dogs (>25 kg) limited to 30 mg every 12 hours. The dose is slowly decreased by 25-30% over several weeks to months. Budesonide (3 mg/m^2 daily), with its high first-pass metabolism, may be associated with lesser systemic effects and, therefore, may be a more suitable option for diabetic animals or large dogs, although side effects such as polyuria, polyphagia, and steroid hepatopathy can still be observed with budesonide.[9] For steroid-refractory cases or when steroid side effects are insufferable, ciclosporin or chlorambucil are alternatives. Prior to reaching for a second immunosuppressive agent in perceived steroid-refractory disease, the clinician should revisit the dietary history to ensure that a wide variety of dietary trials have been employed. Supportive care measures, as described for dogs with acute gastritis, can complement diagnostic evaluations and treatment trials.

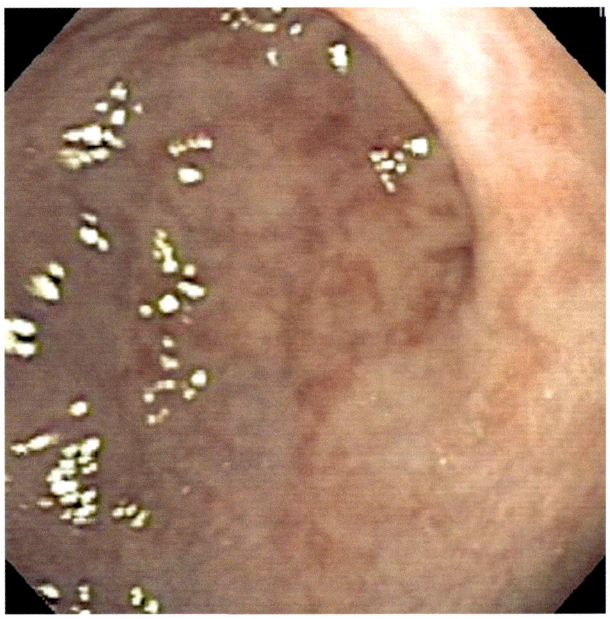

FIG. 46.1 Gastroscopic view of a dog with lymphocytic–lymphoplasmacytic gastritis. Image courtesy of Patricia Secoura.

Gastric ulceration

Dogs with GI ulceration can present with overt clinical signs including melena, hematemesis, hematochezia, abdominal pain, anemia, and hypoproteinemia or they can present with nonspecific signs such as lethargy or altered appetite. As coagulopathies can also cause GI bleeding, it is important to rule out disorders of primary or secondary hemostasis alongside the evaluation for GI ulceration.

Common causes of GI ulceration in the dog include NSAID or glucocorticoid administration, neoplasia, sharp/abrasive foreign bodies, GDV, and high-intensity activity in working dogs.[10] NSAID administration is reported to be the most common cause of severe gastric ulceration in the dog. This type of ulceration usually occurs in the gastric body and pyloroantral regions. NSAIDs can be harmful to the gut in two ways: they are weak acids that can be directly cytotoxic, and they inhibit the synthesis of cytoprotective prostaglandins that bolster the GI mucosal barrier.

Consideration of the dog's breed and age helps to prioritize causes of GI ulceration. Young dogs are more likely to have foreign body, parasitic, and other infectious causes of GI ulceration, while the etiology in older dogs is more often gastric neoplasia.

Diagnostic approach to gastric ulceration

Dogs with diagnosed or suspected gastric ulceration require immediate examination and stabilization simultaneously with diagnostic assessment. The severity and chronicity of bleeding can be determined through review of the historical, physical examination, and blood work (i.e., complete blood count, serum biochemistry) findings.

Physical examination findings may reveal pale mucous membranes, a painful abdomen, appreciable abdominal masses or foreign objects, or evidence of hypovolemic shock. A rectal examination showing hematochezia or melena supports the diagnosis, though lack of these findings does not rule out GI bleeding. Common laboratory findings in dogs with GI ulceration include normocytic, normochromic anemia, hypoalbuminemia, and chronic GI bleeding may present with a mild to moderate microcytic, hypochromic anemia, indicating iron deficiency. A euhydrated dog with a serum blood urea nitrogen to creatinine ratio >27:1 (and which is not being fed a high-protein diet) raises concern of bleeding due to GI ulceration, though this ratio has low sensitivity but warrants further investigation.[11] Fecal occult blood tests can detect smaller amounts of hemoglobin than required to induce melena; however, they can have low sensitivity and specificity. Diet may have less of an effect when using o-tolidine-based tests on canine fecal samples. Survey radiography rarely diagnoses gastric ulceration directly but can identify large abdominal masses or foreign objects as well as peritoneal effusions or tracking gas. Abdominal ultrasound may confirm gastric mucosal abnormalities compatible with ulceration and perforation such

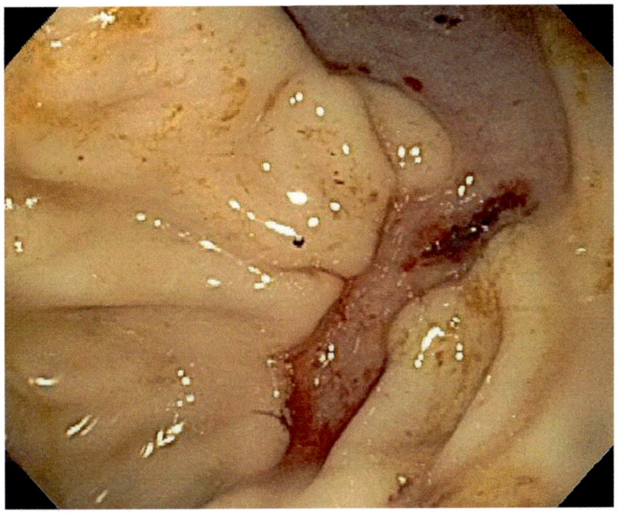

FIG. 46.2 Gastroscopic view of a dog with a gastric ulcer in the body of the stomach. Image courtesy of Patricia Secoura.

as peritoneal fluid and gas tracking through the GI wall or even free gas if perforation has occurred. However, complete ultrasonographic gastric examination is often limited by the stomach's location and intraluminal gas or ingesta, potentially causing ulcerative lesions to be missed. Abdominal computed tomography (CT) has similar sensitivity to ultrasonographic examination for detecting non-perforating GI ulcers in dogs.[12] Video capsule endoscopy offers a less invasive option for detecting gastric and small intestinal mucosal lesions including erosions and ulcers. The technology may be particularly helpful to identify lesions in larger dogs where endoscopy has a limited reach and ultrasonographic examination may prove difficult. Nevertheless, upper GI endoscopy is preferred because of the ability to both visualize and sample abnormal lesions (Fig. 46.2; see also Chapter 22).

For dogs with gastric ulceration without any history of ulcerogenic drug use, additional diagnostic tests should be considered based on the signalment of the dog and the initial test results. These tests may include fecal centrifugal flotation and parasite antigen evaluation, hypoadrenocorticism testing, fasting serum gastrin concentration to evaluate for gastrinoma, bile acid tolerance testing, regionally appropriate infectious disease testing, or abdominal CT angiography.

Therapeutic approach to gastric ulceration

Treatment and prognosis depend on the underlying etiology and severity of the ulceration. Surgical intervention should be pursued in animals with or at risk for perforation. Parenteral or oral administration of proton pump inhibitors (PPIs) is usually advised; however, a constant rate infusion of famotidine is also an effective option for hospitalized dogs (Table 46.2).[13] For NSAID-induced ulceration, misoprostol, a prostaglandin E_1 analog, can complement PPI therapy. Esomeprazole or omeprazole should be orally administered twice daily 30 minutes prior to feeding for approximately

TABLE 46.2 Drugs commonly used for the treatment of gastric diseases in the dog.

Category	Drug	Class	Dosage	Indications	Adverse effects and comments
Antiemetic	Maropitant	NK_1 receptor antagonist	2 mg/kg PO or 1 mg/kg IV or SC every 24 h	Vomiting	Pain at injection site
	Metoclopramide	5-HT_3 receptor antagonist	0.25–0.5 mg/kg IV, SC, IM, or PO every 12 h, or 1–2 mg/kg/day CRI		—
	Dolasetron		0.6 mg/kg PO or IV every 24 h		Poor bioavailability with oral administration
	Ondansetron		0.5–1.0 mg/kg PO or IV every 8–12 h		Sedation, fecal incontinence
Gastric acid suppressant	Famotidine	H_2 receptor antagonist	1 mg/kg PO, IV, or SC every 12 h 8 mg/kg/day CRI (for severe disease)	Exercise-induced GI bleeding, bilious vomiting syndrome	Renal excretion
	Omeprazole Esomeprazole Pantoprazole	PPI	1 mg/kg PO or IV every 12 h	Exercise-induced GI bleeding, gastroduodenal ulceration, esophagitis, bilious vomiting syndrome	Long-term use should be avoided
Cytoprotectant	Sucralfate	Coating agent	0.25 (small dogs)–1.0 g (large dogs) slurry PO every 6–8 h	Gastroduodenal ulceration, esophagitis	Constipation
	Barium	Coating agent	1–2 mL/kg PO every 8–12 h		Fatal if aspirated
Prostaglandin analog	Misoprostol	PGE_1 analog	3 μg/kg PO every 8-12 hours	NSAID toxicity	—
Prokinetic	Cisapride	5-HT_4 receptor agonist	0.1–0.5 mg/kg PO every 8–12 h	Gastric dysmotility, ileus	Diarrhea
	Metoclopramide	D_2 receptor antagonist, 5-HT_3 receptor antagonist	0.25–0.5 mg/kg IV, SC, IM, or PO every 12 h, or 1–2 mg/kg/day CRI		Diarrhea
	Erythromycin	Macrolide antibiotic	0.5–1.0 mg/kg PO every 8–12 h		High doses may result in vomiting

5-HT_3, serotonin type 3; 5-HT_4, serotonin type 4; CRI, constant rate infusion; D_2, dopamine type 2; H_2, histamine type 2; IM, intramuscular; IV, intravenous; NK_1, neurokinin-1; PGE_1, prostaglandin E_1; PO, per os; PPI, proton pump inhibitor; SC, subcutaneous.

3–4 weeks for the outpatient treatment of dogs with NSAID-induced ulceration. In hospitalized animals with severe gastric ulceration, either intravenously administered esomeprazole or a famotidine constant rate infusion are preferred by the author over the administration of pantoprazole. Famotidine should not be co-administered with the PPI when treating gastric ulceration as this practice does not enhance the acid suppressant effect compared to the PPI alone.
Depending on the underlying etiology, acid suppressant therapy may not always resolve the gastric ulceration and will not improve healing in the intestine. Monitoring response to treatment is important so that when clinical signs or laboratory abnormalities persist and other approaches such as clot stabilizers may be required. Prophylactic gastroprotective drugs are not indicated unless the dog has multiple risk factors for ulceration or bleeding. Orally administered sucralfate may help provide some pain relief but should not be used as the sole therapy for esophagitis or ulceration or for pain, and its administration must be separated from the administration of any PPIs by 1–2 hours. Dietary management for acute gastric ulceration typically includes a highly digestible, low residue, reduced fat, high moisture diet with fed in small volumes across multiple meals.

Gastric obstruction

Common functional causes of gastric obstruction include foreign material, benign (e.g., adenomatous polyps) or malignant neoplasms, and pyloric gastropathies. Clinical signs of gastric obstruction can include vomiting, regurgitation, dysorexia, lethargy, weight loss, abdominal distension, early satiety, dehydration, and abdominal pain. The severity of the clinical signs depends on the cause and the degree and duration of the obstruction. Dogs with gastric obstruction can have severe fluid deficits and electrolyte and acid-base disturbances. The diagnosis is often made with abdominal radiography or ultrasound and confirmed by gastroscopy.

Gastric foreign bodies

Gastric foreign material (e.g., bones, baby supplies, toys, needles, clothing, trash, plant material, fishhooks) is a common cause of vomiting, especially in young dogs. These foreign bodies can partially or completely obstruct the stomach. Severe obstruction can lead to bowel ischemia and perforation. Dogs with linear foreign bodies often have more severe clinical signs and prolonged hospitalization and should receive prompt intervention.[14] Small, discrete gastric foreign bodies can often be extracted endoscopically, whereas large or linear foreign bodies might require surgical removal. Bony foreign bodies identified incidentally may not cause complications and can be left to dissolve over time in asymptomatic dogs.[15] Rocks (Fig. 46.3) or metallic sharp-pointed straight foreign bodies (e.g., nails, pins, needles) can also be managed conservatively in asymptomatic dogs if endoscopic or surgical removal is not an option. These objects have an average GI transit time of approximately 60 hours.[16] Close monitoring of clinical signs that might be related to the foreign body or to obstruction and perforation is recommended in case of conservative management of any GI foreign body.

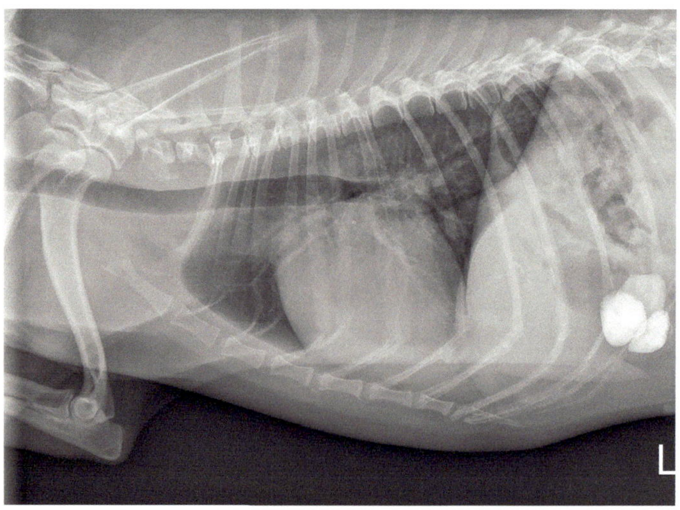

FIG. 46.3 Incidental finding of rocks in a dog's stomach during radiographic evaluation for left-sided cardiac enlargement.

Hypertrophic gastropathy

Hypertrophic gastropathy is a rare condition that may cause diffuse mucosal hypertrophy in the absence of any inflammation. Long-term use (years) of PPIs can lead to gastric mucosal hypertrophy. It can also develop spontaneously as localized hypertrophy of the antral mucosa resulting in intermittent or chronic pyloric obstruction. The condition has been termed chronic hypertrophic pylorogastropathy (CHPG) and is overrepresented in middle-aged, small-breed dogs, especially the Pekingese, Lhasa Apso, and Shih Tzu, and has a possible male sex predisposition. Clinical signs of CHPG reflect slow emptying of the stomach, causing marked abdominal distension, vomiting, dysorexia, and lethargy. While vomiting is the predominant sign, some dogs may experience regurgitation when severe gastric distension overcomes the lower esophageal sphincter's pressure differential.
Radiographically, dogs with CHPG typically show a fluid- or gas-filled stomach. Contrast radiography helps to identify outflow obstruction, while ultrasound documentation of increased pyloric wall thickness supports the diagnosis. Definitive diagnosis requires endoscopic or surgical identification of enlarged mucosal folds that impede pyloric intubation. Surgical resection of the affected area is the preferred treatment; a Y-U pyloroplasty and submucosal resection is the most common procedure. Microscopically, the condition is characterized by pyloric antral mucosal hypertrophy, with or without concurrent muscular hypertrophy.

Giant hypertrophic gastritis

Chronic gastritis and chronic foreign bodies (Fig. 46.4) can cause hypertrophy, but with inflammation. A breed predisposition for idiopathic giant hypertrophic gastritis (GHG) in Basenjis and Drentsche Patriijshond dogs has been identified. Diffuse gastric mural thickening due to foveolar and glandular hyperplasia, loss of chief and parietal cells, and varying degrees of inflammatory cell infiltration characterize GHG. This condition is often incorrectly labeled Ménétrier's or Ménétrier-like disease. In humans, GHG is also recognized, but the name Ménétrier's disease is limited to rugal hypertrophy caused by overgrowth of mucus cells without inflammation.

Gastric polyps

Benign gastric polyps, which are discrete, variably sized nodules that arise from the gastric mucosa and extend into the gastric lumen, can also rarely cause gastric outflow obstruction in dogs (Fig. 46.5). These polyps may be identified incidentally in older dogs but can occasionally

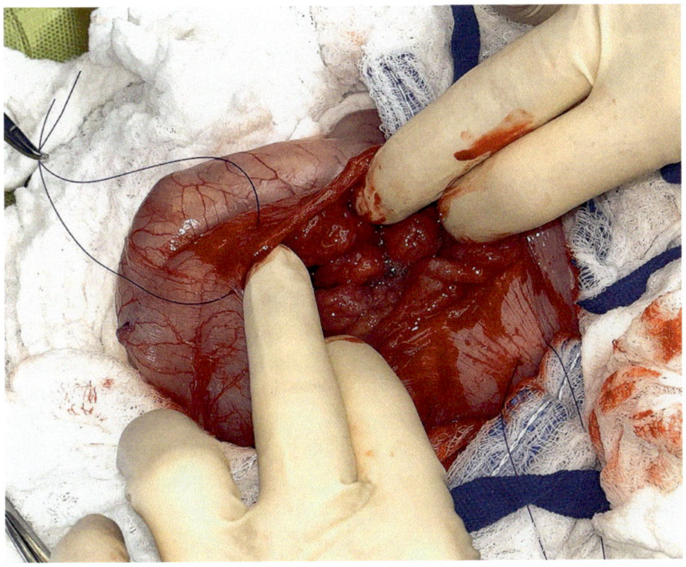

FIG. 46.4 Giant hypertrophic gastritis due to a chronic foreign body.

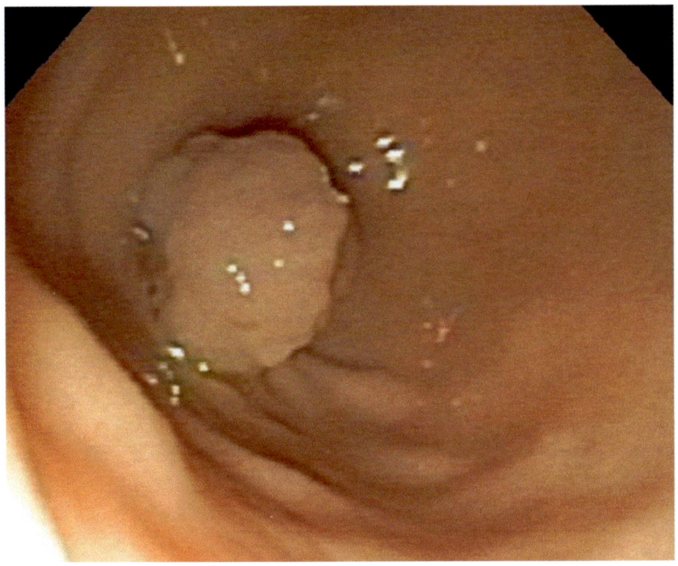

FIG. 46.5 Gastroscopic view of a large polyp in the pyloric antrum of a dog.

disrupt wall layering as observed on ultrasonographic examination. They are not associated with regional lymphadenopathy. Surgical resection and histopathologic examination of the tissue is required for a definitive diagnosis.

Gastric metaplasia and neoplasia

Gastric metaplasia and neoplasia are uncommonly reported in the dog, with the exception of a few predisposed breeds (collies, Staffordshire Bull Terrier, Tervueren Belgian Shepherd). However, gastric metaplasia can be easily overlooked with standard white light endoscopy. Narrow-band imaging has been used to identify metaplastic lesions in Tervueren dogs, so it should be considered in at-risk breeds.[17] Gastric carcinomas, including adenocarcinoma, squamous cell carcinoma, and undifferentiated carcinomas, are the most frequent solid gastric tumors in the dog. Other, less commonly reported canine gastric tumors include mast cell tumor, leiomyoma/sarcoma, extramedullary plasmacytoma, GI stromal tumor, fibrosarcoma, and histiocytic sarcoma. Gastric carcinomas are often identified at the lesser curvature or pyloric antrum in middle-aged to older dogs, with males being overrepresented.

Presenting clinical signs in animals with gastric carcinomas include vomiting, dysorexia, weight loss, abdominal pain, ptyalism, diarrhea, hematemesis, and melena. In a 2019 study, investigators demonstrated that dogs with gastric carcinomas were more likely to be >8 years old and underconditioned and have a serum C-reactive protein >25 mg/L and a low serum folate compared to dogs with chronic gastritis.[8] Most carcinomas exfoliate well or can be found in ulcerated regions and, therefore, can often be diagnosed with examination of a sample from either an ultrasound-guided fine needle aspirate or endoscopic biopsy. B-mode and contrast-enhanced ultrasound might help in the differentiation of gastritis from gastric neoplasia (see Chapter 21). However, gastric carcinomas are often diagnosed at a late stage and can be missed on ultrasonographic examination.[18]

Gastric carcinomas are often poorly responsive to chemotherapy and highly metastatic at the time of diagnosis, with a survival time of <3 months after the diagnosis. Surgery and adjuvant chemotherapy only slightly improve the median survival time to approximately 6 months. Although additional studies are needed to determine if there is a true benefit to adjuvant chemotherapy in dogs with gastric carcinoma, the current treatment of choice, especially for patients without distant metastasis, is surgical resection and postoperative chemotherapy. Common sites of metastasis include the gastric lymph nodes, esophagus, duodenum, spleen, liver, omentum, adrenal glands, and lungs.

Gastric motility disorders

The time it takes for the canine stomach to empty of food can vary considerably between and within individuals, but the majority of meals should pass completely into the duodenum within eight hours. Dogs showing gastric distension or vomiting of food more than 8 to 12 hours after eating may have gastric dysmotility, classified as either mechanical or functional. Mechanical disorders physically impede the passage of gastric contents into the small intestine and include masses, torsion, pyloric stenosis, and foreign objects. Functional, non-obstructive gastric motility disorders can be caused by both local (e.g., inflammatory, neurogenic) and secondary (e.g., opioid administration, metabolic disease, critical illness, abdominal surgery) conditions.[19] Gastric dysmotility lengthens hospitalization time and increases patient morbidity and mortality.

Clinical presentations of dogs with delayed gastric emptying include vomiting or regurgitation but may also feature changes in appetite and/or pica, excessive salivation, belching, abdominal pain or distension, or increased thirst. Abdominal palpation may be unremarkable but may trigger eructation or regurgitation and identify abdominal distension, pain, or an underlying anatomical cause like a mass.

While history and physical examination often suggest gastric motility disorders, evaluating gastric emptying can help to diagnose the disorder and to monitor the response to treatment. Methods that can be used in practice include contrast radiography, barium-impregnated polyethylene spheres, ultrasound, computed tomography, magnetic resonance imaging, and wireless motility capsules (see Chapter 43).

Comprehensive assessment should evaluate both fasting and fed motility phases with solids and liquids, as disorders are not always detectable when evaluating only one phase. Age, body size, test meal composition, assessment method, and procedural stress can all influence gastric emptying times. Contrast radiography (Fig. 46.6), computed tomography, or magnetic resonance imaging can help detect structural disease, but dogs with solid-phase gastric emptying disorders can have normal emptying of liquids, and the stress of restraint and an unfamiliar environment may delay gastric emptying in animals without a true gastric emptying disorder. Abdominal ultrasound offers a non-invasive, real-time assessment of gastric contractions and intestinal motility, helping differentiate structural from functional causes. Using a single, skilled ultrasonographer reduces subjectivity. Examining standing animals may minimize stress and gas-related visualization issues.

Mechanical obstruction should be considered from the information gathered from signalment, history, and physical examination, and ruled in/out via imaging before exploring functional disorders. This approach is most important in young dogs with the likelihood of foreign object ingestion. Older or critically ill animals warrant blood tests alongside abdominal imaging, with potentially additional testing for infectious diseases, hypoadrenocorticism, and exploratory laparotomy, as indicated.

Bilious vomiting syndrome typically occurs as vomiting after prolonged fasting, usually in the early morning, but without other clinical signs. While its etiology remains unknown, it may involve duodenogastric reflux-induced gastric irritation because of low intragastric pressure. Late-night feeding with or without acid suppressants typically improves the frequency of episodes. Despite the diminished efficacy of famotidine with repeated dosing, it is often still effective in dogs with bilious vomiting syndrome that is responsive to acid suppression. This is likely because the drug is acting through a different mechanism, or because potent acid suppression is not required to control the clinical signs.

Treatment success requires identifying and addressing underlying causes. Functional disorders without a clear etiology or secondary to critical illness often need multimodal therapy including prokinetics and nutritional support. In dogs with severe gastric emptying disorders, prokinetic drugs (e.g., cisapride, erythromycin, metoclopramide) may be indicated (see Chapter 31). These drugs should be given intravenously when possible, but if oral administration is necessary, liquid formulations are recommended. Various medications may help: cisapride, a serotonin ($5HT_4$) receptor agonist, particularly affects gastric antral motility. A prolonged QT interval is a reported side effect of cisapride administration in people but has not been reported in dogs, in which the most common adverse effect is diarrhea.

Metoclopramide hydrochloride is a dopamine (D_2) receptor antagonist (at low doses), a serotonin ($5HT_3$) receptor antagonist (at high doses), and a selective serotonin ($5HT_4$) receptor agonist. Like cisapride, metoclopramide enhances acetylcholine release at postsynaptic sites, albeit more weakly than cisapride. Metoclopramide also antagonizes the inhibitory effect of dopamine on intestinal transit, leading to enhanced intestinal smooth-muscle contractions. Metoclopramide transiently increases fasting gastric contractions but has limited effect during feeding. It should be dosed 30 minutes before meals when given intermittently but its short half-life means it is likely to be more effective when given as a constant rate infusion.

Erythromycin is a macrolide antibiotic that, when administered at low doses (0.5–1.0 mg/kg), enhances gastric emptying in dogs. Higher doses (10–20 mg/kg), such as those required for antimicrobial activity, can cause vomiting. Chronic administration of macrolides (>2 weeks) in humans leads to diminished efficacy. Erythromycin is metabolized by the cytochrome P450 system. It should be noted that the use of chronic low doses of erythromycin is contrary to good antibiotic stewardship.

Ranitidine was considered to promote gastric motility promotion but failed to shorten gastric emptying times in healthy dogs when given orally.[20] Furthermore, there is a lack of studies evaluating its effects in dogs with gastric dysmotility. Moreover, ranitidine is no longer available in Europe.

Mirtazapine, at a dose of 2 mg/kg orally, may improve gastric emptying, based on studies in healthy dogs[21] whilst lubiprostone, a chloride channel activator, has also shown accelerated postprandial gastric emptying in healthy dogs.[22] Additional supportive measures include correcting electrolyte abnormalities (avoiding both deficiencies and excesses), judicious fluid therapy (maintaining hydration without causing gut edema), and regular ambulation when possible. Novel therapies such as intragastric L-arginine and L-glutamate have shown improvement in gastric emptying and accommodation.

The concept of "bowel rest" is no longer universally recommended. For many patients, early enteral nutrition, defined as nutrition provided within 48–72 hours of hospitalization, is well tolerated, has few complications, and leads to improved outcomes; therefore, it is recommended as part of a multimodal approach to the management of GI motility disorders. Early enteral nutrition may benefit the patient through the following proposed mechanisms: improved mucosal blood flow to the GI tract, decreased intestinal bacterial translocation, stimulation of GI motility, and secretion of GI hormones, growth factors, and bicarbonate. Most dogs with dysmotility can be orally offered or given assisted feeding at 15–25% of their resting energy requirement. Caloric intake is then gradually increased if the patient tolerates the feeding.

Nasoenteric, esophageal, and gastric feeding tubes are commonly utilized in patients with GI motility disorders. The measurement of gastric residual volumes (GRVs) before the next feed to evaluate for gastric intolerance to enteral nutrition may guide veterinarians to make clinical decisions about whether to delay or stop enteral nutrition. However,

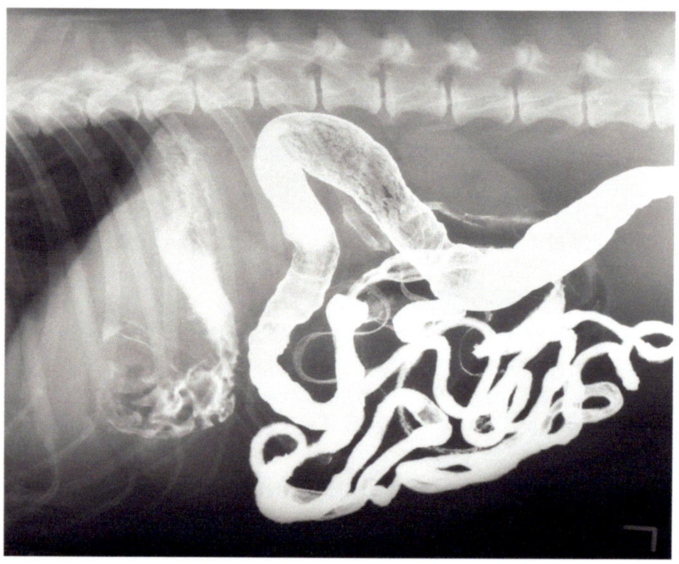

FIG. 46.6 Radiograph showing possible rugal fold enlargement and delayed gastric passage of contrast material in a dog with delayed gastric emptying. The contrast medium was orally administered 5 hours before this radiograph was obtained.

this practice is not recommended based on guidelines provided by the Society of Critical Care Medicine and the American Society for Parenteral and Enteral Nutrition.[23] Another randomized study, comparing continuous versus bolus naso-enteric feeding found no association between gastric residual volume and adverse GI events.[24] This suggests that stopping enteral nutrition due to high gastric residual volume may be unnecessary when other clinical signs such as abdominal distension, vomiting, regurgitation, or pain are absent. Post-pyloric feeding methods, like naso-jejunal tubes, can benefit patients which do not tolerate gastric feeding. For patients with severe GI dysmotility, supplemental parenteral nutrition should be considered to meet nutritional requirements.

The optimal diet for managing GI dysmotility will depend on the patient's dietary history, any comorbidities, and the imaging findings. Generally, the diet should be reduced-fat and high-moisture with low soluble fiber, as highly digestible foods facilitate faster GI transit because of easier digestion, and absorption. Patients with GI dysmotility should have regular nutritional assessment and adjustments to their feeding plan to ensure optimal nutritional support.

Gastric dilatation and volvulus

Gastric dilatation-volvulus (GDV) is an acute life-threatening condition. It primarily affects large, deep- or narrow-chested dogs and involves gastric dilatation with clockwise rotation along the mesenteroaxial axis. If not quickly identified and corrected, GDV results in compromised blood supply and decreased venous return, leading to GI necrosis, shock, and death. The overall mortality rate in dogs with GDV is 11–36%.[25] Risk factors for development of this condition include deep-chested breeds, dietary habits (e.g., rapid eating, dry food, elevated food bowl position, or large food volume), thin body condition, older age, nervous temperament, and a family history of GDV. Previous splenectomy is not a consistent risk factor for GDV.[26] Clinical presentations include a distended tympanitic abdomen, although this is not always obvious in deep-chested dogs. Other signs include excessive salivation, unproductive retching, weakness, breathing difficulties, restlessness, cardiac arrhythmias, and various indicators of shock such as abnormal mucous membrane color, delayed capillary refill, bradycardia, depression, and temperature abnormalities.

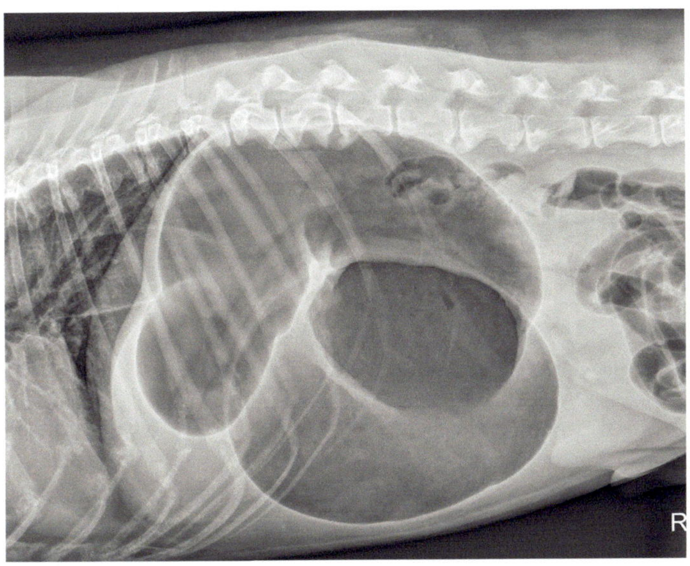

FIG. 46.7 Abdominal radiograph of a dog with gastric dilatation–volvulus and esophageal distension from aerophagia.

A GDV diagnosis is initially suspected based on compatible signalment, history, and physical examination findings as patient stabilization should precede any abdominal imaging. Confirmation then comes from imaging, identifying pyloric malposition with gastric air entrapment ("Popeye arm" or "double bubble" sign) with compartmentalization of the stomach on a right lateral radiograph. Very rarely, organoaxial volvulus with a distended but normally positioned stomach may be revealed by ultrasonographic examination. Radiography or ultrasound may reveal abdominal effusion or air in cases with hemoabdomen or gastric perforation respectively. (see also Chapter 21).

Laboratory abnormalities may include hemoconcentration, acid-base imbalances, hypokalemia, and coagulation disorders including disseminated intravascular coagulation. Negative prognostic indicators include delayed intervention with persistent hyperlactatemia (>6 mmol/L), acute kidney injury, gastric wall necrosis, increased serum myoglobin, and elevated canine pepsinogen A or C-reactive protein..

Effective treatment of a GDV requires prompt intervention: intravenous fluid therapy, gastric decompression and surgery. Stabilization involves placement of large-gauge catheters in veins cranial to the gastric volvulus (i.e., jugular or cephalic veins), followed by aggressive fluid resuscitation with crystalloids and possibly hypertonic saline. After initiation of adequate fluid therapy, gastric decompression is achieved either via percutaneous trocarization or by orogastric tube placement. The former is preferred due to lower risks of rupture and aspiration. Frequent monitoring of vital parameters and biochemical status is essential based on disease severity, but once hemodynamically stable with gastric decompression completed, patients undergo anesthesia for abdominal exploration,

After repositioning of the stomach is achieved, resection or invagination of any areas of devitalized gastric wall is performed as necessary. A permanent gastropexy should always be performed to prevent recurrence. Splenectomy is only performed if its blood flow is compromised. Surgical intervention beyond 3 hours post-admission carries a poorer prognosis, emphasizing the need for rapid stabilization and surgery.

Gastropexy is recommended for all surgically managed GDV cases and at-risk dogs undergoing abdominal surgery for other indications. Various fixation approaches and techniques exist, with the procedure performed on the right abdominal wall near the last rib. While no gold standard technique exists, proper gastropexy placement is critical to minimize complications like partial pyloric obstruction and recurrent bloating. Dietary management modifications—moistened food, smaller frequent meals, avoiding elevated feeding positions, and slow-feeding devices—may help reduce gastric dilatation and GDV risk. Since gastropexy does not eliminate recurrent dilatation risk, ongoing nutritional and environmental management remains essential for successful long-term outcomes. Postoperative management should address pain and any consequences of poor tissue perfusion and ischemia-reperfusion injury, including electrolyte imbalances, arrhythmias, GI ulceration, systemic inflammatory response, kidney injury, and coagulation disorders. Serial lactate monitoring helps determine prognosis and treatment response, while ultrasound monitoring detects potential septic peritonitis.

KEY POINTS

- A normal gastric ultrasound examination does not rule out the presence of gastric pathology, including inflammation or neoplasia.
- Many dogs with chronic idiopathic lymphocytic gastritis have food-responsive disease and do not require steroid therapy.
- Gastric acid suppressants should be reserved for dogs with esophagitis or gastroduodenal ulceration.

References

1. Washabau RJ, Day MJ, Willard MD, et al. Endoscopic, biopsy, and histopathologic guidelines for the evaluation of gastrointestinal inflammation in companion animals. *J Vet Intern Med* 24(1):10–26, 2010.
2. Lidbury JA, Suchodolski JS, Steiner JM. Gastric histopathologic abnormalities in dogs: 67 cases (2002–2007). *J Am Vet Med Assoc* 234(9):1147–1153, 2009.
3. Bastan I, Rendahl AK, Seelig D, et al. Assessment of eosinophils in gastrointestinal inflammatory disease of dogs. *J Vet Intern Med* 32(6):1911–1917, 2018.
4. Husnik R, Klimes J, Kovarikova S, Kolorz M. *Helicobacter* species and their association with gastric pathology in a cohort of dogs with chronic gastrointestinal signs. *Animals (Basel)* 12(10):1254, 2022.
5. Jergens AE, Pressel M, Crandell J, et al. Fluorescence in situ hybridization confirms clearance of visible *Helicobacter* spp. associated with gastritis in dogs and cats. *J Vet Intern Med* 23(1):16-23, 2009.
6. Soderman L, Harkin KR. Gastric *Physaloptera* infection in 27 dogs (1997–2019). *J Am Anim Hosp Assoc* 57(1):8–14, 2021.
7. Billings P, Walton S, Shmalberg J, Santoro D. The use of mefenoxam to treat cutaneous and gastrointestinal pythiosis in dogs: a retrospective study. *Microorganisms* 11(7):1726, 2023.
8. Seim-Wikse T, Skancke E, Nødtvedt A, et al. Comparison of body condition score and other minimally invasive biomarkers between dogs with gastric carcinoma and dogs with chronic gastritis. *J Am Vet Med Assoc* 254(2):226–235, 2019.
9. Dye TL, Diehl KJ, Wheeler SL, Westfall DS. Randomized, controlled trial of budesonide and prednisone for the treatment of idiopathic inflammatory bowel disease in dogs. *J Vet Intern Med* 27(6):1385–1391, 2013.
10. Pavlova E, Gold RM, Tolbert MK, Lidbury JA. Medical conditions associated with gastroduodenal ulceration or erosion in 168 dogs: 2008–2018. *J Vet Intern Med* 35(6):2697–2704, 2021.
11. Safrany B, Holmes AC, Adamantos S, et al. Plasma urea:creatinine ratio as a biomarker of gastrointestinal bleeding in dogs with anaemia. *Vet Med Sci* 9(6):2576–2585, 2023.
12. Fitzgerald E, Barfield D, Lee KC, Lamb CR. Clinical findings and results of diagnostic imaging in 82 dogs with gastrointestinal ulceration. *J Small Anim Pract* 58(4):211–218, 2017.
13. Tolbert MK. Gastroprotective therapy. *Vet Clin North Am Small Anim Pract* 51(1):33-41, 2021.
14. Hobday MM, Pachtinger GE, Drobatz KJ, Syring RS. Linear versus non-linear gastrointestinal foreign bodies in 499 dogs: clinical presentation, management and short-term outcome. *J Small Anim Pract* 55(11):560–565, 2014.
15. Barash NR, Lashnits E, Kern ZT, et al. Outcomes of esophageal and gastric bone foreign bodies in dogs. *J Vet Intern Med* 36(2):500–507, 2022.
16. Crinò C, Humm K, Cortellini S. Conservative management of metallic sharp-pointed straight gastric and intestinal foreign bodies in dogs and cats: 17 cases (2003–2021). *J Small Anim Pract* 64(8):522–526, 2023.
17. Candido MV, Syrjä P, Kilpinen S, Spillmann T. Canine breeds associated with gastric carcinoma, metaplasia and dysplasia diagnosed by histopathology of endoscopic biopsy samples. *Acta Vet Scand* 60(1):37, 2018.
18. Simeoni F, Del Signore F, Aste G, et al. B-mode and contrast enhanced ultrasonography features of gastric inflammatory and neoplastic diseases in dogs. *Animals (Basel)* 11(3):670, 2021.
19. Husnik R, Gaschen F. Gastric motility disorders in dogs and cats. *Vet Clin North Am Small Anim Pract* 51(1):43–59, 2021.
20. Lidbury JA, Suchodolski JS, Ivanek R, et al. Assessment of the variation associated with repeated measurement of gastrointestinal transit times and assessment of the effect of oral ranitidine on gastrointestinal transit times using a wireless motility capsule system in dogs. *Vet Med Int.* 2012:938417, 2012.
21. Yin J, Song J, Lei Y, et al. Prokinetic effects of mirtazapine on gastrointestinal transit. *Am J Physiol Gastrointest Liver Physiol.* 306(9):G796–801, 2014.
22. Song J, Yin J, Xu X, et al. Prokinetic effects of large-dose lubiprostone on gastrointestinal transit in dogs and its mechanisms. *Am J Transl Res.* 7(3):513–521, 2015.
23. Boullata JI, Carrera AL, Harvey L, et al. ASPEN safe practices for enteral nutrition therapy. *J Parenter Enteral Nutr* 41(1):15–103, 2017.
24. Holahan M, Abood S, Hauptman J, et al. Intermittent and continuous enteral nutrition in critically ill dogs: a prospective randomized trial. *J Vet Intern Med* 24(3):520–526, 2010.
25. Song KK, Goldsmid SE, Lee J, Simpson DJ. Retrospective analysis of 736 cases of canine gastric dilatation volvulus. *Aust Vet J* 98(6):232–238, 2020.
26. Sartor AJ, Bentley AM, Brown DC. Association between previous splenectomy and gastric dilatation–volvulus in dogs: 453 cases (2004–2009). *J Am Vet Med Assoc* 242(10):1381–1384, 2013.

CHAPTER 47

Chronic small intestinal diseases

Sara Jablonski
DVM, PhD, DACVIM (SAIM)

Given its critical roles and the complexity of the tasks it must perform, the small intestine (SI) is uniquely susceptible to a variety of important disorders and states of dysfunction. Of perhaps greatest importance, the SI must be both absorptive and exclusionary. Its functions include mixing and propulsion of ingesta, secretion of water and electrolytes, digestion and absorption, and regulation of blood flow, all while controlling immunological reactions and maintaining tolerance. Proper absorption of vital dietary nutrients and fat- and water-soluble vitamins requires a healthy SI, as does exclusion and elimination of unwanted antigens, microbes, and waste products. Thus, the most common signs of chronic disease of the SI include diarrhea and weight loss due to malabsorption. The diarrhea is caused primarily by malabsorption and bacterial fermentation of unabsorbed solutes and typically is characterized by an increase in the volume of feces produced with normal to mildly increased frequency and a lack of tenesmus, urgency, blood, or mucus. Small intestinal disease also may cause changes in appetite (ranging from anorexia to polyphagia), coprophagia, pica, vomiting, borborygmi, abdominal pain, melena, and effusions/edema, among other signs (Box 47.1).

In many cases, careful consideration of the signalment of the dog in addition to a thorough history and physical examination will go a long way toward discovering the cause of its SI disorder (see Chapter 1). The need for additional diagnostic testing (see below) will vary on a case-by-case basis but may prioritize fecal examination for pathogens, minimum database, evaluation of serum or fecal biomarkers, and imaging studies, with or without the need for endoscopy with intestinal biopsy. Management of disease may involve nonspecific and specific dietary and drug therapies depending on the disorder. This chapter provides an overview of the common features and complications of SI disease, followed by the general information, specific diagnostics, targeted therapies, and prognoses for the most common SI disorders in the dog, where available.

Box 47.1 Clinical signs associated with small intestinal disease.

- Diarrhea
  - Hematemesis or melena possible
- Vomiting
- Weight loss
  - Cachexia possible
- Alterations in appetite
  - Polyphagia
  - Hyporexia
  - Anorexia
  - Changes in food preferences
  - Coprophagia
  - Pica
- Borborygmi or flatus
- Halitosis
- Abdominal discomfort
- Complications of hypoalbuminemia
  - Peritoneal effusion
  - Pleural effusion
  - Peripheral edema
- Compensatory polydipsia

Features and complications of chronic SI disease

Malabsorption

Malabsorption is defined as the defective absorption of a dietary constituent resulting from interference with the digestive and/or absorptive processing of that molecule. Malabsorption is a common consequence of a variety of SI diseases, and the lack of nutrient uptake and the loss of nutrients in the feces commonly lead to diarrhea, weight loss, and alterations in appetite. However, in some cases, the distal SI and colon can compensate for a diseased upper SI and prevent diarrhea.

Malabsorption due to SI disease occurs most commonly as a consequence of reductions in the absorptive surface area of the SI (e.g., due to villous atrophy), direct damage to enterocytes, and/or infiltrates of inflammatory or neoplastic cells into the intestinal mucosa. Other causes of malabsorption include rapid intestinal transit time (i.e., hypermotility), brush-border enzyme deficiencies, vascular compromise (e.g., due to vasculitis or portal hypertension), intestinal lymphatic disease, and exocrine pancreatic insufficiency (EPI).[1] Cobalamin malabsorption secondary to reduced expression or function of the receptor (considered to be secondary to mucosal disease) and/or dysbiosis is a common and important complication of chronic SI disease. Cobalamin malabsorption also can occur due to an inherited abnormality of the cobalamin–intrinsic factor receptor or to EPI. Both protein and cobalamin malabsorption are of vital importance to identify and address because dogs with these deficiencies will have difficulty repairing intestinal damage, which could lead to self-perpetuating states of disease.[2]

Dysbiosis and bile acid dysmetabolism

Dysbiosis is defined as changes in the structure, function, and/or diversity of the intestinal microbiome. Dysbiosis and related bile acid dysmetabolism are generally considered to be consequences of SI disease, but in some cases it is theorized that intestinal dysbiosis may be the initiator of SI disease. Because the intestinal microbiota is responsible for many functions critical to the maintenance of gastrointestinal (GI) health, dysbiosis can have significant consequences. For example, a healthy intestinal microbiota directly competes with intestinal pathogens, providing a form of defense against their invasion; educates and modulates the immune system through a variety of mechanisms; promotes tight junction formation, thus enhancing the intestinal barrier; and is critical to a number of important metabolic pathways. Thus, dysbiosis can contribute to impaired host defenses against pathogens; impaired gut immune system responses; disruption of the epithelial barrier, which can lead to translocation of toxins, pathogens, and dietary antigens; and detrimental effects on a variety of metabolic pathways. Of note, dysbiosis can lead to a reduction in bile acid conversion, particularly when *Peptacetobacter* (*Clostridium*) *hiranonis* is depleted, leading to an increase in primary bile acids in the colon, which can have proinflammatory effects, impair the gut immune system, and contribute to diarrhea. Impaired fermentation of short-chain fatty acids is another important consequence of dysbiosis because short-chain fatty acids have roles in mucosal defense, help to regulate intestinal motility, and have anti-inflammatory properties. The complex interactions between the intestinal microbiome, mucosal defense and the host immune system, and metabolic processes suggest that, like malabsorption, dysbiosis can have serious deleterious and self-perpetuating effects on SI health and disease.[3]

Alterations in motility

Normal intestinal motility depends on healthy intestinal smooth muscle and enterocyte gap junctions, coordination between the digestive and central nervous systems, and excitatory and inhibitory signals from the enteric (local) nervous system. Additionally, some GI hormones, such as motilin and gastric inhibitory peptide, as well as interstitial cells of Cajal (pacemakers of intestinal motility) influence normal patterns of motility. Motility in the fasted state cycles through three phases—the quiescent phase, minor contractile activity, and short migrating (motor) complexes meant to sweep away undigested food, desquamated cells, and other substances. Motility in the fed state is characterized by both mixing and propulsive activity and is influenced by the luminal contents.[1]

Alterations in motility commonly occur secondary to chronic SI disease. Primary motility disorders are less common. When hypomotility occurs, the stasis of luminal contents may result in increased bacterial fermentation, resulting in diarrhea. Hypermotility can impair nutrient and water absorption in the intestine, leading to malabsorption and watery diarrhea. In cases of alterations of motility secondary to chronic SI disease, treatment of the underlying disorder will often resolve the alterations in motility. When the dog has a primary motility disorder, treatment can be more challenging[1] (see Chapter 43).

Protein-losing enteropathy

Protein-losing enteropathy (PLE) is a syndrome that can occur as a consequence of a wide variety of SI diseases. It is characterized by the excessive loss of protein through a diseased or damaged SI mucosa due to alterations in intestinal permeability, direct mucosal damage, and/or dilated or dysfunctional intestinal lymphatics. Up to 20% of dogs with chronic SI disease develop PLE, and dogs with PLE are at risk of life-threatening fluid accumulations and thromboembolic disease and have a poorer prognosis than dogs with chronic SI disease and normal serum protein concentrations. Dogs with PLE complicating SI disease have certain different considerations for diagnosis and therapeutic management when compared with dogs with SI disease without PLE[4] (see the section "Protein-losing enteropathy syndrome"; see also Chapter 13).

Specific chronic SI diseases

Congenital diseases

Anatomical congenital abnormalities of the SI are uncommon in dogs. Reported abnormalities include random duplications of SI segments (Fig. 47.1), blind-ended intestinal diverticula, arteriovenous fistulae of the SI, nonrotation of the midgut during embryonic development, intestinal stenosis, intestinal atresia (i.e., agenesis of a segment of intestine), and short bowel syndrome. Congenital short bowel syndrome refers to a lack of development of a major segment of the small bowel. Intestinal stenosis or atresia often results in failure to thrive and poor growth from intestinal obstruction or the inability to properly absorb nutrients. High neonatal mortality is observed in these conditions. If segmental atresia or stenosis of the SI is properly identified through imaging studies or during surgical

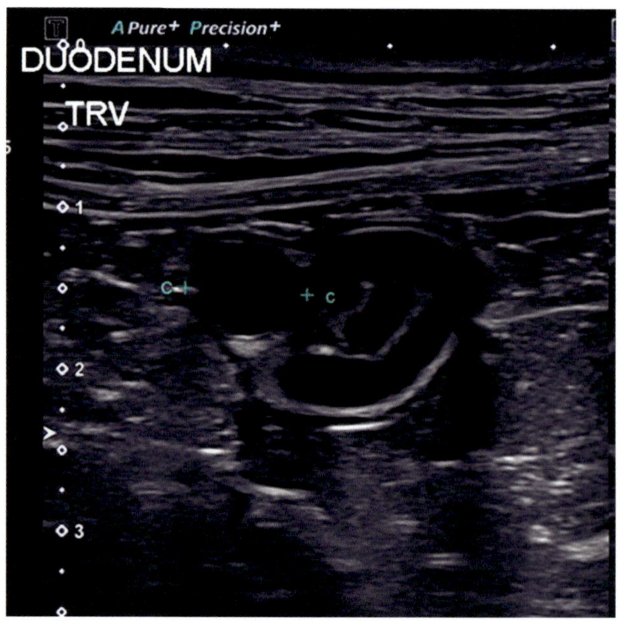

FIG. 47.1 Suspected mid-duodenal enteric duplication cyst (calipers) in a 2-year-old male castrated standard poodle. The cyst was considered clinically incidental.

exploration, it may be possible to treat it with removal of the affected segment of bowel. Affected dogs can compensate for congenital short bowel syndrome as long as 30–40 cm of small intestine is present but may require that a highly digestible diet is fed to maintain body weight and limit diarrhea.[5] Random duplications of the enteric tract and blind-ended intestinal diverticula are often discovered incidentally but can rarely result in GI hemorrhage, intestinal obstruction due to foreign-body entrapment, perforations, or nonspecific clinical signs.[1]

Selective cobalamin malabsorption due to inherited abnormalities of the cobalamin–intrinsic factor receptor affect specific breeds of dogs. These disorders are critical to identify because without treatment, dogs will die due to metabolic derangements and immunodeficiency.[2,6,7] The breeds of dogs affected and the specific details of their disorder are outlined in Table 47.1. Dogs with inherited cobalamin deficiency are often presented as juveniles due to diarrhea, inappetence, failure to thrive, and/or neurological signs. Laboratory abnormalities are common and include normocytic, normochromic nonregenerative anemia, neutropenia, hypoglycemia, hyperammonemia, and ketosis, among others. Clinical signs often improve within 24–48 hours of initiating treatment, whereas hematological abnormalities may take weeks to resolve. Both parenteral and oral therapies have been shown to be successful. Reports of successful parenteral therapy have described dosing intervals of once weekly, once every other week, once monthly, and every 2 months.[2]

Although brush-border enzyme deficiencies have been described in dogs, they appear to be rare and their clinical significance unclear. For example, other peptidases appear to compensate in dogs with congenital absence of the brush-border enzyme aminopeptidase N.[1] Lactase deficiency also may occur under some conditions but similarly does not appear to be clinically significant.

Congenital disorders of the SI should be considered in young dogs presented with clinical signs of failure to thrive or nonspecific SI signs. Of particular importance is the recognition of breeds that have been identified as having selective cobalamin malabsorption (Table 47.1) so that when a young dog of one of those breeds is presented, the possibility of cobalamin deficiency is quickly considered and tested for, because failure to recognize this disorder could have fatal consequences for the dog. A number of other conditions of the SI are suspected to have a genetic basis given breed associations, but in many cases the predisposing factors are unknown, and the signs of disease are not present from birth. Suspected or known genetic predispositions and, where known, associated mutations will be discussed under these specific disorders.

Chronic enteropathies

Overview

Chronic enteropathy (CE) is a broad term used to define disorders resulting in chronic GI signs of >3 weeks' duration. This term can be applied once other causes of GI signs, including extraintestinal disease, infectious etiologies, and solid neoplasms, have been ruled out or are considered unlikely. Chronic enteropathy is often further classified according to treatment response. The treatment response categories include food-responsive enteropathy (FRE), steroid- or immunosuppressant-responsive enteropathy (SRE/IRE), or, historically, antimicrobial-responsive enteropathy (ARE). It was recently proposed that the category ARE should be updated to microbiota-related modulation-responsive enteropathies (MrMRE).[8] This new term would better reflect the varied therapies that may result in improvement in these types of cases and discourage the use of antimicrobial agents to treat CE. Although these classifications based on treatment response can be useful, the clinical signs typically overlap, and histopathology does not appear to differ between subgroups. In addition, it is important to recognize that this classification system may not reflect the complexity of all cases of CE. It is suspected that most forms of CE involve complex interactions between host genetics, the immune system, and the constituents of the intestinal microenvironment (e.g., dietary antigens and the host microbiota). Thus, some animals may require a combination of therapies to control disease. In fact, some clinicians propose that these categories simply reflect a single disease process of increasing severity considering the prevailing hypothesis behind the etiopathogenesis of CE.[9] Importantly, most dogs with CE will be responsive to food; thus, FRE is the most common type of CE. In one study of 203 dogs with CE, 64% were classified as having FRE, 19.2% as having SRE/IRE, and 16.2% as having ARE.[10]

When sequential treatments with diets and therapies to modulate the microbiota are not successful, histopathological evaluation of intestinal biopsies is typically recommended. When intestinal inflammation has

TABLE 47.1 Canine selective cobalamin malabsorption disorders.

Breed	Clinical features	Genetic mutation
Giant schnauzer	■ Chronic inappetence, failure to thrive, neutropenia with hypersegmentation, anemia with anisocytosis and poikilocytosis, and megaloblastic changes of the bone marrow	*AMN* mutation
Border collie	■ Clinical signs are as typical but may be mild. ■ Onset of clinical signs may not occur until adulthood. ■ Hematologic abnormalities are uncommon.	Exon 53 frameshift mutation in *CUBN*
Chinese shar-pei	■ Appears to largely affect the gastrointestinal tract—diarrhea, vomiting, weight loss	None identified
Beagle	■ Lethargy, anorexia, failure to thrive, diarrhea ■ Degenerative liver disease	Exon 8 frameshift mutation in *CUBN*
Australian shepherd	■ Failure to thrive, inappetence, weakness, nonregenerative anemia, neutropenia	*AMN c.3G>A* mutation
Yorkshire terrier	■ Hypoglycemia, lethargy, seizures	None identified
Komondor	■ Failure to thrive, inappetence, vomiting and/or diarrhea, and weakness, dyshematopoiesis	*CUBN* intron 55 splice donor consensus sequence mutation

AMN, amnionless; *CUBN*, cubulin

been documented histologically in a dog with CE, the term *chronic inflammatory enteropathy* (CIE) can be applied. Although *inflammatory bowel disease* (IBD) is often used synonymously with CIE in veterinary medicine, use of the term IBD requires documentation of inadequate response to appropriately designed and implemented trials (e.g., dietary, microbiota modulating, and anthelmintic) and clinical response to anti-inflammatory or immunosuppressive agents. Thus, the term CIE is considered more inclusive. Additionally, IBD is a human term, and human conditions of IBD are considerably different from conditions in dogs. Thus, use of the terms CE (when intestinal inflammation has not been documented) and CIE (when intestinal inflammation has been documented) is preferred.

Clinical signs in dogs with CE include diarrhea, weight loss, changes in appetite, and vomiting. In some cases clinical signs are chronic and progressive, and in other cases the signs may be intermittent but have been occurring for 3 weeks or longer. Importantly, a significant number of dogs and cats presenting for the evaluation of GI signs lasting ≥3 weeks will be reported to be otherwise stable. In other words, these patients maintain normal appetite, body weight, and energy levels despite ongoing diarrhea and/or vomiting. In other cases, dogs may display alterations in appetite, lethargy, weight and muscle loss, and intractable vomiting and diarrhea.

Types

Food-responsive enteropathy (FRE)

Up to 65% of dogs with CE will be responsive to a diet change alone; therefore, it is the most common type of CE. Studies suggest that dogs with FRE tend to be younger than dogs that require glucocorticoids to control disease and tend to have a lower canine CE clinical activity index score (CCECAI)[8,11] (Table 47.2).

Dogs with CE may respond to specific dietary changes for a variety of reasons, including improved digestibility and nutrient absorption, reduced exposure to dietary antigens, and provision of a beneficial amount and source of dietary fiber, among others. Therefore, there are a number of diet types that may have a beneficial effect in dogs with CE. In fact, published studies have shown benefits for hydrolyzed diets, diets providing a new protein and carbohydrate source (novel), fiber-enriched diets, highly digestible diets, and home-prepared diets (see Chapters 25 and 41). There is little evidence to suggest which diet may be most beneficial in an individual dog with CE; therefore, multiple types of dietary trials ideally should be attempted before it is concluded that the dog will not be responsive to food alone.[12]

TABLE 47.2 Canine chronic enteropathy activity index and classification of cumulative score.

Category	Score
Attitude/activity	0, normal 1, slightly decreased 2, moderately decreased 3, severely decreased
Appetite	0, normal 1, slightly decreased 2, moderately decreased 3, severely decreased
Vomiting frequency	0, normal 1, mild (1×/week) 2, moderate (2–3×/week) 3, severe (>3×/week)
Fecal consistency	0, normal 1, slightly soft feces 2, very soft feces 3, watery diarrhea
Defecation frequency	0, normal 1, slightly increased (2–3×/day) 2, moderately increased (4–5×/day) 3, severely increased (>5×/day)
Weight loss	0, none 1, mild (<5%) 2, moderate (5–10%) 3, severe (>10%)
Serum albumin concentration	0, albumin >2.0 g/dL (20 g/L) 1, albumin 1.5–1.9 g/dL (15–19.9 g/L) 2, albumin 1.2–1.4 g/dL (12–14.9 g/L) 3, albumin <1.2 g/dL (12 g/L)
Ascites and peripheral edema	0, none 1, mild ascites or peripheral edema 2, moderate ascites or peripheral edema 3, severe ascites, pleural effusion, or peripheral edema
Pruritus	0, none 1, occasional episodes of itching 2, regular episodes of itching, not when sleeping 3, dog regularly wakes up because of itching

Classification of cumulative score – Severity of disease (Score)
Insignificant (0–3); Mild (4–5); Moderate (6–8); Severe (9–11); Very severe (≥12)

Gluten-sensitive enteropathy in Irish setters

Gluten-sensitive enteropathy of the Irish setter is an inherited (autosomal recessive) condition of immune-mediated intolerance of gluten, similar to celiac disease in humans. It results in partial villous atrophy and lymphoplasmacytic intestinal inflammation. Clinical signs typical of CE will develop in young to middle-aged Irish setters and will resolve with the feeding of a gluten-free diet.[13]

Paroxysmal gluten-sensitive dyskinesias

Border terriers and Maltese dogs have been described to have a constellation of clinical signs that can resolve with the feeding of a gluten-free diet. The hallmark clinical signs of these disorders include episodic tremors, dystonia, and involuntary movements of limbs and facial muscles (i.e., chorea or ballism), with or without a loss of consciousness. Dogs often also display signs consistent with CE, such as diarrhea, vomiting, borborygmi, and flatulence. The diagnosis of these disorders is based on breed, compatible clinical history, presence of serum anti-canine transglutaminase-2-IgA,[14] and resolution of clinical signs in response to being fed a gluten-free diet.[14,15]

Microbiota-related modulation-responsive enteropathy (MrMRE)

This category of CE includes dogs responsive to therapies that may modulate the gut microbiota. In the past, antimicrobial agents were by far the most common therapy prescribed for this indication, and publications have reported that 15–35% of CE cases were responsive to antimicrobial agents.[9] However, in several of these studies, dogs also were treated with diet and, in some cases, other drugs, which limits interpretation of those results. Additionally, responses were rarely durable, with high rates of relapse reported. In one study evaluating long-term outcomes of 814 dogs with CE, 341 dogs were treated with antibiotics, and only eight of 814 (1%) responded solely to antibiotic therapies long term.[16]

Considering this, concerns that have been raised about the development of antimicrobial resistance and the effects that long-term antimicrobial use can have on an individual dog's microbiome health, it is suggested to use therapies other than antimicrobial agents where possible to modulate the microbiota. Examples of such therapies include prebiotics, probiotics, synbiotics, fiber-enriched and hydrolyzed diets, and fecal microbiota transplantation (FMT) (see Chapters 25–27). The evidence and effectiveness for many of these therapies for the maintenance of long-term clinical remission of CE have not been thoroughly investigated or reported. In one randomized, controlled trial, dogs with CIE were given either FMT or a sterile saline enema in addition to prednisolone and a hydrolyzed diet. CCECAI scores improved significantly in both groups, but there was no difference between the groups.[17] Further investigations are needed. Nonetheless, when these therapies are successful in a dog with CE because of a suspected or confirmed improvement in the microbiota, it can be classified as an MrMRE.

Steroid- or Immunosuppressive responsive enteropathy (SRE/IRE)

Approximately 20–25% of dogs with CE appear to require glucocorticoids (e.g., prednisone, prednisolone, or budesonide) or immunosuppressants (e.g., ciclosporin, chlorambucil, or azathioprine) to control their clinical signs. When dogs respond to these therapies after previous inadequate responses to dietary therapies or therapies to modulate the microbiota, the terms SRE or IRE are applied. Several randomized clinical trials have provided high-quality evidence to support the assertion that glucocorticoids can be effective in dogs with CE.[9]

Diagnostic approach

The approach to a dog with clinical signs of CE first should involve consideration of the patient's signalment, clinical history, and degree of illness. Regard also should be paid to age and breed-related disorders, which may change the diagnostic approach (e.g., exocrine pancreatic insufficiency in German Shepherds and Rough Collies).[18] Clinical history taking should include a careful account of current and previous diets fed and questions aimed at determining whether the problem appears to be small, large, or mixed bowel in origin. A fecal scoring system is useful to establish a baseline and for monitoring (Fig. 47.2).

A thorough physical exam should be performed that includes careful assessment of hydration status, body and muscle condition, and evaluation for the detection of ascites, abdominal pain, or lymphadenopathy (see Chapter 17). A thorough evaluation for evidence of dermatological disease should be performed because the presence of cutaneous signs may support an underlying food sensitivity. Finally, digital rectal examination should be performed in all cases for assessment of intra- or extraluminal, anal sac, or prostatic disease and for assessment of fecal consistency, color, and the presence of blood.

CE remains a diagnosis of exclusion. Historical and recent attempts to develop specific assays for the diagnosis of this disorder have been unsuccessful.[19] An overview of the diagnostic approach to a dog with chronic diarrhea can found in Chapter 12. In brief, the initial diagnostic approach for CE involves the exclusion of systemic causes (e.g., renal, hepatic, or endocrine disease) of GI signs, which typically can be achieved with history, physical exam, complete blood count, chemistry profile, and urinalysis. Depending on the level of clinical suspicion, blood work to exclude pancreatic disease (e.g., canine serum trypsin-like immunoreactivity assay to evaluate for EPI) and testing for endocrine disorders may be indicated. Screening for hypoadrenocorticism is reasonable in all dogs with chronic GI signs. A baseline cortisol concentration ≥55 nmol/L (2 µg/dL) excludes hypoadrenocorticism as the cause of the dog's clinical signs.[20] Baseline cortisol concentrations <55 nmol/L (<2 µg/dL) require an adrenocorticotropic hormone stimulation test be performed to exclude or confirm the diagnosis of hypoadrenocorticism. Helminth infections including those from roundworms, tapeworms, and hookworms can cause chronic diarrhea in dogs. Thus, all dogs should have fecal testing performed (e.g., fecal flotation), including specific testing for *Giardia* spp. Regardless of the result, administration of a broad-spectrum anthelmintic (e.g., fenbendazole) is recommended in patients with clinical signs suggestive of CE.

In dogs with mild illness (i.e., dogs maintaining normal appetite, body weight, and energy levels despite ongoing diarrhea and/or vomiting), it would be reasonable at this juncture to consider therapeutic trials (see below) in lieu of additional diagnostics. Sequential therapeutic trials with dietary therapies and medications to modulate the microbiota are commonly performed in dogs with mild illness before further diagnostics are pursued. For dogs with a clinical suspicion of dysbiosis, the dysbiosis index (DI) is a polymerase chain reaction (PCR)–based quantitative assay that can help assess the dog's microbiome health (see Chapter 20). The DI quantifies the fecal abundance of seven bacterial taxa (including *Peptacetobacter (Clostridium) hiranonis*) and correlates negatively with species richness. In other words, the higher a patient's DI, the lower is the microbial diversity and the worse the dysbiosis. The results of this assay can help to decide whether therapies aimed at mitigating dysbiosis in patients may be successful. It is important to note, however, that patients may benefit from therapies aimed at correcting dysbiosis even if their DI is in the healthy range.

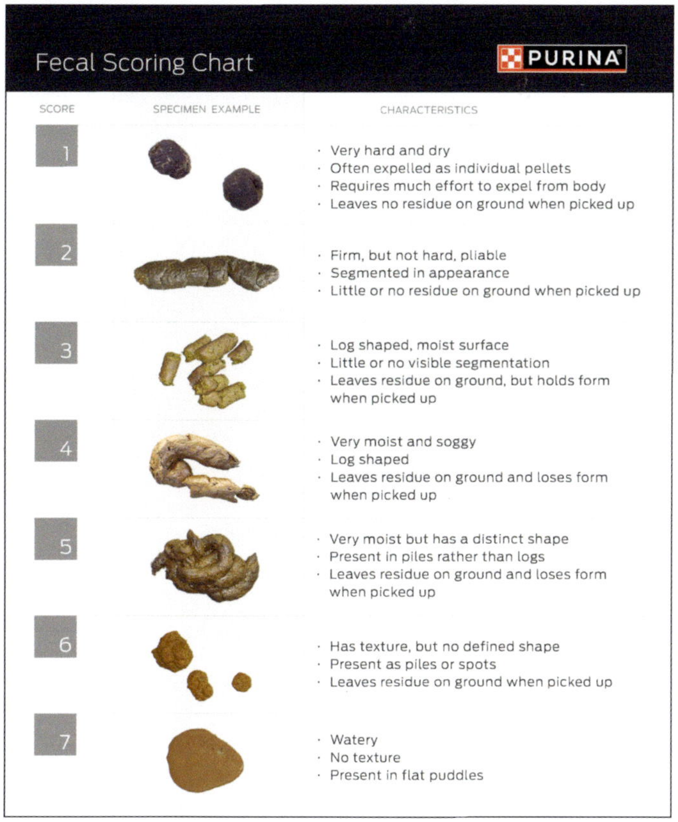

FIG. 47.2 Example of a fecal scoring chart from Nestlé Purina Petcare (with permission).

Dogs with more serious illness (e.g., experiencing lethargy, weight loss, and concerning changes in appetite, such as decreases, increases, or an absence of appetite) deserve more extensive diagnostic investigations such that the cause of their clinical signs is ideally identified and subsequently addressed rapidly. Next steps to be considered in the clinically unwell patient with CE include diagnostic imaging (e.g., abdominal radiographs, abdominal ultrasound, and thoracic radiographs); measurements of serum cobalamin, folate, pancreatic lipase enzyme activity, and trypsin-like immunoreactivity; and specific testing for miscellaneous infectious agents that may be suspected based on signalment, history, comorbid conditions, and geographical location. Which tests are selected and the order in which they are pursued depend on the case and the rank order of the various differential diagnoses. Importantly, low vitamin B_{12} (hypocobalaminemia) may limit the patient's ability to respond to treatment for the underlying disease, so it is important that it be screened for and, if identified, treated appropriately (see Chapter 20). If the results of these tests fail to show a specific cause and thus the diagnosis is considered idiopathic CE, intestinal biopsy with histopathological evaluation can be considered as a next step. Biopsy samples can be collected via endoscopy, laparotomy, or laparoscopy, although endoscopy is generally preferred. Surgical biopsies are only preferred in the presence of focal disease. An advantage of endoscopy is the ability to directly visualize the SI mucosa. Diffuse or segmental gross abnormalities that can be observed include friability, granularity (Fig. 47.3), hyperemia, erosions/ulcerations, and white villous tips (Fig. 47.4), which can support a diagnosis of intestinal lymphangiectasia.[21] Endoscopic scoring systems are available.[22] Because pathology sometimes can differ between the duodenum and ileum, it is recommended to perform both esophagogastroduodenoscopy (upper) and rectocolonoileoscopy (lower) endoscopy. A minimum of six to eight biopsy samples each should be collected from the stomach, duodenum, ileum, and colon. However, if the samples are marginal, 10–15 biopsies per site may be necessary to make a diagnosis. Samples are evaluated for morphological changes including crypt dilation, lacteal dilation, villus blunting, mucosal fibrosis, and inflammatory infiltrates (e.g., lymphoplasmacytic, eosinophilic, neutrophilic, or other). In many cases, a diagnosis can be made with just routine histological evaluation. Occasionally, further characterization of intestinal tissue with immunophenotyping, PCR assay for antigen receptor rearrangement, or fluorescent *in situ* hybridization (FISH) for detection of adherent or invasive bacteria may be necessary (see Chapter 23). It is important to recognize that histopathology of the intestine has limitations, and some chronic SI disorders may lack histopathological abnormalities.[1] Use of the World Small Animal Veterinary Association GI Standardization Group criteria or a recently proposed simplified scoring system may help improve interobserver variation.[23] If advanced diagnostics are declined in dogs that have failed a series of properly implemented dietary trials or in dogs that have serious illness and a refusal to accept the recommended diets, empirical treatment with glucocorticoids can be implemented following counseling of owners of the potential risks (see below).

Therapeutic management

Following exclusion of the various other causes of chronic GI signs in a dog, a diagnosis of CE can be made. At this time, a stepwise approach to therapy is recommended. Because most dogs with CE are considered food responsive, therapeutic diet trials are typically recommended first. Exceptions to this would be in a patient that is severely clinically affected or anorexic and therefore may not accept a dietary change and may benefit from a more aggressive initial approach. A number of dietary strategies are available for patients with CE, and there is not enough robust evidence to suggest that one dietary approach is better than another. In addition, except for a few discrete circumstances, there are no good predictors of which specific diet or dietary approach may be best in an individual patient. Dietary considerations include type of diet (hydrolysate vs limited ingredient vs novel protein vs elemental vs home cooked), fiber content, fat content, and digestibility (see Chapter 25). A diet lower in fat and fiber may be best in patients with signs of gastropathy (e.g., vomiting and gastric distension) to hasten gastric emptying. A fiber-enriched diet may be better for dogs exhibiting mixed or predominately large bowel signs, flatulence, and/or with a strong suspicion of dysbiosis as the primary driver of disease. Previous studies have demonstrated clinical improvement in dogs with CE

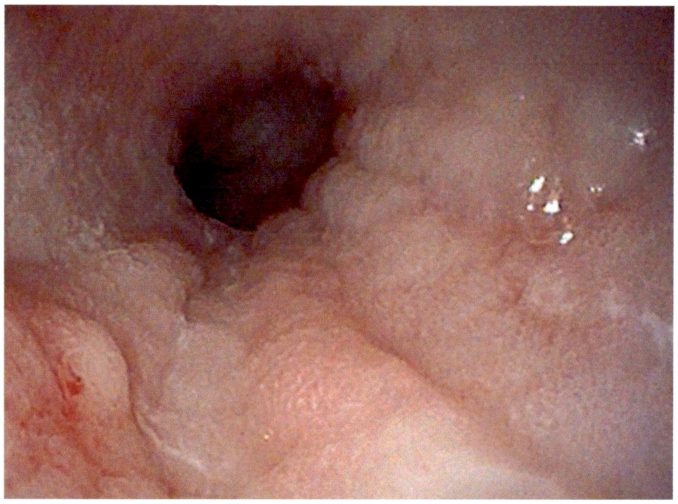

FIG. 47.3 Increased granularity in the duodenum of a 2-year-old female spayed Pembroke Welsh Corgi with moderate lymphoplasmacytic enteritis with fibrosis and villous blunting.

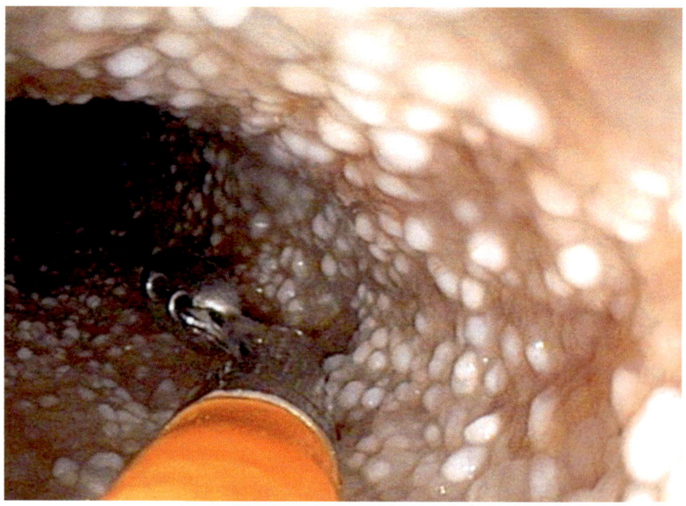

FIG. 47.4 Presence of duodenal pinpoint to coalescing white spots consistent with dilated lacteals in a 5-year-old female spayed Soft Coated Wheaten Terrier with histologically diagnosed marked intestinal lymphangiectasia and the clinical syndrome of protein-losing enteropathy.

in response to hydrolysate, highly digestible, fiber-enriched, single-source protein, and amino acid–based diets; thus, dogs with CE can be responsive to a variety of diets. Home-cooked diets formulated by a board-certified veterinary nutritionist also have been used successfully in cases of CE. Improvement in clinical signs is typically seen within 7–14 days when a food trial is going to be successful.[12]

Although dysbiosis may occur in any patient with CE, it may be a cause or contributing factor particularly in certain breeds (e.g., German Shepherds), in dogs with a history of antimicrobial use, and perhaps in dogs with certain clinical signs (e.g., large bowel diarrhea and flatulence). To screen for dysbiosis, submission of a DI can be considered. Treatments for dysbiosis include switching to a highly digestible diet, antimicrobial agents, prebiotics, probiotics or synbiotics, or FMT. Antimicrobial agents are considered the least desirable of the therapies for dysbiosis because they can cause long-term, severe fecal dysbiosis and tend not to result in durable treatment responses. First-line therapies directed at resolving dysbiosis may include unflavored probiotics or prebiotics such as psyllium fiber.[3]

If dietary therapies and therapies directed toward treatment of dysbiosis are not successful and intestinal inflammation has been documented, treatment with anti-inflammatory or immunosuppressive doses of prednisone or prednisolone, budesonide, or ciclosporin can be instituted depending on the case. Prednisone or prednisolone may be preferred to budesonide in cases where the side effect of increasing appetite may be desired. Budesonide may be preferred to prednisone or prednisolone in cases where the systemic side effects of steroids are best avoided or if a patient has previously been intolerant to prednisone or prednisolone therapy. Ciclosporin may be preferred in cases where it is ideal to avoid steroids altogether (e.g., a patient with concurrent diabetes mellitus) or in a patient that is steroid responsive but the side effects are intolerable at the doses at which a response is seen. In some cases, the use of chlorambucil also may be considered.[24]

In cases where standard treatments have not produced improvements in clinical or biochemical parameters, the disease process may be classified as a nonresponsive enteropathy (NRE). A review of the literature on canine CE found that 5–27% of cases of canine CE are classified as NRE depending on the study.[8] In these cases, there are a number of things to consider. First, it's possible that traditional therapies still may be successful. There is a tendency in clinical practice to consider dogs to be nonresponsive to food after a single trial with one type of diet, and often the validity of these trials cannot be determined. In fact, in one of the earliest studies evaluating the effect of a hydrolyzed protein diet on dogs with chronic GI disease, dogs that responded to the hydrolyzed diet had previously been considered nonresponsive to food based on previous attempts at management with various diets. Thus, some cases of FRE may be misclassified as NRE due to a lack of appropriate or adequate dietary trials. One study described the use of an elemental diet in dogs with chronic inflammatory enteropathies previously refractory to various therapies, including other therapeutic GI diets. The diet was found to be palatable in 95% of the dogs included in the study and induced clinical remission in 73% of dogs (16 of 22 dogs).[25] In summary, regardless of what dietary approach is taken initially, if there is no response, it is recommended to try at least one other approach before classifying the patient as nonresponsive to food. An alternative immunosuppressive approach also could be considered. One study of dogs with steroid-refractory CE found that ciclosporin administered at 5 mg/kg/day induced clinical remission in 12 of 14 dogs.[26]

In patients not obtaining relief from clinical signs despite a multitude of traditional therapies, FMT can be considered, even in patients without documented evidence of dysbiosis (see Chapter 27). *Fecal microbiota transplantation* is defined as the transfer of feces from a healthy donor into the GI tract of a diseased recipient. It can be delivered via enema (**Fig. 47.5**), colonoscopy, duodenoscopy, feeding tube, or administration of oral capsules. In one study, clinical improvement was noted in 24 of 33 dogs with NRE after one to five (the majority received three) FMT treatments delivered via rectal enema.[27] Various procedures for the administration of FMT have been described. Of utmost importance is the careful selection of both recipient and donor. Donor dogs should have no history of significant GI disease, no recent antimicrobial administration, and no signs of systemic disease. Donor feces must be screened for parasites and enteropathogens. Evaluation of the DI is recommended in healthy dogs because it is important that donor feces contain adequate amounts of *Peptacetobacter hiranonis*, crucial for conversion of primary bile acids to secondary bile acids. The most common route for FMT delivery is via rectal enema. To perform this, ~5 g of donor feces per kilogram of recipient body weight is blended in 60 mL of 0.9% NaCl until homogenized. The stool is then administered into the proximal colon via a 12- or 14-inch French red rubber catheter with a 60-mL catheter-tip syringe attached. Typically, the recipient dog does not need to be sedated. It is recommended to restrict food and activity for 4–6 hours after the procedure to avoid a bowel movement in the immediate post-transplantation period. Dogs that experience improvement following FMT typically do so within 2–3 days. However, it is common for them to relapse, and multiple treatments may be necessary.[28]

Dysfunction of bile acid metabolism can occur because of dysbiosis. When bile acid dysmetabolism occurs in patients with CE, it may lead to refractory diarrhea due to decreased production of secondary bile acids and increased electrolyte and water secretion, mucosal permeability, and colonic motility. Dogs with bile acid dysmetabolism are expected to have significantly decreased fecal abundance of the bile acid–converting bacteria, *Peptacetobacter hiranonis*. In these cases, short-term treatment with cholestyramine (0.5–2.0 g per dog PO q12–24h), a bile acid sequestrant, may be beneficial.[27]

Finally, it must be remembered that the etiology of CE is likely multifactorial in most cases. Thus, in cases of NRE, one may need to combine various therapies to see a response rather than simply relying on a single therapy to produce clinical improvement in a patient.

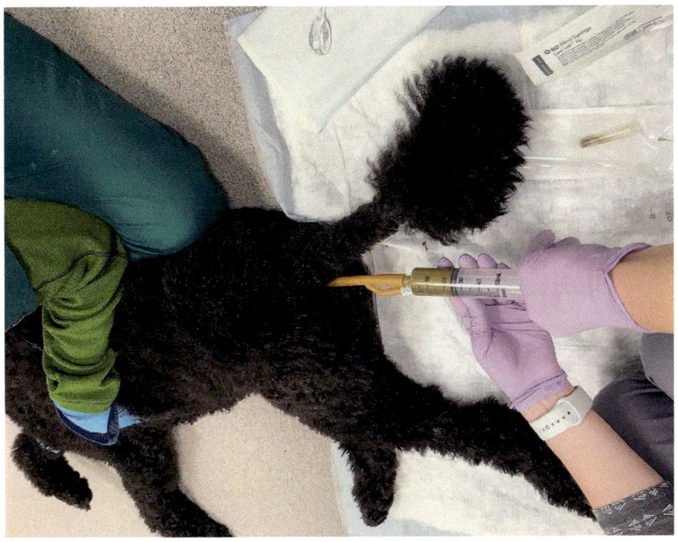

FIG. 47.5 Photograph of a dog receiving a fecal microbial transplant via rectal enema. Photo credit: Jenessa Winston, DVM, PhD, DACVIM (SAIM).

Intestinal lymphatic disorders

Intestinal lymphangiectasia

Intestinal lymphangiectasia (IL) is characterized by intestinal lymphatic vessel dilation with or without lymphangitis, lymphatic obstruction, and lymphatic rupture. Dilated and disordered intestinal lymphatics may subsequently leak lipoprotein-rich lymph, leading to loss of protein and lipid through the intestinal lumen. IL appears to be largely an acquired condition caused by increased hydrostatic or venous pressure. Increased hydrostatic pressure can be a consequence of inflammatory or neoplastic intestinal infiltrates, but, theoretically, increased venous pressure can be secondary to pericardial disease, right-sided heart failure, and portal hypertension. Additionally, several breeds of dogs are consistently reported to have IL (Table 47.3), suggesting that there are perhaps congenital abnormalities of the intestinal lymphatics in some cases or at least a genetic susceptibility to developing abnormalities of the intestinal lymphatic vasculature. However, leakage of lymph into the intestinal wall can recruit inflammatory infiltrates, causing an inflammatory reaction in the intestine, and inflammation can cause obstruction and dilation of lymphatics. Thus, the determination of whether the IL came first or is a secondary finding sometimes can be difficult.[29]

IL is typically diagnosed in dogs with PLE (see below). Most often these dogs are presented for chronic diarrhea with or without weight loss. Endoscopic examination and abdominal ultrasound can increase the suspicion for IL. Endoscopy may reveal white spots[21] (Fig. 47.3) that are thought to represent villi distended by lymph fluid, and in some cases, lymph leakage may be observed. Dogs with IL may have hyperechoic mucosal striations of the SI wall visualized during abdominal ultrasound (Fig. 47.6); the striations may represent dilated lacteals (Video 47.1).[30] However, the definitive diagnosis of IL is via histopathology of the SI, though it is important to recognize that IL can be regional and segmental and can affect the lymphatics not just at the villus but in deeper parts of the intestinal wall. The specific sectioning of the SI and orientation of the tissue sometimes may limit a pathologist's ability to evaluate IL (see Chapter 23). In addition, if IL is confined to the submucosal, muscularis, or serosal layers of the SI or limited to an area not accessible via endoscope (e.g., the jejunum), endoscopic biopsies may not be entirely representative.[29]

A fat-restricted diet is the most critical aspect of the management of IL in dogs. Conventional low-fat diets in dog contain 16–25 g of fat per 1,000 kcal, but some dogs with IL may benefit from diets considered ultra-low-fat at ≤15 g of fat per 1,000 kcal. If dogs have additional diagnoses, such as chronic inflammatory enteropathy (see above), they may have additional dietary requirements. Additional information on nutritional therapy for GI disorders can be found in Chapters 25 and 41. Because IL can lead to lymphangitis and secondary intestinal inflammation, treatment with a glucocorticoid is often indicated. However, it is important to note that there is currently no evidence of an autoimmune pathogenesis of IL in dogs; thus, anti-inflammatory doses (0.5–1 mg/kg PO q24h or divided q12h, not to exceed 60 mg/day) of prednisone or prednisolone are recommended. Dogs with IL also will likely require other therapies common to dogs with other causes of PLE (see below). Importantly, despite being first recognized more than 60 years ago, IL in dogs remains poorly understood and is sometimes challenging to treat.[29] Octreotide (10 µg/kg SC q8-12h) can be considered as a generally safe supplemental therapy for dogs with histologically documented IL failing to respond to appropriate dietary and glucocorticoid therapy, although a direct benefit has not been documented.[31]

TABLE 47.3 Suggested breed predispositions for canine intestinal lymphangiectasia and protein-losing enteropathy.

Breed	Disease
■ Yorkshire Terrier	Lymphangiectasia ± various degrees and types of inflammation ± crypt lesions
■ Shar Pei ■ Maltese ■ Rottweiler ■ Norwegian Lundehund	Lymphangiectasia ± various degrees and types of inflammation
■ Soft Coated Wheaten Terrier	Inflammatory enteritis, lymphangiectasia, lymphangitis
■ Basenji	Immunoproliferative enteropathy (inflammatory infiltrates, hyperglobulinemia, ± gastric hypertrophy)
■ German Shepherd ■ Border Collie ■ Boxer	Chronic enteropathies

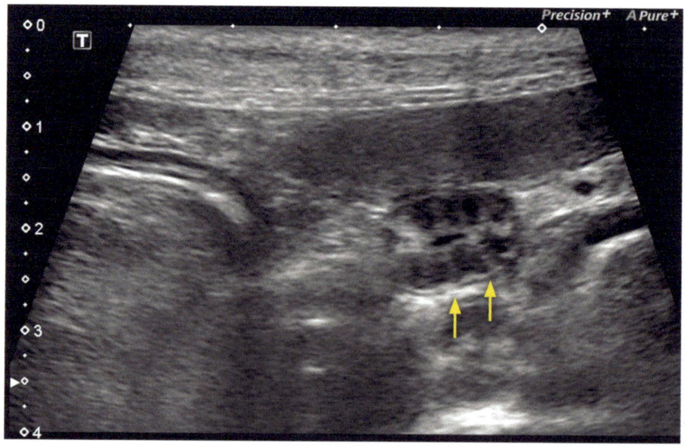

FIG. 47.6 Small intestinal hyperechoic mucosal striations (arrows) in a 3-year-old male castrated Labrador Retriever with moderate intestinal lymphangiectasia and mild lymphoplasmacytic enteritis and the clinical syndrome of protein-losing enteropathy.

Video 47.1

Endoscopic evaluation of the upper gastrointestinal tract in a 5-year-old male castrated American cocker spaniel with protein-losing enteropathy. The video begins at the lower esophageal sphincter and progresses to the gastric antrum, followed by a view of the pyloric sphincter. The endoscope enters through the sphincter into the duodenum. On entering the duodenum, the mucosa appears moderately granular, and multiple white spots suggestive of lacteal dilation are visible. The video completes as the endoscope travels distally through the duodenum.

Lipogranulomatous lymphangitis

Focal intestinal lipogranulomatous lymphangitis is a discrete form of intestinal lymphatic disease in dogs. This disorder is characterized by the documentation of a small intestinal (typically distal jejunal or ileal) mass that may involve the adjacent mesentery. Histological evaluation reveals transmural granulomatous inflammation with marked formation of lipogranulomas predominately involving the muscularis and serosal layers of the SI as well as the adjacent mesentery. Surgical excision of the mass may be curative, but some dogs may have more diffuse IL and require treatment with a fat-restricted diet with or without glucocorticoids postoperatively and long term.[32]

Intestinal lymphatic hypoplasia

Intestinal lymphatic hypoplasia is a human disorder characterized by the presence of significantly fewer or absent intestinal lymphatics with no obvious lymphangiectasia or lymphatic obstruction. It is typically recognized in infancy.

Immunohistochemical labeling of intestinal lymphatics revealed an absence of villous lacteals in three dogs with PLE, and the authors hypothesized that dogs, uncommonly, may be affected by intestinal lymphatic hypoplasia, similar to the human disorder.[33] The significance of this possible disorder in dogs is unclear, but it is possible it is underrecognized because routine immunohistochemical labeling of intestinal lymphatics is not performed in dogs.

TABLE 47.4 Causes of protein-losing enteropathy in dogs.

Diseases that alter intestinal permeability and/or cause mucosal injury	Lymphatic disease

■ Chronic enteropathies
■ Intestinal ulceration
■ Infectious enteropathies
  ■ Fungal (histoplasmosis, pythiosis)
  ■ Parasitic (hookworm, schistosomiasis)
  ■ Viral (parvovirus)
  ■ Bacterial, *rare* (*Campylobacter, Salmonella*)
■ Chronic obstruction of the intestine
  ■ Foreign body
  ■ Intussusception
■ Neoplasia
  ■ Intestinal lymphoma (solitary or diffuse)
  ■ Intestinal adenocarcinoma
■ Intestinal crypt disease (unknown if primary disorder or secondary change)
■ Hypoadrenocorticism (Addison's disease)
	■ Primary lymphangiectasia (suspected genetic predisposition)
	■ Secondary lymphangiectasia:
	  ■ Chronic enteropathies, *common*
	  ■ Intestinal neoplasia, *common*
	  ■ Right heart failure, *suspected* (unconfirmed in veterinary medicine)
	  ■ Constrictive pericarditis, *suspected* (unconfirmed in veterinary medicine)
	  ■ Portal hypertension, *suspected* (unconfirmed in veterinary medicine)
	■ Focal lipogranulomatous lymphangitis

PLE syndrome

Overview and clinical findings

Canine PLE is a life-threatening clinical syndrome characterized by uncompensated protein loss across the intestinal mucosa. There are numerous causes of PLE syndrome in dogs (Table 47.4), but the most common are CIE and IL. Importantly, CIE and IL can occur together in dogs, with one study finding that 76% of dogs with PLE and CIE also had histological evidence of IL.[34]

Although several breed predispositions for PLE have been described (Table 47.3), heritability has not yet been established. Breeds reportedly affected by PLE most frequently over the last 30 years include Yorkshire Terrier, Crossbreed , Border Collie, German Shepherd, Rottweiler, Maltese, Toy Poodle, Dachshund, Shetland Sheepdog, English Springer Spaniel, and Soft Coated Wheaten Terrier. Dogs with PLE are most often presented with a history of chronic relapsing or progressive GI signs (e.g., diarrhea, weight loss, decreased appetite, vomiting) and clinical signs associated with hypoalbuminemia (e.g., ascites, pleural effusions, peripheral edema). Diarrhea, weight loss, and decreased appetite are the most common GI signs reported; vomiting is less common. Overt diarrhea may be absent in 5–10% of cases, but in those cases, the dogs are likely to have other signs consistent with SI disease. Signs associated with hypoalbuminemia include abdominal distension due to ascites, increased respiratory rate, cough, and respiratory difficulty due to pleural effusion and peripheral edema (Fig. 47.7). Uncommon clinical signs include tremors, facial rubbing and/or seizures (secondary to

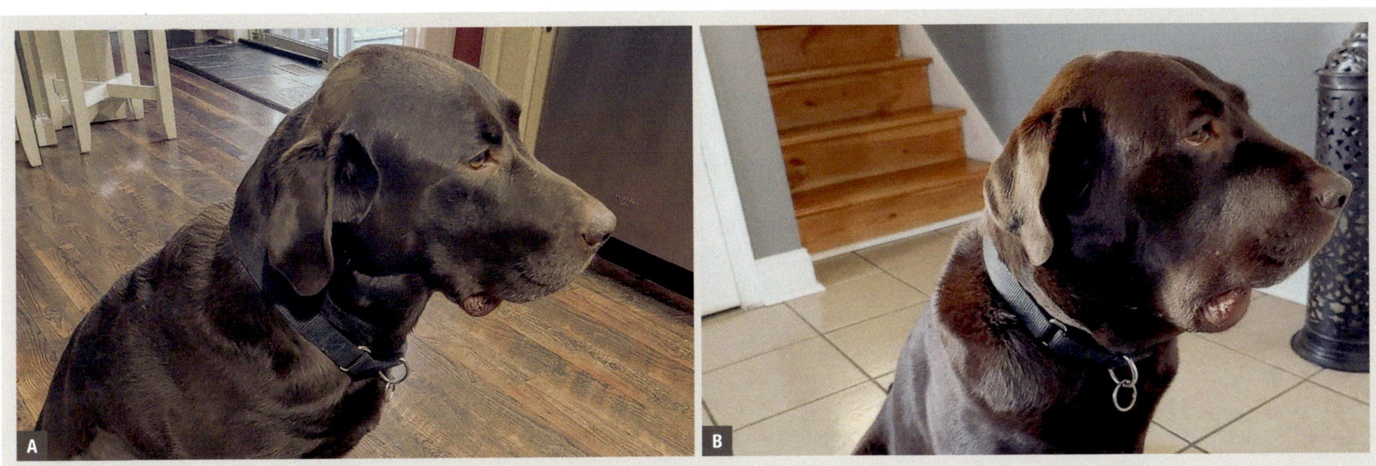

FIG. 47.7 Photographs of a 5-year-old male castrated Labrador Retriever before (A) and after (B) the onset of protein-losing enteropathy. Peripheral edema affecting the lower lip and cervical area secondary to hypoalbuminemia can be observed in the image on the right.

TABLE 47.5 Common biochemical abnormalities in dogs with protein-losing enteropathy.

Complete blood count	Chemistry profile	Other
■ Normochromic, normocytic, non regenerative anemia ■ Lymphopenia ■ Leukocytosis ■ Thrombocytosis	■ Hypoalbuminemia (hallmark finding) ■ Hypo-, normo-, or hyperglobulinemia ■ Hypocholesterolemia ■ Decreased creatinine ■ Increased liver enzyme activity ■ Hypocalcemia ■ Hypomagnesemia	■ Ionized hypocalcemia ■ Hypocobalaminemia (decreased B_{12}) ■ Hypofolatemia (decreased B_9) ■ Increased canine pancreatic lipase immunoreactivity ■ Hypovitaminosis D (decreased vitamin D) ■ Hyperfibrinogenemia

ionized hypocalcemia), signs related to thromboembolic disease (e.g., respiratory, neurological, or musculoskeletal), polyuria/polydipsia, and melena. Physical examination may reveal poor body condition and/or muscle loss due to malnutrition, but findings are variable and range from unremarkable to severe changes. Physical exam also may reveal signs related to the consequences of hypoalbuminemia, including abdominal distension and a palpable fluid wave in a dog with ascites, decreased lung sounds in dogs with pleural effusion, and occasionally detection of peripheral edema. A complete rectal exam should be performed and may reveal thickened/irregular rectal mucosa and diarrheic stool.

Hypoalbuminemia is the hallmark biochemical abnormality in dogs with PLE. Hypoglobulinemia is also commonly observed, but normal or even increased serum globulin concentrations do not exclude PLE. Additional common findings on complete blood count, serum biochemistry, and other analyses can be found in Table 47.5. Viscoelastic testing has demonstrated a hypercoagulable state in dogs with PLE, and thromboelastographic variables associated with hypercoagulability have been correlated with hyperfibrinogenemia and decreased antithrombin activity.[35] However, these findings have not been directly correlated with the development of thromboembolism in dogs with PLE.

Diagnostic approach

The diagnostic approach for dogs with suspected PLE is outlined in Chapter 13. In brief, the approach should first definitively exclude other causes of hypoalbuminemia (especially protein-losing nephropathy and liver insufficiency), then identify the specific cause of PLE, and screen for complications and comorbidities. All dogs should have fecal testing and administration of appropriate anthelmintic therapy prior to pursuing advanced diagnostics. Exclusion of hypoadrenocorticism as the cause of clinical signs and hypoalbuminemia is recommended prior to performing intestinal biopsies. If there is a supportive travel history or any clinical suspicion for histoplasmosis, examination of the fundus, rectal scrape with cytology, and urine antigen testing should be performed (see Chapter 38). Thoracic radiographs can be performed to screen for evidence of fungal disease, metastasis, or pleural effusion. Abdominal radiographs should be performed if ascites is not severe and there is concern for a chronic SI obstruction resulting in hypoalbuminemia. Abdominal ultrasound may be more helpful in excluding focal or extraluminal lesions that may change the diagnostic approach. Additionally, in some cases fine-needle aspiration of masses or abnormal lymph nodes may lead to the ability to make a diagnosis without needing a tissue biopsy. Peritoneal effusion may be observed, and if present, fluid could be collected for analysis. A pure transudate is expected in cases of PLE. Hyperechoic mucosal striations (Fig. 47.6) observed on abdominal ultrasound are supportive of but not specific for the diagnosis of IL.

If at this juncture a cause for the PLE has not been discovered, biopsy with histopathology will be necessary. Biopsy can exclude infectious (e.g., histoplasmosis) or neoplastic (e.g., intestinal lymphoma) causes of PLE. Biopsy also will help to determine whether the dog is affected by CIE, IL, or both and, if both, which process appears to predominate. Surgical exploration for biopsies provides the advantages of identifying focal areas of disease to biopsy and the ability to biopsy all segments of intestine as well as other tissues as indicated (e.g., liver and lymph nodes). However, flexible endoscopy is generally the preferred biopsy method and offers several advantages over surgical biopsies. Advantages for dogs with PLE include less morbidity associated with the procedure, shorter postbiopsy recovery time, ability to directly visualize the mucosa, targeted collection of abnormal tissue, and the ability to sample from several regions of intestinal segments. The visualization of white spots on the mucosa (Fig. 47.4) has been associated with IL. Because pathology can differ between sections of the intestine,[36] it is recommended that both esophagogastroduodenoscopy (upper GI endoscopy) and ileocolonoscopy (lower GI endoscopy) be performed. The quality of endoscopic biopsies can impact the ability to make an accurate diagnosis, and it is important to recognize that pathology can be missed because the jejunum typically cannot be sampled, and it is possible that there may be important lesions deeper in the intestinal wall that endoscopic biopsies will not detect. Additionally, interobserver variation exists in the interpretation of intestinal biopsy samples. Guidelines are available for the interpretation of inflammatory and morphological changes in the GI mucosa of dogs and may help to limit some of the variation.[23] It is important to note that histopathological findings have not been consistently correlated with clinical signs and response to treatment. Some of the responsibility rests with the interpreting clinician to fully review the histopathology report and to use their clinical judgment, particularly if samples are inadequate (see Chapter 23).

The most frequently reported histopathological findings in dogs with PLE include IL (Fig. 47.8), mucosal edema, various types and degrees of

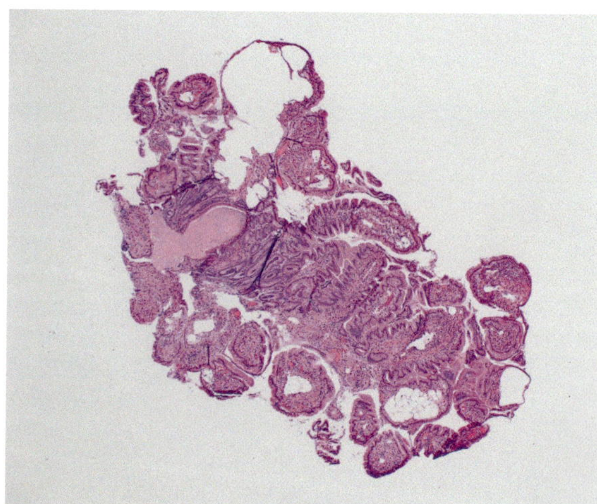

FIG. 47.8 Low-power photomicrograph of marked intestinal lymphangiectasia and moderate lymphoplasmacytic, neutrophilic, and eosinophilic duodenitis in a 5-year-old female spayed soft-coated Wheaten Terrier with protein-losing enteropathy. Image courtesy of Victoria Watson, DVM, PhD, DACVP.

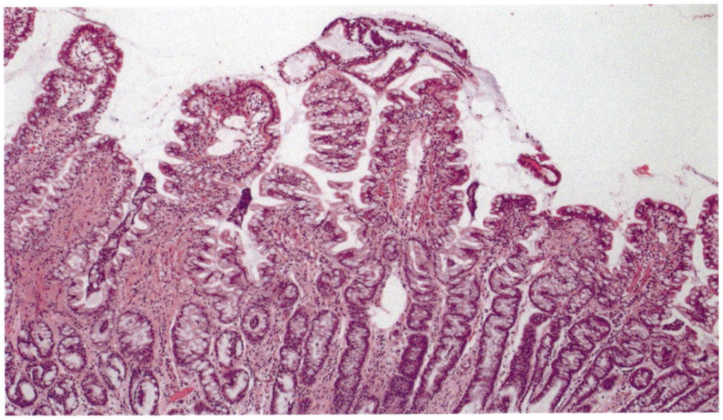

FIG. 47.9 Photomicrograph of mild to moderate lymphoplasmacytic enteritis in a 12-year-old female spayed Airedale Terrier with chronic diarrhea. Image courtesy of Victoria Watson, DVM, PhD, DACVP.

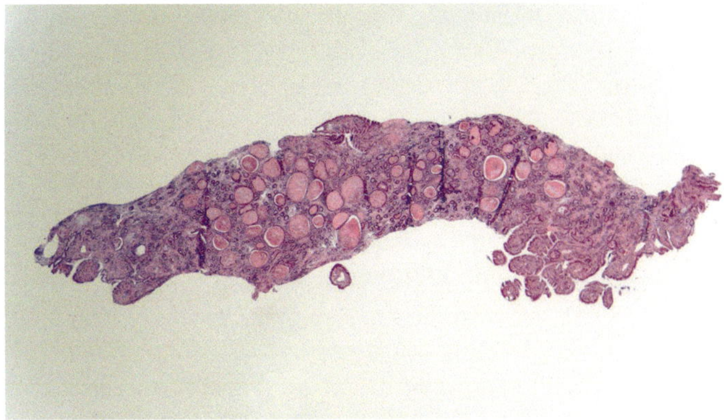

FIG. 47.10 Low-power photomicrograph of markedly dilated crypts with degenerate inflammatory cells intermixed with eosinophilic necrotic debris and mucus in a 6-year-old male castrated small mixbreed dog with protein-losing enteropathy. Image courtesy of Victoria Watson, DVM, PhD, DACVP.

inflammatory infiltrates (Fig. 47.9), and dilated, cystic crypts (Fig. 47.10). IL has been detected in the villus, underlying lamina propria, and submucosa in endoscopic intestinal biopsies.[37] Therefore, it is important for pathologists to evaluate for lymphangiectasia in each of these areas. Immunolabeling of lymphatic endothelial cells may help distinguish dilated lymphatics from mucosal edema. Crypt lesions seem to be especially common in Yorkshire terriers.[38] If concern for bacterial adherence/invasion arises from biopsy evaluation, FISH can be considered to evaluate for bacteria within formalin-fixed tissue. In some cases, immunohistochemistry and PCR for antigen receptor rearrangements may be necessary to help distinguish intestinal lymphoma from inflammatory infiltrates.

Therapeutic management

Treatment of PLE syndrome is specific to the underlying cause/driver of the enteric protein loss. Treatment of CIE and IL is as described earlier, but many dogs with PLE have a combination of CIE and IL, which may complicate therapeutic choices.

Dietary management is the cornerstone of therapy for dogs with PLE. Diet has been shown to be successful as both a monotherapy and a rescue therapy for dogs failing glucocorticoid and immunosuppressive therapies. Dogs with PLE that are responsive to food as a monotherapy are likely to be less unwell, with CCECAI scores of ≤8.[39] In addition, treatment with diet alone has been associated with a positive outcome in several studies. The ideal diet for dogs with PLE is highly digestible with adequate amounts of protein. For dogs with at least moderate IL, the diet should be fat restricted (low fat = 16–25 g of fat per 1,000 kcal; ultralow fat ≤ 15 g of fat per 1,000 kcal). Dogs with CIE as the predominant cause of PLE may benefit from a diet that is hydrolyzed or novel in its protein and carbohydrate sources. Hydrolyzed low-fat diets may be the best choices for dogs with histological evidence of both CIE and IL and in cases where intestinal biopsies have not been performed and thus the underlying etiology is not known. Some dogs with PLE that do not experience improvement in response to traditional extruded and canned-food diets seem to improve clinically in response to a home-cooked (or commercially available fresh-frozen) diet. The reason for this is not fully understood but may involve improved digestibility, the absence of certain ingredients contained in extruded or canned diets, and/or the ability to provide an ultralow fat (≤15 g of fat per 1,000 kcal) and novel protein diet, especially in cases with both CIE and IL. A temporary diet to test responsiveness could be a lean novel protein such as cod or tilapia combined with white rice or pasta and sweet potato in three equal parts by body weight. If the dog is responsive, follow up with a board-certified veterinary nutritionist is ideal for long-term management. Lack of response to one dietary approach or to diet as a monotherapy does not mean that diet will not play an important role in management of the disease. Two separate studies have shown that ~80% of dogs with PLE and incomplete control of disease despite treatment with steroids and other immunosuppressive agents will benefit from a diet change.[40,41] Thus, controlled diets always should be part of the management of dogs with PLE secondary to CIE and IL. Additional information regarding nutritional management of SI conditions can be found in Chapters 25 and 41.

Glucocorticoids are indicated in many cases of PLE for anti-inflammatory and immunosuppressive effects (see Chapter 34). Anti-inflammatory or immunosuppressive doses of prednisone or prednisolone (0.5–2.0 mg/kg PO q24h or divided and administered q12h, not to exceed 60 mg/day) are recommended for dogs with PLE in which CIE appears to be the predominant problem. Dosing of glucocorticoids by body surface area can be considered for large dogs.[42] There is no evidence of an immune pathogenesis for IL; thus, anti-inflammatory doses of prednisone or prednisolone (0.5–1.0 mg/kg PO q24h or divided and administered every 12 hours, not to exceed 60 mg/day) are recommended for dogs with PLE in which IL appears to be the predominant problem. Budesonide (3–7 kg give 1 mg PO q24 h; 7.1–15 kg give 2 mg PO q24 h; 15.1–30 kg give 3 mg PO q24 h; or >30 kg give 3–4 mg PO q24 h) may be considered as an alternative glucocorticoid with a high affinity for intestinal steroid receptors and high first-pass effect. Glucocorticoids worsen the catabolic and hypercoagulable states of dogs with PLE; thus, the lowest effective dose should be used. Therefore, the author does not exceed 1.0 mg/kg/day or 60 mg total per dog in any case of PLE and has not observed a beneficial effect above 1 mg/kg/day. The initial dose should be maintained for 21 days, if tolerated, and then a tapering schedule of 25% at 2- to 3-week intervals can be attempted. Some dogs can be tapered off glucocorticoids successfully and maintained on diet alone. Dogs may benefit from switching to budesonide if they are steroid responsive but experience relapse with tapering or have significant prednisolone or prednisone adverse effects from glucocorticoids at the dosages required to control their disease. If response to glucocorticoids at appropriate doses is inadequate, immunosuppressive medications such as ciclosporin (5 mg/kg PO q24h) can be considered.

Ciclosporin treatment has been shown to be effective in some dogs with steroid-refractory disease.[26] Mycophenolate mofetil is generally not recommended due to its potential to cause significant adverse GI effects. Of note, a recent retrospective study found that treatment with steroids and other immunosuppressive agents offered no survival advantage when compared with steroids alone in dogs with PLE.[43]

Dogs with PLE also may need management of complications and supportive care. Cobalamin deficiency should be treated, and supplementation of folic acid also can be considered in dogs with folate deficiency (see Chapter 20). Clinical ionized hypocalcemia, manifested by muscle twitching or tremors and facial rubbing, should be treated with parenteral 10% calcium gluconate (0.5–1 mL/kg *slowly* IV over 10–30 minutes while monitoring heart rate and, optimally, the electrocardiogram). Oral calcium carbonate (25–50 mg/kg PO q24h or divided PO q12h of elemental calcium) also may be beneficial. Many dogs with ionized hypocalcemia have low 25-hydroxyvitamin D levels and may benefit from treatment with a vitamin D supplement, but the ideal formulation and dose are not known. It is also unknown at this time whether dogs with decreased 25-hydroxyvitamin D and normocalcemia may benefit from vitamin D supplementation. Dogs with PLE are classified as at high risk for thrombosis based on the 2022 Consensus on the Rational Use of Antithrombotics and Thrombolytics in Veterinary Critical Care (CURATIVE) guidelines, and thromboprophylaxis is recommended.[44] Many dogs are administered clopidogrel at 2–3 mg/kg PO q24h, but the use of factor Xa inhibitors (e.g., apixaban or rivaroxaban) for thromboprophylaxis also could be considered.

Draining of abdominal or thoracic effusions is only recommended when the effusion is causing discomfort or respiratory difficulty. The use of diuretics is discouraged. Crystalloid therapy should be judicious due to hypoproteinemia. The volume of plasma needed to increase a patient's albumin concentration is substantial and typically not practical. Colloids, such as hydroxyethyl starches, are most useful for improving edema (see Chapter 24). Human albumin is not recommended for dogs due to the risk of fatal anaphylaxis. A canine albumin product may be available and is anecdotally effective in dogs with PLE. Finally, dogs with PLE often can benefit from other supportive care, such as medications to reduce vomiting and nausea (e.g., maropitant 2 mg/kg PO q24h).

Some dogs with PLE have absent to minimal improvement in response to immunosuppressive doses of steroids and second-line immunosuppressive agents. In these cases, the author recommends tapering these medications and focusing on adjusting the diet (ideally with the consultation of a board-certified veterinary nutritionist), treating deficiencies, and preventing complications. Some dogs with refractory PLE caused by IL may improve in response to octreotide (10 μg/kg SC q8–12h).[31] This medication appears to be generally safe, but its efficacy in the treatment of IL is unknown.

If a histological diagnosis of the cause of PLE is not obtained due to patient or client factors, other causes of hypoalbuminemia should be excluded definitively. Subsequently, every effort should be made to ensure that infectious, mechanical, and neoplastic causes of PLE are unlikely. In such cases, treatment should be approached as if both IL and CIE are present, with consideration of the best approach to manage both conditions concurrently.

Disease-associated death occurred in 54.2% of 445 cases of canine PLE.[4] Improving our understanding of the heterogeneous nature of this disease and the need for individualized therapy may be leading to improvements in outcomes. Despite the guarded prognosis, some dogs with PLE have excellent responses to treatment. It is important to note that even in patients that respond initially, relapse is always possible, and treatment is often lifelong.

Motility disorders

Overview

Inhibition of normal propulsive activity of the intestine due to functional causes is known as *ileus*. Before diagnosing ileus, mechanical obstruction of the SI needs to be excluded. In dogs, ileus most often occurs because of another condition or process. Some of the most common causes of ileus are pancreatitis, parvovirus enteritis, peritonitis, hypokalemia, and hypothyroidism. In these cases, treatment of the underlying process will help to resolve the ileus, but nonspecific therapies to improve intestinal motility also may be necessary. Abdominal surgery and opioid administration are common iatrogenic causes of ileus.[1] Dysautonomia, intestinal pseudo-obstruction, and IBS-like syndromes are uncommon causes of ileus in dogs. Prokinetic agents including 5-HT_4 receptor antagonists (e.g., cisapride), dopaminergic antagonists (e.g., metoclopramide), and, less commonly, motilin-like drugs or acetylcholinesterase inhibitors can be beneficial. Further information on these medications is available in Chapters 31 and 43. Providing nutritional support to dogs with ileus is recommended.

Dysautonomia

Dysautonomia is a generalized autonomic neuropathy characterized by gastric and SI dilation and hypomotility, urinary bladder distension, bradycardia unresponsive to atropine, pupillary dysfunction, and reduced tear dysfunction, among other signs. Megaesophagus is common in cats with dysautonomia but uncommon in canine dysautonomia because of the predominance of striated muscle. The etiology of dysautonomia is unclear, but neurotoxins and xenobiotics have been suspected as the cause. In cats and horses, but not dogs, a possible association with *Clostridium botulinum* neurotoxin has been described. Dysautonomia is typically diagnosed based on history and physical examination findings. The prognosis is generally considered poor, with one retrospective review reporting survival in 32% of dogs. Notably, some dogs survived >2 years, so some long-term survival is possible.[45]

Intestinal pseudo-obstruction

Intestinal pseudo-obstruction describes a variety of conditions that cause chronic, marked intestinal dilation and dysmotility. These conditions include disorders of the enteric smooth muscle (i.e., myopathies) and the enteric nervous system (i.e., neuropathies). Intestinal pseudo-obstruction can occur secondary to other disorders but most often occurs without obvious explanation.

Dogs with intestinal pseudo-obstruction are often presented due to abdominal distension, abdominal discomfort, excessive belching and/or flatulence, and diarrhea. Abdominal radiographs will reveal marked intestinal dilation with no evidence of manual obstruction (Fig. 47.11). Other causes of ileus as described earlier should be considered and excluded. To evaluate for intestinal myopathies or neuropathies, full-thickness biopsies of the intestine are needed. Histological lesions in dogs with chronic intestinal pseudo-obstruction include intestinal leiomyositis, mesenteric plexus vacuolar degeneration, atrophy and fibrosis of the tunica muscularis, and reduced expression of alpha–smooth muscle actin in the tunica muscularis. The prognosis is generally considered guarded to grave in most cases, but long-term survival has been reported. In at least one case, immunosuppressive doses of glucocorticoids appeared to be beneficial.[46]

IBS-like syndromes

Humans with IBS have recurrent abdominal pain, abdominal bloating, and colonic dysmotility/changes in bowel habits with no histopathological

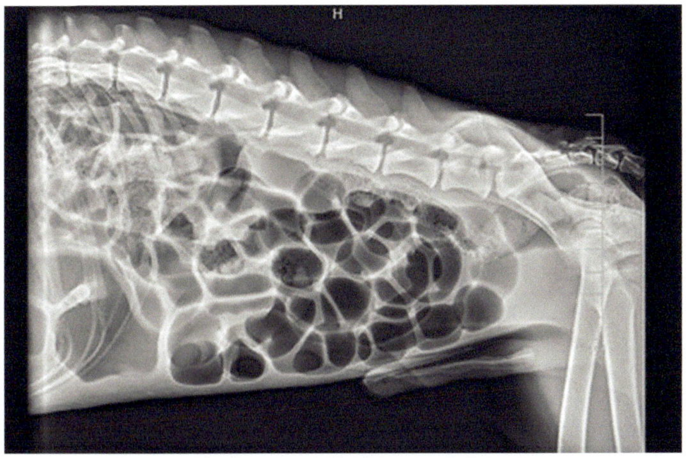

FIG. 47.11 Left lateral abdominal radiograph showing diffuse, severe gas distension of the gastrointestinal tract in a 1-year-old male Gordon setter with suspected intestinal pseudo-obstruction.

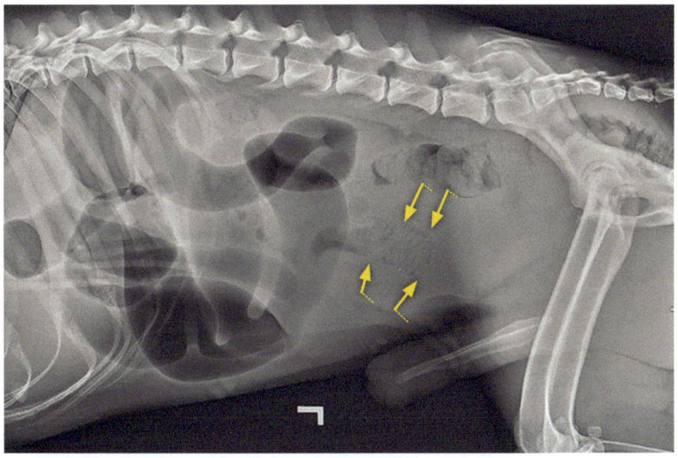

FIG. 47.12 Severe small intestinal dilation/mechanical obstruction secondary to a small intestinal foreign body (arrows) in a 3-year-old male mixed-breed dog with a >1 week history of vomiting and poor appetite. Laparotomy confirmed a midjejunal corn cob foreign body.

evidence of intestinal disease. Altered gut motility and stress and psychological abnormalities are suspected to play a role in this condition, but the etiopathogenesis is unclear.

Some dogs may have a similar syndrome defined primarily by recurrent abdominal distension/bloating and pain and in some cases accompanied by vomiting, diarrhea, and/or constipation. These dogs also may have an absence of intestinal histopathological abnormalities. It is suspected that both anxiety and stress (psychological and physical) may play a role in this condition, and strategies to mitigate these should be attempted, if identified. Additionally, feeding a highly digestible low-fat food may be beneficial. Low- or high-fiber diets also may be helpful on a case-by-case basis. Anti-inflammatory or immunosuppressive therapies do not appear to benefit these patients.[47]

Surgical disorders of the alimentary tract

SI obstruction

Although SI obstructions are commonly acute, it is important to recognize that they also can be chronic. Chronic obstructions are often partial, wherein some nutrients can still pass by the site of obstruction. Obstructions can be the result of intraluminal (most common), extraluminal, or intramural lesions. They are most often caused by foreign objects but also can be caused by intestinal neoplasia, granulomas, hematomas, strictures, intussusceptions, and parasites. Young and large-breed dogs are overrepresented in most case series of foreign-body obstructions, and in one review of 174 cases, latex nipples, plastic and rubber balls, stones, and strings were the most common foreign bodies documented causing obstruction.[48] Clinical signs are highly varied, depending on the degree and site of obstruction and whether perforation, peritonitis, and/or sepsis is present. However, the most common clinical signs are vomiting, abdominal pain, anorexia, and lethargy/depression. Chronic partial obstructions also may result in diarrhea. The most important diagnostic tool in identifying SI obstructions in dogs is plain abdominal radiographs (Fig. 47.12). Pathological dilation of an intestinal loop is defined by a serosal-to-serosal width of the small bowel that exceeds 1.6 times the height of the body of L_5 at its narrowest point (see Table 21.1). Chronic partial small obstructions may cause accumulation of insoluble granular material in the SI, known as the *gravel sign*. If perforation has occurred, peritoneal free gas may be observed and is best visualized dorsally and outlining the diaphragm craniodorsal to the liver margin. Although plain abdominal radiographs will identify most SI obstructions, contrast radiography and/or abdominal ultrasound may be necessary in some cases. The most common laboratory findings in dogs with SI obstructions include hypochloremia, metabolic alkalosis, hyperlactatemia, hypokalemia, and hyponatremia.[48]

The prognosis following surgical correction is often good but will depend on whether perforation with or without peritonitis has occurred, the viability of the intestine, and the cause of the obstruction. For simple foreign-body obstructions, reported survival rates are between 83 and 99%.[1]

SI strangulation and volvulus

Rarely, loops of SI can become incarcerated in tears in the mesentery or in hernias (umbilical or inguinal) resulting in strangulation of the bowel. Adhesions and intraabdominal lipomas also can rarely entrap portions of small bowel resulting in strangulation. Strangulation of the small bowel can result in intestinal ischemia, obstruction, and perforation. Surgery is the treatment of choice, and reperfusion injury is a possible postoperative complication. Intestinal volvulus is an uncommon disorder where the intestines rotate around the root of the mesentery. Ischemia of the distal duodenum, jejunum, ileum, cecum, and ascending and proximal colon occur due to occlusion of the cranial mesenteric artery. This widespread ischemia can quickly result in bowel necrosis, leading to shock and, if not addressed quickly, death.

Dogs with bowel strangulation or intestinal volvulus often present with abdominal pain and weakness and may display vomiting and diarrhea. German shepherds are the breed most reported to develop intestinal volvulus, but it also has been reported to occur in Labrador Retrievers, Great Danes, Neapolitan Mastiffs, and Bloodhounds among others.[49] Dogs with intestinal volvulus are typically severely clinically affected and often will be presented with a distended abdomen and signs of shock, that is, pale mucous membranes, tachycardia, bounding pulses, and hypotension. Abdominal radiographs are the diagnostic test of choice and typically will reveal marked, diffuse distension of the SI (Fig. 47.13). Surgery to correct the volvulus is necessary, but the mortality rate is typically very high. One previous report suggested that prompt surgical intervention may limit mortality.[49]

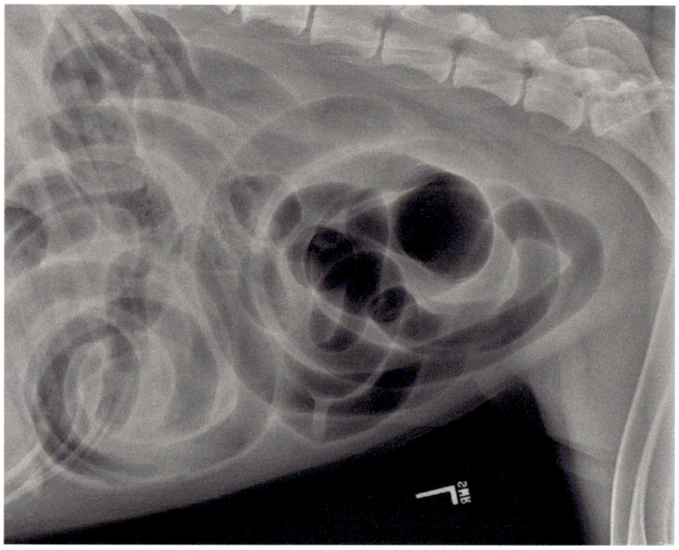

FIG. 47.13 Lateral caudal abdominal radiograph revealing severe small intestinal dilation with characteristic spiraled appearance and suspected cecal displacement in a 5 year-old female spayed German Shepherd with a surgically confirmed mesenteric volvulus.

SI perforation

The most common causes of intestinal perforation and subsequent peritonitis are NSAID administration and ingestion of foreign materials. Foreign bodies most likely to cause perforation are sharp, nondigestible objects such as needles and cocktail sticks. Perforation also can occur if the diagnosis of an SI foreign body is delayed. Other causes of intestinal perforation include neoplastic masses, granulomas, and bowel ischemia.

Short bowel syndrome

Short bowel syndrome (SBS) is characterized by nutrient malabsorption and protein–calorie malnutrition and develops secondary to surgical resection of more than two thirds of the small bowel. Surgical resections of this degree are sometimes necessary due to multiple intestinal perforations (e.g., caused by linear foreign bodies) or when there are severe adhesions. Although some dogs can tolerate resection of large amounts of the SI with minimal effects, others will experience severe clinical disease. Resection of the ileocecocolic valve can create significant problems for several reasons. Resection of the valve can result in loss of regulation of reflux between the colon and ileum. This may result in ileal colonization with colonic bacteria, which can contribute to bile acid dysmetabolism. Additionally, if the terminal ileum is resected along with the valve, bile salt and cobalamin malabsorption may also occur.[50]

Dogs with SBS develop weight loss and diarrhea secondary to malabsorption. Multiple small meals of a highly digestible and fat- and fiber-restricted diet may help limit diarrhea. The use of proton pump inhibitors is generally recommended to reduce gastric acidity. If the ileum has been resected, supplementation of cobalamin is recommended, and supplementation of fat-soluble vitamins also may be necessary. Bile salt malabsorption also can occur in dogs that have had ileal resections, and in these cases, administration of the bile salt–binding resin cholestyramine may be helpful. Loperamide and octreotide also can be considered in dogs failing to respond to the above-mentioned therapies. In some cases, dogs with SBS can undergo adaptive hyperplasia of their remaining small bowel, leading to subsequent clinical improvement with time.[51]

Solid neoplasms of the small intestine

Overview

Although a number of neoplasms can involve the SI, adenocarcinomas, smooth muscle tumors (e.g., leiomyoma, leiomyosarcoma, and GI stromal tumors [GISTs]), and intestinal lymphoma (see Chapter 42) are most common in dogs. Less common tumors of the SI include neuroendocrine tumors, fibrosarcoma, and carcinoids, among others. Clinical signs are similar to other causes of SI disease, but, importantly, intestinal tumors also may result in obstruction or significant bleeding. Most are suspected based on abdominal ultrasound findings, but cytological or histological evaluation of the tissue is necessary for a definitive diagnosis.[1]

Intestinal adenoma and adenocarcinoma

Intestinal adenomas and adenocarcinomas are found more commonly in the large intestine than in the SI in dogs. When they do affect the SI, they tend to be found in the duodenum. Adenomas are typically polypoid, whereas adenocarcinomas typically grow as plaques or annular stenotic lesions and are locally invasive. Adenocarcinomas can extend into the surrounding serosa and mesentery and can metastasize to local lymph nodes, the peritoneal cavity (carcinomatosis), or to other regions of the body via hematogenous metastasis.

The mean age of dogs diagnosed with intestinal adenocarcinoma is 9 years.[52] Common clinical signs include weight loss, lethargy, changes in appetite (usually hyporexia or anorexia), vomiting, and diarrhea. Some dogs will be presented with clinical signs suggestive of partial or complete intestinal obstruction with evidence of peritonitis if rupture has occurred. Adenocarcinomas also may cause mucosal erosion and GI bleeding, resulting in melena and pallor. In these cases, a regenerative or nonregenerative (due to chronic bleeding and development of iron deficiency) anemia is often identified on complete blood count. Abdominal ultrasound is usually adequate to identify the mass lesion (Fig. 47.14), and an ultrasound-guided fine-needle aspiration of the mass with cytological analysis may be able to provide a definitive diagnosis. If not, surgical biopsies may be necessary. The treatment of choice for adenoma or adenocarcinoma of the SI is surgical resection. Median

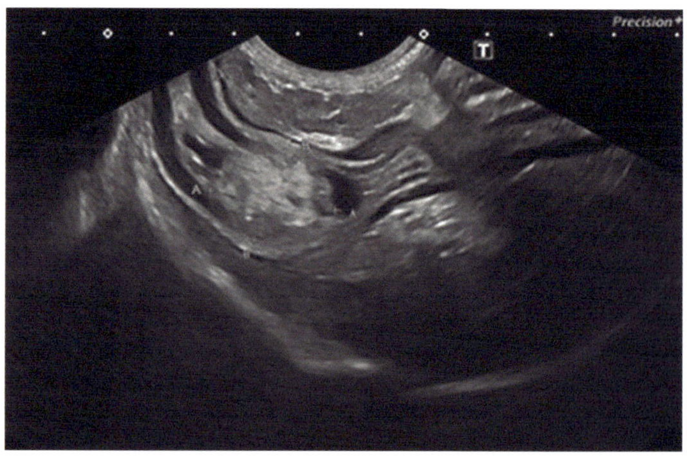

FIG. 47.14 Ultrasound still image of a small intestinal mass at the pyloroduodenal junction in a 15-year-old male castrated beagle. Fine-needle aspirate of the mass was suspicious for intestinal adenocarcinoma.

postoperative survival times for dogs with intestinal adenocarcinoma and no evidence of metastatic spread at the time of surgery is 15 months. If metastasis has already occurred, the median survival time is 3 months. In a recent retrospective review of dogs undergoing surgical treatment for intestinal adenocarcinoma, those aged <8 years had longer survival times compared with those aged ≥8 years, and lymph node metastasis was not associated with survival time.[52]

Smooth muscle and stromal cell tumors

Smooth muscle tumors of the canine SI, including leiomyoma and leiomyosarcoma, are rare. They are typically located on the antimesenteric border of the intestine and are found most commonly in the jejunum or cecum. Leiomyosarcomas have low potential for metastatic spread. GISTs that arise from the interstitial cells of Cajal are similarly rare and also have low potential for metastatic spread.

The clinical signs associated with smooth muscle and stromal cell tumors are like those of other solid intestinal neoplasms. A unique clinical manifestation of smooth muscle tumors is paraneoplastic hypoglycemia, which can result from tumor production of insulin-like growth factor 2 peptide. Leiomyosarcomas also can cause erythrocytosis due to amplification of an erythropoietin-like molecule. Smooth muscle tumors and GISTs are typically identified by abdominal ultrasound. Histologically, leiomyomas and leiomyosarcomas may be difficult to distinguish from one another but can be distinguished from GISTs with immunohistochemical labeling. Surgical resection is the treatment of choice for all tumors. Most GISTs express a transmembrane receptor with a tyrosine kinase component known as c-kit (CD117), whereas smooth muscle tumors will be c-kit negative.[53]

Surgical resection is the treatment of choice for intestinal smooth muscle tumors and GISTs. The prognosis is excellent following surgical removal of leiomyomas and good for leiomyosarcomas, with median survival times of 21 months reported for dogs that have had complete surgical resection of a leiomyosarcoma.[54] Survival times are longer for dogs with surgically resected cecal versus SI GISTs, but good overall with a median survival time of 18 months postoperatively.[55] Dogs with surgically resected GISTs may benefit from adjunctive tyrosine kinase inhibitors.[56] Tyrosine kinase inhibitors also may be beneficial for dogs with unresectable disease.

Miscellaneous solid intestinal neoplasms

Hamartomatous polyps, fibrosarcoma, osteosarcoma, schwannoma, hemangiosarcoma, and carcinoid tumors can affect the SI in dogs but are all very uncommon. These tumors are locally invasive, and clinical signs associated with these tumors are similar to those of other intestinal tumors. Extramedullary plasmacytomas rarely occur in the SI and can be associated with the presence of a monoclonal gammopathy.[1]

Diffuse, infiltrative tumors of the alimentary tract

Alimentary lymphoma typically infiltrates the whole SI and can cause PLE syndrome (see Chapter 42). Malignant histiocytic infiltration of the SI is very rare and not amenable to any treatment.

KEY POINTS

- Clinical manifestations of chronic disease of the small intestine (SI) include diarrhea and weight loss due to malabsorption.
- Dysbiosis and related bile acid dysmetabolism are generally considered to be consequences of SI disease, but in some cases it is theorized that intestinal dysbiosis may be the initiator of SI disease.
- Alterations in motility commonly occur secondary to chronic SI disease. When a dog has a primary motility disorder, treatment can be more challenging.
- Specific chronic SI diseases include anatomical congenital abnormalities, chronic enteropathies, intestinal lymphatic disorders, motility disorders, surgical disorders, and solid neoplasms.
- Reported congenital abnormalities include random duplications of SI segments, blind-ended intestinal diverticula, arteriovenous fistulae of the SI, nonrotation of the midgut during embryonic development, intestinal stenosis, intestinal atresia (i.e., agenesis of a segment of intestine), and short bowel syndrome.
- Chronic enteropathies are often classified according to treatment response. The treatment response categories include food-responsive enteropathy, steroid- or immunosuppressant-responsive enteropathy, and, microbiota-related modulation-responsive enteropathy. Clinical signs in dogs with chronic enteropathy include diarrhea, weight loss, changes in appetite, and vomiting. Following exclusion of the various other causes of chronic gastrointestinal signs in a dog, a diagnosis of chronic enteropathy can be made. At this time, a stepwise approach to therapy is recommended.
- Intestinal lymphatic disorders include intestinal lymphangiectasia, lipogranulomatous lymphangitis, and intestinal lymphatic hypoplasia, and can cause protein-losing enteropathy (PLE).
- There are numerous causes of PLE syndrome in dogs. The diagnostic approach should first definitively exclude other causes of hypoalbuminemia (especially protein-losing nephropathy and liver insufficiency), then identify the specific cause of protein-losing enteropathy, and screen for complications and comorbidities.
- Motility disorders include dysautonomia, intestinal pseudo-obstruction, and irritable bowel syndrome–like disorders. Treatment involves addressing the underlying process, but nonspecific therapies to improve intestinal motility also may be necessary.
- Surgical disorders include SI obstruction, SI strangulation and volvulus, SI perforation, and short bowel syndrome. Surgery is often the treatment of choice.
- Solid neoplasms of the SI include adenomas and adenocarcinomas, smooth muscle and stromal cell tumors, and miscellaneous other solid neoplasms. Clinical signs are similar to other causes of SI disease, but intestinal tumors also may result in obstruction or significant bleeding. Most are suspected based on abdominal ultrasound findings, but cytological or histological evaluation of the tissue is necessary for a definitive diagnosis. Treatment is most often surgical.

References

1. Jablonski SA, Cridge H. Diseases of the small intestine. In: Ettinger SJ, Feldman EC, Cote E (eds.). *Ettinger's Textbook of Veterinary Internal Medicine*. 9th ed. Elsevier; 2024. pp. 1683–1728.
2. Kather S, Grützner N, Kook PH, et al. Review of cobalamin status and disorders of cobalamin metabolism in dogs. *J Vet Intern Med*. 34(1):13–28, 2020.
3. Suchodolski JS. Diagnosis and interpretation of intestinal dysbiosis in dogs and cats. *Vet J*. 215:30–37, 2016.
4. Craven MD, Washabau RJ. Comparative pathophysiology and management of protein-losing enteropathy. *J Vet Intern Med*. 33(2):383–402, 2019.
5. Guilford W, Center S, Strombeck D. *Small Animal Gastroenterology*. 3rd ed. Saunders; 1996.
6. Kook PH, Drögemüller M, Leeb T, et al. Degenerative liver disease in young beagles with hereditary cobalamin malabsorption because of a mutation in the cubilin gene. *J Vet Intern Med*. 28(2):666–671, 2014.
7. Fyfe JC, Giger U, Hall CA, et al. Inherited selective intestinal cobalamin malabsorption and cobalamin deficiency in dogs. *Pediatr Res*. 29(1):24–31, 1991.
8. Dupouy-Manescau N, Méric T, Sénécat O, et al. Updating the classification of chronic inflammatory enteropathies in dogs. *Animals (Basel)*. 14(5):681, 2024.
9. Makielski K, Cullen J, O'Connor A, Jergens AE. Narrative review of therapies for chronic enteropathies in dogs and cats. *J Vet Intern Med*. 33(1):11–22, 2019.
10. Allenspach K, Culverwell C, Chan D. Long-term outcome in dogs with chronic enteropathies: 203 cases. *Vet Rec*. 178(15):368, 2016.
11. Allenspach K, Wieland B, Gröne A, Gaschen F. Chronic enteropathies in dogs: evaluation of risk factors for negative outcome. *J Vet Intern Med*. 21(4):700–708, 2007.
12. Tolbert MK, Murphy M, Gaylord L, Witzel-Rollins A. Dietary management of chronic enteropathy in dogs. *J Small Anim Pract*. 63(6):425–434, 2022.
13. Hall EJ, Batt RM. Dietary modulation of gluten sensitivity in a naturally occurring enteropathy of Irish setter dogs. *Gut*. 33(2):198–205, 1992.
14. Lowrie M, Hadjivassiliou M, Sanders DS, Garden OA. A presumptive case of gluten sensitivity in a border terrier: a multisystem disorder? *Vet Rec*. 179(22):573, 2016.
15. Polidoro D, Van Ham L, Santens P, et al. Phenotypic characterization of paroxysmal dyskinesia in Maltese dogs. *J Vet Intern Med*. 34(4):1541–1546, 2020.
16. Holmberg J, Pelander L, Ljungvall I, et al. Chronic enteropathy in dogs—epidemiologic aspects and clinical characteristics of dogs presenting at two Swedish animal hospitals. *Animals (Basel)*. 12(12):1507, 2022.
17. Collier AJ, Gomez DE, Monteith G, et al. Investigating fecal microbial transplant as a novel therapy in dogs with inflammatory bowel disease: a preliminary study. *PLoS One*. 17(10):e0276295, 2022.
18. Cridge H, Williams DA, Barko PC. Exocrine pancreatic insufficiency in dogs and cats. *J Am Vet Med Assoc*. 262(2):246–255, 2024.
19. Langlois DK, Pritchard JC, Tolbert MK, et al. Clinical utility of an immunoglobulin A–based serological panel for the diagnosis of chronic enteropathy in dogs. *J Vet Intern Med*. 37(2):446–454, 2023.
20. Gold AJ, Langlois DK, Refsal KR. Evaluation of basal serum or plasma cortisol concentrations for the diagnosis of hypoadrenocorticism in dogs. *J Vet Intern Med*. 30(6):1798–1805, 2016.
21. García-Sancho M, Sainz A, Villaescusa A, et al. White spots on the mucosal surface of the duodenum in dogs with lymphocytic plasmacytic enteritis. *J Vet Sci*. 12(2):165–169, 2011.
22. Slovak JE, Wang C, Sun Y, et al. Development and validation of an endoscopic activity score for canine inflammatory bowel disease. *Vet J*. 203(3):290–295, 2015.
23. Washabau RJ, Day MJ, Willard MD, et al. Endoscopic, biopsy, and histopathologic guidelines for the evaluation of gastrointestinal inflammation in companion animals. *J Vet Intern Med*. 24(1):10–26, 2010.
24. Dandrieux JRS, Noble PJM, Scase TJ, et al. Comparison of a chlorambucil-prednisolone combination with an azathioprine-prednisolone combination for treatment of chronic enteropathy with concurrent protein-losing enteropathy in dogs: 27 cases (2007–2010). *J Am Vet Med Assoc*. 242(12):1705–1714, 2013.
25. Manchester AC, Dow S, Chow L, et al. Efficacy of an elemental diet in achieving clinical remission in dogs with chronic enteropathy. *J Vet Intern Med*. 37(6):2322–2333, 2023.
26. Allenspach K, Rüfenacht S, Sauter S, et al. Pharmacokinetics and clinical efficacy of cyclosporine treatment of dogs with steroid-refractory inflammatory bowel disease. *J Vet Intern Med*. 20(2):239–244, 2006.
27. Toresson L, Spillmann T, Pilla R, et al. Clinical effects of faecal microbiota transplantation as adjunctive therapy in dogs with chronic enteropathies—a retrospective case series of 41 dogs. *Vet Sci*. 10(4):271, 2023.
28. Chaitman J, Gaschen F. Fecal microbiota transplantation in dogs. *Vet Clin North Am Small Anim Pract*. 51(1):219–233, 2021.
29. Jablonski SA. Pathophysiology, diagnosis, and management of canine intestinal lymphangiectasia: a comparative review. *Animals (Basel)*. 12(20):2791, 2022.
30. Sutherland-Smith J, Penninck DG, Keating JH, Webster CRL. Ultrasonographic intestinal hyperechoic mucosal striations in dogs are associated with lacteal dilation. *Vet Radiol Ultrasound*. 48(1):51–57, 2007.
31. Jablonski SA, Mazepa ASW, Tolbert MK. Use of octreotide for the treatment of protein-losing enteropathy in dogs: retrospective study of 18 cases. *J Vet Intern Med*. 38(1):145–151, 2024.
32. Watson VE, Hobday MM, Durham AC. Focal intestinal lipogranulomatous lymphangitis in 6 dogs (2008–2011). *J Vet Intern Med*. 28(1):48–51, 2014.
33. Malatos JM, Kurpios NA, Duhamel GE. Small intestinal lymphatic hypoplasia in three dogs with clinical signs of protein-losing enteropathy. *J Comp Pathol*. 160:39–49, 2018.
34. Jablonski Wennogle SA, Priestnall SI, Webb CB. Histopathologic characteristics of intestinal biopsy samples from dogs with chronic inflammatory enteropathy with and without hypoalbuminemia. *J Vet Intern Med*. 31(2):371–376, 2017.
35. Jablonski Wennogle SA, Olver CS, Shropshire SB. Coagulation status, fibrinolysis, and platelet dynamics in dogs with chronic inflammatory enteropathy. *Vet Intern Med*. 35(2):892–901, 2021.
36. Procoli F, Mõtsküla PF, Keyte SV, et al. Comparison of histopathologic findings in duodenal and ileal endoscopic biopsies in dogs with chronic small intestinal enteropathies. *J Vet Intern Med*. 27(2):268–274, 2013.
37. Jablonski Wennogle SA, Priestnall SL, Suárez-Bonnet A, et al. Lymphatic endothelial cell immunohistochemical markers for evaluation of the intestinal lymphatic vasculature in dogs with chronic inflammatory enteropathy. *J Vet Intern Med*. 33(4):1669–1676, 2019.
38. Simmerson SM, Armstrong PJ, Wünschmann A, et al. Clinical features, intestinal histopathology, and outcome in protein-losing enteropathy in Yorkshire terrier dogs. *J Vet Intern Med*. 28(2):331–337, 2014.
39. Nagata N, Ohta H, Yokoyama N, et al. Clinical characteristics of dogs with food-responsive protein-losing enteropathy. *J Vet Intern Med*. 34(2):659–668, 2020.
40. Okanishi H, Yoshioka R, Kagawa Y, Watari T. The clinical efficacy of dietary fat restriction in treatment of dogs with intestinal lymphangiectasia. *J Vet Intern Med*. 28(3):809–817, 2014.
41. Jablonski Wennogle SA, Stockman J, Webb CB. Prospective evaluation of a change in dietary therapy in dogs with steroid-resistant protein-losing enteropathy. *J Small Anim Pract*. 62(9):756–764, 2021.
42. Sri-Jayantha LS, Doornink MT, Urie BK. Increased risk of select glucocorticoid adverse events in dogs of higher body weight. *Can Vet J*. 63(1):32–38, 2022.
43. Salavati Schmitz S, Gow A, Bommer N, et al. Diagnostic features, treatment, and outcome of dogs with inflammatory protein-losing enteropathy. *J Vet Intern Med*. 33(5):2005–2013, 2019.
44. deLaforcade A, Bacek L, Blais MC, et al. 2022 Update of the Consensus on the Rational Use of Antithrombotics and Thrombolytics in Veterinary Critical Care (CURATIVE) domain 1—defining

populations at risk. *J Vet Emerg Crit Care (San Antonio)*. 32(3):289–314, 2022.

45. Clarke KE, Sorrell S, Breheny C, et al. Dysautonomia in 53 cats and dogs: retrospective review of clinical data and outcome. *Vet Rec*. 187(12):e118, 2020.
46. Murtagh K, Oldroyd L, Ressel L, Batchelor D. Successful management of intestinal pseudo-obstruction in a dog. *Vet Record Case Rep*. 1(1):e000025, 2013.
47. Cerquetella M, Rossi G, Spaterna A, et al. Is irritable bowel syndrome also present in dogs? *Tierarztl Prax Ausg K Kleintiere Heimtiere*. 46(3):176–180, 2018.
48. Hayes G. Gastrointestinal foreign bodies in dogs and cats: a retrospective study of 208 cases. *J Small Anim Pract*. 50(11):576–583, 2009.
49. Junius G, Appeldoorn AM, Schrauwen E. Mesenteric volvulus in the dog: a retrospective study of 12 cases. *J Small Anim Pract*. 45(2):104–107, 2004.
50. Fernández Y, Seth M, Murgia D, Puig J. Ileocolic valve resection in dogs and cats: 17 cases (2001–2014). In: *British Small Animal Veterinary Association Congress*; 2015:431–432.
51. Gorman SC, Freeman LM, Mitchell SL, Chan DL. Extensive small bowel resection in dogs and cats: 20 cases (1998–2004). *J Am Vet Med Assoc*. 228(3):403–407, 2006.
52. Smith AA, Frimberger AE, Moore AS. Retrospective study of survival time and prognostic factors for dogs with small intestinal adenocarcinoma treated by tumor excision with or without adjuvant chemotherapy. *J Am Vet Med Assoc*. 254(2): 243–250, 2019.
53. Russell KN, Mehler SJ, Skorupski KA, et al. Clinical and immunohistochemical differentiation of gastrointestinal stromal tumors from leiomyosarcomas in dogs: 42 cases (1990–2003). *J Am Vet Med Assoc*. 230(9):1329–1333, 2007.
54. Cohen M, Post GS, Wright JC. Gastrointestinal leiomyosarcoma in 14 dogs. *J Vet Intern Med*. 17(1):107–110, 2003.
55. Irie M, Tomiyasu H, Tsujimoto H, et al. Prognostic factors for dogs with surgically resected gastrointestinal stromal tumors. *J Vet Med Sci*. 83(9):1481–1484, 2021.
56. Berger EP, Johannes CM, Jergens AE, et al. Retrospective evaluation of toceranib phosphate (Palladia) use in the treatment of gastrointestinal stromal tumors of dogs. *J Vet Intern Med*. 32(6):2045–2053, 2018.

CHAPTER 48

Large intestinal diseases

Florent Duplan
DVM, MSc, AFHEA, DECVIM-CA, MRCVS

Guillaume C. Ruiz
DVM, CEAV-MI, DECVIM-CA, MRCVS

The large intestine (LI) is the continuation of the small intestine (SI). It starts at the ileocolic junction, comprises the cecum, colon, and rectum, and terminates at the anus. Histologically, the structure of the LI is similar to that of the SI, with four layers: mucosa (subdivided into epithelial layer, lamina propria containing fibroblasts, inflammatory cells, vascular network, and lymphatics, and muscularis mucosa with smooth muscle fascicles), submucosa, muscularis, and serosa. The LI mucosa does not contain any villi, unlike the SI mucosa. Epithelial cells secrete almost no digestive enzymes, but goblet cells, a type of epithelial cell, produce mucus, which protects the wall against excoriation and bacterial activity and contains bicarbonates that protect against the acids formed by bacteria in the feces.

The two main functions of the LI are the reabsorption of water and electrolytes from the chyme to form solid feces (mainly in its proximal half) and the storage of feces in its distal half until voluntary defecation occurs. When a healthy dog defecates, the whole colon is often evacuated, so the final part of the stool is typically softer than the first part passed. The LI contains a large population of bacteria which can digest cellulose and provide metabolites, some vitamins (K, B_1, B_2, B_{12}), and gases (e.g., carbon dioxide, hydrogen, methane, and, particularly if there is malabsorption, sulfur-containing gases and volatile fatty acids). Consequently, any disease affecting the LI can lead to impaired reabsorption of water and electrolytes (diarrhea), impaired storage of feces (fecal incontinence), excessive gas production (flatulence and malodor), or reduced elimination of feces (constipation).

Large bowel diarrhea is typically of small volume, has liquid/mucoid content, and is characterized by straining and an urgency to defecate, leading to increased frequency of defecation. Due to the distal position of the LI, mucosal bleeding will manifest as the presence of fresh blood in the feces (hematochezia) rather than digested blood (melena) (Fig. 48.1). When the rectum is affected, there is often dyschezia (difficult or painful elimination of feces) and/or tenesmus (ineffective straining or discomfort after defecation).

Many disease processes affecting the SI will also affect the LI. When a condition is restricted to the LI, dogs typically remain in good body condition and systemically well. Abdominal palpation may identify discomfort, an intussusception, or a colonic mass. Digital rectal examination is essential to assess the rectal wall, anal glands, and fecal content and consistency.

Congenital malformations

A rectovaginal fistula is a communication between the ventral wall of the rectum and the dorsal wall of the vagina and is generally associated with an imperforate anus (atresia ani). Clinical signs generally appear after weaning, during the change from a liquid to a solid diet, and include, beyond the absence of the anus, passage of feces through the vulva, tenesmus, constipation, megacolon, abdominal distension, and signs of cystitis (e.g., hematuria, pollakiuria). Concurrent tail agenesis has been reported in some cases.[1] Surgical treatment is generally successful, although fecal incontinence, tenesmus, constipation, stenosis, anal gland odor, or urinary incontinence are possible complications.

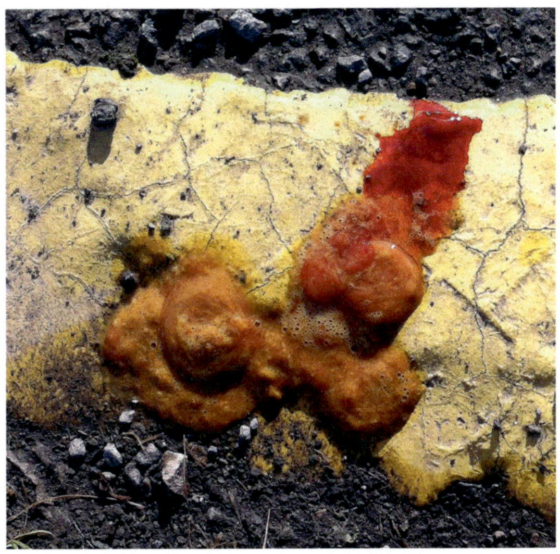

FIG. 48.1 Large intestinal diarrhea and hematochezia in a dog presented for chronic colitis. The dog had increased urgency to defecate. Note the small volume of stool and the presence of mucus.

Acute diseases

Acute colitis

Definition and clinical presentation

Acute colitis can result from a wide range of causes, leading to the development of large bowel diarrhea. Although hematochezia is also frequently reported, in many cases this only reflects superficial damage to the colonic mucosa by the underlying process, and therefore fresh blood in the feces is not necessarily a sign of disease severity. When inflammation is limited to the LI, there are generally no other clinical signs and the dogs remain clinically well otherwise (no vomiting, normal appetite and activity levels). The inciting cause is generally not identified, but dietary indiscretion, ingestion of putrid/rotten material, or toxin exposure are commonly suspected. Infectious agents (viral, bacterial, parasitic) are other possible causes.

Clinicopathological findings

In the absence of systemic clinical signs, further diagnostics are rarely required. Checking the worming status of the dog by performing a fecal analysis on pooled samples (flotation, *Giardia* ± *Cryptosporidium* antigen test) will allow treatment of specific parasites if present. Fecal culture can be considered if the dog is raw fed, if the diarrhea persists beyond a few days, or if there are systemic consequences to the diarrhea (e.g., fever).

Box 48.1 Dietary fibers.

Definition

Dietary fibers are essential for maintaining digestive function. Soluble, fermentable fibers soften the feces, decrease gut transit time and fecal bulk, and are metabolized by the microbiota, resulting in the formation of short-chain fatty acids that are important for gastrointestinal health. Fibers with low fermentability and solubility remain intact in the gastrointestinal tract, so they stimulate gut motility and make defecation easier. There is typically an overlap between fiber fermentability and solubility. Pectins are highly fermentable and soluble, while cellulose has low fermentability and solubility.[47] The reader is referred to Chapter 25 for further information.

Use of fibers in dogs with large intestinal disease

High-fiber veterinary diets are ideal to treat fiber-responsive disorders, such as colitis (acute or chronic) and constipation, as they are complete and balanced diets with different specific fiber sources (e.g., soluble, insoluble, prebiotic). Adding fiber to a complete, balanced diet might be an alternative if commercially available diets cannot be used (e.g., during a diet trial with a hypoallergenic hydrolyzed protein diet). However, this is considered less suitable because typically only one source of fiber is used. In a retrospective study, the reported median dose of soluble fibers (psyllium husk) was two tablespoons for the management of chronic idiopathic large bowel diarrhea and provided a very good to excellent response. The dose ranges from a quarter of a tablespoon to six tablespoons per day.[17] The dose should be gradually increased to avoid side effects such as bloating, abdominal cramps, or flatulence. Other dose recommendations are empirical. There is a great variability in the response to fibers, and therefore their use should be tailored to each animal.

Treatment

Management is mainly supportive. In many cases, the clinical signs will spontaneously resolve once the inciting cause has been withdrawn. An easily digestible diet can accelerate recovery and will allow appropriate nutrition of the intestinal tract. Whilst some studies support a beneficial effect of fibers (psyllium in particular, see Box 48.1)[2] or probiotics added to the diet, others failed to show a significant benefit of these over a diet change alone.[3] A course of fenbendazole (50 mg/kg PO every 24 h for 3–5 days) can be considered, particularly if the dog is not regularly wormed or if a parasite is identified on fecal analysis.

Metronidazole administration as part of the management of dogs with acute colitis used to be a common practice. Multiple studies have since shown that the use of this drug leads to significant dysbiosis. Along with the raising concerns associated with antimicrobial resistance in both human and veterinary medicine, a recent study showed that the use of metronidazole actually delayed recovery in dogs with acute colitis compared to administration of an easily digestible diet alone.[3] Therefore, the use of metronidazole in dogs with acute colitis is no longer recommended. If the patient becomes systemically unwell (e.g., dehydration, pyrexia, inappetence), specific assessment and management are required (see Chapter 35).

Colonic intussusception

An intussusception involving the ileum (ileocolic), colon (colocolic), cecum (ceco-colic/cecal inversion), or rectum (colorectal), or a combination of the above, is an important differential diagnosis for acute colitis. Multiple causes have been reported, including proliferative disorders (e.g., lymphoma, hamartomatous ganglioneuromatosis, carcinoid tumor, plasmacytoma),[4–7] infections, and inflammatory conditions. Sometimes, however, no underlying cause is identified.[8]

Clinical signs are similar to those of acute colitis, although abdominal discomfort and the presence of a caudal mass on abdominal palpation can be expected. In some cases, the intussusception can be chronic or intermittent and may not completely prevent the passage of fecal material.

Diagnosis requires abdominal imaging, more specifically ultrasound or computed tomography. Treatment is generally surgical, although anecdotally medical management can be successful.[8]

Intestinal angiodysplasia

Angiodysplasia (vascular ectasia) is a vascular malformation that can lead to intestinal blood loss and anemia (Fig. 48.2A). The underlying causes are still unknown, even in human medicine, but chronic obstruction of submucosal veins, congestion, or chronic steroid use have been reported. In a recent study using videocapsule endoscopy, the majority of dogs with confirmed gastrointestinal (GI) angiodysplasia had lesions in the colon, and this technique was more sensitive than abdominal ultrasound, endoscopy, or histopathology.[9] However, narrowband imaging (see Chapter 22) can enhance visualization of the source of bleeding if the lesion is within reach of a flexible endoscope with this technology (Fig. 48.2B).

Treatment can be surgical resection or argon plasma coagulation if a specific area can be identified and is associated with significant blood loss. Most commonly, however, management is supportive by discontinuing drugs that can cause GI ulceration (e.g., corticosteroids, nonsteroidal

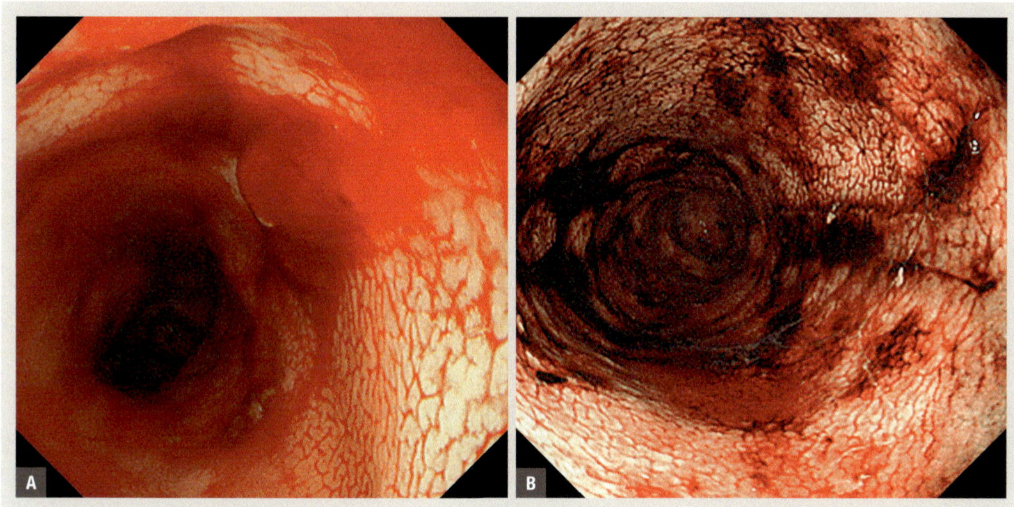

FIG. 48.2 Colonoscopic images of angiodysplasia in a Staffordshire Bull Terrier with severe hematochezia. (**A**) Under white light, diffuse bleeding (red areas) is seen. (**B**) With narrowband imaging, several bleeding points (black areas) can be identified.

anti-inflammatory drugs) and administering blood transfusions and iron supplementation as needed. In human medicine, thalidomide, hormonal therapy, angiogenesis inhibitors, and somatostatin analogs have been successfully used.[10] In dogs, literature is sparse, but case reports have documented a good success with a combination of estrogen and progesterone.[11]

Chronic noninfectious conditions

Idiopathic chronic colitis

Definition

Idiopathic chronic colitis (ICC) is a disorder characterized by chronic large intestinal diarrhea of more than 3-week's duration and inflammation detected on histopathology of colonic biopsies, without a specific cause identified. This disease is typically seen as part of a diffuse chronic inflammatory enteropathy (CIE), formerly known as inflammatory bowel disease, affecting both the SI and LI.

The exact pathophysiology of ICC is unknown, but it is suspected to be due to a combination of genetic predisposition, defective mucosal barrier, abnormal immune system, and intestinal dysbiosis, leading to a loss of tolerance to luminal bacteria and food antigens and secondary inflammation (see also Chapter 47).

Clinical presentation

ICC most commonly affects middle-aged dogs. Although some breed-specific forms of inflammatory bowel disease have been described, any breed may be affected by ICC. The disease typically causes large bowel diarrhea due to inflammation of the colonic mucosa. Anorexia, abdominal pain, and lethargy are noticed during acute exacerbations. Vomiting and weight loss are typically identified when the patient suffers from a diffuse disease also affecting the SI.

Clinicopathological findings

Hematology and biochemistry are typically unremarkable in dogs with ICC. Severely affected animals may have an inflammatory leukogram due to systemic inflammation, nonregenerative anemia due to chronic disease or GI bleeding, panhypoproteinemia due to intestinal loss, or increased liver enzymes due to a reactive hepatopathy. Serum cobalamin and folate determination is helpful to identify concurrent SI involvement. Basal cortisol and trypsin-like immunoreactivity should be measured to exclude hypoadrenocorticism and exocrine pancreatic insufficiency, respectively. Fecal parasitology, *Giardia* ELISA antigen test, and fecal culture are essential to investigate infectious causes of colitis (see below).

Diagnostic imaging findings and other diagnostic procedures

Lower GI endoscopy is recommended because histopathologic examination of the colonic mucosa is necessary to reach a final diagnosis. Assessment of the distal ileum, and rectum and cecum if there is evidence of malabsorption (e.g., concurrent hypocobalaminemia), is also pertinent. At least eight endoscopic biopsies per area are required, as the lesions may be patchy. Bacterial culture of colonic biopsies is useful if an infectious cause is suspected (e.g., granulomatous colitis). The reader is referred to Chapters 21–23 for detailed information on imaging and endoscopic biopsy of the lower GI tract.

Determining the severity of the inflammation and the type of inflammatory cells identified in the colonic lamina propria is essential to reach a final diagnosis, according to the World Small Animal Veterinary Association (WSAVA) guidelines.[12] Lymphocytic–plasmacytic inflammation of the colonic mucosa (i.e., lymphoplasmacytic colitis) is the most common form of chronic colitis and falls under the umbrella term CIE. Eosinophilic colitis is another, less frequent, form of CIE and may suggest intestinal parasitism or food-responsive enteropathy. Suppurative colitis (neutrophilic inflammation), sometimes associated with a concurrent granulomatous component (infiltrate of macrophages), can be suggestive of an infectious cause. Bacterial culture, special staining (periodic acid–Schiff [PAS]), and fluorescence *in situ* hybridization (FISH) of colonic biopsies are recommended in these cases (see below).

Morphological criteria and immune cell populations should be interpreted on histopathology. Surface epithelial injury and mucosal fibrosis and atrophy are signs of severe inflammation. Crypt hyperplasia is suggestive of regeneration secondary to inflammation, while crypt dilation and distortion are seen with chronic inflammatory damage.[12] Due to the difficulty of measuring the number of goblet cells in colonic biopsies (falsely decreased during biopsy procedure), assessment of the abnormal number of goblet cells was not included in the WSAVA guidelines. This is a significant limitation, as goblet cells play an important role in mucus production and prevention of bacterial invasion, and correlate with the presence of granulomatous colitis, severity of lymphoplasmacytic colitis, and response to treatment.

Treatment

As ICC is typically part of a more diffuse CIE, management is similar to that described in Chapter 47. However, additional therapeutic strategies specific for the management of chronic colitis are detailed below.

The use of a high-fiber diet or the addition of fiber (e.g., psyllium husk) to a hydrolyzed protein diet are common dietary strategies for the management of ICC. The response to fibers should be tailored to each individual and assessed after a minimum of 2 weeks.

Antibiotics such as metronidazole, tylosin, and oxytetracycline were previously used for the management of ICC. This strategy is no longer recommended, as antimicrobials can significantly alter the intestinal microbiota; therefore, they should only be used when a specific bacterial infection is confirmed or when all other treatment options have failed.[13]

Fecal microbiota transplantation has gained interest over the past few years and can be considered if intestinal dysbiosis is suspected to contribute to the clinical signs (see Chapter 27).

Budesonide, being 15 times more potent than prednisolone, is an alternative to systemic glucocorticoids. The gastroresistant, slow-release formulation and the extensive first-pass metabolism in the liver in people make budesonide a suitable local anti-inflammatory for Crohn's disease in the ileum and colon, with reduced systemic side effects. However, the efficacy of budesonide is variable amongst dogs, and suppression of the hypothalamic–pituitary–adrenal axis has been described. The recommended dose is 1 mg (small dog), 2 mg (medium dog), or 3 mg (large dog) orally once a day.[14]

Sulfasalazine is a local nonsteroidal anti-inflammatory drug. It is converted into 5-aminosalicylic acid by colonic bacteria, leading to a high concentration of the drug in the colon, inhibiting prostaglandin and leukotriene synthesis. Monitoring tear production at the start and during therapy is required, as sulfasalazine may cause irreversible keratoconjunctivitis sicca if not withdrawn promptly. The dosage ranges from 10 to 30 mg/kg every 8-12 hours, and maximum effect is expected after 10–14 days. Sulfasalazine should not be used alongside glucocorticoids or when there is concurrent small intestinal inflammation.

Prognosis

Prognosis of ICC depends mainly on the severity of the clinical signs and the response to treatment. Young dogs that respond to dietary manipulation have a more favorable prognosis than elderly dogs refractory to therapy.

Irritable bowel syndrome

Definition and clinical presentation

Irritable bowel syndrome is a common symptom-based condition in human medicine characterized by chronic, recurrent episodes of acute abdominal pain or discomfort, associated with constipation, diarrhea, or a combination of both, in the absence of another disease to account for the clinical signs. Histopathology of the colon often shows no or minimal changes.[15] The pathogenesis is complex and multifactorial and is still an area of ongoing research. Psychosocial distress, food intolerance, previous infectious enteritis, use of antibiotics, altered gut immune activation, heightened colonic sensation, and increased colonic permeability are all components that have been identified in affected patients. The condition is diagnosed based on compatible clinical presentation and exclusion of other diseases.[15]

Similar clinical presentations in dogs have raised interest of researchers as to whether irritable bowel syndrome exists in these animals.[16] A study recruited dogs based on clinical signs (increased frequency of defecation, presence of mucus, tenesmus) and absence of an underlying cause identified on blood work, fecal analysis, diagnostic imaging, colonoscopy and histopathology.[17] These dogs were diagnosed with "chronic idiopathic large bowel diarrhea" (CILBD), which may be the canine counterpart to human irritable bowel syndrome. Interestingly, abnormal personality traits and potential environmental stress factors (e.g., people visiting the household, travel, visit to the veterinarian, separation anxiety) were identified in almost 40% of the dogs, although a direct relationship with the incidence of diarrhea could not be established in this retrospective study. A link between CIE and compromised emotional health was also suggested in a recent abstract,[18] with significantly higher scores on negative activation (frustration-related behavior, fear, anxiety) noted in dogs with CIE compared to control dogs.

Treatment

In humans, the management of irritable bowel syndrome is multimodal and is tailored to the patient's clinical presentation (e.g., abdominal pain, bloating, diarrhea, constipation). It can include regular exercise, dietary manipulation (gluten-free diet, reduced fermentable carbohydrates), fiber supplements, multistrain probiotics, laxatives, motility modifiers (Table 48.1), antidepressants, and psychological therapy.[15]

In the study on dogs with CILBD mentioned above, the addition of soluble fiber (psyllium) to a highly digestible diet led to a very good to excellent and sustained response in 85% of the cases.[17] This response to soluble fiber (Box 48.1) was also reported in another study in which fiber was part of a hydrolyzed diet given with probiotics.[19] Response to probiotics in dogs with CILBD has also been documented using a multistrain blend dissolved in drinking water as the sole therapeutic intervention.[20] The time to clinical remission (resolution of diarrhea and tenesmus) in this study was a median of 23 days. The authors hypothesized that the use of probiotics altered the dogs' microbiota, which in turn reduced the number and activity of mucosal mast cells, leading to improved colonic motility, secretion, and immune homeostasis.

Another study looked at the effects of a structured exercise program set up by a canine rehabilitation therapist in sedentary dogs with chronic enteropathy for which the management was otherwise standardized.[21] Interestingly, dogs undergoing low to moderate training with aerobic and resistance activities showed a significant improvement in their clinical scores after 6 weeks of exercise. Further investigations are required to determine which dogs may benefit from such interventions; however, a multimodal therapeutic approach to these patients, in addition to more conventional therapies, may help to control clinical signs.

Given the prevalence of altered personality or increased stressors in dogs having large intestinal signs,[16,18] further research on the benefit of environmental modifications and the use of behavior-modifying drugs (e.g., alpha-casozepine, L-tryptophan, clomipramine, fluoxetine) is warranted in the future. Symptomatic drugs are also commonly used in dogs despite limited studies that objectify their effects (see Chapters 28 and 31–33).

TABLE 48.1 Recommended dosages of intestinal motility modifiers used in dogs.

Type	Drug	Dosage	Notes
Spasmogenic	Loperamide	0.04–0.2 mg/kg PO every 8–12 h	Do not use in dogs with intestinal obstruction or mutation of the multidrug resistance (*MDR*) gene (e.g., collies)
	Diphenoxylate	0.05–0.1 mg/kg PO every 6–8 h	Do not use in dogs with intestinal obstruction
Spasmolytic	Butylscopolamine (hyoscine)	0.5 mg/kg PO every 12 h	—

Bile acid diarrhea

Definition and clinical presentation

Bile acids are produced and conjugated in the liver before being released into the SI, where they are converted to secondary bile acids and form micelles, which facilitate the absorption of lipids.[22] The vast majority (95%) of bile acids are reabsorbed in the distal ileum and undergo enterohepatic recycling. A small proportion of bile acids reach the colon and undergo bacterial deconjugation. In human medicine, it has been shown that conditions affecting bile acid reabsorption in the ileum lead to an increased amount of unconjugated bile acids in the colon, stimulating electrolyte and water secretion and shortening colonic transit time, leading to large bowel diarrhea.

There has been an increased interest in canine fecal bile acids over recent years. A study showed a decreased amount of secondary fecal unconjugated bile acids in dogs with inflammatory bowel disease compared to healthy dogs, and this was correlated with a reduced abundance of *Peptacetobacter hiranonis* (formerly called *Clostridium hiranonis*), which belongs to the normal intestinal flora and is known to convert primary bile acids into secondary bile acids.[23] As secondary fecal unconjugated bile acids inhibit the secretion of inflammatory cytokines IL-1β and IL-8, their reduction can have pro-inflammatory effects.

It is suspected that bile acid diarrhea occurs in dogs and may be associated with inflammatory enteropathies, neoplasia, dysbiosis, and possibly other conditions as described in humans (e.g., cholecystectomy, pancreatic insufficiency, genetic disorders).

Treatment

Bile acid diarrhea is treated with bile acid sequestrants in humans. In veterinary medicine, a recent study reported the successful treatment of two dogs using cholestyramine (0.04–0.06 g/kg PO every 12 h) for more than a year.[24] Since then, the same author has reported a positive response to treatment in 14 other dogs.

Whilst dogs with reduced abundance of *P. hiranonis* and increased primary fecal bile acids are more likely to respond to bile acid sequestrants, no definitive test is currently available to confirm the diagnosis. It is therefore suggested that this treatment is reserved for dogs with chronic refractory diarrhea after full investigations and conventional treatment options (i.e., multiple dietary trials, multistrain probiotics, corticosteroids and other immunosuppressants, fecal microbiota transplantation) have failed to improve clinical signs. The potential side effects of long-term treatment with cholestyramine in dogs remain unknown.

Infectious conditions

Infectious causes of large intestinal inflammation encompass a wide range of viral, bacterial, fungal, and protozoal agents. The increased popularity of raw diets has been regularly associated with reports of infectious enteritis. Easy access to extensive fecal screening from external laboratories has also increased the number of positive results and the temptation for practitioners to treat. However, whilst some infectious agents cause clinical signs related to their direct presence (fungi, protozoa), the actual effects of other agents (viruses, bacteria) on the gut are disputed. This has resulted in a shift from the concept of "antibiotic-responsive enteropathy" to alternative means to influence a dysregulated microbiota, including dietary manipulation, use of fibers, development of probiotics, and ongoing research on fecal microbiota transplantation. See Chapters 36–40 for further information on the diagnosis of bacterial, viral, and parasitic enteritis.

Escherichia coli-associated granulomatous colitis

Definition

Previously called histiocytic ulcerative colitis, granulomatous colitis was considered to be an incurable immune-mediated disease. Advanced molecular techniques (e.g., FISH) have since shown that granulomatous colitis is actually caused by an intracellular infection with *Escherichia coli*. The disease most commonly affects young Boxers and French Bulldogs, but it has also been reported in other breeds (e.g., Alaskan Malamute, Mastiff).

Clinical presentation

Granulomatous colitis mainly affects the colon, although a recent report described the involvement of the ileum, causing a protein-losing enteropathy. Clinical signs of severe colitis are frequent, including mucoid diarrhea, hematochezia, urgency, and tenesmus. Weight loss is also common. Physical examination is typically unremarkable, except decreased body and muscle conditions and presence of blood and mucus on rectal examination.

Clinicopathological findings

Evaluating hematology, biochemistry, and urinalysis is recommended to exclude extra-GI diseases. Fecal parasitology and culture should be performed to look for *Giardia*, *Salmonella*, or *Campylobacter* infection. Rectal scraping for cytology helps to evaluate infectious causes of colitis (see Chapter 38).

Diagnostic imaging findings and other diagnostic procedures

Abdominal ultrasound may be unremarkable or show evidence of diffuse thickening of the colonic mucosa. Colonoscopy is required to diagnose granulomatous colitis. The colonic mucosa is typically ulcerated, and biopsies should be collected for histopathology, bacterial culture, and FISH analysis.

Histopathology reveals mucosal ulceration, lymphocytic and macrophagic inflammation, and loss of goblet cells. The presence of

PAS-positive material within macrophages is pathognomonic for granulomatous colitis. Intracellular *E. coli* within PAS-positive macrophages is confirmed by FISH analysis. Bacterial culture is recommended to guide antimicrobial use.

If the pet owner's finances are limited, it is acceptable to perform a blind biopsy of the colonic wall for histopathology and bacterial culture in patients with suspected granulomatous colitis. In this case, practitioners should be mindful about the risks of colonic perforation.

Treatment

Fluoroquinolones (e.g., enrofloxacin 5 mg/kg PO q12–24h) are typically prescribed for 4–8 weeks. The infection is usually cleared after one course of antibiotics, but recurrence may occur in some dogs. There is growing evidence of multiresistant strains of *E. coli*, which is why bacterial culture and sensitivity testing of colonic biopsies is important.[25]

Repeat colonic biopsies for histopathology, bacterial culture, and FISH analysis are recommended if the dog fails to improve on antibiotics in order to confirm the persistence of granulomatous colitis and guide treatment.

Prognosis

Prognosis depends on the response to antibiotics. Some reports describe complete remission within 30 days of starting fluoroquinolones, lasting up to 102 months.[25] However, partial responses and relapses are well documented, requiring repeat endoscopy, biopsy, and bacterial culture and ultimately a change of antibiotics.[25,26] Long-term symptomatic treatment, including dietary management, fiber supplementation, and sulfasalazine administration, is typically helpful to control colitis-related clinical signs.[25] Empirical use of enrofloxacin prior to definitive diagnosis has been significantly associated with antimicrobial resistance and poor clinical outcome.[27] Despite reaching an appropriate diagnosis, some dogs are euthanized due to multiresistant *E. coli* infection leading to refractory colitis.

Other infectious granulomatous colitis

Other infectious agents have been reported in association with neutrophilic and/or macrophage-rich infiltrates in the LI. *Leishmania* amastigotes, *Histoplasma capsulatum* yeasts, *Neospora caninum* tachyzoites, *Prototheca* spp., or *Pythium* spp. are pathogens that have been reported in case reports as inclusions within intracolonic macrophages on histopathology, on regular or special stains, or by PCR (Fig. 48.3).[28–30] Etiologic treatment of these infections resulted in clinical improvement in some cases. Additional tests (e.g., special stains, culture, PCR) on colonic biopsies of dogs diagnosed with granulomatous and/or neutrophilic infiltrates must be adapted based on the geographic area.

Neoplastic conditions

General concepts

Definition and introduction

Neoplastic proliferations of the LI can be benign or malignant, and they can present diffusely within the wall or as a demarcated mass. There is limited information regarding the prevalence and types of colorectal tumors in dogs, with many reports being more than 30 years old. In a 2017 study documenting colonoscopic and histological features of rectal masses in dogs,[31] the most common lesions were benign polyps or adenomas (64%), followed by adenocarcinomas (26.6%), plasmacytomas (4.6%), and lymphomas, mucosal hyperplasia, and leiomyomas (1.6% each). As this study focused on masses, not all infiltrative diseases were necessarily included, so the proportion of round cell tumors may have been underestimated. The lesions observed were very often distal, mainly affecting the rectum. Interestingly, the histopathologic diagnosis from endoscopic biopsies was identified as more differentiated in some cases as compared to histopathology obtained following subsequent surgical excision of the lesions, potentially underdiagnosing malignancy. Neurofibromas, ganglioneuromatosis, hemangiosarcomas, leiomyosarcomas, and gastrointestinal stromal tumors (GISTs) have also been reported to affect the LI.[32–34] Of note, the majority of GISTs were found in the cecum in one study.[33]

Clinical presentation

Clinical signs of large intestinal tumors are nonspecific,[35] and they are associated with damage to the intestinal wall (hematochezia, tenesmus, less commonly diarrhea or abdominal pain) or with the mass effect of the lesion within the lumen (constipation, obstipation, rectal prolapse).

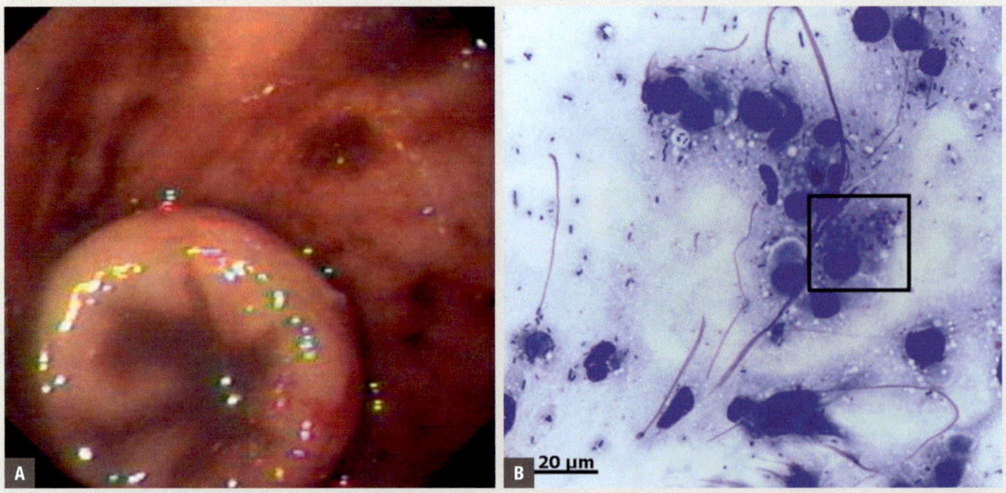

FIG. 48.3 Visceral leishmaniasis in an 18-month-old Labrador crossbreed presented for 4 months of hemorrhagic diarrhea and vomiting. (A) Endoscopic image showing extensive mucosal hemorrhage in the proximal colon near the ileocolic junction. Histopathology was consistent with moderate to severe chronic lymphoplasmacytic and histiocytic inflammation and erosion of the mucosal epithelium. (B) Imprint cytology from a colonic biopsy obtained by endoscopy (May–Grünwald–Giemsa stain, ×100 magnification). *Leishmania* amastigotes can be seen in the cytoplasm of a macrophage (square).

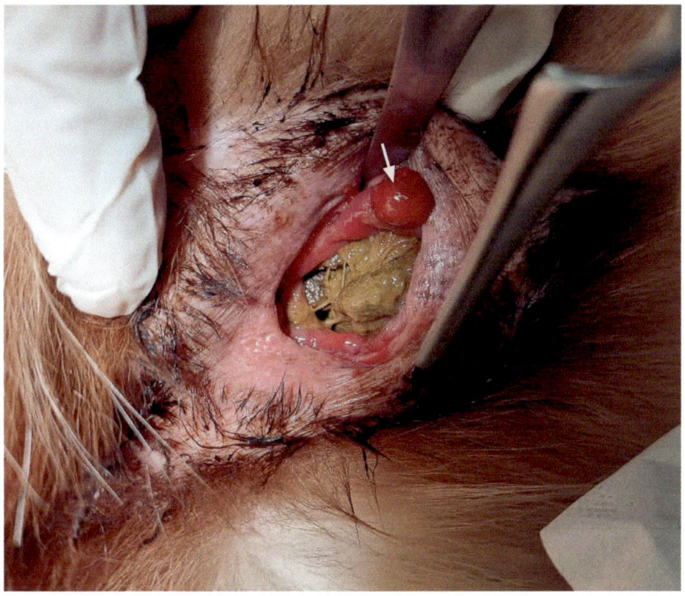

FIG. 48.4 Rectal mass (arrow) causing hematochezia identified during rectal examination in a dog. Use of a speculum allowed better direct assessment of the lesion. Histopathology following surgical excision identified a carcinoma *in situ*.

Hematochezia appears more frequently than diarrhea in dogs with a demarcated mass, so hematochezia in the absence of diarrhea should raise the suspicion of a mass.[31,35] The pattern of hematochezia is worth assessing; a delimited mass (e.g., polyp, carcinoma) will tend to produce a linear trace of fresh blood on the feces, whilst in case of a diffuse lesion (e.g., lymphoma) fresh blood will generally cover all the stool. Constipation can occur in the absence of luminal obstruction due to the pain associated with feces passing through the lesioned area. Conversely, paradoxical diarrhea can occur in dogs with intestinal obstruction when excessive straining leads to mucus hypersecretion. In this case, the volume of diarrhea is usually small, and a large amount of feces remains in the colon and can be identified by abdominal palpation. Digital rectal examination is crucial in assessing the rectum, as many masses can be identified, sublumbar lymph nodes assessed, and the presence of blood confirmed (Fig. 48.4).

Diagnostic imaging findings and other diagnostic procedures

General concepts on the benefits of the different imaging modalities (radiographs, ultrasound, computed tomography) can be found in Chapter 21. Interestingly, a recent study in dogs with small intestinal neoplasia reported some contrast computed tomography features which may help to differentiate between adenocarcinoma, lymphoma, and spindle cell sarcoma,[36] and similar findings may apply to the LI. Thoracic imaging is pertinent to evaluate for metastatic disease, particularly in case of carcinoma, although local spread is more common.[31] Endoscopy of the lower intestinal tract following appropriate preparation allows direct assessment and sampling of the lesions, evaluation of associated strictures, and polypectomy or resection if needed (see Chapter 22). This technique is an important part of the investigations of a lower intestinal neoplasm even if biopsies are superficial and lack information on deeper infiltration of the tumor.[31] Whilst a single mass is identified in most cases, multiple lesions have been reported in approximately 7% of dogs in one study.[31]

Benign colorectal polyps and adenomas

Definition and clinical presentation

Benign inflammatory polyps are characterized by an inflammatory infiltrate associated with lamina propria fibromuscular hyperplasia.[37] Benign adenomas are often considered similar to inflammatory polyps in their macroscopic aspect, clinical behavior, and management, but they differ histologically in that focal proliferating epithelial cells are present. West Highland White Terriers are overrepresented in a recent European study,[35] whilst a longitudinal Japanese study reported that Miniature Dachshunds are predisposed and their polyps have specific histopathological features.[37] The origin of these polyps is likely multifactorial, with chronic inflammation being suspected as an inciting cause.

Treatment

The most common treatment options include surgical excision (pull out, colectomy) or endoscopic diathermy resection; argon plasma coagulation has also been reported.[35,37] In some Miniature Dachshunds with multiple polyps associated with granulomatous tissue and a mixed inflammatory infiltrate within the lamina propria, an immune-mediated mechanism has been suggested, and these dogs seem to respond to immunosuppression (prednisolone, ciclosporin, chlorambucil, alone or in combination).[38]

Prognosis

The abovementioned Japanese study in Miniature Dachshunds with inflammatory polyps reported that 52% of dogs had recurrent lesions following initial excision, and in 56% of these cases the lesions had neoplastic features on histopathology (adenoma or adenocarcinoma), raising suspicion that inflammatory polyps, at least in this breed, may progress into neoplastic lesions.[37] Regular monitoring following excision is therefore recommended.

Colorectal lymphoma

Lymphoma of the LI is reported in dogs, but prognosis is more favorable than that of lymphoma affecting the SI.[39] See Chapter 42 for detailed information on intestinal lymphoma.

Adenocarcinomas

Definition and clinical presentation

Adenocarcinomas are more common in the LI than in the stomach or SI. They usually occur in the descending colon and rectum and mainly affect middle-aged or older male dogs (mean of 7 years).[40,41] In a study in dogs with colorectal epithelial tumors, a significantly different fecal microbiota profile was reported compared to control dogs.[42] Further studies are needed to determine if specific taxa, such as those identified in this study, could contribute to the development of adenocarcinomas, similar to what is reported in humans.

Diagnostic imaging findings

Abdominal ultrasound documents changes (thickened colonic wall, enlarged lymph nodes) in a minority of cases. Diagnosis commonly relies on endoscopic biopsies.

Treatment

Surgical excision is the treatment of choice for adenocarcinomas, with different techniques reported depending on the location of the tumor and surgeon's preference.

Prognosis

Prognosis is generally good (73% overall survival after 5 years in one study), although minor complications, such as transient dyschezia and tenesmus, are common and recurrence possible (approximately 30% of cases).[43]

Mesenchymal tumors

Definition and clinical presentation

Leiomyomas and leiomyosarcomas arise from smooth muscle, whilst GISTs arise from interstitial cells of Cajal. Both tumor types used to be confused until immunohistochemistry allowed differentiation between them. GISTs occur more frequently in the cecum and LI than leiomyomas or leiomyosarcomas. Paraneoplastic hypoglycemia, erythrocytosis, and metastatic disease have been associated with smooth muscle tumors and GISTs. Septic peritonitis due to cecal rupture is a reported complication of GISTs.

Treatment and prognosis

Treatment of mesenchymal tumors is mainly surgical and leads to a similar overall median survival time of about a year, although dogs with GISTs surviving the postoperative period appear to live longer than dogs with leiomyosarcomas or undifferentiated sarcomas.[33] Whilst tyrosine kinase inhibitors as adjunctive or palliative treatment for GIST have been shown to have biological activity on the tumor, their actual benefit on survival and disease progression remains to be fully evaluated.[44]

Constipation, obstipation, and megacolon

Definition

Constipation is the absence or reduced evacuation of feces, which become hard and dry due to prolonged stasis in the colon. Obstipation is the consequence of fecal impaction preventing defecation. It is not uncommon for dogs to present with dyschezia and tenesmus secondary to constipation. See Chapter 15 for the differential diagnosis of and diagnostic approach to constipation.

Megacolon is a very rare condition in dogs characterized by partial or complete progressive distension of the colon and loss of motility, causing chronic constipation. The disease can be congenital due to aganglionosis (called Hirschsprung's disease in humans) or secondary to prolonged obstipation due to partial imperforate anus, pelvic fracture, stricture, diet low in fiber or containing bones, prostatic enlargement (often benign prostatic hypertrophy), perineal hernia, or chronic constipation. Diagnosis is made by lateral abdominal radiographs, typically comparing the diameter of the colon, the pelvic width, and the length of the lumbar vertebrae L2 and L7 (see Chapter 21).

History and signalment

It is essential to document the duration of the clinical signs, the frequency of defecation, and the animal's ability to defecate; indeed, obstipation requires urgent medical management. The diet should be thoroughly evaluated to assess the quantity of dietary fiber and indigestible elements (e.g., bones, hair). A history of pelvic trauma or abdominal surgery should not be overlooked, as loss of colonic motility can be insidious.

Physical examination

A thorough physical examination is an essential part of the diagnostic approach to constipation. The abdomen might be tense or painful on abdominal palpation, and therefore palpation of the colon and abdominal lymph nodes might not be possible. The presence of anal furunculosis (Fig. 48.5) or masses should be assessed. Digital rectal examination should then be performed under sedation to identify a mass, foreign body, stricture, pelvic fracture, sublumbar lymphadenomegaly, prostatomegaly, or perineal hernia. The appearance of the feces retrieved during rectal examination may reveal the presence of blood, mucus, or pus. Finally, inspection of the anal glands is required to evaluate for impaction, abscessation, or abnormal content.

Clinicopathological and diagnostic imaging findings and other diagnostic procedures

Hematology and biochemistry can assess for azotemia, hypokalemia, or other electrolyte disturbances predisposing to constipation. Abdominal radiographs can be performed to evaluate the severity of constipation and identify a pelvic fracture, foreign body, prostatomegaly, or lymphadenomegaly. The ratio of maximum colonic diameter to the length of the L2 vertebral body is 1.05 ± 0.30 in normal dogs, and megacolon is diagnosed when the ratio of maximum colonic diameter to the length of the L7 vertebral body is above 1.5.[45,46] Abdominal ultrasound is typically of low yield due to the pelvis and the presence of gas and dry fecal material in the colon, limiting the assessment of the colonic mucosa. However, ultrasound-guided aspiration of an inflammatory or neoplastic lesion might be possible. Computed tomography can provide additional useful information (Fig. 48.6).

Endoscopy is an essential step of the diagnostic investigations once secondary causes of constipation have been ruled out. First, after manual removal of feces, a proctoscopy is recommended for evaluation

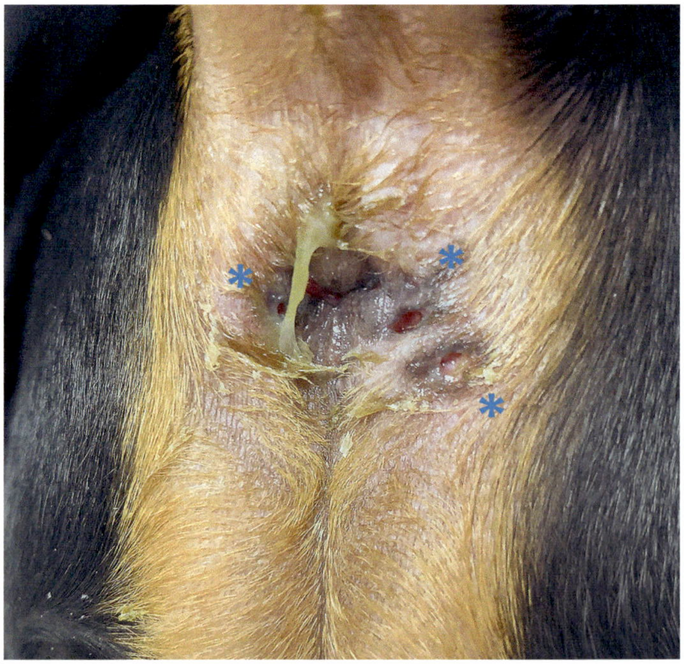

FIG. 48.5 Anal furunculosis in a dog (tract openings identified by asterisks), causing painful defecation and leading to constipation. Successful treatment of the anal furunculosis allowed for resolution of constipation.

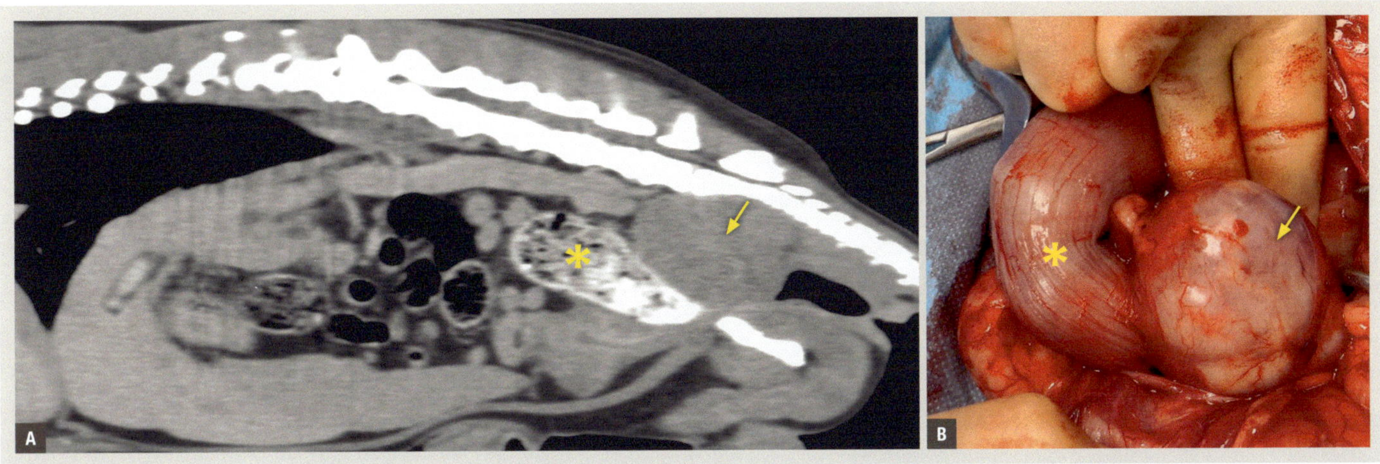

FIG. 48.6 Dog with chronic and worsening constipation. (A) Sagittal postcontrast computed tomography image of the abdomen showing a distal colonic mass (arrow) narrowing the colonic lumen (*), leading to accumulation of fecal material. (B) Perioperative image of the colonic mass (arrow) obstructing the lumen and causing distension of the colon proximal to the lesion (*). Surgical excision of the mass allowed resolution of the clinical signs. Histopathology was consistent with a fully excised leiomyoma.

of the rectum; this can be performed with a speculum, a light source, and direct visualization. Any abnormal lesion should be biopsied. A colonoscopy is then recommended to investigate proximal intraluminal lesions. The animal should receive osmotic laxatives (polyethylene glycol–based) for 24 hours prior to the procedure and a warm enema on the day of the procedure. The clinician should evaluate the aspect of the mucosa (heterogeneous hyperemia or "blotchy appearance" can reflect active inflammation) and the presence of a stricture or a mass. Multiple endoscopic biopsies are recommended, as there is a poor correlation between the macroscopic aspect of a lesion and histological diagnosis. Finally, electrodiagnostics can be considered to evaluate neuromuscular causes of constipation.

Treatment

Mild constipation

Symptomatic treatment of constipation includes dietary manipulation and use of laxatives (Table 48.2) and prokinetics (Table 48.3). Prokinetics are not recommended in case of intestinal obstruction. A good-quality, highly digestible diet should be given, as it provides the dog with appropriate nutrition whilst limiting the amount of residue. Fiber supplementation is also an important strategy for dogs with persistently reduced colonic motility (Box 48.1).[47] Regular walks and exercise are also essential to stimulate gut peristalsis and fecal elimination. Recurrent episodes of constipation should prompt the clinician to look for an underlying cause.

TABLE 48.2 Recommended dosages of laxatives used in dogs.

Type	Mechanism of action	Agent	Dosage
Bulk forming	Fiber added to diet that is poorly absorbed and distends the colon	Wheat bran	■ 1–2 tablespoons per dog, mixed with food, once or twice a day
		Psyllium	■ 1–4 teaspoons per dog per meal, mixed with food
Emollient	Anionic surfactants that rehydrate feces	Dioctyl sodium sulfosuccinate (DSS), docusate sodium, docusate calcium	■ 250 mg per dog once rectally ■ 50–200 mg per dog PO once a day or divided doses up to 4 times a day
Lubricant	Facilitation of passage of feces	Mineral oil (liquid paraffin)	■ 10–20 mL per dog PO, mixed with food, twice a day ■ Generally not recommended due to the risk of lipid pneumonia ■ Do not use in combination with DSS
Osmotic	Polysaccharides that are poorly absorbed, leading to water retention in the colon	Lactulose	■ 0.5–1 mL/kg PO every 8–12 h ■ 5–10 mL/kg (mix 3 parts of lactulose and 7 parts of warm water) once rectally
		Polyethylene glycol (PEG) 3350	■ 0.5–2 teaspoons per dog PO once a day
Stimulant	Stimulation of colonic smooth muscle contractions	Bisacodyl	■ 1–3 tablets per dog PO once a day
Microenema	Softening of feces and induction of defecation	Sodium citrate, sodium alkylsulfoacetate	■ 1 pipette (5 mL) per dog once rectally

PO, per os.

TABLE 48.3 Recommended dosages of gastrointestinal prokinetics used in dogs.

Type	Mechanism of action	Drug	Dosage
Serotonergic 5-HT_4 receptor agonist	Contraction of gastrointestinal smooth muscle	Cisapride	■ 0.1–0.5 mg/kg PO every 8–12 h
		Prucalopride	■ 0.01–0.2 mg/kg PO every 12 h
Motilin receptor stimulant	Initiation of migrating motor complexes	Erythromycin	■ 0.5–1 mg/kg PO every 8 h ■ Not recommended due to risk of development of antimicrobial resistance

Metoclopramide has no prokinetic effect on the large intestine. See also Chapter 31. 5-HT_4, serotonin type 4; PO, per os.

Box 48.2 Suggested protocol for performing an enema in a constipated dog.

Equipment required

- Isotonic fluid or tap water warmed to 37°C (alternatively, mix 3 parts of lactulose with 7 parts of warm water)
- Lubricant
- Bowl
- Soft rubber tube, size adapted to dog's weight (12 Fr or 4 mm if <10 kg, 22 Fr or 7 mm if 10–20 kg, 30 Fr or 10 mm if >20 kg)
- Waterproof apron
- Gloves
- 20 mL syringes

Procedure

First, make sure the patient is fully hydrated. The procedure should be performed in an area that is easy to clean and with the dog anesthetized and intubated. The rubber tube should be well lubricated and advanced gently into the descending colon, up to the level of the last rib, while slowly administrating warm fluid through the tube (10–20 mL/kg). If resistance is felt, the tube should be redirected to reach the desired location; rolling the tube between the fingers can help to advance further. Rigid tubes or forceful movements should be avoided, as they can lead to colonic perforation.

If it is not possible to place the rubber tube up to the level of the last rib, a smaller tube should be used to go past the site of impaction and deliver the fluid; a feeding tube can sometimes be used for this. It is necessary to wait several minutes after fluid administration so that the feces soften. Gentle transabdominal colonic massaging can be performed to break down impacted feces, but care must be taken to avoid damaging abdominal organs. The goal is to move smaller and softer feces into the rectum so that they can be removed by digital extraction. This procedure might need to be repeated several times in severely affected dogs. Use of sponge forceps might be necessary to remove impacted feces or bones, preferably under direct visualization to avoid damage to the colon.

Additional considerations

It is important to administer the fluid slowly into the colonic lumen, as fast instillation may cause abdominal pain, vomiting, or colonic perforation. It may not be possible to remove all the impacted stool, but the dog may pass the rest of the feces with appropriate management using laxatives and prokinetics after the procedure. Alternatively, the procedure might be repeated the next day depending on the severity of the clinical signs. Antibiotics (e.g., amoxicillin with clavulanic acid) should be considered in patients with a significantly ulcerated colonic mucosa due to the risk of bacterial translocation; however, they are rarely required.

Moderate to severe constipation or megacolon

When constipation is more severe and associated with dehydration, prerenal azotemia, or electrolyte disturbances, hospitalization and intravenous fluid therapy are recommended. Enemas are necessary when constipation/obstipation is severe and should be performed once the patient is clinically stable and rehydrated (Box 48.2). Dietary management and use of laxatives and prokinetics are recommended (see above). Fiber supplementation, however, should not be utilized for management of megacolon due to the absence of colonic motility. Laxatives should not be administered long-term, as they irritate the colonic mucosa and can cause constipation. In refractory cases, subtotal colectomy is recommended.

Prognosis

In a retrospective study, the median survival time of dogs with colonic impaction medically managed was 2 years. In this study, the degree of colonic dilation was not related to the long-term outcome.[48]

KEY POINTS

- Large intestinal diseases are common in dogs. Acute colitis rarely requires diagnostic investigations and generally responds to symptomatic treatment within a few days.
- Chronic inflammatory enteropathies are generally diffuse and affect both the small and large intestine. Refractory cases may benefit from bile acid sequestrants, as occurs in humans with bile acid diarrhea. Neutrophilic and/or granulomatous colitis require additional infectious testing, as different conditions will require specific medications.
- Further research is needed to confirm the existence of a syndrome in dogs similar to human irritable bowel syndrome. It is, however, worth considering alternative and less conventional approaches to the management of chronic large intestinal diarrhea, hematochezia, or tenesmus in dogs if no significant anomalies have been identified on blood work, fecal analysis, diagnostic imaging, colonoscopy, and histopathology.
- Benign and malignant cancerous processes present similarly, and their treatment is generally surgical, except for intestinal lymphoma.
- Constipation is not uncommon in dogs, and further investigations and management depend on the severity and recurrence of the clinical signs.

References

1. Rahal SC, Vicente CS, Mortari AC, et al. Rectovaginal fistula with anal atresia in 5 dogs. *Can Vet J* 48(8):827–830, 2007.
2. Lappin MR, Zug A, Hovenga C, et al. Efficacy of feeding a diet containing a high concentration of mixed fiber sources for management of acute large bowel diarrhea in dogs in shelters. *J Vet Intern Med* 36(2):488–492, 2022.
3. Rudinsky AJ, Parker VJ, Winston J, et al. Randomized controlled trial demonstrates nutritional management is superior to metronidazole for treatment of acute colitis in dogs. *J Am Vet Med Assoc* 260(S3):S23–S32, 2022.
4. Thomsen BJ, Ulfelder EH. A case of colonic–colonic intussusception in a dog secondary to lymphoma treated with colonic resection and anastomosis. *Can Vet J* 63(9):957–961, 2022.
5. Jaffe M, Alexander K, Ryan M, et al. Colonic hamartomatous ganglioneuromatosis in a 4 mo old puppy. *J Am Anim Hosp Assoc* 59(5):224–228, 2023.
6. Yoon S, Lee SK, Lee J, et al. Dual-phase computed tomography angiography of intestinal carcinoid tumor as a lead point for cecocolic intussusception in a dog. *J Vet Med Sci* 81(6):928–932, 2019.
7. Bellezza E, Bianchini E, Pettinelli S, et al. Intestinal plasmacytoma causing colocolic double intussusception in an adult dog. *J Small Anim Pract* 57(12):718, 2016.
8. Moores AL, Urraca CI, de Sousa RJR, et al. Nonsurgical reduction of prolapsed colocolic intussusception in 2 puppies. *J Vet Emerg Crit Care (San Antonio)* 31(5):656–660, 2021.
9. Defarges A, Stiller J, Solomon JA. Gastrointestinal angiodysplasias diagnosed using video capsule endoscopy in 15 dogs. *J Vet Intern Med* 37(2):428–436, 2023.
10. Gkolfakis P, Fostier R, Tziatzios G, et al. Efficacy of pharmacologic treatment for treating gastrointestinal angiodysplasias-related bleeding: a systematic review and meta-analysis. *Eur J Gastroenterol Hepatol* 34(10):1021–1030, 2022.
11. Goldman CK, Parnell NK, Holland CH. Hormone therapy for treatment of colonic vascular ectasia in 2 dogs. *J Vet Intern Med* 22(4):1048–1051, 2008.
12. Washabau RJ, Day MJ, Willard MD, et al. Endoscopic, biopsy, and histopathologic guidelines for the evaluation of gastrointestinal inflammation in companion animals. *J Vet Intern Med* 24(1): 10–26, 2010.
13. Jergens AE, Heilmann RM. Canine chronic enteropathy—Current state-of-the-art and emerging concepts. *Front Vet Sci* 9:923013, 2022.
14. Dye TL, Diehl KJ, Wheeler SL, Westfall DS. Randomized, controlled trial of budesonide and prednisone for the treatment of idiopathic inflammatory bowel disease in dogs. *J Vet Intern Med* 27(6):1385–1391, 2013.
15. Chey WD, Kurlander J, Eswaran S. Irritable bowel syndrome: a clinical review. *JAMA* 313(9):949–958, 2015.
16. Cerquetella M, Rossi G, Spaterna A, et al. Is irritable bowel syndrome also present in dogs? *Tierarztl Prax Ausg K Kleintiere Heimtiere* 46(3):176–180, 2018.
17. Leib MS. Treatment of chronic idiopathic large-bowel diarrhea in dogs with a highly digestible diet and soluble fiber: a retrospective review of 37 cases. *J Vet Intern Med* 14(1):27–32, 2000.
18. Ludvigsson U, Heath S, Heath S, et al. Chronic enteropathy and emotional health in dogs—a prospective comparative pilot study. Abstract. *J Vet Intern Med* 38(1):802–803, 2024.
19. Rossi G, Cerquetella M, Gavazza A, et al. Rapid resolution of large bowel diarrhea after the administration of a combination of a high-fiber diet and a probiotic mixture in 30 dogs. *Vet Sci* 7(1):21, 2020.
20. Rossi G, Gioacchini G, Pengo G, et al. Enterocolic increase of cannabinoid receptor type 1 and type 2 and clinical improvement after probiotic administration in dogs with chronic signs of colonic dysmotility without mucosal inflammatory changes. *Neurogastroenterol Motil* 32(1):e13717, 2020.
21. Huang HP, Lien YH. Effects of a structured exercise programme in sedentary dogs with chronic diarrhoea. *Vet Rec* 180(9):224, 2017.
22. Walters JR, Pattni SS. Managing bile acid diarrhoea. *Therap Adv Gastroenterol* 3(6):349–357, 2010.
23. Guard BC, Honneffer JB, Jergens AE, et al. Longitudinal assessment of microbial dysbiosis, fecal unconjugated bile acid concentrations, and disease activity in dogs with steroid-responsive chronic inflammatory enteropathy. *J Vet Intern Med* 33(3):1295–1305, 2019.
24. Toresson L, Steiner JM, Suchodolski JS. Cholestyramine treatment in two dogs with presumptive bile acid diarrhoea: a case report. *Canine Med Genet* 8(1):1, 2021.
25. Manchester AC, Dogan B, Guo Y, Simpson KW. *Escherichia coli*-associated granulomatous colitis in dogs treated according to antimicrobial susceptibility profiling. *J Vet Intern Med* 35(1):150–161, 2021.
26. Cochran L, Hill S, Lotti U, et al. Clinical characteristics and long-term outcome of *E. coli*-associated granulomatous ileocolitis in dogs: five cases (2010–2014). *J Small Anim Pract* 62(7):588–598, 2021.

27. Craven M, Dogan B, Schukken A, et al. Antimicrobial resistance impacts clinical outcome of granulomatous colitis in boxer dogs. *J Vet Intern Med* 24(4):819–824, 2010.
28. Ruiz G, Laloy E, Benchekroun G. Chronic gastritis and enterocolitis associated with *Leishmania* infection in an 18-month-old, intact female dog. *Vet Q* 35(4):236–239, 2015.
29. Schumacher LL, Love BC, Ferrell M, et al. Canine intestinal histoplasmosis containing hyphal forms. *J Vet Diagn Invest* 25(2):304–307, 2013.
30. Curtis B, Harris A, Ullal T, et al. Disseminated *Neospora caninum* infection in a dog with severe colitis. *J Vet Diagn Invest* 32(6):923–927, 2020.
31. Adamovich-Rippe KN, Mayhew PD, Marks SL, et al. Colonoscopic and histologic features of rectal masses in dogs: 82 cases (1995–2012). *J Am Vet Med Assoc* 250(4):424–430, 2017.
32. Iwata et al. - Case Report Rapport de cas.pdf.
33. Russell KN, Mehler SJ, Skorupski KA, et al. Clinical and immunohistochemical differentiation of gastrointestinal stromal tumors from leiomyosarcomas in dogs: 42 cases (1990–2003). *J Am Vet Med Assoc* 230(9):1329–1333, 2007.
34. Schöniger S, Summers BA. Localized, plexiform, diffuse, and other variants of neurofibroma in 12 dogs, 2 horses, and a chicken. *Vet Pathol* 46(5):904–915, 2009.
35. Méric T, Issard J, Maufras T, et al. Recurrence and survival in dogs with excised colorectal polyps: A retrospective study of 58 cases. *J Vet Intern Med* 37(6):2375–2384, 2023.
36. Lee S, Hwang J, Kim H, et al. Computed tomographic findings may be useful for differentiating small intestinal adenocarcinomas, lymphomas, and spindle cell sarcomas in dogs. *Vet Radiol Ultrasound* 64(2):233–242, 2023.
37. Saito T, Chambers JK, Nakashima K, et al. Histopathologic features of colorectal adenoma and adenocarcinoma developing within inflammatory polyps in Miniature Dachshunds. *Vet Pathol* 55(5):654–662, 2018.
38. Murakami A, Shibahashi A, Iwasaki R, et al. Combination chlorambucil/firocoxib or chlorambucil/prednisolone treatment for inflammatory colorectal polyps in Miniature Dachshunds. *J Am Anim Hosp Assoc* 54(3):161–166, 2018.
39. Desmas I, Burton JH, Post G, et al. Clinical presentation, treatment and outcome in 31 dogs with presumed primary colorectal lymphoma (2001–2013). *Vet Comp Oncol* 15(2):504–517, 2017.
40. Spużak J, Ciaputa R, Kubiak K, et al. Adenocarcinoma of the posterior segment of the gastrointestinal tract in dogs—clinical, endoscopic, histopathological and immunohistochemical findings. *Pol J Vet Sci* 20(3):539–549, 2017.
41. Ohmi A, Ohno K, Chambers JK, et al. Clinical and histopathological features and prognosis of gastrointestinal adenocarcinomas in Jack Russell Terriers. *J Vet Med Sci* 83(2):167–173, 2021.
42. Herstad KMV, Moen AEF, Gaby JC, et al. Characterization of the fecal and mucosa-associated microbiota in dogs with colorectal epithelial tumors. *PLoS One* 13(5):e0198342, 2018.
43. Cantatore M, Jimeno Sandoval JC, Das S, et al. Submucosal resection via a transanal approach for treatment of epithelial rectal tumors—a multicenter study. *Vet Surg* 51(3):397–408, 2022.
44. Berger EP, Johannes CM, Jergens AE, et al. Retrospective evaluation of toceranib phosphate (Palladia®) use in the treatment of gastrointestinal stromal tumors of dogs. *J Vet Intern Med* 32(6):2045–2053, 2018.
45. Unterer S, Werner M. Diseases of the large intestine. In: Ettinger SJ, Feldman EC, Côté E (eds.). Ettinger's Textbook of Veterinary Internal Medicine, 9th ed. Elsevier; pp. 1729–1753, 2024.
46. Lee R, Leowijuk C. Normal parameters in abdominal radiology of the dog and cat. *J Small Anim Pract* 23(5):251-269, 1982.
47. Moreno AA, Parker VJ, Winston JA, Rudinsky AJ. Dietary fiber aids in the management of canine and feline gastrointestinal disease. *J Am Vet Med Assoc* 260(S3):S33–S45, 2022.
48. Tzimtzimis E, Papazoglou L, Patsikas M, et al. Colonic impaction in dogs: a retrospective study of 58 cases (1996 to 2014). *J Small Anim Pract* 60(7):444–449, 2019.

Index